T0133791

Routledge International Handbook of Qualitative Nursing Research

Qualitative research, once on the fringes, now plays a central part in advancing nursing and midwifery knowledge, contributing to the development of the evidence base for health care practice. Divided into four parts, this authoritative handbook contains over forty chapters on the state of the art and science of qualitative research in nursing.

The first part begins by addressing the significance of qualitative inquiry to the development of nursing knowledge, and then goes on to explore in depth programs of qualitative nursing research. The second section focuses on a wide range of core qualitative methods, from descriptive phenomenology, through to grounded theory and to ethnography, and narrative research. Part III highlights key issues and controversies in contemporary qualitative nursing research, including discussion of ethical and political issues, evidence-based practice and Internet research. Finally, Part IV takes a unique look at qualitative nursing research as it is practiced throughout the world with chapters on countries and regions from the UK and Europe, North America, Australasia, Latin America, to Japan, China, and Korea.

With an international selection of established scholars contributing, the *Routledge International Handbook of Qualitative Nursing Research* is an essential overview and will help to propel qualitative research in nursing well into the twenty-first century. It is an invaluable reference for all nursing researchers.

Cheryl Tatano Beck is Distinguished Professor in the School of Nursing at the University of Connecticut, USA.

Routledge International Handbook of Qualitative Nursing Research

Edited by Cheryl Tatano Beck

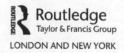

Routledge
Taylor & Francis Group

LONDON AND NEW YORK

First published in paperback 2016

First published 2013
by Routledge
2 Park Square, Milton Park, Abingdon, Oxon OX14 4RN

and by Routledge
711 Third Avenue, New York, NY 10017

Routledge is an imprint of the Taylor & Francis Group, an informa business

British Library Cataloguing in Publication Data
A catalogue record for this book is available from the British Library

Library of Congress Cataloging in Publication Data
Routledge international handbook of qualitative nursing research / edited by Cheryl Beck.
    p. ; cm.
  International handbook of qualitative nursing research
  Includes bibliographical references.
  I. Beck, Cheryl Tatano. II. Title: International handbook of qualitative nursing research.
[DNLM: 1. Nursing Research—methods. 2. Qualitative Research. WY 20.5]
  610.73072¢1—dc23
            2012037182

ISBN: 978-0-415-67356-3 (hbk)
ISBN: 978-1-138-95523-3 (pbk)
ISBN: 978-0-203-40952-7 (ebk)

Typeset in Bembo
by Keystroke, Station Road, Codsall, Wolverhampton

To my family:
my husband Chuck, son Curt and daughter Lisa for all
their understanding and support of my professional career

Contents

List of figures   xi
List of tables   xii
About the editor   xiv
Notes on contributors   xv
Acknowledgments   xxix

1   Introduction to qualitative nursing research   1
    Cheryl Tatano Beck

PART I
What does qualitative nursing research do?   **11**

2   The development of qualitative nursing research   13
    Janice M. Morse

3   Building on "grab," attending to "fit," and being prepared to "modify":
    how grounded theory "works" to guide a health intervention for abused
    women   32
    Judith Wuest, Marilyn Ford-Gilboe, Marilyn Merritt-Gray, and Colleen Varcoe

4   The power of qualitative inquiry: traumatic experiences of marginalized
    groups   47
    Joanne M. Hall

5   Learning about the nature of fatigue   64
    Karin Olson

6   Using a qualitative method to describe the experiences of living with
    chronic pain syndrome   75
    Siv Söderberg

7   Qualitative research program in the care of ventilator-dependent ICU
    patients   86
    Mary Beth Happ

Contents

8   Cultural aspects of Latino early childhood obesity   103
    Lauren Clark, Susan L. Johnson, Mary E. O'Connor, and Jane Lassetter

9   Bringing visibility to an invisible phenomenon: a postpartum depression
    research program   119
    Cheryl Tatano Beck

PART II
Qualitative research methods   **131**

10 Descriptive phenomenology   133
    Cheryl Tatano Beck

11 Interpretive phenomenology   145
    Patricia L. Munhall

12 Glaserian grounded theory: the enduring method   162
    Phyllis Noerager Stern

13 Strauss' grounded theory   169
    Juliet Corbin

14 New directions in grounded theory   183
    Rita Sara Schreiber and Wanda Martin

15 Traditional ethnography   203
    Pamela J. Brink

16 Ethnonursing method of Dr. Madeleine Leininger   213
    Marilyn A. Ray, Edith Morris, and Marilyn McFarland

17 Critical ethnography   230
    Karen Lucas Breda

18 Institutional ethnography   242
    Janet M. Rankin

19 Historical research in nursing: a current outlook   256
    Sandra B. Lewenson

20 Narrative inquiry   268
    Patricia Hill Bailey, Phyllis Montgomery, and Sharolyn Mossey

21 Discourse analysis   282
    Michael Traynor

22 Interpretive description   295
    Sally Thorne

23 Focus groups   307
    Denise Côté-Arsenault

24 Participatory Action Research: a new science for nursing?   319
    Lynne E. Young

25 Metasynthesis   331
    Barbara Paterson

26 Synthesizing qualitative and quantitative research findings   347
    Margarete Sandelowski, Corrine I. Voils, Jamie L. Crandell, and Jennifer Leeman

PART III
Contemporary issues in qualitative nursing research methods   357

27 Ethical issues in qualitative nursing research   359
    Wendy Austin

28 Politics and qualitative nursing research   371
    Joy L. Johnson

29 Internet qualitative research   380
    Eun-Ok Im and Wonshik Chee

30 Secondary qualitative data analysis   393
    Sally Thorne

31 Evidence-based practice: contributions and possibilities for qualitative
    research   405
    Barbara Bowers

PART IV
International qualitative nursing research: state of the science   417

32 International qualitative nursing research: state of the science in England,
    Wales and Scotland   419
    Dawn Freshwater and Jane Cahill

33 Qualitative nursing research in Ireland: an overview of the journey to date   437
    Carolyn L. Tobin

Contents

34 Qualitative nursing research in Canada: state of the science   451
    Joan M. Anderson with Sheryl Reimer-Kirkham, Patricia Rodney, and
    Heather McDonald

35 Australia and New Zealand qualitative nursing research   468
    Jennieffer Barr

36 Qualitative nursing research in Latin America: the cases of Brazil,
    Chile, Colombia, and Mexico   478
    María Claudia Duque-Páramo, Maria Itayra Padilha,
    Olivia Inés Sanhueza-Alvarado, María Magdalena Alonso Castillo,
    Fabiola Castellanos Soriano, Karla Selene López-García, and
    Yolanda Flores-Peña

37 Qualitative nursing research in Spain: an evolving strategy of resistance   500
    Andreu Bover Bover, Denise Gastaldo, Margalida Miró, and Concha Zaforteza

38 State of science of qualitative nursing research in Portugal   514
    Marta Lima-Basto

39 Finland and Sweden: qualitative research from nursing to caring   527
    Terese Bondas

40 Qualitative nursing research in Norway, Denmark and Iceland:
    state of the science   546
    Marit Kirkevold

41 Qualitative nursing research in the Netherlands and Flanders   560
    Maria Grypdonck, Marijke C. Kars, Ann Van Hecke, and Sofie Verhaeghe

42 Qualitative nursing research in Korea   577
    Kyung Rim Shin, Miyoung Kim, and Seung Eun Chung

43 Qualitative nursing research in Japan: a state of the science and
    indications for future directions   597
    Shigeko Saiki-Craighill

44 Qualitative nursing research in South–East Asia, China and Taiwan   610
    David Arthur

45 Future directions in international qualitative nursing research   623
    Cheryl Tatano Beck

Index   *628*

Figures

1.1   Narrowing the focus of qualitative research   2
3.1   Theory of Strengthening Capacity to Limit Intrusion (SCLI)   41
5.1   Revised Edmonton Fatigue Framework   70
7.1   Model of technological access during critical illness   89
7.2   Ventilator weaning event sequence   92
8.1   Infant silhouettes developed by Kramer et al. (1983) and those commissioned
        for this research study   108
9.1   The four-stage process of teetering on the edge   121
9.2   Four perspectives involved with postpartum depression   124
9.3   Example of a completed content validity rating form   126
9.4   Second modification of teetering on the edge: Stage 1   127
14.1 Example of a positional map   189
20.1 Framework for narrative analysis   274
21.1 Dimensions of discourse analysis   288
32.1 Conceptual map of discourse development   431
33.1 Research output and funding   441
33.2 Research focus   442
33.3 Research approach   443
33.4 Recasting hope   445
33.5 Interrelationship of proposed categories   447
42.1 Qualitative research published in *JKAN* and *JQR*   580
42.2 Type of research undertaken   581
42.3 Keywords found in research   582
42.4 Categories of research participants   583
42.5 Number of research participants   584
42.6 Research evaluation   584
43.1 A comparison of the growth in university nursing programs with the
        number of qualitative research articles in the health sciences   598

Tables

2.1	Qualitative nursing research methods books, by type, date, and country	17
2.2	Level of research developing nursing phenomenon: the example of caring	24
8.1	Basic outline of focus group questions for parents/grandparents about childhood feeding and weight	107
8.2	Parents' and grandparents' freelisted responses to the question, "Why are Mexican or Mexican-American children overweight?"	113
8.3	Parents' and grandparents' freelisted responses to the question, "What are some behaviors that protect Mexican and Mexican-American children from becoming overweight?"	114
9.1	Comparison of phenomenological and grounded theory studies on postpartum depression	120
9.2	Development of selected PDSS items from qualitative data	125
10.1	Descriptive phenomenological methods used in 20-year period by country	135
10.2	Comparison of three phenomenological methods	136
10.3	Example of extracting significant statements	141
10.4	Fundamental structure of the phenomenon	141
11.1	International interpretive phenomenological nursing studies: a random sample	146
16.1	Dissertations analyzed for the meta-ethnonursing study using Leininger's theory	224
20.1	Limited genre story elements	273
20.2	"Just before the crisis story"	276
23.1	Advantages and disadvantages of focus groups	309
23.2	Suggested ground rules	312
23.3	Essential ingredients of focus groups	313
24.1	Guidelines for rating participatory research	322
25.1	Metasynthesis methods	334
26.1	Types of research synthesis studies by mode and object of synthesis	350
26.2	Comparison of research synthesis logics	351
26.3	Comparison of designs for mixed research synthesis studies	353
29.1	Ten sample studies that were reviewed	384
32.1	Qualitative approaches in nursing research	422
35.1	A brief outline of the contribution of key professional bodies	469
35.2	Types of qualitative methodologies and methods in Queensland Nursing Council applications, 1996–2000	470
35.3	Examples of additional studies	474
37.1	The main topics of studies, with example publications	504

37.2   Main methodological topics in publications, with examples, 2000–2011   506
37.3   International journals in which Spanish authors have published, 2000–2011   507
37.4   Main Spanish journals for qualitative nursing research publications, 2000–2011 508
38.1   Landmarks in the development of nursing education and research in Portugal   515
38.2   Frequency of areas of study   517
38.3   Clinical areas of study before and after 2009   518
38.4   Frequency of research designs   518
38.5   Frequency of qualitative methods in inductive and mixed studies   519
38.6   Categorization of central concepts, in decreasing order   519
42.1   Methods of data analysis   583
43.1   Number of articles by qualitative method   600
43.2   Breakdown of articles attributed to grounded theory approach in the
        Ichushi database   603
43.3   Articles that used grounded theory approach sorted by year and
        appropriateness of methodological rationale   604
43.4   Adequacy of citation   604
43.5   Explanation and usage of steps of analysis   606

About the editor

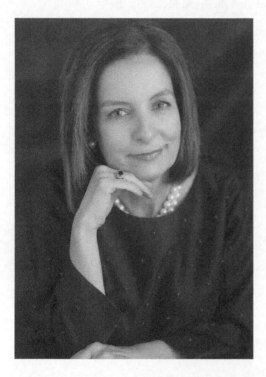

Dr Beck is a Distinguished Professor at the University of Connecticut, School of Nursing. She also has a joint appointment in the Department of Obstetrics and Gynecology at the School of Medicine. Her Bachelor of Science degree in Nursing is from Western Connecticut State University. She received her Master's degree in maternal-newborn nursing from Yale University. Cheryl is a certified nurse-midwife. She received her certificate in nurse-midwifery also from Yale University. Her Doctor of Nursing Science degree is from Boston University. She is a fellow in the American Academy of Nursing. She has received numerous awards, such as the Association of Women's Health, Obstetric, and Neonatal Nursing's Distinguished Professional Service Award, Eastern Nursing Research Society's Distinguished Researcher Award, the Distinguished Alumna Award from Yale University and the Connecticut Nurses' Association's Diamond Jubilee Award for her contribution to nursing research. She has been appointed to the President's Advisory Council of Postpartum Support International.

Over the past 30 years Cheryl has focused her research efforts on developing a research program on postpartum mood and anxiety disorders. Based on the findings from her series of qualitative studies, Cheryl developed the Postpartum Depression Screening Scale (PDSS), which is published by Western Psychological Services. She is a prolific writer who has published over 135 journal articles, including such topics as phenomenology, grounded theory, narrative analysis, metasynthesis, and qualitative secondary analysis. Cheryl is co-author with Dr. Denise Polit of the textbook *Nursing Research: Generating and Assessing Evidence for Nursing Practice*. Editions of this text received both the 2007 and the 2011 American Journal of Nursing Book of the Year Award. Cheryl also co-authored with Dr. Jeanne Driscoll another book, entitled *Postpartum Mood and Anxiety Disorders: A Clinician's Guide*, which received the 2006 American Journal of Nursing Book of the Year Award.

Contributors

María Magdalena Alonso Castillo PhD, MPH, RN with a major in Psychology from the Universidad Autónoma de Nuevo León in Monterrey, México is a professor and Graduate Director of the School of Nursing at the Universidad Autónoma de Nuevo León. She is president of the Consejo Mexicano para la Acreditación de Enfermería (Mexican Council for Nursing Accreditation [COMACE]). She is Coordinator of the Cuerpo Académico de Prevención de Adicciones (Academic Body of Addiction Prevention). She has received funding support for research projects in the phenomenon of drugs. She has published scientific articles and book chapters, is a member of the Sistema Nacional de Investigadores (National Research System) (SNI-Level I), and is a member of the Sigma Theta Tau Association, Chapter Tau Alpha.

Joan M. Anderson PhD, RN is a Professor Emerita in the School of Nursing at the University of British Columbia, Canada. An internationally recognized health and social scientist, Dr. Anderson has conducted extensive research in the areas of culture, gender, migration, health, and inequities in health and health care through the lens of critical feminist inquiry, postcolonial inquiry, and, more recently, critical humanism. The Medical Research Council of Canada/the Canadian Institutes of Health Research, and the Social Sciences and Humanities Research Council of Canada have funded some of her research, which has been widely disseminated in a number of academic journals. Dr. Anderson's active scholarship now includes writing in the areas of social justice, critical humanism and decolonization. A UBC Killam Award for Excellence in Mentoring in 2004 for the outstanding mentorship of graduate students is among the awards and recognitions she has received.

David Arthur PhD, MEd, BEd Studies, BAppSci, RN is an Australian who, after nearly 20 years of nursing in Australia, spent 12 years as an Associate Professor/Professor at the Hong Kong Polytechnic University where he worked with numerous colleagues and students in the Asia Pacific region helping to develop nursing scholarship and research in the exciting developmental period 1995 to 2006. He became the foundation head of the first Bachelor of Nursing program in Singapore in 2006 and left the "ivory towers" in 2009 to practice nursing in communities in the Philippines while also helping to develop nursing scholarship in several universities. He currently also pursues his passions of organic farming, freelance writing, and enjoying the peace and beauty of unspoiled environments in the tropics with his wife Lynneth, and family. The highlights of his career were: helping to produce the first home-grown PhD nurse in China; starting new PhD programs in the Philippines; taking a senior appointment in Singapore; and resigning from the same.

Wendy Austin PhD, MEd, RN is a Professor and Canada Research Chair (*Relational Ethics in Health Care*) in the Faculty of Nursing and the Dossetor Health Ethics Centre, University of Alberta, Canada. Wendy's research is interdisciplinary in nature and encompasses exploring relational ethics issues in health care, developing a relational ethics perspective on research ethics, and identifying ways to better prepare health care practitioners and researchers for ethical action. She teaches a graduate interdisciplinary course in health ethics and has taught a doctoral-level course in research ethics. Wendy has served as a member of the Canadian Nurses Association's Ethics Committee, the Board of the International Academy of Law and Mental Health, and the Board of the Health Law Institute, University of Alberta. She is currently an International Board Member of the Canadian Unit of the International Network of the UNESCO Chair in Bioethics.

Patricia Hill Bailey PhD, MHSc, BScN, RN is a nurse researcher and professor. She teaches courses in nursing inquiry and knowledge creation at both undergraduate and graduate levels. Her research interests using narrative inquiry include persons living with enduring health challenges.

Jennieffer Barr PhD, BN, RN, RM is the Director of Higher Degrees Research Training at Southern Cross University, Australia. She has research experience in both qualitative and quantitative research approaches. Typically, she uses qualitative approaches to understand the experiences of others and this heightened awareness aids in the identification of well-defined variables for use in quantitative research projects. Her research interests lies in primary health care, with the focus on how to prevent illness but also how to maximize well-being when one is ill. She is particularly interested in women and has competitive grants in examining issues such as minimizing the impact of postpartum depression and cardiac and diabetic events in women following menopause. The world trend of increasing morbidity is of concern to Dr Barr, not just for women but also in nursing itself. A recent national competitive research grant has been awarded for a national survey to examine the health and well-being of nurses in Australia. Other current funded work includes experiences of nurses and patients addressing chronic pain, exploration of specific mental illness diagnosis for those with postpartum depression, and a randomized clinical trial feasibility study for a novel intervention for women who have postpartum depression.

Terese Bondas PhD, LicNSc, MNSc, PHN, RN is a Professor, University of Nordland, Faculty of Professional Studies, Bodö, Norway, and Adjunct Professor in methodological questions, University of Eastern Finland, Department of Nursing Science, Finland. Terese has worked as a nurse and researcher pursuing qualitative research in both Finland and Sweden for several years. She leads two large research networks, both of which started as a collaboration between Finnish and Swedish researchers: "The qualitative research network: Childbearing in Europe" (www.uin. no/bfin), as well as the research network for Health Care Leadership (www.uin.no/niv). Terese belongs to the Finland-Swedish minority and her native language is Swedish, while the second native language in her bilingual family is Finnish. Her unique inside/outside perspective, may enable her to look at the development in Finland and Sweden with openness and respect, chairing a full professorship in another Nordic neighboring country, Norway. Moreover, Terese is well known in the university systems in both countries and she has a lively interest in pursuing qualitative nursing research, particularly in relation to caring, maternal care and nursing leadership, and in recent years for qualitative metastudies.

Andreu Bover Bover PhD, MA, BScBio, RN is Associate Professor at the Faculty of Nursing and Physiotherapy at the University of Balearic Islands (UIB) (Spain). His academic work focuses on community health and social determinants of health, critical theory and qualitative health research. As a researcher, he is currently developing several projects funded by the FIS, the Spanish Ministry of Health, in the areas of gender, generation, migration, and policy as social determinants of health. He is the director of the Critical Health Research Group: Policy, Practice and Citizenship at UIB.

Barbara Bowers PhD, RN, FAAN is a Professor of Nursing and Associate Dean for Research at the University of Wisconsin-Madison. Her research has focused on long-term care, particularly workforce development and organizational models of service delivery. Dr. Bowers has participated in many policy advisory committees at the state and federal levels as well as in Australia, New Zealand and Japan.

Karen Lucas Breda PhD, MSN, BSN, RN is a tenured Associate Professor at the University of Hartford in West Hartford, Connecticut, USA. Breda holds a doctorate (PhD) in anthropology from the University of Connecticut, in Storrs, Connecticut, and a bachelor's degree (BSN) and a Master's degree (MSN) from Boston University School of Nursing, in Boston, Massachusetts. First, as a Fulbright Scholar to Italy and later, as a fellow with the Giovanni Agnelli Foundation in Turin, Italy, Breda studied the political economy of health care in the Italian national health system. Her interests in cross-national health care, globalization, and the world system have infused her scholarship and teaching for nearly two decades. Additionally, her specialization in critical political economy and cultural anthropology allows her to bring multidisciplinary analyses to her work. The volume *Nursing and Globalization in the Americas: A Critical Perspective* is an outcome of these efforts. Breda's clinical background is in pediatrics, mental health, and culturally competent community nursing. Breda brings a critical and anthropological lens to her teaching and scholarship. Dr. Breda is project director of Project Horizon, a community service learning initiative at the University of Hartford. Project Horizon links students, faculty and staff from across the university with community partners to co-create health, social and cultural advocacy initiatives. She is a local, national and international presenter, a successful grant writer, and an advocate for urban families and children living in poverty. She maintains her areas of expertise through reading, conference attendance and presentation, and professional networking, especially with colleagues from diverse professions and disciplines.

Pamela J. Brink PhD, RN, FAAN is a Professor Emerita at the University of Alberta. Her academic career was divided between nursing and anthropology, teaching medical anthropology and nursing research. Her research career was divided between research on successful weight losers and ethnographic field research with the Pyramid Lake Paiute of Nevada and the Annang in rural Nigeria. Her first book, *Transcultural Nursing* (1976, Prentice Hall) provided articles by nurses and anthropologists on using anthropological theory and methods in nursing. She has co-authored two nursing research texts (*Basic Steps in Planning Nursing Research* and *Advanced Design in Nursing Research*), and founded and edited the *Western Journal of Nursing Research*.

Jane Cahill MA Hons, PhD is currently in post as a senior research fellow at the Leeds School of Healthcare. She has published widely in the field of psychological therapy effectiveness research, having worked at the Psychological Therapies Research Centre in Leeds for nine years before being appointed to the School. Jane continues to work and publish within the field of mental health: her current program of research supports the mental health research program within the School, having a special focus on the therapeutic alliance, practice-based evidence approaches, workforce mental health issues, and complementary and alternative approaches to mental health. Jane has recently secured funding to carry out a knowledge transfer partnership (KTP) project, which concerns the development and validation of a model of employment support for mental health service users. This project is in collaboration with Leeds Partnership NHS Foundations Trust and has strong service user involvement and representation.

Fabiola Castellanos Soriano PhD, MSc, RN is Associate Professor and Director of the Department of Collective Health at the School of Nursing in the Pontificia Universidad Javeriana in Bogotá, Colombia. She has a PhD in nursing and received her Master´s degree in Education. She leads the research group on conceptualization and nursing practice on topics related to chronic diseases and nursing care of the elderly. She has conducted qualitative research studies and has several publications on nursing care and disability of the elderly.

Wonshik Chee PhD is Research Associate Professor at University of Pennsylvania. He received his PhD in mechanical engineering from the University of California at Berkeley in 1997 and did his postdoctoral fellowship at the same institution. His expertise is control algorithm development including fuzzy logic control and Internet web programming, and his previous industrial and academic experiences were closely related to development of adaptive robust control systems for various mechatronic systems and web application development in research projects. Dr. Chee has closely worked with Dr. Im in her series of Internet studies, and he has provided his expertise in computer and Internet technologies for her Internet studies.

Seung Eun Chung PhD, RN is Professor of the Department of Nursing at the Korea National University of Transportation, Korea. She is Editor of the *Journal of Qualitative Research* (Medical Love) of the Academy of Qualitative Research, the Korea Center for Qualitative Methodology, and on the editorial board of *Qualitative Health Research* (Sage). She was an organizing and scientific advisory board member of the Global Congress for Qualitative Health Research, 2011–2012. She has been interested in qualitative inquiry since she was a visiting professor (2002–2003) at the International Institute for Qualitative Methodology, University of Alberta, Canada. She currently teaches Adult Health Nursing based on clinical setting and Qualitative Research Methodology in the Master's Program. She is the author of many articles and books on qualitative research methods about health for the elderly and for women, and simulation-based education for nursing students.

Lauren Clark PhD, RN, FAAN is Professor in the College of Nursing, University of Utah. She is a nurse-anthropologist with two decades of funded research among Mexican Americans in the Southwest US. Her research complements her public health nursing clinical interests in the social determinants of health and cultural understandings of health and illness. She serves on the editorial boards of *Qualitative Health Research* and *Journal of Specialists in Pediatric Nursing* and is a fellow of the American Academy of Nursing and the Society of Applied Anthropology.

Juliet Corbin PhD, RN received her BSN from Arizona State University, her MSN from San Jose State University, and her DNSc from University of California, San Francisco. Following her doctorate, she did a postdoctorate in the Department of Social & Behavioral Sciences also at UCSF under the direction of Dr. Anselm Strauss with whom she collaborated in research and writing for 15 years until his death in 1996. Areas of research collaboration with Dr. Strauss included chronic illness, biography, and the sociology of work. It was while working with Dr. Strauss and sitting in on his method classes that the idea for writing *Basics of Qualitative Research* was born. The book is now in its third edition with the fourth in process and has been translated into many different languages including Arabic, Farsi, Chinese, Japanese, Korean, Spanish, and German. Dr. Corbin also taught nursing at San Jose State University for many years. She also guided many Master's and doctoral students with their research projects in grounded theory. Dr. Corbin has presented keynote addresses in the U.S., Canada, and other European and Asian countries, and published many papers with Dr. Strauss on chronic illness and grounded theory. Since her retirement, she has taught numerous workshops on grounded theory in various countries around the world.

Denise Côté-Arsenault PhD, RNC, FNAP is currently Professor and Chair of the Department of Parent and Child Nursing at the University of North Carolina at Greensboro School of Nursing. She has conducted focus groups in her own research on women's experiences of pregnancy after perinatal loss, as well as serving as moderator or consultant in the research of others. Her work includes several qualitative and mixed methods design studies.

Jamie L. Crandell PhD is Research Assistant Professor in the School of Nursing and Department of Biostatistics at the University of North Carolina at Chapel Hill. Her main areas of research include Bayesian methods and the modeling of longitudinal data. Recent projects have focused on the application of Bayesian methods to synthesize qualitative and quantitative research findings.

María Claudia Duque-Páramo PhD, MSc, RN is a full Professor at the School of Nursing in the Pontificia Universidad Javeriana in Bogotá, Colombia. She has a PhD in anthropology, received her bachelor's degree in nursing, her Master's degree in community psychology and has completed a specialization in pediatric nursing. She has a longstanding experience as an educator, researcher, writer, and national and international speaker on issues related to childhood and migration, children's health, health and culture, and indigenous health. Related to her current research on childhood and migration, she is a member of national and international networks, and works on promoting policies and programs for children and their families.

Yolanda Flores-Peña PhD, RN graduated from Universidad de São Paulo in Ribeirão Preto, Brazil. She is a full Professor in the College of Nursing at the Universidad Autónoma de Nuevo León in Monterrey, México. Her focus of research is cognitions, lifestyles, and socio-demographics of maternal and child's factors related to obesity. She participated as Director of Dissertations and Master's Theses. Her research activities have produced over 20 manuscripts and book chapters. She is a member of the Sistema Nacional de Investigadores (National System of Researchers (CONACYT-México), and member of the Sigma Theta Tau Association.

Marilyn Ford-Gilboe PhD, RN, FAAN is a Professor and Echo Chair in Rural Women's Health Research in the Arthur Labatt Family School of Nursing at the University of Western Ontario. Her research and scholarship focus on reducing health inequities and promoting the health of marginalized women and families, particularly those affected by violence, using diverse methodological and analytic approaches. She is currently studying violence among women living in rural communities, and testing novel nursing and health care interventions designed to improve the health, safety and quality of the life of women who have experienced intimate partner violence.

Dawn Freshwater PhD, RNT, RN, BA (Hons) FRCN is Pro-Vice-Chancellor for Staff and Organizational Effectiveness, Professor of Mental Health and former Head of the School of

Healthcare, University of Leeds, UK. Her research interests span mental health, offender health and psychological therapies. Her research uses a variety of approaches, most notably narrative, reflexivity and discursive methodology. She has developed a body of work around leadership and workforce planning using appreciative inquiry in change management. In her role as PVC, she is leading on the Equality Strategy for the University of Leeds and has recently been successful in Athena Swan Women in Science awards. Dawn has supervised 15 PhD students to completion and has earned over £2m in grant income. She is the author of 15 books, over 100 papers and has contributed widely to academic discourse around research methods and is currently the Editor of the *Journal of Psychiatric Mental Health Nursing*. She is also a Fellow of the Royal College of Nursing and Elected Representative for England on the Council of Deans Executive Nursing.

Denise Gastaldo PhD, MA, BScN is Associate Director at the Centre for Critical Qualitative Health Research and Associate Professor at the Bloomberg Faculty of Nursing, University of Toronto. She is also cross-appointed to the Doctorate Program, Faculty of Nursing and Physiotherapy, University of Balearic Islands, Spain. Since 1998 she has collaborated with Spanish colleagues in different roles, such as co-investigator, teacher, mentor and supervisor. Her research focuses on health equity issues, such as migration and gender as social determinants of health. She has co-edited two books about Ibero-American qualitative health research, co-organized international conferences, and taught qualitative methods in several countries.

Maria Grypdonck PhD, RN is Professor Emerita of Ghent University and the University of Utrecht. She obtained a PhD degree from the University of Manchester, and was Professor of Nursing Science at the universities of Leuven, Ghent and Utrecht. Since 1988, she has been engaged in qualitative research, mostly on the lived experience of patients with chronic illness and their family members, has supervised many dissertations using qualitative methods and obtained several grants to conduct qualitative studies. She won the Leadership award from the International Institute of Qualitative Methodology in 2005.

Joanne M. Hall PhD, RN, FAAN is a Professor in the College of Nursing, University of Tennessee Knoxville (UT) who practiced for more than 20 years as a mental health nurse. Having earned a Master's degree in nursing at University of Iowa, a PhD from the University of California, San Francisco, Dr. Hall completed a postdoctoral fellowship under the mentorship of Dr, Afaf Meleis. Her program of research has been an exploration of risks and thriving in marginalized populations. A lesbian and proponent of liberation philosophies, Hall uses narrative approaches to research. She is a Co-Director of the UT Cooperating Site of the International Institute of Qualitative Methodology and a Fellow in the American Academy of Nursing. Currently she is also learning to play the Irish button accordion.

Mary Beth Happ PhD, RN, FAAN is the Nursing Distinguished Professor of Critical Care Research at the Ohio State University College of Nursing. Her research focuses on understanding and improving communication with seriously ill hospitalized adults and older adults who are unable to speak. With more than 16 years of sustained external research funding, her program of research includes studies of prolonged mechanical ventilation in the ICU, interventions to improve patient communication during mechanical ventilation, treatment decision-making, and symptom communication in the ICU. Dr. Happ has expertise in qualitative and mixed methods research approaches and has published and presented internationally on research methodology.

Eun-Ok Im PhD, PHH, RN, CNS, FAAN is Professor and Marjorie O. Rendell Endowed Professor at the University of Pennsylvania. Her expertise is international cross-cultural women's health issues including menopause, cancer pain, and breast cancer. She has conducted more than 20 studies on international cross-cultural women's health issues and authored more than 100 articles published or accepted for publication in refereed journals. Since 1999, she has conducted a series of Internet studies that were funded by multiple funding agencies including the National Institute of Health and the Oncology Nursing Foundation. She has been on dozens of research review panels (NIH study sections), is on the editorial boards of three top nursing journals and is on the editorial review boards of 10 journals.

Joy L. Johnson PhD, RN, FCAHS is a Professor in the School of Nursing at the University of British Columbia. Drawing on a broad array of theoretical perspectives, her research focuses on the social, structural and individual factors that influence health behaviour. A major thrust of her work focuses on sex and gender issues in substance use and mental health. Dr. Johnson also serves as the Scientific Director of the Canadian Institutes of Health Research, Institute of Gender and Health. In this role she works with the gender, sex and health research community and stakeholders to identify research priorities, develop research funding opportunities, strengthen research capacity, build partnerships and translate research evidence to improve the health of Canadians.

Susan L. Johnson PhD is Associate Professor and Director of the Healthy Youth and Families Initiative, Department of Pediatrics, University of Colorado School of Medicine. She is Associate Editor of *Journal of Nutrition Education and Behavior* and a member of the Colorado Nutrition Network. Her research focuses on factors that influence the development of children's food intake and eating patterns. As the Director of the Children's Eating Laboratory at the University of Colorado, she has a facility to investigate the effects of child-feeding practices on children's food preferences, energy intake patterns, and weight outcomes.

Marijke C. Kars PhD, RN is Assistant Professor at the Department of Medical Humanities of the Faculty of Medicine of the University of Utrecht. Subsequent to her career as a pediatric nurse, as a nurse scientist her research focuses on chronically ill children and their families, as well as on pediatric palliative care. She has conducted several nationally funded qualitative studies. She teaches methods of qualitative research at the Department of Clinical Health Sciences of the University of Utrecht. She supervises several research projects using a qualitative design.

Miyoung Kim PhD, RN is presently an Associate Professor in the Division of Nursing Science, College of Health Sciences at Ewha Womans University, Korea. She is majoring in nursing administration; currently serves as a Director of the Korea Center for Qualitative Methodology and the Academy of Qualitative Research; and is a Board Member of the Korean Nurses Association. She has translated many books related to the qualitative research such as *Basics of Qualitative Research: Techniques and Procedures for Developing Grounded Theory* (3rd ed.) and *Developing Grounded Theory: The Second Generation.*

Marit Kirkevold EdD, MA, MEd, RN is Professor of Nursing Science at the Institute for Health and Society, University of Oslo, Norway, and Director of Research Center for Habilitation and Rehabilitation Models and Services (CHARM). She is also Professor of Nursing Science at the University of Aarhus, Denmark. Kirkevold conducts research on issues related to living with and adjusting to chronic illness and aging, and explores ways nursing care can promote adjustment and psychosocial well-being. She has also published a number of articles and textbooks on the issue of knowledge translation and the application of research knowledge in nursing practice.

Jane Lassetter PhD, RN is an Associate Professor in the College of Nursing, Brigham Young University. She has worked as a pediatric nurse for many years. Her research focuses on childhood obesity in Pacific Islanders. She serves as President of the Iota-Iota Chapter at Large of Sigma Theta Tau International and is a manuscript reviewer for *Qualitative Health Research* and *ICAN: Infant, Child, and Adolescent Nutrition*.

Jennifer Leeman DrPH, MDiv is an Assistant Professor at the University of North Carolina at Chapel Hill (UNC-CH) School of Nursing and a fellow in the UNC-CH Mentored Career Development Program in Comparative Effectiveness Research (K12 HS019468, 07/1/10 –06/30/13). Her research is focused on ways effectively to translate, disseminate, and implement findings from research to improve practice related to health behaviors. She is currently co-PI of a Centers for Disease Control and Prevention-funded Center (U48 DP000059, 2004–2014) for translating and disseminating evidence to support public health practitioners' obesity prevention efforts nationwide. Dr. Leeman has published multiple systematic reviews identifying factors related to disseminating and implementing change in practice.

Sandra B. Lewenson EdD, RN, FAAN is a Professor of Nursing at the Lienhard School of Nursing, College of Health Professions, Pace University, located in Pleasantville, New York. Her research includes the history of nursing education, the history of nursing's political activity, and the history of public health nursing. She teaches courses on nursing history and integrates historical research into the other courses she teaches in the Master's program. Her book, *Taking Charge: Nursing, Suffrage, and Feminism in America, 1873–1920*, received the American Association for the History of Nursing Lavinia Dock Award for Historical Scholarship and Research in Nursing. She also received the *American Journal of Nursing* Book of the Year Awards for *Capturing Nursing History: A Guide to Historical Methods in Research* and *Decision-Making in Nursing: Thoughtful Approaches for Practice*. Dr. Lewenson is a member of the American Academy of Nursing and Sigma Theta Tau International Honor Society. She co-edited two books, *Public Health Nursing: Practicing Population-Based Care* (2nd edition) and *Nursing Interventions Through Time: History as Evidence*.

Marta Lima-Basto PhD, MSc, RN is "Coordinating Professor" retired from Escola Superior de Enfermagem de Lisboa but still active in the profession. At present, she is a member of the Scientific Committee (executive body) of the Doctoral Program in Nursing of the University of Lisbon and a researcher at the Unidade de Investigação & Desenvolvimento em Enfermagem. She supervises doctoral theses and coordinates a seminar for doctoral students. She is a Scholar of the European Academy of Nursing Science and continues to study and publish about knowledge developed and used by nurses and change in professional behavior.

Karla Selene López-García PhD, RN graduated from the School of Nursing at Ribeãro Preto, Universidad de São Paulo, Brazil. She is a full-time Professor of the School of Nursing at the Universidad Autónoma de Nuevo León in Monterrey, México. She has authored about 20 articles. She is a member of the Cuerpo Académico de Prevención de Adicciones (Academic Body of Addiction Prevention) of the Universidad Autónoma de Nuevo León and of the Sigma Theta Tau International, chapter Tau Alpha. She also is member of the Sistema Nacional de Investigadores (National Research System) (SNI-Level I), and is an assembly member of the

Consejo Mexicano para la Acreditación de Enfermería (Mexican Council for Nursing Accreditatio)n (COMACE).

Wanda Martin PhD(c), RN is a PhD Candidate in Nursing at the University of Victoria, Canada. She holds a Canadian Institutes of Health (CIHR) Doctoral Research Award. Her dissertation focuses on public health in the area of food security, using a complexity science framework. She is also a co-investigator on a complexity science knowledge synthesis project and a research associate on programmatic CIHR grant on reducing health inequities. Her interests are in reducing food insecurity and health inequities.

Marilyn McFarland PhD, RN, FNP-BC, CTN-A is Professor of Nursing at the University of Michigan-Flint. She is a board-certified Family Nurse Practitioner and has a longstanding involvement in transcultural nursing as an author, researcher, presenter, consultant, and educator. Her research on the care of people from diverse cultures has been conducted with the ethnonursing research method and guided by the Culture Care theory.

Marilyn Merritt-Gray MN, RN is a well-published honorary research associate and retired professor at the Faculty of Nursing, University of New Brunswick, New Brunswick, Canada. Her practice and research interests are health program design, women's physical and mental health, particularly for women with trauma histories who are rurally located. She has extensive experience working at a governance level within the not-for-profit service sector.

Margalida Miró PhD, BScPsy, RN is Associate Professor at the Faculty of Nursing and Physiotherapy at the University of Balearic Islands (Spain). She is member of the Critical Health Research Group: Policy, Practice and Citizenship and of the Qualitative Research Network in Spain (REDICS). She has taught qualitative research and critical theory at undergraduate, Master's and doctoral levels. Currently, she is conducting research projects in the areas of professional boundaries and power relations in health care teams supported by poststructuralist theories.

Phyllis Montgomery PhD, MScN, BScN, RN is an advanced practice nurse and qualitative researcher interested in mental health among women made vulnerable by their circumstances. Many of her research projects focus on women's effort to craft a life in the presence of adversity.

Edith Morris PhD, RN, PNP-BC is a Clinical Associate Professor of Nursing at the University of Cincinnati College of Nursing. Additionally, she is an Advanced Practice Nursing Education Consultant at Cincinnati Children's Hospital Medical Center. She has conducted several research studies using the ethnonnursing method, including her dissertation study on adolescent gangs which has been published. She has chaired dissertation committees where her students have chosen to use the ethnonursing method, as well as assisted nurses in using the method for clinical research.

Janice M. Morse PhD (Nurs), PhD (Anthro), FAAN is a Professor and holds a Presidential Endowed Chair at the University of Utah College of Nursing, and is Professor Emerita, University of Alberta, Canada. She was the founding Director and Scientific Director of the International Institute for Qualitative Methodology, University of Alberta, founding editor of the *International Journal of Qualitative Methods*, and presently serves as the founding editor for *Qualitative Health Research* (Sage). From 1998 to 2007 she was the editor for the Qual Press, and is currently editor for the series *Developing Qualitative Inquiry, The Basics of Qualitative Inquiry* (Left

Coast Press). Dr. Morse is the recipient of the Lifetime Achievement in Qualitative Inquiry, from the International Center for Qualitative Inquiry (2011), the International's Nurse Researcher Hall of Fame, the Episteme Award (Sigma Theta Tau), and honorary doctorates from the University of Newcastle (Australia) and Athabasca University (Canada). She is the author of 370 articles and 18 books on qualitative research methods, suffering, comforting and patient falls.

Sharolyn Mossey MScN, BScN, RN teaches in a humanistic educative undergraduate nursing program with an emphasis on praxis. Her clinical research interests, using qualitative inquiry, focus on persons living with enduring health challenges in a northern and rural context.

Patricia L. Munhall EdD, ARNP, PsyA, FAAN is presently the President of the International Institute for Human Understanding and head of MiamiTherapy.com, located in Miami, Florida. She has held academic appointments in nursing for 30 years. As a phenomenologically oriented author she has just completed the fifth edition of *Nursing Research: A Qualitative Perspective* and has been the author of two series of phenomenologies: one series, on women's experiences, the other series, on experiences of women, family and men in the twenty-first century. She has also authored a text on revisioning phenomenology. She prescribes to phenomenological philosophy as a way of "being-in-this-world" and practices psychoanalysis in private practice from that perspective. Additionally Patricia gives workshops and consultations on phenomenology, nationally and internationally.

Mary E. O'Connor MD, MPH is Professor of Pediatrics, University of Colorado School of Medicine. She is a general pediatrician at Westside Family Health Center at Denver Health where she cares for a multi-ethnic group of low-income patients. She has been involved in breastfeeding education and research for over 20 years and is the lead author of the website BreastfeedingBasics at www.BreastfeedingBasics.org. She has published numerous articles on breastfeeding and other topics related to general pediatrics. She is active in the American Academy of Pediatrics.

Karin Olson PhD, RN is a Professor in the Faculty of Nursing at the University of Alberta. She holds certification in palliative care nursing from the Canadian Nurses Association and is the author of *Essentials of Qualitative Interviewing* (2011). Dr. Olson's program of research focuses on fatigue, primarily in individuals with cancer.

Maria Itayra Padilha PhD, MSc, RN is a Post-Doctor in History of Nursing at University of Toronto, Doctor in Nursing at Universidade Federal do Rio de Janeiro (Federal University of Rio de Janeiro)/Brazil, and tenured Professor of Department of Nursing at Universidade Federal de Santa Catarina (Federal University of Santa Catarina), Brazil. She is Editor of *Text & Context Nursing Journal* at UFSC. She is the author of over 100 articles, chapters and books, and a Leader of the Research Group of Nursing History in Santa Catarina/Brazil. She is a member of the American Association of Nursing History (AANH) and Sigma Theta Thau Association of Brazil. She is a researcher on the National Council for Scientific and Technological Development (CNPq).

Barbara Paterson PhD, RN, 3M Fellow was the lead author of a 2001 text about metastudy, a metasynthesis method. Since that time, she has participated in several metasynthesis research projects, including a multimillion-dollar-funded project to investigate inquiry learning in science education. She is the author of more than a dozen articles or book chapters about metasynthesis and has provided workshops and keynote speeches on metasynthesis across the globe. Currently, she is the Dean of the Thompson Rivers University School of Nursing in British Columbia, Canada.

Janet M. Rankin PhD, RN is an Assistant Professor in the Faculty of Nursing at the University of Calgary. She has been working in a variety of nursing specialties since 1979. Her doctoral work used institutional ethnography to study nurses' work in contemporary hospitals. Published as *Managing to Nurse: Inside Canada's Health Care Reform*, the research explicated tensions embedded in managerial technologies being used to streamline and coordinate nurses' work. Currently Dr. Rankin is chair of the Institutional Ethnography Division of the Society for the Study of Social Problems. She is supporting a number of graduate students using institutional ethnography and is lead facilitator of an "IE Working Group" that uses free electronic media to meet once a month. Her own program of institutional ethnographic research rests at the intersections of nursing practice and nursing education.

Marilyn A. Ray PhD, MSN, MA (Anthro), RN, CTN-A, Fellow, SfAA is a Professor Emerita at Florida Atlantic University, Christine E. Lynn College of Nursing, Boca Raton, Florida, holds a diploma from St. Joseph Hospital, Hamilton, Canada, BSN and MSN degrees from the University of Colorado, an MA degree in cultural anthropology from McMaster University, a PhD in transcultural nursing from the University of Utah, and an honorary degree from Nevada State College. As a certified transcultural nurse and scholar of the Transcultural Nursing Society, Ray was mentored by Dr. Madeleine Leininger. She is a Fellow of the Society for Applied Anthropology. Ray held faculty positions at the Florida Atlantic University, University of Colorado, McMaster University, University of California San Francisco, and University of San Francisco. Ray retired as a Colonel in 1999 from the United States Air Force Reserve Nurse Corps after a 30-year career in aerospace nursing. As one of the first nursing researchers to advance the study of caring in complex cultural organizational systems, she was awarded charter membership in the International Association for Human Caring. She is committed to transcultural nursing and caring as the essence of nursing. Throughout her career Ray has researched and published on the subjects of caring in organizational cultures developing the Theory of Bureaucratic Caring, caring methodology, technological and economic caring, transcultural caring and ethics, complex caring dynamics, and complexity sciences, and military health care. She received the Federal Nursing Award for excellence in research. Her books include: *Transcultural Caring Dynamics in Nursing and Health Care: A Study of Caring within an Institutional Culture*, *The Discovery of the Theory of Bureaucratic Caring* and with her colleagues Davidson and Turkel, *Nursing, Caring, and Complexity Science: For Human-Environment Well Being*.

Shigeko Saiki-Craighill PhD, RN is Professor of Pediatric Nursing at Keio University. She received her doctorate in nursing sciences from the University of California, San Francisco, in 1994. For her doctoral dissertation, she interviewed mothers who had recently lost a child to cancer to find what their coping strategies are and how the journey from diagnosis to grieving had transformed them. Since then she has been exploring various aspects of the medical culture surrounding pediatric oncology, including its effect on other members of the family, the community, and the health professionals themselves. Earlier, she worked on establishing focused and well-organized support groups for grieving mothers. This led to a research focus on issues of disclosure and communication as it applies to children and their families, and more recently how notions of professionalism incorporate the emotional labor of extremely stressful situations.

She also frequently gives seminars and workshops on qualitative research, and has published several books on grounded theory techniques for Japanese researchers.

Margarete Sandelowski PhD, RN, FAAN is Cary C. Boshamer Distinguished Professor at the University of North Carolina at Chapel Hill School of Nursing. She has numerous publications in the areas of qualitative and mixed methods primary research and research synthesis, including the *Handbook for Synthesizing Qualitative Research* (Springer, 2007). She is currently multiple PI (with Kathleen Knafl) of a five-year study funded by the National Institute of Nursing Research (1R01NR012445, 09/01/2011–06/30/2016) for the project "Mixed-Methods Synthesis of Research on Childhood Chronic Conditions and Family."

Olivia Inés Sanhueza-Alvarado PhD, MSc, RN received her Doctor in Nursing at the University of São Paulo, Brazil. She is a Tenured Professor of Nursing at Universidad de Concepción, Chile, and Director of the International Centre of Nursing Research (CIIENF) of the Chilean Association for Nursing Education (ACHIEEN). She is the author of around 60 articles and chapters in books. A member of the Nursing Care Research Group and member of the Multidisciplinary Gender Studies Program (PROMEG) at the Universidad de Concepción. She has become the First Research Vocal at the Latinoamerican Nursing Faculties and Schools Association (ALADEFE). Also a member of New York University Sigma Theta Tau, and a reviewer for the National Fund for Health Research (FONIS).

Rita Sara Schreiber DNS, RN is a Professor and Coordinator of the nurse practitioner program at the School of Nursing, University of Victoria. She has conducted, and supervised, a number of grounded theories on topics including women's experiences with depression, treatment, and recovery; mental health nurses dealing with ethical issues; and nurse anaesthesia practice. She is a convener of the Grounded Theory Club, an ongoing advanced research seminar at the University of Victoria. With Phyllis Stern, she is co-editor of *Using Grounded Theory in Nursing* (Springer).

Kyung Rim Shin EdD, FAAN is presently a Professor of College of Health Sciences at Ewha Womans University; a member of the 19th National Assembly, Republic of Korea; and the Chief vice President at Korean National Council of Women. She was the former President of the Korean Nurses Association; Chair of the Board of Directors, Korean Accreditation Board of Nursing; and a Chair of the Board of Directors, National Health Personnel Licensing Examination Board. She currently serves as Associate Editor of *Nursing & Health Sciences* (Wiley-Blackwell, Asia). Dr. Shin does not restrict her influence to Asia. In the US, she serves on the editorial board of *Qualitative Health Research* (Sage). She is a Fellow of the American Academy of Nursing, and as the past president (2002–2004) of the International Council of Women's Health Issues, has hosted an international congress in Korea.

Siv Söderberg PhD, RNT is a registered nurse and Professor in Nursing at the Division of Nursing, Department of Health Science, Luleå University of Technology, Luleå, Sweden. Her research is conducted in the fields, e.g. living with illness, patient safety, health promotion/prevention and eHealth. Her main research topic concerns what it means to be ill with a focus on personal needs. The research topic also focuses on other subjects such as being met and received by others, transitions in illness, fatigue, pain, women's health, and well-being. In this area of research she is tutoring several doctoral students. She has extensive experience of research in the area of eHealth.

Phyllis Noerager Stern PhD, LLD (hon.), FAAN, Professor Emerita of Indiana Perdue University at Indianapolis School of Nursing, learned grounded theory during her doctoral work in the mid-1970s from its originators, Barney Glaser and Anselm Strauss, and has been explaining the method to her colleagues and students ever since. She edited the journal *Health Care for Women International* for 20 years and moved it from a maternity focus to an international status with the broader lens of overall health conditions for women. In 1983, she accepted the position of Director of the School of Nursing at Dalhousie University in Halifax, Canada. From that base, she established the International Council on Women's Health Issues in 1984. This society holds Congresses all over the world. In 2003 she received an honorary doctorate from Dalhousie, for "Changing the face of nursing in Eastern Canada." In 2008, she was named a "Living Legend" by the American Academy of Nursing for her research using grounded theory and her work pertaining to women's health.

Sally Thorne PhD, RN, FAAN, FCAHS is Professor of Nursing at the University of British Columbia. Her program of substantive research has been in the field of chronic illness and cancer experience, with a particular focus on the human interface of care delivery processes. She holds leadership positions and serves on policy boards related to cancer care, nursing advocacy, and research development. A widely published author, including scholarly papers and books on qualitative research methodology, she serves as Editor-in-Chief for the journal *Nursing Inquiry*.

Carolyn L. Tobin PhD, RM, RNT, RN was born in Dublin, Ireland, and undertook nursing and midwifery education to Master's level in the UK. She returned to Ireland with her family in 1997 where she worked as a lecturer at Trinity College Dublin for one year before starting a six-year appointment as midwife teacher at the Rotunda Hospital, Dublin. She completed her doctoral degree at Trinity College Dublin, in 2010. She is currently an Assistant Professor in the Department of Nursing at the University of New Hampshire, USA. Carolyn's primary research interests are in the area of women's health with a particular focus on vulnerable populations.

Michael Traynor PhD, MA, RHV, RGN studied English Literature at Cambridge, then completed general nursing and health visiting training in the UK. He has worked at the Royal College of Nursing, the London School of Hygiene & Tropical Medicine and is currently Trevor Clay Professor of Nursing Policy at Middlesex University, London. He researches professional identity and the application of discourse analysis and approaches from literary theory and psychoanalysis to nursing policy and health care issues. He is Editor of the journal *Health: An Interdisciplinary Journal for the Social Study of Health, Illness, and Medicine*.

Ann Van Hecke PhD, RN joined the staff of Ghent University in 2004 as researcher and is now Professor in the Nursing Science Department, Ghent University. Her research mainly concerns self-management in patients with a chronic illness using qualitative and mixed methods. Currently, she is supervising several dissertations and PhD theses and leads several funded projects on this topic using a qualitative research approach.

Colleen Varcoe PhD, RN is a Professor in the School of Nursing at the University of British Columbia. Her research focuses on women's health, concentrating on violence and inequity and the culture of health care, with an emphasis on ethics, and aims to promote ethical practice and policy in the context of violence and inequity. Her research includes a number of studies in partnership with Aboriginal communities. She is currently leading a study of an intervention for Aboriginal women who have experienced violence.

Sofie Verhaeghe PhD, MSc, RN started her work at Ghent University in 1998 and did a PhD based on the principles of grounded theory. She is now head of the Department of Nursing Science at Ghent University and is involved in research focusing on family nursing, and interpersonal relationships between patients, nurses and family members. Most of this research is situated in the areas of oncological nursing, psychiatric nursing and neurological nursing. She teaches qualitative research methodology and supervises research projects and PhD theses.

Corrine I. Voils PhD is a research scientist at the Durham Veterans Affairs Medical Center and an Associate Professor in the Department of Medicine at Duke University Medical Center. Her research is focused on treatment adherence. She is currently multiple PI (with William Yancy Jr.) of three studies: a randomized controlled trial to evaluate the impact of genetic testing on health behaviors (IBD 09-039 from VA HSR&D, 04/01/10–03/31/13), a randomized controlled trial to evaluate a weight loss maintenance intervention (IIR 11-040 from VA HSR&D, 01/01/12–06/30/15), and a descriptive study to develop a self-report measure of medication adherence and to examine longitudinal trajectories of medication adherence (1R21AG035233, 07/01/10–06/30/12).

Judith Wuest PhD, RN is Professor Emerita at the University of New Brunswick, Faculty of Nursing in Fredericton, New Brunswick, Canada. Her research interests are in the field of women's health, particularly intimate partner violence and women's caregiving. She is internationally known as a qualitative grounded theorist; however, research questions emerging from her grounded theory analysis have led to quantitative theory testing and intervention development. She is currently leading a feasibility study on implementing the grounded theory-based Intervention for Health Enhancement after Leaving with existing domestic violence outreach services in New Brunswick.

Lynne E. Young PhD, RN is a Professor in the University of Victoria School of Nursing, Victoria, BC, Canada. Health promotion is her primary theoretical area of interest with her research focused on generating knowledge to promote the cardiovascular health of women.

Concha Zaforteza PhD, BA, RN is Associate Professor at the Faculty of Nursing and Physiotherapy, University of Balearic Islands (Spain). She is a member of the Critical Health Research Group: Policy, Practice and Citizenship and of the International Collaboration on Participatory Health Research. She teaches qualitative research and critical theory on Master's and doctoral programs. As a researcher, she employs participatory approaches to develop projects, funded by the FIS, Spanish Ministry of Health, in the areas of clinical practice transformation and knowledge translation. She is the author of several articles in this field.

Acknowledgments

It was truly a privilege and an honor to have worked with all the distinguished qualitative nursing scholars from around the globe who have graciously contributed these cutting-edge chapters to the *Routledge International Handbook of Qualitative Nursing Research*. I especially would like to thank Janice Morse for her insightful guidance with envisioning the outline for this first ever handbook and also for her invaluable help in identifying contributors. I would like to express my gratitude to Grace McInnes, Routledge Senior Editor, Health and Social Care, for inviting me to be the editor of this handbook. James Watson, Editorial Assistant, Health and Social Care, has been a joy to work with, along with Routledge's entire production team. While it was not possible to include chapters representing all the countries around the world where qualitative nursing research is being conducted, I hope that the second edition of this handbook will represent these other cultures and their traditions. This handbook is an initial step in helping to bring together international qualitative nursing researchers to advance our discipline.

Introduction to qualitative nursing research

Cheryl Tatano Beck

Qualitative nursing research: a subdiscipline

Morse (2010) asked: "How different is qualitative health research from qualitative research? Do we have a subdiscipline?" (p. 1459). Her answer was yes. Morse (2012) defined qualitative health research "as a research approach to exploring health and illness as they are perceived by the people themselves, rather than from the researcher's perspective" (p. 21). Morse argued that the context, the participants in the research, and the nature of the research questions investigated in qualitative health research are distinct. She made the case (p. 1463) that researchers who conduct qualitative health research required special skills and qualifications as "insiders":

- Health professionals are "street smart," knowing the rules, regulations, and norms for working in a hospital or other health care contexts.
- Health professionals, with some working knowledge of the patient population, can recognize appropriate research questions.
- Because of their knowledge of the signs of fatigue and experience with illness, health professionals can monitor their patient participants throughout data collection.
- From their completed projects, health professionals can more readily make realistic recommendations for practice.

When conducting qualitative health research, a variety of health care professionals can be considered "insiders," such as nurses, physicians, respiratory therapists, social workers, dieticians, and physical therapists, to name but a few. Each of these qualitative health researchers can make a unique contribution to their respective disciplines and to health care, providing understanding and meaning to our research agendas.

Kuzel (2010) agreed with Morse that "insiders" are generally better than "outsiders" to conduct believable qualitative research. Eisner (1998, p. 39) stressed that "qualitative research becomes believable because of its coherence, insight, and instrumental utility." He called on qualitative researchers to have an enlightened eye, that is, "the ability to see what counts is what distinguishes novices from experts" (p. 34). Kuzel believed that experts in their respective fields are better suited to deliver these qualities that Eisner highlighted.

To begin this first ever *International Handbook of Qualitative Nursing Research*, I will ask the question: Is qualitative nursing research a subdiscipline of qualitative health research? Following

Morse's line of argument that qualitative health research is a subdiscipline of qualitative research, I believe qualitative nursing research *is* a subdiscipline of qualitative health research, and is particularly important for the advancement of nursing science. Many of Morse's arguments for why qualitative health research is a subdiscipline are pertinent to making the case for narrowing again the focus of qualitative research, this time to qualitative research in the discipline of nursing (Figure 1.1).

Qualitative health researchers need to be connoisseurs of the phenomena they are studying. These researchers are not connoisseurs in all health care-related disciplines. Phenomena studied in nutritional sciences, for example, are different than phenomena in medicine or social work or occupational therapy, including human behaviors associated with the physical phenomena. Nutrition, for instance, focuses on eating behaviors; medicine with symptom responses, compliance, and responses to therapy; occupational therapy to coping, and so forth. Each health care discipline can be considered a culture unto itself, with its own norms and perspectives. Medicine and these other disciplines do not have a subdiscipline of qualitative research yet but nursing does.

Members of each health care discipline can be considered as "insiders" while members of the other disciplines can be viewed as "outsiders." Nursing is a culture different from the other "cultures" in health care. Nurse researchers are the "insiders" who have the required special skills and qualifications: (1) to conduct qualitative research on phenomena in the discipline of nursing; and (2) to develop a specific body of knowledge known as qualitative nursing research.

In this introductory chapter, the emergence of qualitative inquiry in nursing is described. The remainder of the chapter describes the four parts of this handbook: Part I: What does qualitative nursing research do?, Part II: Qualitative research methods, Part III: Contemporary issues in qualitative nursing research methods, and Part IV: International qualitative nursing research: State of the science.

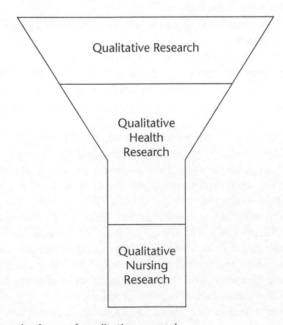

Figure 1.1 Narrowing the focus of qualitative research

Emergence of qualitative nursing research

In the 1960s, the federal nurse scientist program started and provided nurses opportunities to obtain doctoral degrees in the social sciences. Methods courses in anthropology and sociology were available for nurses to enroll in. Nurses studied with qualitative scholars such as Barney Glaser, Anselm Strauss, and Leonard Schatzman, to name but a few. At universities such as the University of California at San Francisco and Columbia University, nurses were educated in qualitative research methods. Jeanne Quint Benoliel, one of nursing's first qualitative scientists, was educated in this first wave. Until that time many nurses who had undertaken doctoral studies obtained their degrees in education and psychology where quantitative research was the prevailing method.

In the 1970s and early 1980s, tensions occurred in the discipline of nursing between the predominant quantitative researchers and the qualitative researchers who were in the minority. Qualitative research was viewed as "soft science." Hutchinson (2001) recounted how in the mid-1980s she and a few other qualitative nurse researchers who were members of the Council of Nursing and Anthropology met every year at the American Anthropology Association where they would present their qualitative papers. They would share with each other the high rejection rate of their qualitative manuscripts from journals that had rejected them for the wrong reasons. Reviewers not educated in qualitative methods would reject their manuscripts for reasons, such as small sample size and lack of random sampling. Hutchinson went on to tell how she and those few qualitative colleagues started on a mission to contact editors of journals to request that they add qualitative reviewers. Their efforts met with success in such journals as *Western Journal of Nursing Research*, *Advances in Nursing Science*, and *Image: Journal of Nursing Scholarship*. In the mid-1980s qualitative research textbooks in nursing were beginning to be published. Examples of these textbooks include Field and Morse's (1985) *Nursing Research: The Application of Qualitative Approaches*, Parse, Coyne, and Smith's (1985) *Nursing Research: Qualitative Methods*, Leininger's (1985) *Qualitative Research Methods in Nursing*, and Munhall and Oiler's (1986) *Nursing Research: A Qualitative Perspective*.

In 1986, Munhall astutely asked why had our nursing scholarship "evolved into a search for structural truth rather than dynamic meaning?" (p. 1). Why must nursing scholarship be polarized into two distinct positions of quantitative and qualitative research? Munhall argued (p. 5) that:

- our different angles enlarge our promise;
- are to be summative not negating;
- but engaging us in our community of endeavors.

Janice Morse in 1988 held a think tank for nurse leaders in qualitative research. Issues relevant to qualitative research were discussed. Morse published four edited volumes on qualitative research issues that were an outgrowth of these series of think tanks. The first volume was entitled *Qualitative Nursing Research: A Contemporary Dialogue* (Morse, 1991), followed by *Critical Issues in Qualitative Research Methods* (Morse, 1994). The third and fourth volumes were entitled *Completing a Qualitative Project* (Morse, 1997) and *The Nature of Qualitative Evidence* (Morse, Swanson, & Kuzel, 2001), respectively.

As the decade of the 1980s was coming to a close, the numbers of qualitative research manuscripts being published increased. Though progress was being made in the acceptance of qualitative research in our discipline, this was accompanied by a potential problem. There were not enough qualitative reviewers with expertise in different qualitative methods to review the influx of manuscripts. As a result, some sloppy qualitative research was being published. Research which included "method slurring" (Baker, Wuest, & Stern, 1992) of qualitative methods in a study was being published in top tier nursing journals. Reviewers, lacking substantive under-standing of qualitative methods, used rule-bound checklists as criteria for reviews, whether the criteria were appropriate for the methods they were reviewing or not.

In 1991, Janice Morse launched the first issue of the journal *Qualitative Health Research*. At that time the journal had four issues per year with six articles in each issue. It took six years for *Qualitative Health Research* to be referenced in Medline. Its niche market and readership have grown tremendously so much so that 22 years later there are now 12 issues a year with about 12 articles in each issue.

Next in this introductory chapter the four parts of this first ever international handbook of qualitative nursing research are introduced.

Part I: What does qualitative nursing research do?

Part I consists of eight chapters. This first section of the handbook will feature the "so what" of qualitative nursing research. In Chapter 2, Janice Morse addresses the significance of qualitative inquiry to the development of nursing knowledge. The other seven chapters in Part I feature exemplars of qualitative nursing research programs.

In Chapter 3, Judith Wuest, Marilyn Ford-Gilboe, Marilyn Merritt-Gray, and Colleen Varcoe discuss the processes, challenges, and advantages of translating their grounded theory, "Strengthening Capacity to Limit Intrusion," into a primary health care intervention for women who have left their abusive partners. Translation of grounded theories by researchers is crucial to facilitating their utilization in the clinical area.

In Chapter 4 the power of a program of qualitative research is clearly illustrated by Joanne Hall with her studies on traumatic experiences of marginalized groups. She examines the complex interrelated experiences, such as interpersonal violence, substance misuse, and racism in traumatized women.

Karin Olson in Chapter 5 describes her program of research on fatigue using qualitative research in conjunction with quantitative approaches. She and her team used their qualitative findings to reconceptualize fatigue, explore the social construction of fatigue, and develop the Edmonton Fatigue Framework.

In Chapter 6, Siv Söderberg presents her program of research on experiences of living with chronic pain syndrome that emerged from personal narrative interviews. By means of her research Söderberg illustrates that in order to preserve people's dignity within the health care system, clinicians need to be aware of the vulnerability of persons with chronic pain and their dependence on the power of health care providers to meet their individual needs.

Mary Beth Happ's qualitative research program in the care of ventilator-dependent ICU patients is highlighted in Chapter 7. Using a variety of qualitative and mixed methods Happ's research helped to explicate the social and cultural context and processes of interaction during critical care treatment of ventilator-dependent patients. Her research trajectory moved from descriptive theory building to intervention development and testing and then on to qualitative program evaluation.

In Chapter 8, Lauren Clark, Susan Johnson, Mary O'Connor, and Jane Lassetter describe their series of qualitative studies aimed at filling in the gaps of clinicians' understanding of Latino families' cultural values and patterns of infant feeding that result in normal weight or childhood obesity. Their focused ethnography helped to identify the mismatch between Latino parents and clinicians' cultural construction of childhood obesity, and in turn to develop effective childhood obesity prevention with Latino families.

In Chapter 9, Cheryl Tatano Beck's program of research on postpartum depression illustrates a line of scientific inquiry that was knowledge-driven and not limited to either qualitative or quantitative research methods. Her series of qualitative studies using phenomenology and grounded theory provided the conceptual basis for the development of her instrument, the Postpartum Depression Screening Scale (PDSS). All the items on the PDSS were developed from her qualitative findings.

Part II: Qualitative research methods

Seventeen chapters comprise Part II of the handbook which concentrates on various qualitative research methods. Some of these chapters on different qualitative research methods start with a brief history of that method's use in nursing research. Philosophical or theoretical underpinnings of the qualitative research method are discussed when appropriate. An advanced level discussion of the method and any various approaches to that method are addressed as well as any current debates or controversies regarding the method. A review of published studies over the past 20 years in which nurse researchers used that particular qualitative research method is included which leads to presentation of the state of the science of qualitative nursing research in regards to the method. Highlights of particular nursing research studies using that method and their analyses are included. Chapters end with a summary of the contributions of qualitative nursing research using this method, and future directions of this qualitative research method in nursing.

The first two chapters in Part II focus on phenomenology. In Chapter 10, Cheryl Tatano Beck describes the state of the science of descriptive phenomenology in nursing research. Published descriptive phenomenological studies conducted by nurse researchers across the globe over the past 20 years are reviewed. Trends in the methods used by nurse researchers and also the phenomena studied are identified.

Next, in Chapter 11, Patricia Munhall addresses interpretive phenomenology not only as a research method but also as a way of being-in-the-world. She helps the reader inquire how one should use an interpretive phenomenological philosophy as a research approach. Munhall describes her own approach to interpretive phenomenological inquiry. Exemplars of international interpretive phenomenological studies are identified.

Grounded theory is the focus of the next three chapters. In Chapter 12, Phyllis Noerager Stern presents classic Glaserian grounded theory supplemented with excellent examples from her own grounded theory studies. Next in Chapter 13 Juliet Corbin addresses Strauss' grounded theory method. The philosophy underlying Strauss' method and some of the criticisms directed at his method are described. A summary of studies using Strauss' method conducted by nurse researchers over the past 20 years is presented.

New directions in grounded theory are presented in Chapter 14 by Rita Schreiber and Wanda Martin. Some of the areas where grounded theorists are currently pushing the boundaries of the method are described, such as constructivist grounded theory, situational analysis, and complex adaptive systems perspective to ground theory. Examples from nursing research of each of these methods are highlighted.

The next four chapters concentrate on ethnography. First, in Chapter 15, Pamela Brink addresses traditional ethnography. She begins with the history of traditional ethnography in both anthropology and nursing, following this with a discussion of the basic requirements of this method. Some of the misunderstandings found in nursing literature regarding ethnography are identified. Her chapter ends with a review of some traditional ethnography nursing publications over the past 20 years.

In Chapter 16, Leininger's ethnonursing method is presented by Marilyn Ray, Edith Morris, and Marilyn McFarland. These authors address the philosophical and human science foundations of Leininger's ethnonursing method and the progression of her transcultural theory of culture care diversity and universality. Leininger's method is outlined and highlighted in terms of complexity science, complex caring dynamics, and translational science. Nursing research studies incorporating the ethnonursing method are highlighted. The chapter concludes with a description of the new meta-ethnonursing research method.

Karen Breda in Chapter 17 describes the historical evolution, value and relevance of critical ethnography within the family of critical qualitative research methodologies. She analyzes the nursing literature using critical ethnography, including controversial applications of this research method. Breda's chapter concludes with a discussion of the future directions of critical ethnography in nursing.

Institutional ethnography is the topic of Chapter 18 by Janet Rankin. This chapter includes a discussion of the philosophical and theoretical underpinnings of institutional ethnography and its methodological fit for nursing research. Selected examples of this type of ethnography conducted by nurse researchers are described in addition to examples from Rankin's own research which are presented to demonstrate the pragmatics of formulating an institutional ethnographic project.

Historical research in nursing is the focus of Chapter 19 by Sandra Lewenson. In this chapter the meaning and significance of historical research, and the impact various organizations, centers, and archives have had on the advancement of research on nursing history are addressed.

In Chapter 20, Patricia Hill Bailey, Phyllis Montgomery, and Sharolyn Mossey discuss narrative inquiry in nursing. The chapter begins by describing this method from the perspective of the major authors in this area. Next common classifications and features of stories and models of narrative analysis are presented. The authors discuss the ongoing controversy of the legitimacy of narrative as a research method. The state of narrative inquiry in nursing research concludes the chapter, along with an example of this method.

Discourse analysis is the featured topic of Chapter 21 by Michael Traynor. There are three main components of this chapter: (1) the range of practices that come under the title of discourse analysis and some of these differing assumptions about human subjectivity; (2) the different focus of discourse analysis by nurse researchers; and (3) the relationship between subjectivity and language.

In Chapter 22, Sally Thorne presents the interpretive description approach she has developed. The origins and development of this applied methodological approach that capitalizes on the perspective that nursing brings to rigorous qualitative inquiry are described. An exemplar of a nursing research study using the interpretive description is included to illustrate the method.

Denise Côté-Arsenault addresses focus groups in Chapter 23 where she provides a brief history of this method along with its use in nursing. Key aspects and considerations when using focus groups are described to help avoid common misuse of focus groups. Also included in this chapter are current controversies with focus groups. The chapter concludes with a review of published nursing research using focus groups from 2000 to 2010.

Participatory Action Research (PAR) is the focus of Chapter 24 by Lynne Young. She begins with defining PAR as a moving target as she differentiates it from Action Research. With PAR's roots in the social and political sciences and in organizational change literature, Young discusses how it is well suited to questions relevant to nursing. She provides examples of research that align with the principles of PAR to illustrate how these designs have been used by nurse researchers. Challenges and issues facing PAR researchers along with future directions are addressed in this chapter.

In Chapter 25, Barbara Paterson provides a historical and methodological overview of metasynthesis as a research approach. She highlights the major schools of thought in the field. Some of the most commonly used metasynthesis methods are described while comparing and contrasting their epistemological and methodological underpinnings. The chapter also includes critiques of metasyntheses that are identified in the literature and the challenges facing nurse researchers conducting metasyntheses.

In Chapter 26, the final chapter in Part II of this handbook, Margarete Sandelowski, Corrine Voils, Jamie Crandell, and Jennifer Leeman address mixed research synthesis. An overview is presented of the challenges of and approaches to conducting an integration of results from primary qualitative, quantitative, and mixed methods studies in a specific domain of research.

Part III: Contemporary issues in qualitative nursing research methods

Part III of the *Routledge International Handbook of Qualitative Nursing Research* targets some contemporary issues in the field. This third part consists of five chapters.

Chapter 27 focuses on ethical issues in qualitative nursing research and is authored by Wendy Austin. The more subtle risks in qualitative research, such as the emotional and social risks, are highlighted, along with particular ethical issues that can arise in dynamic and emergent qualitative research designs and that cannot be predicted with certainty. In this chapter, current policies and practices of research ethics are also addressed. Austin's approach of relational ethics is key in this chapter.

Joy Johnson considers the overlapping spheres of politics and qualitative nursing research in Chapter 28. Five related areas are addressed: the politics of evidence, the politics of research funding, the politics of grant writing and peer review, the politics of policy-making, and the politic of partnerships. Johnson draws on examples from her experiences in relation to her work with the Canadian Institutes of Health Research.

In Chapter 29, issues of Internet qualitative research are explored by Eun-Ok Im and Wonshik Chee. Characteristics of Internet research are reviewed, followed by general types of Internet qualitative research. A review of literature related to issues in Internet qualitative research in nursing is presented.

Sally Thorne considers secondary qualitative data analysis as it is currently applied within nursing in Chapter 30. She first presents its history and tradition in the qualitative nursing research context. Significant issues are addressed that nurse researchers must wrestle with and work out before a viable qualitative secondary analysis can be undertaken. Thorne describes five secondary research approaches: analytic expansion, retrospective interpretation, armchair induction, cross-validation, and amplified sampling. Issues in writing and reporting results from a qualitative secondary analysis are discussed in this chapter.

In the final chapter in Part III of the handbook, Chapter 31, Barbara Bowers explores the contributions and possibilities for qualitative nursing research in evidence-based practice. Questions are raised regarding what qualitative methodologies have to offer as nurse researchers develop evidence to support clinical practice. Challenges facing qualitative nurse researchers and the unrealized potential of qualitative research for our discipline are addressed.

Part IV: International qualitative nursing research: state of the science

In each of the 14 chapters in Part IV the focus is on the state of the science of qualitative nursing research in a particular country. Based on a review of literature of studies conducted in that country for the past 20 years, each chapter includes a brief history of qualitative nursing research in that country and describes what qualitative research methods are used most frequently by nurse researchers in that country. Specific contributions of qualitative nursing research in that country and to the nursing profession as a whole are addressed, along with highlights of some exemplars of the country's qualitative nursing research. The chapters end with a discussion of future directions of qualitative nursing research in that specific country. This fourth part of the handbook is the most unique and valuable addition to qualitative nursing research as nursing scholars from across the globe can see the state of the science of qualitative nursing research internationally.

In Chapter 32, Dawn Freshwater and Jane Cahill provide a state of the science of qualitative nursing research in England, Wales, and Scotland. The chapter begins with the historical context of nursing research in these three countries. Based on their literature review, these two authors describe the most frequent qualitative methods used in these countries by nurse researchers. Also research centers of excellence that focus on qualitative approaches in these countries are identified, along with their contributions to the field. Exemplars of cutting-edge qualitative nursing research are highlighted.

Qualitative nursing research in Ireland is the focus of Chapter 33, written by Carolyn Tobin. A history of nursing research in the Irish Republic in which the fundamental innovations that provided the building blocks for the increased research productivity over the past 15 years is described. Results of a literature review of qualitative nursing research conducted in the Irish Republic identify trends, research productivity, and focus over the past 15 years. Exemplars of qualitative research conducted by nurse researchers in Ireland are presented.

In Chapter 34, Joan Anderson considers the state of the science of qualitative nursing research in Canada. She begins by presenting the context of the development of qualitative research in Canada. Following this, she presents her interpretation of the intersecting factors influencing the development of qualitative nursing research by means of exemplars from Canadian nurse scholars, who have used different qualitative perspectives, in order to highlight the breadth of the theories and methodologies being used in Canada. Anderson concludes the chapter with a reflection on some broader questions based on her experience conducting qualitative research for 30 years.

Jennieffer Barr considers the state of qualitative nursing research in the countries of Australia and New Zealand in Chapter 35. She begins with the history of research development of Australasian nurses. The qualitative research methods most frequently used by nurse researchers are discussed, followed by the contribution that Australasian nurse researchers have made to the discipline of nursing. Suggestions for future research endeavors are included.

In Chapter 36, qualitative nursing research in four countries in Latin America (Brazil, Chile, Colombia, and Mexico) is presented. The authors of this chapter are María Claudia Duque-Páramo, Maria Itayra Padilha, Olivia Inés Sanhueza-Alvarado, María Magdalena Alonso Castillo, Fabiola Castellanos Soriano, Karla Selene López-García, and Yolanda Flores Peña. Their analysis reflects the different processes and characteristics of qualitative nursing research in these four countries. An in-depth literature review is also supplemented by interviews with researchers. For each Latin American country the following questions are addressed: the historical context; current purposes and contributions; methods, perspectives, approaches, tools; challenges and limitations; and future directions.

Qualitative nursing research in Spain is the focus of Chapter 37 written by Andreu Bover Bover, Denise Gastaldo, Margalida Miró and Concha Zaforteza. In this chapter the authors describe the movement that led to an increase in Spanish qualitative nursing research. Major trends in qualitative nursing research in Spain over the past decade are identified by means of a review of studies published by Spanish scholars in nursing. Qualitative nursing research in Spain represents a political opportunity to re-position nursing as a profession that produces scientific knowledge and engages with research in both academic and health care settings. Challenges facing qualitative nurse researchers in Spain are addressed.

Portugal is the focus of Chapter 38 which is authored by Marta Lima-Basto. The chapter begins with a historical background highlighting landmarks in the development of nursing research. Included is an analysis of doctoral theses conducted by Portuguese nurse researchers. The impact that qualitative studies have had in Portugal is reflected on.

In Chapter 39, Terese Bondas considers the qualitative methodological developments over the past two decades in nursing and caring science in Finland and Sweden. On the basis of an extensive literature review, Bondas classifies qualitative nursing research in these two countries in three eras: the trembling years, years of steady growth, and coming of age.

Qualitative nursing research in Norway, Denmark, and Iceland is addressed in Chapter 40 by Marit Kirkevold. After a brief historical overview of nursing research in these three countries, Kirkevold uses Kim's description of the structure of nursing knowledge to reveal how qualitative research in these countries has contributed to nursing in the areas of normative/ethical knowledge, situated/hermeneutical knowledge, transformative/critical hermeneutical understanding knowledge, aesthetic knowledge, and inferential/generalized knowledge.

Maria Grypdonck, Marijke Kars, Ann Van Hecke, and Sofie Verhaeghe consider qualitative nursing research in the Netherlands and Flanders in Chapter 41. The similarities and differences in the history of nursing research in these two countries are presented in the first section of the chapter. Qualitative methodologies used by nurse researchers in the Netherlands and Flanders are described with supporting examples of published studies.

In Chapter 42, qualitative nursing research in Korea is addressed by Kyung Rim Shin, Miyoung Kim, and Seung Eun Chung. The historical background of qualitative nursing research in Korea for the past 20 years is briefly examined. Published qualitative studies by Korean nurse researchers are reviewed from 1991 to 2010 and analyzed for trends and suggested future research directions.

Shigeko Saiki-Craighill presents the state of the science of qualitative nursing research in Japan in Chapter 43. Framed by the historical context, she provides an overview of both the quantity and quality of qualitative research conducted by nurse researchers in Japan. An in-depth analysis of one particular representative method, grounded theory, is performed.

In Chapter 44, David Arthur considers qualitative nursing research in South-East Asia, China, and Taiwan. He describes the development of qualitative research by nursing scholars in these countries. Next, the quantity and quality of qualitative research in these countries are addressed followed by some exemplars. Arthur highlights some methodological issues in these countries and the future of qualitative research in nursing.

The final chapter, by Cheryl Tatano Beck, looks at the future directions in international qualitative nursing research. Chapter 45 is a compilation of the directions for future qualitative research around the globe that the nursing contributors of this handbook have identified and merit our attention in order to advance qualitative research in our discipline.

References

Baker, C., Wuest, J., & Stern, P. N. (1992). Method slurring: The grounded theory/phenomenology example. *Journal of Advanced Nursing, 17*, 1355–1360.

Eisner, E. W. (1998). *The enlightened eye: Qualitative inquiry and the enhancement of educational practice.* Upper Saddle River, NJ: Bobbs Merrill.

Field, P. A., & Morse, J. M. (1985). *Nursing research: The application of qualitative approaches.* Rockville, MD: Aspen Publishers.

Hutchinson, S. A. (2001). The development of qualitative health research: Taking stock. *Qualitative Health Research, 11*, 505–521.

Kuzel, A. J. (2010). Commentary 1: The importance of expertise. *Qualitative Health Research*, *20*, 1464–1465.

Leininger, M. M. (Ed.). (1985). *Qualitative research methods in nursing*. Orlando, FL: Grune & Stratton, Inc.

Morse, J. M. (Ed.). (1991). *Qualitative nursing research: A contemporary dialogue*. Newbury Park, CA: Sage.

Morse, J. M. (Ed.). (1994). *Critical issues in qualitative research methods*. Thousand Oaks, CA: Sage.

Morse, J. M. (Ed.). (1997). *Completing a qualitative project: Details and dialogue*. Thousand Oaks, CA: Sage.

Morse, J. M. (2007). What is the domain of qualitative health research? *Qualitative Health Research*, *17*, 715–717.

Morse, J. M. (2010). How different is qualitative health research from qualitative research? Do we have a subdiscipline? *Qualitative Health Research*, *20*, 1459–1464.

Morse, J. M. (2012). *Qualitative health research: Creating a new discipline*. Walnut Creek: CA: Left Coast Press.

Morse, J. M., Swanson, J., & Kuzel, A. (Eds.). (2001). *The nature of qualitative evidence*. Thousand Oaks, CA: Sage.

Munhall, P. L. (1986). Methodological issues in nursing research: Beyond a wax apple. *Advances in Nursing Science*, *8*, 1–5.

Munhall, P., & Oiler, C. (Eds.). (1986). *Nursing research: A qualitative perspective*. Norwalk, CT: Appleton-Century-Crofts.

Parse, R. R., Coyne, A. B., & Smith, M. J. (1985). *Nursing research: Qualitative methods*. Bowie, MD: Brady Communications Company.

Sandelowski, M., & Barroso, J. (2007). *Handbook for synthesizing qualitative research*. New York: Springer.

Part I

What does qualitative nursing research do?

The development of qualitative nursing research

Janice M. Morse

Nursing care is neither easily taught, nor easily learned. Most difficult, is researching nursing care: documenting the art of nursing, describing and eliciting the nurse–patient interaction, the meaning of care to the patient, and the effects and outcomes of such care. Such description requires introspective understanding, interpretative insight, and the creation of theories; it requires identification of interventions, the production of evidence that reveals effectiveness, and it thereby furthers the development of nursing practice. This is what we call qualitative nursing research.

People say, "soft science is harder," meaning that engaging in the science of an art is more difficult than bench science or quantitative research. It is more difficult because qualitative researchers study subjective experiences rather than hard concrete facts. We are using humanistic methods, examining subjectively, inductively and inferentially, rather than using discrete measures. And as nurses, our participants are those who are suffering, who are at the edge of what they know and understand, and facing their greatest fears and losses. They are vulnerable in the extreme.

Qualitative methods provide researchers with a way of seeing, and a way to understand; a way of listening, and a way to hear; ways of accessing and empathetically knowing the most intimate parts of the other. Our methods are humanistic, gentle and kind, in our empathetic interaction with our participants. Our nursing selves—with the skills that nurses have learned clinically, working with those in pain, ill or dying—facilitate our ability to collect data, to observe, to interview, to know, and to subsequently analyze and disseminate the research and identify interventions.

Qualitative researchers have no concrete measures, no yardsticks to verify what people feel, no monitors to quantify their agonies and to add credence to our research. The quality of qualitative inquiry can only be shown in the quality of the results, in the richness and accuracy of the description, in the essence of the interpretation, in the recognition of the situation or what it implies, and in the elegance of the theory and its ramifications. And when qualitative researchers reveal the experiences of such suffering or the struggles to regain health, such disclosure is often not very pleasant. Many people find it so painful read that it is easier to ignore, than to face what we write.

In this chapter, I will describe the development of qualitative nursing research, both as a method and in the substantive areas that we study; I will also discuss the global dissemination of this method. In doing so, I will explain why qualitative research is so essential to molding our profession, and to improving health and health care to society in general.

What is qualitative nursing research?

Qualitative nursing research is a recent research paradigm in nursing—so new, in fact, that many established nurse researchers may have never taken a course in qualitative inquiry, and know little of its various methods and strategies, assumptions, principles, and contributions. In fact, as with all innovations, qualitative methods are not uniformly distributed, accepted or equally incorporated into the curriculum. In some nursing programs they are standard and accepted, but in others—and sometimes in quite influential schools of nursing—they are absent. These schools argue that qualitative inquiry is not justified in their program because it may be considered "unfundable" by our national granting agencies (that is, unsuited for funding because of its unorthodox methods and different standards), and their goal is to train career nurse researchers, whose quantitative skills will be fundable. Thus, these schools do not offer qualitative courses and no qualitative research is conducted in these programs. This position, of course, will change dramatically in the future, as qualitative nurse researchers increase in number, as the number of publications using qualitative methods increase, and as the number of qualitative researchers on national funding boards balance the present quantitative researcher majority. It is now inevitable that qualitative nursing research will become an essential component of nursing programs at the doctoral level (or earlier), and that qualitative inquiry will become critical for the development of nursing knowledge. This volume gives credence to this position, in helping move qualitative nursing research one step forward.

The development of qualitative research

In this section, I will provide an overview of the development of qualitative methods in general, and then discuss the later development of qualitative inquiry in nursing.

The first phase (1900–1960): The development of qualitative methods

Observation and interviewing have always contributed to the development of knowledge. For instance, in medicine, there was the development of the compendia of signs and symptoms and basic anatomy, as developed from observation and pattern recognition over the past several centuries. In the early 1900s, qualitative methods developed in the "modern" form, from several disciplines, in different ways. In anthropology, Malinowski developed methods of fieldwork and ethnography—methods that were further developed by his students, including Margaret Mead, Ruth Benedict, and Evans-Pritchard. With other early anthropologists, ethnography was established, and the normative way to study culture was by living with the group being studied, learning their languages, and observing, interviewing, and recording field notes.

A second strand of inquiry emerged from the European phenomenological philosophers, mainly Husserl (1859–1938) who worked through phenomenological reductionism, intentionality, consciousness and "bracketing" and Heidegger (1889–1976), related to the essence of "being in the world" and the experiences associated with being. In psychology, the phenomenologist Merleau-Ponty (1908–1961), a student of both Husserl and Heidegger, developed the notion of "consciousness as the source of all knowledge," of perception, and embodiment. Also from psychology is also the work of Jean Piaget (1896–1980), who used microanalytic observational methods, observing his own two infants, and developing a theory of cognitive development.

The work of these early researchers formed the basis of qualitative methods as we know them today. Although the number of strategies have increased and been formalized within each method, and different forms (or styles) of each method have emerged, these early researchers must be credited with the development of qualitative research.

During this period in nursing, apart from the epidemiological efforts of Florence Nightingale, research was virtually absent. Without qualitative research methods, early nursing theorists used their own experiences of nursing to develop nursing frameworks for practice, writing from what they already knew or had learned themselves in the process of providing care. This is the case for our greatest early nurses, such as: Florence Nightingale's *Notes on Nursing* (1859/1960), Virginia Henderson's collaborative work with Harmer and Henderson (1939) and Henderson's (1966), *The Nature of Nursing*; Hildegard Papleau's (1952) *The Interpersonal Relations in Nursing*; and Dorothea Orem's (1971) *Nursing: Concepts of Practice*. Their nursing "theories" were not actually theories, but rather conceptualizations of practice. Using their own knowledge of nursing practice, they described ways to organize care and to give it a particular perspective. These nurses made a tremendous contribution to nursing, considering they did not have the research tools and supports that we now have in the twenty-first century.

The second phase: Recognition of the essentialness of nursing concepts, 1950–present

After these "framework theorists," beginning about the 1950s, it was realized that new concepts were essential if we were to describe nursing practice. Hildegard Papleau invited Carl Rogers to Keynote at the America Nurses Association Annual Convention in 1957. He described empathy in his address, and this concept was immediately adopted into nursing (Morse, Anderson, Bottorff, et al., 1992). But borrowing concepts from other disciplines was only a partial solution (and often an unsatisfactory solution) for nursing. Often concepts developed for another discipline were not always a good fit for nursing phenomena. Subsequently, in 1973, a group of 11 nurses formed the Committee of the Whole of the Nursing Development Conference Group (NDCG, 1973) to discuss concepts and their development. About this time, several edited books appeared, with each chapter written about a particular concept of interest to nurses and nursing education (Carlson, 1970; Norris, 1982). Note that while nursing was struggling with these efforts, other disciplines, particularly anthropology and sociology, were conducting qualitative research and publishing monographs to develop their concepts.

The demand for *nursing concepts* continues to this time, with several approaches to concepts development available to nurses (e.g. Walker & Avant, 1983; Knafl & Rodgers, 2000). Unfortunately, this important task is conducted by students as a part of their first doctoral class, rather than being approached seriously by competent nurse researchers, so progress in developing our profession has been hobbled.

The third phase (1960–1985): The emergence of qualitative health research

In the third phase, qualitative methods began to cluster in various university departments by types of methods. In these units, a professor with a particular type of methodological expertise, with a group of students, formed a *cluster*, a team investigating particular topics. The earliest example was at the University of California at San Francisco, where Barney Glaser and Anselm Strauss, sociologists hired by the University of California School of Nursing, wrote their classic methods book, *The Discovery of Grounded Theory* (Glaser & Strauss, 1967). In addition to developing grounded theory, they conducted studies on dying in hospitals (Glaser & Strauss, 1965, 1968), and later, collaborating with their students, studies on the comfort work of nurses (Corbin & Strauss, 1988). These were strong studies with mid-range theory, and clinical application to nursing and health care. As Glaser and Strauss' students graduated, they continued to conduct research in health care, to mentor students of their own, and to publish both methods texts and studies of health illness, thus promulgating grounded theory across the United States and beyond.

In the1960s, recognizing the importance of nursing research and the need for doctorally prepared nurses, the NCNR NIH Nurse Scientist Program provided funding to support nurses to attend doctoral programs in disciplines outside of nursing. Many selected bench science programs, but a few chose anthropology and sociology. Nurses who selected sociology and anthropology learned qualitative methods, and brought them back into nursing, primarily through the study of culture and health—and later to develop transcultural nursing (Leininger, 1978). Through the American Anthropological Association, they developed an interest group, the Council of Nursing and Anthropology (CONAA), supporting the development of transcultural nursing and qualitative inquiry nationally. Although transcultural nursing remained the primary vehicle for qualitative methods for some time, eventually qualitative inquiry moved beyond "culture" to explore the subjective domains of nursing. In 1985, Leininger published the first qualitative methods book, applying qualitative inquiry from culture and health to nursing in general.

We owe a tremendous debt to this cadre of nurses who fought for the introduction of qualitative research into nursing. Margarita Kay, Eleanor Bowen, Pam Brink, Noel Chrisman, and Melanie Dreher prepared course outlines, and taught the first courses. They monitored journal editors, insisting on fair reviews by qualified reviewers. And by their presence they provided an appreciative audience for our meetings, which was mentorship *par excellence*!

The fourth phase: qualitative nursing methods: Coming of age, 1990–present

In the mid-1990s, qualitative research "came of age." Qualitative researchers received NIH funding. They examined nursing phenomena, both micro- and macroanalytically, and it is these topics that are combining with ongoing work to form the theoretical foundation of nursing.

Etching a new and different research approach into academia and into nursing was a relatively slow and arduous process. Despite resistance, qualitative inquiry is now making a distinct contribution to nursing and to health care, filling a necessary void that cannot be filled by quantitative research. Articles describing methods added to our understanding of qualitative inquiry, albeit in short "bites" given the limitations of the 15-page article, and these become increasingly common from the 1990s. Presently, *Qualitative Health Research* is the primary venue for qualitative nursing research, with many supporting journals such as *Nursing Inquiry*, *Journal of Advanced Nursing*, *Western Journal of Nursing Research*, and *Research in Nursing and in Health*. A journal, *Global Qualitative Nursing Research*, is planned for 2013 (Sage, online), and other nursing journals routinely publish qualitative inquiry. The International Institute for Qualitative Methodology (IIQM) holds annual Qualitative Health Research conferences. The recently established Global Congress for Qualitative Health Research will present its third convention in Thailand, in 2013. Qualitative nurse researchers also attend multidisciplinary qualitative conferences (such as the International Congress for Qualitative Inquiry (ICQI)) where they stand shoulder-to-shoulder with researchers from other disciplines.

In 1985, the first qualitative research texts written especially for nursing appeared (Leininger; Field & Morse; Morse & Field; Parse, Coyne, & Smith) (see Table 2.1). Shortly afterwards, the first edition of Munhall's classic series appeared (Munhall & Boyd, 1987), and this edited book has been continuously in print since that time; it is now in its fifth edition (Munhall, 2012). These "overview" books were generally used in introductory courses, and are detailed and comprehensive; much of the content is specific to the context of nursing, illustrating how qualitative inquiry may enhance care. The publication dates of these books closely resemble the establishment of doctoral programs internationally, and it is probable that the demand for such texts by doctoral students was a factor in their publication.

A proliferation of single method books closely trailed the overview texts, with grounded theory forming the strongest and earliest cadre of collaborators (Table 2.1). The single method books tend to be used for more advanced courses or by researchers needing more detailed information.

There are also "special topics" books, which address particularly difficult aspects of qualitative inquiry. The appearance of these books indicates that nurse researchers have something useful, and even insightful, to add to the growing debates in qualitative inquiry, and attacking special problems—certainly a sign of qualitative maturity.

Table 2.1 Qualitative nursing research methods books, by type, date and country

Title	Author(s)	Date	Country
General			
Nursing research: The application of qualitative approaches (trans. Finnish, Korean, German, Japanese)	Field & Morse Morse & Field	1st ed. 1985 2nd ed. 1995	Canada
Qualitative research methods in nursing	Leininger	1985	USA
Nursing research: Qualitative methods	Parse, Coyne, & Smith	1985	USA
Qualitative health research	Morse	1992	Canada
Nursing research: A qualitative perspective	Munhall & Boyd Munhall	1st ed. 1987 2nd ed. 1993 3rd ed. 2000a 4th ed. 2006 5th ed. 2012	USA
Qualitative research for nurses *Qualitative research for nurses* *Qualitative research for nursing and health care*	Holloway & Wheeler	1st ed. 1996 2nd ed. 2002 3rd ed. 2010	Great Britain
Qualitative research in nursing: Advancing the humanistic perspective	Streubert & Carpenter Streubert & Carpenter Speziale & Carpenter Speziale & Carpenter Streubert & Carpenter	1st ed. 1995 2nd ed. 1999 3rd ed. 2003 4th ed. 2007 5th ed. 2011	USA
Pesquisa em Enfermagem: Novas Metodologias Aplicadas [Nursing research: New methods]	Gauthier, Santos, Cabral, & Tavares	1998	Brazil
Readme first for a user's guide to qualitative research (trans. Korean, Italian, Japanese)	Morse & Richards Richards & Morse Richards & Morse	1st ed. 2002 2nd ed. 2007 3rd ed. 2012	Canada/ Australia

Table 2.1 Continued

Title	Author(s)	Date	Country
Qualitative Gesundheits- und Pflegeforschung [Qualitative health research and care]	Schaeffer & Müller-Mundt	2002	Germany
Advanced qualitative research for nursing	Latimer	2003	Great Britain
ศิริพร จิรวัฒน์กุล. การวิจัยเชิงคุณภาพในวิชาชีพการพยาบาล. ขอนแก่น: ศิริภัณฑ์ออฟเซท. จำนวน หน้า [Qualitative research in nursing] [Qualitative research in nursing] [Qualitative research in nursing]	Chirawatkul	1st ed. 2003 2nd ed. 2005 3rd ed. 2012	Thailand
질적연구 용어사전 [Qualitative research methodology]	Shin, Kim, Kim, et al.	2003	South Korea
질적연구방법론 [Qualitative research methodology]	Shin, Cho, & Yang	2004	South Korea
Pesquisa Qualitativa em Enfermagem [Qualitative research in nursing]	Matheus & Fustinoni	2006	Brazil
护理质性研究 [Qualitative research in nursing]	Liu	2008	China
Abordagens Qualitativas: trilhas para pesquisadores em saúde e enfermagem [Qualitative approach: Path for researchers in health and nursing]	Teixeira	2008	Brazil
Grounded theory			
From practice to grounded theory	Chenitz & Swanson	1986	USA
Basics of qualitative research (trans. Chinese, Japanese, Arabic)	Strauss & Corbin Strauss & Corbin Corbin & Strauss	1st ed. 1990 2nd ed. 1998 3rd ed. 2007	USA
Grounded theory in practice	Strauss & Corbin	1997	USA
Using grounded theory in nursing	Schrieber & Stern	2001	Canada/USA
Developing grounded theory: The second generation	Morse, Stern, Corbin, Charmaz, & Clarke	2009	USA
Essentials of accessible grounded theory	Stern & Porr	2011	USA/Canada
Ethnography			
Ethnography in nursing research	Roper & Shapira	2000	USA
Interpretative description			
Interpretive description	Thorne	2008	USA

Table 2.1 Continued

Title	Author(s)	Date	Country
Phenomenology			
Interpretative phenomenology	Benner	1994	USA
Revisioning phenomenology: Nursing and health science research	Munhall	1994	USA
Hermeneutic phenomenological research	Cohen, Steeves, & Kahn	2000	USA
현상학적 연구 [Phenomenological research]	Shin & Kong	2001	Korea
Å forske i sykdoms- og pleieerfaringer: Livsfenomenologisk bidrag [Research in sickness- and caring experiences: A life world phenomenological contribution]	Bengtsson	2006	Norway
Reflexive lifeworld research	Dahlberg, Dahlberg, & Nyström	2008	Sweden
Mixed-method			
Mixed-method design: Principles and procedures	Morse & Niehaus	2007	Canada
Special topics			
Qualitative nursing research: A contemporary dialogue	Morse (Ed.)	1989	Canada
Qualitative health research	Morse (Ed.)	1992	Canada
Critical issues in qualitative research methods (trans. Spanish)	Morse (Ed.)	1994	Canada
Completing a qualitative project: Details and dialogue	Morse (Ed.)	1997	Canada
Qualitative research proposals and reports	Munhall	1st ed. 1991 2nd ed. 2000b 3rd ed. 2010	USA
The nature of qualitative evidence	Morse, Swanson, & Kuzel	2001	Canada/USA
O método de análise de conteúdo: uma versão para enfermeiros [Content analysis: Nurses approach]	Rodrigues & Leopardi	1999	Brazil
Handbook for synthesizing qualitative research	Sandelowski & Barroso	2007	USA
Essentials of a qualitative doctorate	Holloway & Brown	2012	Great Britain
Essentials of qualitative interviewing	Olson	2011	Canada
Focus group research	Carey & Ashbury	2012	USA

Global dissemination for qualitative methods for nursing

Compared with the slow and rocky introduction of qualitative research into nursing, the spread of qualitative methods internationally was relatively rapid. New methods were disseminated first by foreign students learning qualitative methods during the course of their doctoral programs in the United States. As these students returned to their own countries to teach qualitative methods and to offer workshops, and supervise students, they published articles and chapters using the particular methods with which they were familiar, and, in time mentored a new generation of qualitative researchers. The original mentor may also have translated the methods book written in English into his or her own language. The final step is the writing of a new qualitative methods book for nursing for their own context, and in their own language.

The international dispersal of qualitative methods in nursing

The introduction of qualitative methods in chapters, written by nurses, in edited books prepared for a larger market, appears before foreign language books; they are more difficult to trace, and I have not cited them here. However, they do provide some evidence of the growth of qualitative inquiry within a particular region. For instance, I could not find a single book written by nurses in Spanish, but Denise Gastaldo has contributed a chapter in a more general text (Mercado, Gastaldo, & Calderón, 2002).

The dispersal of qualitative methods internationally typically follows the publication of books in the United States. First, books published by authors in North America were translated into other languages. These books, written in foreign languages for nurses of a particular country, appeared to be an indicator of "readiness" to learn about and to do qualitative inquiry in schools of nursing.

These translated books were then followed by qualitative methods books, both general and specialist methods, authored by nurses internationally (see Table 2.1). The publication dates of these books provide one indicator of the dissemination of qualitative research methods internationally. They form a pattern of dissemination and indicate the introduction, demand and even the utilization of qualitative methods globally. The list in Table 2.1 contains those books with an author or co-author who is a nurse, and who was writing qualitative methods for nursing students and nurse researchers. The list is probably not complete, and I apologize to those whose books have been omitted. The list also does not reflect the distribution of books in qualitative inquiry written in English (and that were later translated) or, for instance, of books such as Morse and Field's (1995) that was simultaneously published in the US and Great Britain. Note that while the first general qualitative books emerged from the US and Canada in 1985, the first in Great Britain was not until 1995; Sweden, Germany and Australia in 2002; South Korea in 2003; China in 2008; and Thailand in 2011.

Grounded theory made its mark quite early internationally, and the early Strauss and Corbin works have been translated into ten languages. The other major method is phenomenology, and research groups using van Manen's (1990) text are found in Scandinavia, Australia, China, and South Korea, as well as the US.

Nurses' contributions to the development of qualitative methods

As noted in the first part of this chapter, methods of qualitative inquiry developed rapidly, and this trend continues as nurses become major players in the areas of synthesis, qualitative evidence, and qualitatively driven mixed methods design. In nursing, we are expanding beyond our

30-year preoccupation with the development of concepts and theory, to application and the integration of research in two ways: (1) by making our research stronger by synthesizing several similar projects; and (2) in mixed methods, we are becoming stronger by forming a foundation that is then enhanced by quantitative findings or provides a springboard for quantitative inquiry. Qualitative inquiry is becoming essential to knowledge development.

Qualitative methods continue to evolve and be modified, and new methods develop. In nursing we realize that when collecting data in the clinical area, there are constraints to data collection imposed by the hospital environment and by the patients' condition that often require modifications to standard qualitative methods. For instance, in the hospital environment, it may be difficult to find a private, quiet place to conduct an interview. Patients often share rooms, other staff interrupt to check on the patient or to give medications, and the patient has a host of scheduled appointments: X-rays, blood tests, doctors' visits, housekeeping, meals, and relatives' visits all intrude. Recordings may prove difficult—the patient may have a dry mouth, or be fatigued; once, when I placed the recorder on the patient's chest, I found I had recorded the click of artificial heart valves, rather than the interview. Patients may be too shocked, or enduring events or pain, to be able to express themselves; they may be on a ventilator and unable to speak. They may be confused, be cognitively impaired or have amnesia, or feel drowsy from drugs, and thus not be able to be interviewed. In these cases, observational research becomes more important, i.e., "retrospective" interviews conducted once the patient is able to be interviewed, or interviews with the vigilant significant others (Morse, 2012). Shorter hospital stays, and patients being discharged before they are well, transfer some data collection into the home or rehabilitation hospital. There is no doubt that qualitative nurse researchers must be versatile and resourceful.

What do these conditions do to the application of the method? If only inadequate data can be collected by the method planned—for instance, only one, not two of the planned interviews may be obtained from each patient—then the researcher must either increase the sample size or interview observers, that is, other patients, significant others or nurses. Sometimes multiple indicators have to be used to examine the same phenomena. For instance, Kayser-Jones, Kris, Miaskowski, Lyons, and Steve (2006), when needing an indicator of pain intensity experienced by elderly demented nursing home residents, used posturing and grimacing, vocalizations, and the assessment of relatives and nurses.

Have nurses developed qualitative methods? To date, only Leininger has attempted to develop a separate method for nursing, an adaptation of ethnography for nursing, which she called ethnonursing (Leininger, 1997). However, it is not used extensively, and a recent metasynthesis of the findings from these studies revealed only 24 dissertations (McFarland, Wehbe-Alamah, Wilson, & Vossos, 2011).

Other nurses have made contributions to qualitative nursing research. Sandelowski and Barroso (2007) refined methods of synthesizing qualitative findings. Morse and Niehaus (2009) introduced some strategies to refine mixed method design. The latest complete method book was Thorne's (2008) *Interpretative Description*, moving description another step forward by adding methods to eliciting meaning.

The implementation failure of qualitative nursing research?

Qualitative inquiry is still somewhat ignored in the areas of evidence-based practice. Yet qualitative projects are being conducted with greater intensity. What happens to these projects?

These articles fill our journals, and, in turn, are primarily cited by other researchers and students. Not clinicians? I do not think they know what to do with the information at the bedside.

If these studies provide information that assists them to recognize "what is going on" with their patients, it is not making its way back to our conferences or to our literature.

Are the qualitative studies too small, too local? Perhaps they need to be amalgamated. Metasynthesis will facilitate this process, and these are appearing with greater frequency for our more common topics. The recent funding of a five-year project by Kathy Knafl and Margarete Sandelowski to synthesize literature on child health (Anon, 2011) will be a major milestone in this area. The utilization of methods of synthesis will have importance for clinical research, including incorporation of qualitative findings into the Cochrane Database.

Perhaps there is a lack of useful qualitative inquiry because most qualitative researchers are focused on inferential methods, rather than on "harder" data, such as methods of microanalytic description. I made the argument that methods of qualitative inquiry, such as microanalysis of video data, would enable evaluation of much clinical phenomena, such as assessing risk of fall while climbing out of bed (Morse, 2012).

Elsewhere I have argued that our methods of assessing evidence—and even considering the nature of evidence—are narrow and exclude qualitative contributions. Qualitative assessment enables evaluation for less monetary cost, and less risk of harm; and if one includes principles of logic and common sense, such inquiry may not even require data of the actual incident (Morse, 2012). For instance, such qualitative methods with potential may be the assessment of incident reports, with or without harm, and extrapolation of these patterns of causation to the introduction of policy to prevent future incidence. Such use of qualitative research is in aviation, where the human cost of an "incident" is too great to wait until it occurs, and policy changes are based upon near misses (Connell, 2004). It is the ethical, moral and economic way to proceed in many instances, and this approach has great potential for nursing and is already the basis for preventing errors in hospitals, such as medication errors.

What does qualitative research contribute to nursing knowledge?

The discipline of nursing is both a hard science and an art, concerned with both the objective and the subjective—concerned both with the physical body and with all aspects of the person. But qualitative nursing research focuses on the subjective: on health and illness, on birth and dying, on the person, their family, and the community. In nursing, the technical aspects of care are melded with the interpersonal, with the patient as a recipient of care and the attentions of the lay caregiver or the nurse. In nursing, the subjective experiences of illness, rehabilitation and attaining health is as important as the objective measurement inherent in physical assessment. Nursing is focused on the person, yet concerned with populations and, of course with dyads and families. These are areas in which qualitative inquiry should be a key player in research, making major contributions. Has it? Earlier I argued that qualitative research was poorly funded. Studies are small and criticized for their lack of significance. These questions remain: Has qualitative inquiry contributed to nursing knowledge? What has been contributed? And how?

The collectiveness of qualitative knowledge

One criticism of qualitative studies is that they are small and insignificant, because the investigator cannot "manage" large numbers of cases of in-depth data. Even when using a qualitative data program, there are limits to human conceptualization. As a result, qualitative studies tend to be limited in scope and number of participants—usually less than 50 for a study using interview data. While one could argue that such a study may produce significant insights, a single qualitative study, published as a 15-page article, usually has limited impact.

Generally, however, the development of qualitative knowledge does not depend upon one study at a time, but rather upon the accrual of results of many small studies on a similar topic. Despite problems with replication, these studies on diverse topics, on concepts, on changing phenomena, presenting different interpretations, eventually support each other and meld into consensus: knowledge becomes accepted, and extends to form theory. Of course, this does not happen by itself, nor by some magical emergence. It happens through our basic inquiry, our overlapping findings, our beginning inquiry on firm foundations from the research of others, from our metasynthesis, and eventually leading to the acceptance of our concepts and theories.

While patterns of inquiry and research programs differ, these studies are most often conducted by different authors, and are not exactly the same—not replications—but they are overlapping studies that in part endorse each other.

These studies develop general areas of knowledge, following a general trend. The pattern of development falls roughly into eight levels (Morse, 2012):

Level 1: Exploratory, descriptive studies, identifying the phenomenon.
Level 2: From the phenomenon, description and delineating, developing the concept(s).
Level 3: Examining the concept in different contexts or situations.
Level 4: Exploring the concept with other co-occurring concepts.
Level 5: Synthesizing studies about the concept.
Level 6: Model and theory development.
Level 7: Developing assessment and measurement.
Level 8: Clinical applications, evaluation and outcomes.

These levels do not indicate that studies at a higher level are more significant, or more rigorous, than those at a lower level. Although generally descriptive studies must precede inferential ones, and studies developing the concept should precede studies that develop theory, leveling is not associated with contribution nor sophistication of higher level studies (Sandelowski, 2008).

There are numerous broad topics that have been researched by many qualitative nurse researchers, and these have made major contributions following this general pattern of knowledge development. Examples of these topics are: caring, social support, empathy, and nurse–patient relationships. These areas are not inclusive—they are listed because they were primarily the first areas that qualitative researchers addressed, and have therefore a long history of inquiry and had the time to build a strong body of knowledge. These studies incrementally accrue to form a theoretical foundation for nursing science and nursing praxis.

Developing qualitative knowledge: the example of caring

Because it takes time and many, many studies to develop an area of inquiry, I will demonstrate the development of one of the earliest qualitative areas: caring. Paley (2001) noted in frustration that there has been "a small avalanche of publications" on this topic (p. 188), and that these descriptions of caring are "simply added to previous descriptions . . . and the space into which it expands has no effective boundaries" (p. 192). Thus, knowledge piles, often without any acknowledgment of previous work, or advance in knowledge. I disagree that researchers have no boundaries: such boundaries should be enforced by reviewers and editors. Since qualitative inquiry does not directly replicate, if a qualitative study does not contribute anything new, it should be rejected.

However, as Paley (2001) correctly indicates, we are in the midst of a vast collection of studies on caring. Therefore, the ones used in the example below are not especially seminal, but are typical of the studies of each general type for each level.

From the titles of studies listed in Table 2.2, one can clearly see the changes in the focus of the studies by each level. As knowledge is gained, the studies do change in focus, from basic description, to analyzing the concepts, to exploring different settings in which the concepts occur and allied (co-occurring) concepts. By Level 5, there are sufficiently rich and detailed to build a foundation for metasyntheses, then mid-range theories. At this point the research shifts to assessment and measurement, and to clinical application and caring interventions. The research area becomes "mature," and embodied into the discipline and into practice.

Table 2.2 Level of research developing nursing phenomenon: the example of caring

Level of research	Examples of studies
Level 1: Identifying caring	The experience of caring (Forrest, 1986) Noncaring and caring in the clinical setting: patients' descriptions (Reimen, 1986)
Level 2: Describing, delineating and developing the caring as a concept	Comparison of cancer patients' and professional nurses' perceptions of important caring behaviors (Larson, 1987) The caring concept and nurse-identified caring behaviors (Wolf, 1986)
Level 3: Examining caring in different contexts or situations	Importance of nurse caring behaviors as perceived by patients after myocardial infarction (Cronin & Harrison, 1988) Caring needs of women who miscarried (Swanson-Kauffman, 1988)
Level 4: Exploring caring with other co-occurring concepts	How well do family caregivers cope after caring for a relative with advanced disease and how can health professionals enhance their support? (Hudson, 2006) Patients' and nurses' experiences of the caring relationship in hospital: an aware striving for trust (Berg & Danielson, 2007)
Level 5: Synthesizing caring studies	Metasynthesis of qualitative analyses of caring: defining a therapeutic model of nursing (Sherwood, 1997) Metasynthesis of caring in nursing (Finfgeld-Connett, 2007)
Level 6: Developing models and theories of caring	Empirical development of a middle-range theory of caring (Swanson, 1991) The theory of human caring: retrospective and prospective (Watson, 1997)
Level 7: Assessing and measuring caring	Effects of nursing rounds on patients' call light use, satisfaction and safety (Meade, Bursell, & Ketelsen, 2006) Caring in patient-focused care: the relationship of patients' perceptions of holistic nurse caring to their levels of anxiety (Williams, 1997)
Level 8: Clinical application and caring interventions	Caring theory as ethical guide to administrative and clinical practices (Watson, 2005) Nursing as informed caring for the well-being of others (Swanson, 1993)

Patterns of researcher programs in qualitative nursing research

Not all qualitative nursing research is conducted in such an apparently disjointed manner as described above. Some researchers are working on a single problem or areas for large blocks of time—some even for their entire careers. And their research forms a logical sequence of studies, and creates a meaningful contribution. Some of these researchers have contributed review articles of this work to this volume, and other examples are summarized below.

Identifying phenomena (Level 1)

In the course of analyzing data on nurses' responses to patients in agonizing pain in the trauma room, we found data that did not fit empathy as it was presently described: as a feeling towards another's plight. Rather, these data described a physical response in the nurses towards the pain expression and observing injuries experienced in patients, which we labeled *compathy* (Morse & Mitcham, 1997; Morse, Mitcham, & van der Steen, 1998). Compathy was the shared, and therefore contagious, response. The response could mirror the response of the person in pain, be reflected to a lesser degree, or be converted to another somatic response (such as feeling nausea), or be blocked so that the person had no feelings at all and objectified the person.

The response would be triggered by seeing and/or hearing the person in pain, by reading about it, or even thinking about it.

Once compathy was identified from the descriptive data and developed into a concept, examples were evident, and examples were present in the literature—for instance, couvade, the husband's experience of his wife's labor pains, is an example of compathy.

Delineating the concept of fatigue (Level 2)

Karin Olson and her colleagues have been studying the concept of fatigue, concentrating on behavioral indices and ways to circumvent fatigue. First, they explored fatigue in different populations (in illness: cancer care, chronic fatigue syndrome; depressions; and in healthy persons: shift workers and athletes) (Olson & Morse, 2005). Once the symptoms of fatigue were identified in each group, the common characteristics (attributes) of fatigue were identified across groups, and delineated from tiredness and exhaustion.

Olson then extended her research program to explore fatigue in persons with different illness, for instance, lung and colorectal cancer (Olson, Tom, Hewitt et al., 2002); advanced cancer in active treatments and palliative care (Olson, Krawchuk, & Quddusi, 2007); multiple sclerosis and exercise (Smith, Hale, Olson, & Schneiders, 2009); and depression (Porr, Olson, & Hegadoren, 2010). Olson then collaborated with an international team to examine fatigue cross-culturally (Graffigna, Vegni, Barello Olson, & Bosiol, 2011). Finally Olson advanced her research program into measurement, developing the *Adaptive Capacity Index*, or the ability to adapt to multiple stressors that indicate risk for fatigue (Olson et al., 2011), extending her research program, firmly embedded in Level 2 to Levels 7 and 8.

Working horizontally in Levels 2–6

In a research program exploring the experiential and behavioral indices of suffering, Morse conducted a number of studies in various contexts for 20 years. These studies explored the suffering of pain (trauma room, and chronic pain), of dying, of relatives' response to illness and dying. The research delineates enduring, a state in which the emotions are deliberately suppressed to prevent the person from panicking (and therefore not being able to help him or herself, or others). The second stage is emotionally suffering in which the emotions are released in the form of crying, weeping and sobbing, and the person demands to be comforted both behaviorally, by their vocalizations, and requests (Morse, 2010).

The model, the *praxis theory of suffering* (Morse & Carter, 1996; Morse 2001, 2010) is developed from many contexts—from trauma care, hospital care to dying, from the individual's perspective to the family and the community, and in a trajectory from impact to the resolution of suffering. It links the behaviors to the alleviations of suffering through nurse comforting. And comforting behaviors are described from the microanalytic touch (Morse, Solberg, & Edwards, 1993), to interpersonal strategies (Morse & Proctor, 1998).

Such a research program extends from examining suffering at many levels, contexts, and patient states. Yet it is useful to the clinician, for nursing is a profession in which clinicians must respond instantly, and the only indication that they may have is distress. They may not know what is causing the distress, but they must act immediately. Such is the usefulness of clinical frameworks provided by qualitative inquiry.

Metasynthesizing (Level 5)

In the context of developing methods for metasynthesis, Sandelowski and Barroso (2007) conducted metasyntheses on women with HIV/AIDS. These publications draw the work of many researchers together and solidify evidence. This research is one way to increase the scope and sample size in qualitative inquiry, while at the same time increasing the variation, and certainty in patterns identified in the individual studies. For example, exploring the trajectory of minority mothers, substance abuse and the events surrounding substance abuse, Barroso and Sandelowski (2004) were able to follow the course of substance abuse and on the onset of HIV, motherhood and recovery and beyond. In a second study, coping with motherhood in the context of HIV (Sandelowski & Barroso, 2003), they identified a "distinctive kind of maternal practice—virtual motherhood— to resist forces that disrupted their relationships with their children and their ability to care for them, as well as their identities as mothers" (p. 470). In virtual motherhood, there is a reciprocal relationship between the HIV "redefined mother-hood"—the "redefining of treatment" and "eternal motherhood" and "protective mother-hood"—"defensive motherhood" and virtual identify" (p. 475). From such examples we can see that metasynthesis is more than a summary of the findings of numerous studies—it is also a re-analysis and reconceptualization.

Identifying interventions (Level 8)

Identifying interventions in qualitative inquiry is difficult, as the interventions themselves are tangled with the descriptions, the context, and the concept. The event is not usually linear, and the outcome of the intervention may be tangled with the preconditions and the intervention itself. Even more difficult, qualitative researchers are working with small samples, purposefully selected, while managing their own perceptions; hence they are subject to all the accusations that come with poor design and bias. Qualitative design does not intend to prove, so results are not definitive.

In this context, when seeking interventions, the researcher must be well integrated into the topic, including both qualitative research and research in the library. One such program of research is Joanne Hall's research into women who have experienced abuse. She writes convincingly that it is possible that women who have been sexually abused as children could develop an insight that allowed them to believe in themselves enough to recover and become responsible, productive and successful adults (Hall et al., 2009; Hall, 2011). To use narrative methods with such conviction that Hall says it is possible they could spearhead change gives credence to qualitative inquiry. Such change in focus is the most difficult type of change—for it works not by changing policy or rules—but by instigating change of the attitudes deep within others. This is the most important outcome we can ever hope for our research.

Working vertically through most of the levels

Usually developing change from research takes time. One of the first qualitative nursing researchers was Jeanne Quint Benoliel, the first doctoral student at UCSF, supervised by Glaser and Strauss, who became a pioneer in palliative care, and conducted studies within Levels 2 to 4 in death and dying, mainly caring for the dying and their family. She conducted studies for almost 40 years, with her dissertation, *The Nurse and the Dying Patient* (Quint, 1967), her first major qualitative research contribution. She continued to conduct qualitative studies of dying for the next 40 years— studies from the patients', the families' and the nurses' perspective, studies of societal values and norms about death, the ethics of practices surrounding dying, and of loss and bereavement, and her bibliography appears with a tribute to her in *Qualitative Health Research* (Stern, 2012).

How important is her research? Today, in 2012, we argue constantly about the efficacy and impact of research, focusing on impact and outcomes, and with statistics proving effectiveness. But for qualitative studies we do not usually have anything to measure statistically. Yet, although we cannot demonstrate effectiveness, this does not mean that our research is not effective or important. We will let Yale University, who recognized it with an honorary degree, a Doctor of Medical Science in 2002, speak to the effectiveness and impact of Jeanne Quint Benoliel's qualitative research program. The citation from Yale University reads:

> Through your pioneering studies of death and dying, you have helped society understand that death is a part of life. Your work has shown us the value of providing community-based care to those who are dying and the value of comfort when the body will not heal. With an influence felt world-wide, you have encouraged the inclusion of the family in caring for the dying, and you have advocated support and care for the bereaved.
>
> *(Honorary Degrees, Yale Bulletin and Calendar, 2002)*

Acknowledgments

I would like to thank the many people who assisted in the preparation of this chapter: Seung Eun Chung, PhD (Nurs), RN; Carmen de la Cuesta, RN, PhD; Siriporn Chirawatkul, PhD; Elin Dysvik, RN, PhD; Bodil Furnes, PhD; Immy Holloway, PhD; and Rumei (May) Yang.

References

Anon. (2011). Drs. Kathleen Knafl and Margarete Sandelowski receive National Institute of Nursing Research (NINR) funding for mixed-methods synthesis of research on childhood chronic conditions and family. *Journal of Family Nursing*, *17*(4), 515– 517.

Barroso, J., & Sandelowski, M. (2004). Substance abuse in HIV-positive women, *Journal of the Association of Nurses in AIDS Care*, *15*(5), 48–59.

Bengtsson, J. (Ed.) (2006). *Å forske i sykdoms- og pleieerfaringer: Livsfenomenologisk bidrag* [Research in sickness- and caring experiences: A lifeworld phenomenological contribution]. Kristiansand, Norway: Høyskole Forlaget.

Benner, P. (1994). *Interpretative phenomenology: Embodiment, caring, and ethics in health and illness*. Thousand Oaks, CA: Sage.

Berg, L., & Danielson, E. (2007). Patients' and nurses' experiences of the caring relationship in hospital: An aware striving for trust. *Scandinavian Journal of Caring Sciences*, *21*(4), 500–506.

Booker, R., Olson, K., Pilarski, L. M., Noon, J. P., & Bahlis, N. J. (2009). The relationships among physiologic variables, quality of life, and fatigue in patients with multiple myeloma. *Oncology Nursing Forum*, *36*(2), 209–216.

Carey, M. A., & Asbury, J-E. (2012). *Focus group research*. Walnut Creek, CA: Left Coast.

Carlson, C. E. (Ed.). (1970). *Behavioral concepts and nursing intervention*. Philadelphia. PA: J. B. Lippincott.

Chenitz, C., & Swanson, J. (1986). *From practice to grounded theory*. Philadelphia, PA: Prentice-Hall.

Chirawatkul, S. (2003). การวิจัยเชิงคุณภาพในวิชาชีพการพยาบาล [Qualitative research in nursing] (1st ed.). Khon kaen: Siriphan Offset (in Thai).

Chirawatkul, S. (2005). การวิจัยเชิงคุณภาพในวิชาชีพการพยาบาล [Qualitative research in nursing] (2nd ed.). Khon kaen: Siriphan Offset (in Thai).

Chirawatkul, S. (2012). การวิจัยเชิงคุณภาพในวิชาชีพการพยาบาล [Qualitative research in nursing] (3rd ed.). Khon kaen: Siriphan Offset (in Thai).

Cohen, M., Kahn, D. L., & Steeves, R. H. (2000). *Hermeneutic phenomenological research*. Thousand Oaks, CA: Sage.

Connell, L. (2004). Qualitative analysis: Utilization of voluntary supplied confidential safety data in aviation and health care. Paper presented at the Qualitative Health Research Conference, Banff, Alberta, Canada, April/May.

Corbin, J., & Strauss, A. (1988). *Unending work and care: Management of chronic illness at home*. San Francisco, CA: Jossey-Bass.

Corbin, J., & Strauss, A. (2007). *Basics of qualitative research* (3rd ed.). Thousand Oaks, CA: Sage.

Cronin, S. N., & Harrison, B. (1988). Importance of nurse caring behaviors as perceived by patients after myocardial infarction. *Heart & Lung*, *17*(4), 374–380.

Dahlberg, K., Dahlberg, H., & Nyström, M. (2008). *Reflexive lifeworld research*, Lund, Sweden: Studentlitteratur.

Field, P. A., & Morse, J. M. (1985). *Nursing research: The application of qualitative approaches*. London: Croom Helm.

Finfgeld-Connett, D. (2007). Meta-synthesis of caring in nursing. *Journal of Clinical Nursing*, *17*, 196–204.

Forrest, D. (1986). The experience of caring. *Journal of Advanced Nursing*, *14*, 815–823.

Gauthier, J., Santos, I., Cabral, I., & Tavares, C. (1998). *Pesquisa em enfermagem: novas metodologias aplicadas* [Research in nursing: New applied methodologies]. Rio de Janeiro: Guanabara-Koogan.

Glaser, B. G., & Strauss, A. (1965). *Awareness of dying*. Chicago: Aldine.

Glaser, B. G., & Strauss, A. (1967). *The discovery of grounded theory*. Chicago: Aldine.

Glaser, B. G., & Strauss, A. (1968). *Time for dying*. Chicago: Aldine.

Graffigna, G., Vegni, E., Barello, S., Olson, K., & Bosio, C. (2011). Studying the social construction of cancer-related fatigue experience: The heuristic value of ethnoscience. *Patient Education and Counseling*, *82*, 402–409.

Hall, J. (2011). Narrative methods in a study of trauma recovery, *Qualitative Health Research*, *21*(11), 3–13.

Hall, J., Roman, M. W., Thomas, S. P., Travis, C., Brown, P., Powell, J., et al. (2009). Thriving as becoming resolute in narratives of women surviving childhood maltreatment. *American Journal of Orthopsychiatry*, *19*(3), 375–386.

Harmer, B., & Henderson, V. (1939). *Principles and practice of nursing* (3rd ed.). New York: Macmillan.

Henderson, V. (1966). *The nature of nursing: A definition and its implications for practice, research, and education*. New York: Macmillan.

Holloway, I., & Brown, L. (2012). *Essentials of a qualitative doctorate*. Walnut Creek, CA: Left Coast.

Holloway, I., & Wheeler, S. (1996). *Qualitative research for nurses*. Oxford: Blackwell.

Holloway, I., & Wheeler, S. (2002). *Qualitative research for nurses* (2nd ed.). Oxford: Blackwell.

Holloway, I., & Wheeler, S. (2010). *Qualitative research for nursing and health care* (3rd ed.). Oxford: Blackwell.

Honorary Degrees (2002). *Yale Bulletin and Calendar*, *30*(31). Available at: http://www.yale.edu/opa/arc-ybc/v30.n31/story103.html (accessed June 1, 2010).

Hudson, P. L. (2006). How well do family caregivers cope after caring for a relative with advanced disease and how can health professionals enhance their support? *Journal of Palliative Medicine*, *9*(3), 694–703.

Kayser-Jones, J., Kris, A. E., Miaskowski, C. A., Lyons, W. L., & Steve, P. (2006). Hospice care in nursing homes: Does it contribute to higher quality pain management? *Gerontologist*, *46*(3), 325–333.

Knafl, K., & Rodgers, B. (Eds.). (2000). *Concept development in nursing*. Philadelphia, PA: W. B. Saunders.

Larson, P. (1987). Comparison of cancer patients' and professional nurses' perceptions of important caring behaviors. *Heart & Lung, 16*(2), 187–193.

Latimer, J. (Ed.). (2003). *Advanced qualitative research for nursing*. Oxford: Blackwell Science.

Leininger, M. (1978). *Transcultural nursing: Concepts, theories, research and practices*. New York: John Wiley & Sons.

Leininger, M. (Ed.). (1985). *Qualitative research methods in nursing*. Orlando, CA: Grune & Stratton.

Leininger, M. (1997). Overview of the theory of culture care with the ethnonursing research method. *Journal of Transcultural Nursing, 8*(2), 32–52.

Liu, M. (2008). 护理质性研究 [Qualitative research in nursing]. Beijing, China: People's Medical Publishing House (in Chinese).

Matheus, C. C., & Fustinoni, S. M. (2006). *Pesquisa qualitativa em enfermagem* [Qualitative research in nursing]. São Paulo: Livratia Médica Paulista (in Brazilian).

McFarland, M., Wehbe-Alamah, H., Wilson, M., & Vossos, H. (2011). Synopsis of findings discovered within a descriptive meta-synthesis of doctoral dissertations guided by the culture care theory with the use of ethnonursing research method. *Online Journal of Cultural Competence in Nursing & Healthcare, 1*(2), 24–29.

Meade, C. M., Bursell, A. L., & Ketelsen, L. (2006). Effects of nursing rounds on patients' call light use, satisfaction and safety. *American Journal of Nursing, 106*(9), 58–70.

Mercado, F. J., Gastaldo, D., & Calderón, C. (2002). *Metodos, análisis y etica*. Guadalajara, México: Universidad de Guadalajara.

Morse, J. M. (Ed.). (1989). *Qualitative nursing research: A contemporary dialogue*. Rockville, MD: Aspen Press.

Morse, J. M. (Ed). (1992). *Qualitative health research*. Newbury Park, CA: Sage.

Morse, J. M. (Ed.). (1994). *Critical issues in qualitative research methods*. Newbury Park, CA: Sage.

Morse, J. M. (Ed.). (1997). *Completing a qualitative project: Details and dialogue*. Newbury Park, CA: Sage.

Morse, J. M. (2001). Toward a praxis theory of suffering. *Advances in Nursing Science, 24*(1), 47–59.

Morse, J. M. (2010). The praxis theory of suffering. In J. B. Butts & K. L. Rich (Eds.), *Philosophies and theories in advanced nursing practice* (pp. 569–602). Sudbury, MA: Jones & Bartlett.

Morse, J. M. (2012). *Qualitative health research: Creating a new discipline*. Walnut Creek, CA: Left Coast.

Morse, J. M., Anderson, G., Bottorff, J., Yonge, O., O'Brien, B., Solberg, S., & McIlveen, K. (1992). Exploring empathy: A conceptual fit for nursing practice? *Image: Journal of Nursing Scholarship, 24*(4), 274–280.

Morse, J. M., & Carter, B. (1996). The essence of enduring and the expression of suffering: The reformulation of self. *Scholarly Inquiry for Nursing Practice, 10*(1), 43–60.

Morse, J. M., & Field, P. A. (1995). *Qualitative approaches to nursing research* (2nd ed.). London: Chapman & Hall; Thousand Oaks, CA: Sage.

Morse, J. M., & Mitcham, C. (1997). Compathy: The contagion of physical distress. *Journal of Advanced Nursing, 26*, 649–657.

Morse, J. M., Mitcham, C., & van der Steen, V. (1998). Compathy or physical empathy: Implications for the caregiver relationship. *Journal of Medical Humanities, 19*(1), 51–65.

Morse, J. M., & Niehaus, L. (2009). *Mixed-method design: Principles and procedures*. Walnut Creek, CA: Left Coast Press.

Morse, J. M., & Proctor, A. (1998). Maintaining patient endurance: The comfort work of trauma nurses. *Clinical Nursing Research, 7*(3), 250–274.

Morse, J. M., & Richards, L. (2002). *Readme first for a user's guide to qualitative methods*. Thousand Oaks, CA: Sage.

Morse, J. M., Solberg, S., & Edwards, J. (1993). Caregiver–infant interaction: Comforting the postoperative infant. *Scandinavian Journal of Caring Sciences, 7*, 105–111.

Morse, J. M., Stern, P. N., Corbin, J., Bowers, B., Charmaz, K., & Clarke, A. (2009). *Grounded theory: The second generation*. Walnut Creek, CA: Left Coast Press.

Morse, J. M., Swanson, J., & Kuzel, A. (Eds.). (2001). *The nature of qualitative evidence*. Thousand Oaks, CA: Sage.

Munhall, P. (1991). *Qualitative research proposals and reports*. Sudbury, MA: Jones & Bartlett.

Munhall. P. (Ed.). (1993). *Nursing research: A qualitative perspective* (2nd ed.). New York: National League for Nursing.

Munhall. P. (1994). *Revisioning phenomenology: Nursing and health science research*. Sudbury, MA: Jones & Bartlett.

Munhall. P. (Ed.). (2000a). *Nursing research: A qualitative perspective* (3rd ed.). Sudbury, MA: Jones & Bartlett.

Munhall. P. (Ed). (2000b). *Qualitative research proposals and reports* (2nd ed.). Sudbury, MA: Jones & Bartlett.

Munhall. P. (Ed.). (2006). *Nursing research: A qualitative perspective* (4th ed.). Sudbury, MA: Jones & Bartlett.

Munhall, P. (2010). *Qualitative research proposals and reports* (3rd ed.). Sudbury, MA: Jones & Bartlett.

Munhall. P. (Ed.). (2012). *Nursing research: A qualitative perspective* (5th ed.). Sudbury, MA: Jones & Bartlett.

Munhall. P., & Boyd, C. (Eds.). (1987). *Nursing research: A qualitative perspective.* Norwalk, CT: Appleton & Lange.

NDCG (Nursing Development Conference Group). (1973). *Concept formalization in nursing: Process and product.* Boston: Little Brown.

Nightingale, F. ([1859] 1960). *Notes on nursing.* New York: Appleton/Dover.

Norris, C. M. (1982). *Concept clarification in nursing.* Rockville, MD: Aspen.

Olson, K. (2011). *Essentials of qualitative interviewing.* Walnut Creek, CA: Left Coast.

Olson, K., Krawchuk, A., & Quddusi, T. (2007). Fatigue in individuals with advanced cancer in active treatment and palliative settings. *Cancer Nursing, 30*(4): E1–10.

Olson, K., & Morse, J. M. (2005). Delineating the concept of fatigue using a pragmatic utility approach. In J. Cutcliff, & H. McKenna (Eds.), *The essential concepts of nursing* (pp. 141–159). Oxford: Elsevier Science.

Olson, K., Rogers, W. T., Cui, Y., Cree, M., Baracos, V., Rust, T., et al. (2011). Development and psychometric testing of the Adaptive Capacity Index, an instrument to measure adaptive capacity in individuals with advanced cancer. *International Journal of Nursing Studies, 48,* 986–994.

Olson, K., Tom, B., Hewitt, J., Whittingham, J., Buchanan, L., & Ganton, G. (2002). Evolving routines: Managing fatigue associated with lung and colorectal cancer. *Qualitative Health Research, 5,* 655–670.

Orem, D. (1971). *Nursing: Concepts of practice.* St. Louis, MO: Mosby.

Paley, J. (2001). An archaeology of caring knowledge. *Journal of Advanced Nursing, 36*(2), 188–198.

Papleau, H. (1952). *The interpersonal relations in nursing.* New York: G. P. Putman & Sons.

Parse, R., Coyne, A. B., & Smith, M. J. (1985). *Nursing research: Qualitative methods.* Bowie, MD: Brady.

Porr, C., Olson, K., Hegadoren, K. (2010). Tiredness, fatigue and exhaustion in the context of a major depressive disorder. *Qualitative Health Research, 20*(10), 1315–26.

Quint, J. C. (1967). *The nurse and the dying patient.* New York: Macmillan.

Reimen, D. J. (1986). Noncaring and caring in the clinical setting: Patients' descriptions. *Topics in Clinical Nursing, 8*(2), 30–36.

Richards, L., & Morse, J. M. (2007). *Readme first for a user's guide to qualitative methods* (2nd ed.). Thousand Oaks, CA: Sage.

Richards, L., & Morse, J. M. (2012). *Readme first for a students' guide to qualitative research* (3rd ed.). Thousand Oaks, CA: Sage.

Rodrigues, M. S. P., & Leopardi, M. T. (1999). *O método de análise de conteúdo: Uma versão para enfermeiros* [Content analysis: The nurses approach]. Fortaleza: Fundação Cearense de Pesquisa e Cultura (in Brazilian).

Roper, J., & Shapira, J. (2000). *Ethnography in nursing research.* Thousand Oaks, CA: Sage.

Sandelowski, M. J. (2008). Justifying qualitative research, *Research in Nursing & Health,* 31, 193–195.

Sandelowski, M., & Barroso, J. (2003). Motherhood in the context of maternal HIV infection. *Research in Nursing & Health, 26*(6), 470–482.

Sandelowski, M., & Barroso, J. (2007). *Handbook for synthesizing qualitative research.* Philadelphia, PA: Springer.

Schaeffer, D., & Müller-Mundt, G. (Eds.). (2002). *Qualitative Gesundheits- und Pflegeforschung* [Qualitative health research and care]. Bern: Huber.

Schrieber, R. S., & Stern, P. N. (2001). *Using grounded theory in nursing.* Philadelphia, PA: Springer.

Sherwood, G. D. (1997). Meta-synthesis of qualitative analyses of caring: Defining a therapeutic model of nursing. *Advanced Practice Nursing Quarterly, 3*(1), 32–42.

Shin, K., Cho, M. O., & Yang, J. H. (2004). 질적연구방법론 *Qualitative research methodology.* Seoul: Ewha Womans University Press (in Korean).

Shin, K., Kim, G. B., Kim, S. S., Yu, E. K., Kim, N. C., Park, E. S., et al. (2003). 질적연구 용어사전 *Qualitative research methodology.* Seoul: Hyunmoonsa (in Korean).

Shin, K. R., & Kong, B, H. (2001). *Phenomenological research.* Seoul: Hyunmoonsa (in Korean).

Smith, C., Hale, L., Olson, K. M., & Schneiders, A. G. (2009). How does exercise influence fatigue in people with multiple sclerosis? *Disability and Rehabilitation, 31*(9), 685–692.

Speziale, H. S., & Carpenter, D. R. (2007). *Qualitative research in nursing: Advancing the humanistic perspective* (4th ed.). Philadelphia, PA: Lippincott, Williams & Wilkins.

Speziale, H. S. & Carpenter, D. R. (2003). *Qualitative research in nursing: Advancing the humanistic perspective* (3rd ed.). Philadelphia, PA: Lippincott, Williams & Wilkins.

Stern, P. N. (2012). A moment of silence: Jeanne Quint Benoliel, 1920–2012. *Qualitative Health Research*, *22*, 1580–1581.

Stern, P. N., & Porr, C. (2011). *Essentials of accessible grounded theory*. Walnut Creek, CA: Left Coast.

Strauss, A. L., & Corbin, J. (1990). *Basics of qualitative research*. Newbury Park, CA: Sage.

Strauss, A. L., & Corbin, J. (1997). *Grounded theory in practice*. Thousand Oaks, CA: Sage.

Strauss, A. L., & Corbin, J. (1998). *Basics of qualitative research* (2nd ed.). Thousand Oaks, CA: Sage.

Strauss, A., Corbin, J., Fagerhaugh, S., Glaser, B., Maines, D., Suczek, B., & Wiener, C. (1984). *Chronic illness and the quality of life* (2nd ed.). St. Louis, MO: C.V. Mosby.

Streubert, H. J., & Carpenter, D. R. (1995). *Qualitative research in nursing: Advancing the humanistic imperative*. Philadelphia, PA: Lippincott, Williams & Wilkins.

Streubert, H. J., & Carpenter, D. R. (1999). *Qualitative research in nursing: Advancing the humanistic perspective* (2nd ed.). Philadelphia, PA: Lippincott, Williams & Wilkins.

Streubert, H. J. & Carpenter, D. R. (2011). *Qualitative research in nursing: Advancing the humanistic perspective* (5th ed.). Philadelphia, PA: Lippincott, Williams & Wilkins.

Swanson-Kauffman, K.M. (1988). Caring needs of women who miscarried. In M. M. Leininger (ed.). *Care: Discovery and uses in clinical and community nursing*. Detroit, MI: Wayne State University Press.

Swanson, K. (1991). Empirical development of a middle range theory of caring. *Nursing Research*, *40*(3), 161–166.

Swanson, K. (1993). Nursing as informed caring for the well-being of others. *IMAGE*, *25*(4), 352–357.

Teixeira, E. (2008). *Abordagens qualitativas: Trilhas para pesquisadores em saúde e enfermagem* [Qualitative approach: Path for researchers in health and nursing]. Brasilia: Martinari (in Brazilian).

Thorne, S. (2008). *Interpretive description*. Walnut Creek, CA: Left Coast.

Van Manen, M. (1990). *Researching the lived experience*. Albany: State University of New York.

Walker, L., & Avant, K. (1983). *Strategies for theory construction in nursing*. Norwalk, CT: Appleton-Century-Crofts.

Watson, J. (1997). The theory of human caring: Retrospective and prospective. *Nursing Science Quarterly*, *10*(1), 49–52.

Watson, J. (2005). Caring theory as ethical guide to administrative and clinical practices. *Nurse Administrative Quarterly*, *30*(1), 48–55.

Williams, S. A. (1997). Caring in patient-focused care: The relationship of patients' perceptions of holistic nurse caring to their levels of anxiety. *Holistic Nursing Practice*, *11*(3), 61–68.

Wolf, Z. R. (1986). The caring concept and nurse-identified caring behaviors. *Topics in Clinical Nursing*, *8*(2), 84–93.

3

Building on "grab," attending to "fit," and being prepared to "modify"

How grounded theory "works" to guide a health intervention for abused women

*Judith Wuest, Marilyn Ford-Gilboe,
Marilyn Merritt-Gray, and Colleen Varcoe*

Grounded theories have unique potential for influencing clinical practice. The theory has *grab* (Glaser, 1978); it resonates for those who have experienced the situation that the theory explains, or know or practice with those who have. Because grounded theories can explain, interpret, and predict human behavior in specific social contexts, they *work* and have practical utility (Glaser, 1978). A fundamental premise of grounded theory research is that people actively shape the worlds they live in through the process of symbolic interaction and that their viewpoints are vital to generating useful knowledge of process, interaction and social change (Glaser, 1992; Strauss, 1987). "Nursing is a practice discipline whose essence lies in processes" (Stern & Pyles, 1986, p. 1). For clinicians, the theoretical rendering of what is most problematic in the study situation and how it is processed by participants offers insights into how and when a clinician might intervene. Thus grounded theory lends itself to conceptual utilization, that is, a rethinking of situational phenomena that may or may not lead to change in action (Estabrooks, 2001). Indeed, the effects of grounded theories on nursing practice appear to have been minor (Hall & May, 2001; Morse, Penrod, & Hupcey, 2000). Poor uptake is not a problem specific to research evidence with qualitative origin (Estabrooks, 2001). However, translation of grounded theories by researchers is essential to facilitate their utilization in concrete applications such as clinical protocols, decision trees or practice guidelines (Estabrooks, 2001; Sandelowski, 2004). Little has been written about how such purposeful translation takes place. Yet, as Thorne (2011) reminds us, nurses need to understand phenomena "in a way that will be applicable to the diversity of context and complexity within the actual real-time setting" (p. 449). Thorne calls upon researchers to mobilize research toward "meaningful social and pragmatic action" (p. 450). Importantly, with grounded theory, the work of knowledge translation not only makes the theory more accessible to practitioners; it also has potential to add breadth and depth to the original theory through the constant comparative process with multiple sources of new data. In this chapter, we discuss the processes, challenges and advantages of translating our theory Strengthening Capacity to Limit Intrusion (SCLI) (Ford-Gilboe, Wuest, & Merritt-Gray, 2005; Wuest, Ford-Gilboe, Merritt-Gray, & Berman, 2003) into a primary health care intervention, the Intervention for Health Enhancement After Leaving (iHEAL) (Ford-Gilboe, Merritt-Gray, Varcoe, & Wuest, 2011), and conducting initial feasibility studies using the iHEAL with women who have left their abusive partners in the past three years.

Background

Grounded theory is distinctive among qualitative research methods in that its goal is the development of substantive theory, that is, theory that accounts for a human behavior within a particular social context (Glaser, 1978; Glaser & Strauss, 1967).[1] Through constant comparative analysis of data from interviews, observations, documents and/or images, researchers conceptually construct what is most problematic and the social-psychological process by which the problem is addressed. The analytic outcome goes beyond descriptive themes or the recounting of individual narratives to the articulation of a theoretical scheme in which key concepts are identified and defined, and the relationships among them delineated. While some grounded theories are reported in terms of a core category, more commonly they are written as basic social psychological processes (BSP), that is, a core category with at least two sequential stages. Vital to their usefulness is the naming of factors or conditions that influence variation in the core category or BSP, not just by their presence or absence, but also by their degree or intensity (Wuest, 2012). Conditions that influence variation are diverse and may include individual attributes such as age or family history, relational factors such as conflict, support, services and resources, and/or structural influences such as poverty or discrimination. Thus, a grounded theory is a substantive theory that accounts for the heterogeneity in how a basic social process unfolds for individual people in different contexts and suggests possibilities for action that previously may have been invisible (Glaser, 1978; Swanson, 2001). Substantive theory helps us transcend our finite grasp of the specific through its potential transferability to other situations (Glaser, 1978). "Analytic generalization and theoretical transferability are the bases for utility in grounded theory research" (Sandelowski, 2004, p. 1371).

The theory of Strengthening Capacity to Limit Intrusion (SCLI)

In our program of research focusing on women's health after leaving an abusive partner, we conducted a grounded theory study of family health promotion after separation from an abusive partner and developed the theory of Strengthening Capacity to Limit Intrusion (SCLI) (Ford-Gilboe et al., 2005; Wuest et al., 2003). We used a feminist grounded theory approach (Wuest, 1995; Wuest & Merritt-Gray, 2001) and analyzed repeat interview data from 40 mothers, ages 22–48 ($M = 36$) and 11 of their children. The families had been living separately from the abusive partners on average just under four years (range 1–20). As we coded and constructed provisional conceptual categories and the relationships among them, we shared our findings with the women during their second or third interviews, seeking their feedback for modification and confirmation of our emerging theoretical schema. In this way, we identified that the core problem related to health promotion for the families under study was *intrusion*, that is "external control or interference that demands attention, diverts energy away from family priorities and limits choices" (Ford-Gilboe et al., 2005, p. 482). Intrusion stems from ongoing abuse and harassment from the ex-partner (frequently exacerbated by child custody and access issues), physical and mental health problems of women and their children, the "costs" of seeking help (for example, measuring up to criteria imposed by policies, increased surveillance by income assistance workers or family members), and negative changes to daily life (Wuest et al., 2003). Leaving an abusive partner is a risk-taking act to position the family for a better future. However, increasing intrusion after leaving forces families to focus on promoting health by creating stability in day-to-day survival. As stability is achieved, women are able to focus again on positioning for the future, an act which may lead in turn to increased intrusion.

Families spontaneously engaged in the process of SCLI in four ways: (1) providing; (2) rebuilding security; (3) renewing self; and (4) regenerating family (Ford-Gilboe et al., 2005). *Providing* involves meeting basic needs of income, housing, personal energy, food, childcare, recreation, transportation, medication and relief from symptoms. *Rebuilding security* includes safeguarding from threats to physical and emotional safety and cautious connecting with family, friends, services and the larger community. *Renewing self* refers to the process of developing personal capacity to make their personal needs a priority, make sense of the past, consider who they are and who they want to be, and find comfort and relief from day-to-day intrusions and distress. *Regenerating family* entails developing a family storyline to explain their past, increasing predictability in day-to-day life, and naming and using new standards for relationships. Within these sub-processes, the health promotion focus for women shifts from positioning for the future to surviving and back again according to the degree of intrusion the family is experiencing.

Significantly, when we shared the emerging theory with women, they readily connected with the grounded theory conceptualization and offered further data to help refine the theory. Similarly, the theory had grab for other researchers, clinicians, and other helpers. As we presented our work in the community, at professional conferences and in peer-reviewed papers, we discussed the implications of the theory for practice, largely at a level of "conceptual utilization" (Estabrooks, 2001). The theory shaped how we understood women's experiences of leaving and how we individually interacted with women with abuse histories. At the same time, the identification of intrusion from ongoing physical and mental health problems related to abuse helped us to recognize that, despite the dominant belief that leaving an abusive partner is the solution for abused women, little was known about the trajectory of women's health after leaving abusive partners. To address this gap, we conducted a four-year longitudinal study examining changes in women's resources and health after separation from an abusive partner, the Women's Health Effects Study (WHES). Annually, 309 Canadian women who had left abusive partners in the previous three years took part in structured interviews and health assessments (Ford-Gilboe et al., 2009). Baseline data revealed that the women (who had been separated on average 20 months) had significantly poorer physical and mental health and higher rates of service use than Canadian women of similar age with little relief from their symptoms, and that the annual health system costs attributable to violence were approximately $4,969.79 per woman (Ford-Gilboe et al., 2009; Scott-Storey, Wuest, & Ford-Gilboe, 2009; Varcoe et al., 2011; Wuest et al., 2007, 2008, 2009, 2010).

These quantitative results were useful as comparative data for further development of our grounded theory, particularly to expand the concept of intrusion from physical and mental health problems, "costs" of seeking help, ongoing abuse and harassment, and changes in lifestyle (for example, forced moves, income disruption). Despite the lack of attention to constant comparison with quantitative data in grounded theory scholarship today, Glaser and Strauss (1967) asserted that both quantitative and qualitative data are useful, and sometimes necessary, for the generation of grounded theory through constant comparative analysis. Although the WHES was not a grounded theory study, we found the WHES data to be an important source of secondary data for theoretical sampling, that is, purposefully choosing data for comparison in order to augment the original SCLI theory through the refinement of the properties of concepts and the relationships among them (Glaser, 1978).

Our grounded theory and the WHES findings, along with the dearth of existing health interventions for women after leaving, demonstrated the urgent need to develop a community health intervention specifically designed to assist women who had experienced the trauma of abuse to promote their health (Ford-Gilboe et al., 2011). This compelling evidence also helped us to garner financial support and partnerships from funding agencies and decision-makers to develop and examine the feasibility of a health intervention for women after leaving. The theory of Strengthening Capacity to Limit Intrusion was the logical starting point for health intervention development.[2] The scope of the theory provides evidence that survivor health is socially determined. Thus, we decided to design the iHEAL to be delivered collaboratively by a nurse and a domestic violence worker. Based on the SCLI theory, we agreed that the aims of the intervention would be to improve women's health and quality of life after leaving an abusive partner: (1) by reducing intrusion; and (2) by enhancing women's capacity (knowledge, skills, and resources) to limit intrusion (Ford-Gilboe et al., 2011).

Processes and challenges in developing the intervention

Our theory captures the central pattern of health promotion behavior in mother-headed, single-parent families after leaving an abusive male partner, and its consequences (Ford-Gilboe et al., 2005). Importantly, this theoretical rendering captures the naturally occurring and intuitive actions taken by diverse women and their children to strengthen their capacity to manage intrusion at different points in time after leaving, and consolidates the lessons learned from them. A key intervention principle of the iHEAL is that

> women's own experiences of leaving an abusive partner and those of other women, as reflected in the theory of strengthening capacity to limit intrusion, will be a key source of knowledge to help women reflect on, reframe, and name their experiences, concerns, and priorities.
>
> *(Ford-Gilboe et al., 2011, p. 203)*

This principle draws on what Estabrooks (2001) called the persuasive power of research evidence which is akin to Glaser's (1978) *grab*. Stories of others' experiences are important "in evoking, persuading, and provoking; in promoting empathetic, feeling or visceral understandings of the people and events; in moving listeners and readers to act" (Sandelowski, 2004, p. 1373). Grounded theories, because they frequently focus on aspects of human experience that have received little attention, can help to mitigate feelings of isolation and alienation.

The theory, however, is more than individual stories; it captures a pattern of survivors' personal and social behaviors in terms of antecedents, consequences, and influencing factors. The theory then has potential to resonate with women's disparate experiences in different contexts, and to permit diverse women to name their experiences and see new possibilities for limiting intrusion, leading to better health. The SCLI theory presents what women do, with and without help from others, highlighting how contextual factors limit or enable women's growth. Although this theoretical scaffold directs clinicians to draw upon and augment women's expert knowledge and skills in supporting them to strengthen their capacity to limit intrusion, a limitation of the SCLI theory is that it *does not* explicitly explain *how* clinicians might do this. In short, it is not a theoretical construction of how to practice. However, the theory's concepts and the relationships among them can shape the underlying philosophical assumptions and practice principles for an intervention. Further, the process of Strengthening Capacity to Limit Intrusion provides direction for the intervention's structure. Just as the original grounded theory was generated, so the iHEAL was constructed in a series of reflective, strategic, iterative choices about which aspects of the theory should be highlighted in the context of our agenda to improve women's health. The discussion that follows is a reconstruction of key challenges and processes in moving from theory to intervention, from our initial attempts to create a rough outline of goals, components and potential outcomes of the intervention (Ford-Gilboe, Wuest, Varcoe, & Merritt-Gray, 2006) to a more complete rendering some four years later (Ford-Gilboe et al., 2011). As with most retrospective accounts, our discussion reflects a more organized, conscious, and polished process of intervention development than was actually the case. It does not fully capture our false starts, dead ends, and stumbling steps in developing the iHEAL.

Theoretical sensitivity, constant comparison and emergent fit: naming underlying philosophical assumptions and principles of practice

Grounded theory analysis is informed by theoretical sensitivity, that is, the researcher's capacity to use knowledge of theoretical constructions from many disciplines as well as personal and vicarious experiences as a basis for constructing concepts and the relationships between them (Glaser, 1978). Theoretical sensitivity does not drive theory construction but it does open the researcher to theoretical possibilities that are then checked out and refined through theoretical sampling and constant comparison (Wuest, 2012). The philosophical assumptions delineated for the iHEAL reflect the shared perspectives and values that underpinned our program of research (Ford-Gilboe et al., 2011). Our theoretical sensitivity in the grounded theory research that generated the SCLI theory was informed by diverse philosophical assumptions, including a feminist viewpoint of intimate partner violence (Varcoe, 1996), health promotion as a process of enabling people to increase control over and improve their health (World Health Organization (WHO), 1986), health as socially determined (Health Canada, n.d.), and primary health care (WHO, 1978). This sensitivity influenced our theory construction; for example, it enhanced our ability to see women's agency, our recognition of women's health promotion taking place on social, relational and individual levels, and how we theorized "costs" of seeking help. As we scrutinized the theory with practice in view, we quickly identified the applicability of these assumptions for our health intervention, with women's health being socially determined and primary health care being key (Ford-Gilboe et al., 2011).

Some other key assumptions were named much later when the structure of the intervention and activities for the interventionists were under development. Drawing on our theoretical sensitivity, we progressively became aware that some existing expert practice philosophies *fit* with the theoretical scaffold of the iHEAL such as harm reduction (Pauly, 2008), cultural safety (Browne et al., 2009), and trauma-informed care (Elliot, Bjelajac, Fallot, Markoff, & Reed, 2005). In grounded theory, categories are inductively developed through substantive coding and constant comparison such that the category *fits* the data (Glaser, 1978). But not all categories must be new. Emergent fit refers to using constant comparison between pre-existing categories and the data to determine whether it fits the data (Glaser, 1978; Wuest, 2000). Using a process of emergent fit between the practice implications of data from both the SCLI theory as well as the WHES findings and expert practice philosophies, we identified philosophical assumptions true to our theoretical conceptualization and reflective of expert practice beliefs. One example of emergent fit is incorporation of harm reduction (Pauly, 2008) as an underlying philosophical assumption that aligned well with the processes in the theory of SCLI.

Our grounded theory process of *renewing self* conceptualizes how women, relieved from the oppression of abuse, initially relished *living free*, that is, finding release in a wide range of activities, some of which were potentially harmful such as substance use, extensive partying, overinvestment in children or work, and hasty connecting in new relationships (Ford-Gilboe et al., 2005). Most also continued to use some previously learned strategies to find comfort from the trauma of abuse such as smoking, working long hours, eating, sleeping, or using drugs and alcohol. These theoretical findings were supported by the WHES study's findings; of 309 women, at baseline, 44% smoked and 53% were overweight or obese. In the previous 12 months, 27% had used street drugs, 16% overused prescription medication (Wuest et al., 2008) and 26% screened positive for potential high-risk drinking. Just over 3% reported having a sexually transmitted infection in the past month. However, our grounded theory findings also showed that as intrusion levels settled, women found that despite *living free*, they did not feel happy or satisfied and began to position for the future by engaging in the work associated with *living better* (Ford-Gilboe et al., 2005). One way of living better was to begin intentionally to take better care of themselves. The process of *living better* was facilitated by formal and informal support that focused on fortifying women and avoided undermining their dreams. Harm reduction is an intervention philosophy that focuses on engaging non-judgmentally and respectfully with people to help them find ways that they can be safer, healthier and more in control while risk-taking (Pauly, 2008). Our theoretical sensitivity to harm reduction initiated constant comparison with our data for emergent fit. Through constant comparison, we identified harm reduction to be a congruent and important philosophical orientation for supporting women whether they were *living free* or working on *living better*. By making the assumption that risky behaviors are a rational and purposeful response to the trauma and aftermath of abuse, and focusing on supporting women to reduce the health and social harms of such behaviors, we incorporated harm reduction as a key philosophical underpinning of the iHEAL (Ford-Gilboe et al., 2011).

Principles of practice

We also developed intervention principles for the iHEAL, that is, key guidelines to ensure that the intervention built on the practice implications of the theory. For each previous publication and presentation of the theory, we had carefully scrutinized and reflected on the theory, considering particularly how practicing from this theoretical base might differ from "usual" nursing practice. Collectively, we reflected and discussed and argued about meaning for practice over time as we did this scholarly work together and used it to inform our policy work related to the grounded theory and the Women's Health Effects Study. Developing the iHEAL, however, pushed our thinking to another level as we considered how we might articulate interventionist approaches based on the SCLI theory. Although we had worked together successfully for more than ten years, and shared many common values, this exercise made visible differing viewpoints. Notably, individual commitments to the Developmental Model of Health and Nursing (Allen & Warner, 2002) and relational inquiry (Doane &Varcoe, 2005) required intense and lengthy discussion regarding how these nursing approaches might *fit* with the SCLI theory. As well, because the intervention was being developed for delivery by nurses and domestic violence advocates, current best practices in domestic violence advocacy also were considered. Gradually we realized that rather than choosing an existing practice model or philosophy to guide the iHEAL, we needed a set of general practice principles that would fit with our shared assumptions and the theory of SCLI, and would guide practice by both nurses and advocates.

Some principles were identified readily. Principles such as the intervention being women-centered, that is "women will direct the pace, what is given priority and who is involved," and strengths-based, that is "women's strengths and capacities will be recognized, drawn upon, and further developed" (Ford-Gilboe et al., 2011, p. 203) reflected not only our own philosophies of nursing practice but also best practices in the domestic violence intervention sector. Other support for the latter principle stemmed from the SCLI theory demonstrating that survivors habitually had their deficits reinforced by ex-partners, other family members, and helping agencies, yet were consistently demonstrating creative resourcefulness and successful management of complex day-to-day challenges. WHES study findings reinforced this finding, showing that, after leaving, women's scores on standard measures of resilience, mastery and family functioning were comparable to those of other women of the same age.

Some principles of the iHEAL are a direct bridge from philosophical assumptions to a practice approach such as the principle of advocacy stating: "The interventionists will work to reduce intrusion from community services and to advocate for improved system responses to women who are situated in varied contexts of social inequity" (Ford-Gilboe et al., 2011, p. 203). The principle of advocacy translates our stated assumption that intimate partner violence "is sanctioned and enabled by broader social, cultural, and political structures that systematically oppress women, the poor, and those from non-traditional cultural backgrounds" (p. 200). However, further support for this principle was derived through constant comparative analysis with our theoretical findings of intrusion experienced by women who seek help, including having to measure up to criteria to access services by repeatedly recounting stories of abuse, submit to ongoing surveillance as a condition of receiving help, or settle for services that do not match their needs (Wuest et al., 2003) and our WHES findings that services accessed commonly meet women's needs poorly.

Other principles came primarily from scrutiny of the theory and constant comparison to develop a more generalized principle. For example, another practice principle is: "Women will be supported to assess, judge, and take calculated risks necessary for moving forward" (Ford-Gilboe et al., 2011, p. 203). Risk-taking is inherent in the act of leaving an abusive partner in that abuse and harassment intensify after leaving (Canadian Centre for Justice Statistics, 1993; Wuest & Merritt-Gray, 1999). Indeed, 83% of women in the WHES reported ongoing harassment an average of 21 months after leaving (Wuest et al., 2007). Women who left their partners took the risk of experiencing more violence because they wanted a better future for themselves and their children. Thus, leaving is an act of *positioning for the future*, that is "promoting health through proactive, strategic efforts to develop the skills, assets, and strengths needed to realize their family's dreams in the long term" (Ford-Gilboe et al., 2005, p. 483). However, within our data, we found countless examples of women taking diverse risks to position for the future; for example, leaving a stable low-paying job in order to go back to school to gain needed credentials for a career that promised more financial security and fulfillment, buying a house using non-conventional or under-the-table financing in order to build equity for children, or involving children in family decision-making about safety strategies, money, and relationships. In usual practice, clinicians may encourage women to maintain stability through the status quo and discourage taking calculated risks that might lead to further intrusion. However, the SCLI theory suggests the importance of interventionists reinforcing the legitimacy of survivors continuing to take calculated risks in order to build capacity and helping women to contain the potential costs of doing so.

Our initial assumptions and principles offered direction for the subsequent development of the iHEAL, a six-month community-based primary health care intervention to be delivered in 12–14 one-to-one meetings, with the majority of client contact with the nurse (Ford-Gilboe et al., 2011) but were, in turn, refined and expanded in response to our further work. We decided that the theoretical processes of strengthening capacity (*rebuilding security*, *providing*, *renewing self*, and *regenerating family*) would structure the content of the intervention, which we named as components. However, as we began our translation work to develop the components, the need for theory modification became apparent.

Modifying the theory in the process of developing the intervention components

Our work on developing the intervention components began with a review of the original SCLI theory. Often this included returning to the original coded interviews, process tables and memos, particularly to support our choice of language and illustrative examples. Although the WHES study provided additional data for constant comparison, our modification of the theory in response to that data had been largely informal as our common understandings evolved. Thus, as we began our work on the iHEAL, we found ourselves in a process of conscious theory modification in response to theoretical sampling of our WHES findings as well as the original grounded theory data. Modifiability is a key characteristic of grounded theory (Glaser, 1978) and also an aspect of grounded theory application. Glaser and Strauss (1967) noted:

> The person who applies the theory must be enabled to understand and analyze ongoing situational realities, to produce and predict changes in them, and to predict and control consequences . . . As changes occur, his [*sic*] theory must allow him [*sic*] to be flexible in revising his [*sic*] tactics of application and in revising the theory itself if necessary.
>
> *(p. 245)*

Although the original theory had been developed with a sample of women with dependent children who had been separated from abusive partners as long as 20 years, 40% of the WHES sample did not have dependent children (Wuest et al., 2008) and had been separated between three months and three years from their abusive partners. Although women who were mothers were more likely to experience some types of intrusions such as harassment and disabling chronic pain, mothering generally did not account for differences in resources or health patterns found in the WHES. We intend the iHEAL for all women in the early years after leaving abusive partners, believing that early intervention has the potential to prevent or ameliorate many health problems identified in the WHES sample. Thus, data from the WHES helped us to modify the grounded theory for wider applicability.

The original theory has four health promotion sub-processes called *providing, rebuilding security, renewing self,* and *regenerating family* (Ford-Gilboe et al., 2005). *Providing* addressed meeting basic needs including those usually identified such as food, money, housing, and childcare, and also ones not usually named such as medication, energy, leisure, and relief from symptoms. However, the WHES findings related to women's health problems and health service use greatly expanded our conceptual understanding of intrusion related to physical and mental health problems. We learned that women on average reported three current diagnoses by a health professional and 12 current health problems or symptoms, with more than 60% reporting fatigue, difficulty sleeping, back pain, headaches and difficulty concentrating. Rates of high disability chronic pain (35%) (Wuest et al., 2008) and pre-hypertension (42%) (Scott-Storey et al., 2009) were twice as high as those for Canadian women in general in a similar age group. As well, 73% of women had symptoms consistent with clinical depression and 48% reported symptoms consistent with posttraumatic stress disorder (Wuest et al., 2010). Visits in the past month to a physician doctor were more than five times higher than Canadian women in general; and to emergency department 20 times higher (Varcoe et al., 2011). Despite such high levels of service use, women in the WHES appeared to have little relief from their health symptoms. These data enhanced our theoretical understanding of symptom management in the context of intrusion from health problems and increased its primacy in the theory. It also led to our explicitly identifying the principle, "Women's physical, mental, emotional, and spiritual health will be prioritized" (Ford-Gilboe et al., 2011, p. 203).

Consequently, we divided the process of providing into two components: *managing symptoms* and *managing basics*. *Managing symptoms* focuses on supporting women to build confidence in preventing and managing intrusive symptoms through self-management and support from health professionals (Ford-Gilboe et al., 2011). *Managing basics* focuses on "assisting women to build the economic, material, and personal energy resources needed to establish and sustain herself separate from the abuser over time" (p. 207). Using similar processes of comparative analysis with WHES data, we also divided *rebuilding security* into two components: *safeguarding* and *cautious connecting* (Ford-Gilboe et al., 2011). We retained the two processes, *renewing self* and *regenerating family*, as individual components. Thus, the theoretical model used to guide the intervention included six components or ways of strengthening capacity to limit intrusion (see Figure 3.1).

From theoretical process to practice component

Our next challenge was the translation from theoretical process to practice component. Grounded theory processes are very recognizable to those who took part in the study either as participant or investigator because they can see the *fit* between the theoretical concepts and the data or their own experiences (Glaser, 1978). However, these processes may be dense and complex for the interventionist who tries to use them, especially if she/he is not familiar with the study domain or, on the other hand, is an expert in the field with an entrenched practice approach. The conceptualization may be contrary to previous understandings and the language may feel awkward, at least initially. Thus it was important to identify and explain what was unique or different about each component for this population of abused women based on our qualitative data. For example, while the concept of *managing basics* in terms of housing, jobs, childcare and transportation was easily grasped, aspects such as recreation and energy were more unusual. The conceptual understanding that women face the challenge of managing basics while feeling undeserving and often with their energy levels "on empty" is new.

Further, the theoretical construction, not the conceptual indicators from the women's stories, has the broadest applicability clinically. For example, all women struggled with *managing basics* related to intrusion from negative changes to daily life after leaving, such as those related to financial losses. However, a conceptual indicator of how a woman managed her current difficulty in paying hockey registration fees for her teenage son may have little meaning for many women, including those who have no sons of hockey age, or those whose economic circumstances have always precluded children taking part in such activities. However, the broader concepts of determining what *is* basic currently, and the process of *managing without* are recognizable for all. This is not to say that specific examples of women's experiences (conceptual indicators) are inappropriate for illustrating ways of managing particular situations. However, the experience used must be matched to the needs and context of the woman, requiring the interventionist to have a range of diverse examples from which to draw. Those who developed the theory will have in their minds a range of indicators of the concepts from the original data. Alternatively, interventionists attempting to practice from this new theoretical lens will take time to amass a collection of diverse indicators that capture the variation in intrusion and the six components (health promotion processes). Hall and May (2001) asserted that because substantive theory is more specific and complex than practice theory, "more mental agility, and a certain amount of experience and knowledge of the substantive area" may be required for its application (p. 214).

As well, grounded theories often include multiple sub-processes and strategies that may be too layered or complex to be readily useful for an interventionist, especially one who has a novice understanding of the theory. Thus, a re-examination of each of the theoretical processes was necessary to ascertain which elements were core to the process and germane to directing practice

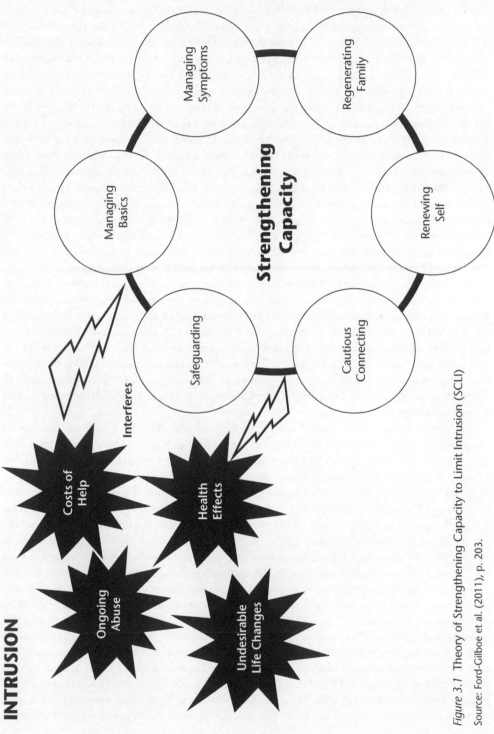

Figure 3.1 Theory of Strengthening Capacity to Limit Intrusion (SCLI)

Source: Ford-Gilboe et al. (2011), p. 203.

to improve health outcomes. We drew on our presentations and publications in our deliberations, particularly the papers focusing on intrusion (Wuest et al., 2003) and the theory overview (Ford-Gilboe et al., 2005). The process of *regenerating family* had been published as a separate paper detailing the varied strategies used by families (Wuest et al., 2004). Interestingly, we had the most difficulty in developing the core elements of the *regenerating family* component, partially because it required modification to apply to women without children but also because once the detail of variation in process or concept has been explicated, it is difficult to set it aside. This latter issue had similarly challenged Wuest and Merritt-Gray in their work developing measures of caregiving concepts from a grounded theory of women's caring where they learned, for example, that the concept of dependency in the care recipient as reason to take on caregiving had broad application, but the conceptual indicators of dependency such as cognitive difficulties or inability to speak English did not (Wuest et al., 2006). The caveat, then, was to use the more abstract concepts, not the conceptual indicators, so that the interventionist would be free to identify a wide range of indicators for each concept, based on personal experience as well as our original work. Over time, as the interventionist delivers the iHEAL, the repertoire of exemplars grows and provides further data for the ongoing refinement of the SCLI theory. In *regenerating family*, we ultimately focused on three core elements that we believed could be most helpful to women: (1) the storyline or how women construct how they have come to be in their current situations; (2) using routines, new roles, and rules in working with others to increase predictability in daily life; and (3) purposefully naming and using new standards for relationships with others.

For each component, the next step was to determine how these core elements could be best translated as a clear guide to practice while staying true to the original conceptualization. We developed a standard template for developing practice modules for each component that included: (1) defining the component; (2) naming expected outcomes; (3) identifying the theoretical and empirical grounding by linking it to the theory of strengthening capacity to limit intrusion but also to existing related research; (4) developing standard required and optional tools to facilitate exploring intrusion, or sharing options; (5) writing an illustrative script for the interventionist to demonstrate an approach for exploring intrusion and sharing options; and (6) identifying potential actions for strengthening capacity.

In doing this work, we guarded against conceptual drift. Despite efforts on the part of grounded theorists to choose conceptual labels that *fit*, the meaning given to words varies widely according to individual contexts and experiences. As we worked together on components, we found that among ourselves our understandings of concepts were sometimes different, and we needed to revisit our analysis of the original data. As well, common disciplinary understandings can intrude. The component of *cautious connecting*, for example, on first glance seems to focus on women's needs for support from family, friends, community and formal services and the interventionist could see the principal focus on helping women make the needed connections. But the theory shows that when women seek support, especially when they have an urgent need for help and few connections, the consequence is often increased intrusion from having to retell their story to justify their need for help, ongoing surveillance from people or agencies, and help that does not match needs well. Thus, some key elements of *cautious connecting* are that it is healthy and important for women to withhold trust from potential helpers until they feel ready, and that agencies and individuals may misinterpret and try to violate the woman's limits. The focus of *cautious connecting* then is supporting women to evaluate the costs and benefits of the connections they have or are thinking of making, with the goal of decreasing conflict and increasing their sense of belonging, emotional support, social interaction, and practical aid. This conceptual focus goes well beyond making referrals. Thus, the illustrative script for *cautious connecting* and the tools developed needed to elaborate and detail this conceptual focus. An information sheet of lessons learned from other women about connecting with others after leaving was developed for exploring intrusion related to *cautious connecting*. Large print showing various reasons women want to connect to others after leaving and a colored table of "costs" of seeking help provide a useful tool to facilitate women exploring the range of possible intrusions from connecting with others. A second tool, a Relationship Map, which is similar to an ecomap, was developed to help women look at the strength and quality of their relationships with people and/or resources that they identify as important to them, first in their "inner circle" and then in the larger community. The illustrative script directs the interventionist to support women to discuss the quality and nature of each relationship and identify which connections are most helpful and which are more intrusive. This sets the stage for a discussion regarding what women might like to change with respect to their connections. A third tool called Options, Tradeoffs and Choices facilitates women's consideration of their options for taking actions to change connections that are most intrusive. Once women determine the action to take, the interventionist then focuses on helping them build capacity. Seven strategies for supporting women to build capacity regardless of the component are: pacing, informing/educating, acknowledging strengths, coaching/guiding, monitoring change or progress, connecting with services or resources, and advocating (Ford-Gilboe et al., 2011). The modules that we developed for each component became the core materials for a training manual for interventionists.

Putting the intervention into practice

We currently are conducting two studies to gain information regarding the feasibility of implementing the iHEAL in diverse community contexts. A key step in moving forward with the feasibility studies was training the interventionists to practice from the theoretical base, and use its language and conceptual rendering in a meaningful way. The *grab* of grounded theory is helpful here, but it is also easy to frame parts of the intervention in usual practice. During the initial training, we oriented interventionists to the SCLI theory and to the assumptions, principles, structures, and activities of the intervention. Mindful discussions about our mutual understandings of abuse and trauma, resources and services, and practice philosophies and strengths set the stage for more specific iHEAL preparation sessions. Differences between the iHEAL and usual practice, as well as potential gaps, were identified and salient clinician expertise was useful for further refinement of the therapeutic approach to fit particular contexts. We found that clinical coaching in regular, scheduled meetings was essential for safe case management and to review, highlight, and ensure consistent application of the theory. Interventionist perspectives are particularly useful for helping us to attend to pragmatic obligation (Thorne, 2011), the interrogation of theoretical findings for their potential to cause harm in practice, by bringing potential problem areas to the surface. Periodic ongoing interventionist development sessions were necessary to uncover problem areas, reflect particular challenges with various components, provide further training, identify issues with services and resources that called for advocacy with decision-makers, and gather data to inform further theory development. The strength of a grounded theory-based intervention is the openness to modification using constant comparative analysis with new data to improve fit.

Within the feasibility studies, we have formally collected data not just through pre- and post-test measures of quality of life, health, capacity, and intrusion, but also through qualitative indicators of the intervention process. The latter include interviews with interventionists early in the intervention process and after the intervention study is completed, interviews with participants about their experiences, and notes reflecting salient points from regular administrative and process-focused meetings with interventionists and/or the research team. Further, clinical file reviews and constant comparative analysis considering the quantitative and qualitative data collected on the corresponding participant are a rich source of insights on the client trajectory, and how the theory was operationalized in the intervention. Together these analyses will lead to further modification of both the intervention and the theory.

Final thoughts

The process of translating the SCLI theory to the iHEAL intervention and conducting two feasibility studies focusing on implementation is complex and demanding. Although our feasibility studies are ongoing, preliminary qualitative and quantitative findings are promising. In particular, the *grab* of the SCLI theory, particularly the concept of *intrusion*, for both the interventionists and the women taking part is convincing evidence that grounded theories are an important starting point for clinical interventions that are useful. The complexity of ensuring conceptual correspondence among the original theory, the iHEAL as written, and the iHEAL as implemented requires detailed knowledge of theory and of the practice field. We have come to understand that intervention development, like grounded theory itself, is an ongoing process open to constant modification. The process of developing and implementing an intervention based on a grounded theory does not result in a fixed intervention. Rather continuing constant comparison, refinement of fit, and emergent fit lead to modification not only of the intervention but also the theory itself which in turn has implications for the intervention. Feedback from interventionists and from women combined with outcomes and chart review all contribute to identify aspects of the intervention and theory that need to be rethought or further refined and confirm the usefulness of others. As we move forward, we are challenged to understand how and why this theory-based intervention works or does not work for women with particular health, abuse, or demographic characteristics in order to sharpen its therapeutic focus for diverse groups of women. Thus, our work, it appears, has barely begun!

Acknowledgments

The research that supported the work described in this chapter was funded by the Canadian Institutes of Health Research (CIHR) New Emerging Team grant 106054 (PI: M. Ford-Gilboe) and Partnership for Health System Improvement Grant #101529, co-funded by the New Brunswick Health Research Foundation (PI: J. Wuest). We also thank the many women who have supported our program of research focusing on women's health after leaving an abusive partner by taking part in our research studies.

Notes

1 For a full discussion of grounded theory as a research method, see Wuest (2012).
2 For a full description of the Intervention for Health Enhancement After Leaving (iHEAL), see Ford-Gilboe, Merritt-Gray, Varcoe, and Wuest (2011).

References

Allen, M., & Warner, M (2002). A developmental model of health and nursing. *Journal of Family Nursing*, 8, 96–135.
Browne, A. J., Varcoe, C., Smye, V., Reimer-Kirkham, S., Lynam, M. J., & Wong, S. (2009). Cultural safety and the challenges of translating critically oriented knowledge in practice. *Nursing Philosophy*, *10*, 167–179.

Canadian Centre for Justice Statistics. (1993). *Violence against women survey highlights and questionnaire package*. Ottawa: Statistics Canada.

Doane, G. H., & Varcoe, C. (2005) *Family nursing as relational inquiry: Developing health promoting practice*. Philadelphia, PA: Lippincott, Williams & Wilkins.

Elliot, D., Bjelajac, P., Fallot, R., Markoff, L., & Reed, B. (2005). Trauma-informed or trauma-denied: Principles and implementation of trauma-informed services for women. *Journal of Community Psychology*, *4*, 461–477.

Estabrooks, C. (2001). Research utilization and qualitative research. In J. Morse, J. Swanson, & A. Kuzel (Eds.), *The nature of qualitative evidence* (pp. 275–298). Thousand Oaks, CA: Sage.

Ford-Gilboe, M., Merritt-Gray, M., Varcoe, C., & Wuest, J. (2011). A theory-based primary health care intervention for women who have left abusive partners. *Advances in Nursing Science*, *34*, 198–214.

Ford-Gilboe, M., Wuest, J., & Merritt-Gray, M. (2005). Strengthening capacity to limit intrusion: Theorizing family health promotion in the aftermath of woman abuse. *Qualitative Health Research*, *15*, 477–501.

Ford-Gilboe, M., Wuest, J., Varcoe, C., Davies, L., Merritt-Gray, M., Hammerton, J., Wilk, P., & Campbell, J. (2009). Modelling the effects of intimate partner violence and access to resources on women's health in the early years after leaving an abusive partner. *Social Science and Medicine*, *68*, 1021–1029.

Ford-Gilboe, M., Wuest, J., Varcoe, C., & Merritt-Gray, M. (2006). Developing an evidence-based health advocacy intervention to support women who have left abusive partners. *Canadian Journal of Nursing Research*, *38*, 147–168.

Glaser, B. (1978). *Theoretical sensitivity*. Mill Valley, CA: Sociology Press.

Glaser, B. (1992). *Basics of grounded theory analysis*. Mill Valley, CA: Sociology Press.

Glaser, B., & Strauss, A. (1967). *The discovery of grounded theory*. Chicago: Aldine.

Hall, W., & May, K. (2001). The application of grounded theory: Issues of assessment and measurement in practice. In R. Schreiber and P. N. Stern (Eds.), *Using grounded theory in nursing* (pp. 211–226). New York: Springer.

Health Canada. (n.d.) What determines health? Available at: http://www.hc-sc.gc.ca/hppb/phdd/determinants/index/html (accessed August 26, 2002).

Morse, J., Penrod, J., & Hupcey, J. (2000). Qualitative outcome analysis: Evaluating nursing interventions for complex clinical phenomena. *Journal of Nursing Scholarship*, *32*, 125–130.

Pauly, B. (2008). Shifting moral values to enhance access to health care: Harm reduction as a context for ethical nursing practice. *International Journal of Drug Policy*, *19*, 195–204.

Sandelowski, M. (2004). Using qualitative research. *Qualitative Health Research*, *14*, 1366–1386.

Scott-Storey, K., Wuest, J., & Ford-Gilboe, M. (2009). Intimate partner violence and cardiovascular risk: Is there a link? *Journal of Advanced Nursing*, *65*, 2186–2197.

Stern, P. N., & Pyles, S. (1986). Using grounded theory methodology to study women's culturally based decisions about health. In P. N. Stern (Ed.), *Women, health and culture* (pp. 1–24). Washington, DC: Hemisphere.

Strauss, A. (1987). *Qualitative analysis for social scientists*. Cambridge: Cambridge University Press.

Swanson, J. (2001). The nature of outcomes. In J. Morse, J. Swanson, & A. Kuzel (Eds.), *The nature of qualitative evidence* (pp. 223–255). Thousand Oaks, CA: Sage.

Thorne, S. (2011) Toward methodological emancipation in applied health research. *Qualitative Health Research*, *21*, 443–453.

Varcoe, C. (1996). Theorizing oppression: Implications for nursing research on violence against women. *Canadian Journal of Nursing Research*, *28*, 61–78.

Varcoe, C., Hankivsky, O., Ford-Gilboe, M., Wuest, J., & Wilk, P., & Campbell. J. C. (2011). Attributing selected costs to intimate partner violence in a sample of women who have left abusive partners: A social determinant of health approach. *Canadian Public Policy*, *37*, 359–380.

WHO (1978). *Declaration of Alma Ata 1978: Primary health care*. Geneva, Switzerland: WHO.

WHO (1986). *Ottawa charter for health promotion*. Ottawa: Health and Welfare.

Wuest, J. (1995). Feminist grounded theory: An exploration of congruency and tensions between two traditions in knowledge discovery. *Qualitative Health Research*, *5*, 125–137.

Wuest, J. (2000). Negotiating with helping systems: An example of grounded theory evolving through emergent fit. *Qualitative Health Research*, *10*, 51–70.

Wuest, J. (2012). Grounded theory: The method. In P. Munhall (Ed.), *Nursing research: A qualitative perspective* (pp. 225–256). Sudbury, MA: Jones & Bartlett.

Wuest, J., Ford-Gilboe, M., Merritt-Gray, M., & Berman, H. (2003). Intrusion: The central problem for family health promotion among children and single mothers after leaving an abusive partner. *Qualitative Health Research, 13*, 597–622.

Wuest, J., Ford-Gilboe, M., Merritt-Gray, M., Varcoe, C., Lent, B., Wilks, P., & Campbell, J.C. (2009). Abuse-related injury and symptoms of posttraumatic stress disorder as mechanisms of chronic pain in survivors of intimate partner violence. *Pain Medicine, 10*, 739–747.

Wuest, J., Ford-Gilboe, M., Merritt-Gray, M., Wilks, P., Campbell, J. C., Lent, B., et al. (2010). Pathways of chronic pain in survivors of intimate partner violence. *Journal of Women's Health, 19*, 1665–1674.

Wuest, J., Hodgins, M., Merritt-Gray, M., Seaman, P., Malcolm, J., & Furlong, K. (2006). Queries and quandaries in developing and testing a measurement instrument derived from grounded theory. *Journal of Theory Construction and Testing, 10*, 26–33.

Wuest, J., & Merritt-Gray, M. (1999). Not going back: Sustaining the separation in the process of leaving abusive relationships. *Violence Against Women, 5*, 110–133.

Wuest, J., & Merritt-Gray, M. (2001). Feminist grounded theory revisited. In R. Schreiber, & P. Stern (Eds.), *Using grounded theory in nursing* (pp. 159–176). New York: Springer.

Wuest, J., Merritt-Gray, M., & Ford-Gilboe, M. (2004). Regenerating family: Strengthening the emotional health of mothers and children in the context of intimate partner violence. *Advances in Nursing Science, 27*, 257–274.

Wuest, J., Merritt-Gray, M., Ford-Gilboe, M., Lent, B., Varcoe, C., & Campbell, J. C. (2008). Chronic pain in women survivors of intimate partner violence. *Journal of Pain, 9*, 1049–1057.

Wuest, J., Merritt-Gray, M., Lent, B., Varcoe, C., Connors, A., & Ford-Gilboe, M. (2007). Patterns of medication use among women survivors of intimate partner violence. *Canadian Journal of Public Health, 98*, 460–464.

4

The power of qualitative inquiry
Traumatic experiences of marginalized groups

Joanne M. Hall

Introduction

What can we accomplish with qualitative research? Qualitative research is increasingly accepted by the scientific community for initial exploration in an area where there is little known, or to gain subjective views (Borreani, Miccinesi, Brunelli, & Lina, 2004). But qualitative inquiry can be more consequential than we have been accustomed to thinking. In this chapter I will explore some of the ways that I and colleagues have used qualitative techniques in a coherent program of scholarship, in which one study follows on needs and questions developed from previous analysis. My program of research has also been grounding for theoretical development, especially of the critical concept of marginalization (Hall, 1999b; Hall & Fields, 2012; Hall, Stevens, & Meleis, 1994). I speak of knowledge development from this emancipatory perspective (Chinn & Kramer, 2008).

I will explore many commonly held tenets and beliefs about qualitative research, raising challenges, in order to persuade qualitative researchers to go further in terms of the breadth and reach, the power, of qualitative work. I will touch on marginalized populations, advocacy, environmental relevance, language, generalizability, causality, funding, and clinical practice. Without intending to raise the timeworn debate about qualitative versus quantitative research, I would argue, however, that qualitative research is not to be set to the sidelines but should be a full partner in knowledge development, providing essential knowledge by distinctive means. I hope to stimulate dialogue and to help qualitative researchers and their study participants to empower themselves in the larger research sphere.

Finding and understanding hidden populations

Throughout my research I have focused on marginalized, stigmatized populations (Hall, 1999a, 2003b; Hall & Fields, 2012; Hall, et al., 2009; Hall & Stevens, 1992; Hall, Stevens, & Meleis, 1992; Stevens & Hall, 2001; Thomas & Hall, 2008). I have focused on resiliencies as well as risks faced by those populations. My dissertation's main research question was, "What is the experience of lesbians in recovery from alcohol problems?" I used critical ethnographic interviews because lesbians in a local community comprise a cultural group. A critical approach was needed because in a hostile, legally unprotected environment, many in the Lesbian, Gay, Bisexual, Transgender and Queer (LGBTQ) group cannot safely expose themselves without social and political risks, including interpersonal violence. However, 1990s activism helped lesbian women be more open, especially in San Francisco. I was in the right place at the right time.

Insider status as a lesbian helped me recruit initially, followed by referral (snowball) sampling within the lesbian recovery community. The sample (n = 30) was a large number, but I sought racial, age, ethnic and socioeconomic diversity within what was a stereotyped, sexually defined group. Marginalized groups are best accessed by inviting them to relate the whole of their life experiences, not only substance recovery. Allowing the participant to talk in research gives them more control, especially when past research has been pathologizing. One participant expressed the urgency and fears she and others felt: "Don't talk *about* us, listen *to* us."

I nearly missed the point when more than half of the sample reported being child sexual abuse (CSA) survivors, in answer to questions about substance recovery. I learned that the agenda changes; trauma becomes central. Participants said that the impact of CSA was so great that it surpassed their discrimination and addiction experiences. The critical ethnographic approach revealed individual experiences, but also sociocultural and political aspects of recovery, such as the dynamics of Alcoholics Anonymous (AA), and psychotherapy (Hall, 1990, 1992, 1993a, 1994a, 1994c). Qualitative research is iconoclastic. Because of the reflexive and interactive nature of an open-ended interview, the researcher is corrected by participants, dismantling false assumptions.

Two core research foci are measures of central tendency (commonalities), and measures of dispersion (diversity). Qualitative dialectical analysis oscillates between individuals' diverse subjectivities and common experiences across the group (Stevens & Hall, 2001). The tension between commonality and diversity creates a discursive space, making a marginalized group visible, vibrant, and multivocal within research process(es).

Taking on the next question

CSA and substance misuse are entangled, each problem complex in itself and potentiating the other. Exploring this, I engaged a population of African American women CSA survivors in very early stages of substance recovery (Hall, 2003b). I built rapport with staff (most of whom were in substance recovery themselves) of several women's treatment halfway houses. *De facto* geographic segregation meant that most of the women in one house were African American, including some who were lesbians. Qualitative research can explore in obscure social realms, which might seem too narrow to try to represent. These women's strategies for successful recovery, however, were very robust, when referenced against those of, e.g., a White middle-class sample. This was useful: if a coping tactic works in the meanest of circumstances, it will likely work in less oppressive circumstances; the converse is not true: the greater resources of the dominant group protect them from the most severe stressors. A participant said, "The skills I learned in poverty work in any setting you are in."

Among recovering women abuse survivors, the centrality of traumatic stress became more evident. I explored trauma more specifically and critiqued extant research concerning abuse survival (Hall, 1996a, 1996b, 1996c, 1999a; Hall & Kondora, 1997). I was challenged by a participant: "Why are you only interested in sexual abuse? Why is it considered OK to beat your children on a daily basis?" Was that the message I had delivered through my focus on CSA? Apparently so. Sexual abuse had become exotic in the 1990s, with celebrities revealing incest histories, etc. But what of the more common physical abuse and neglect? Qualitative research is a dialogue continuing across a program of studies; participants teach us about our exclusivity and bias. I began to collect stories of women, regardless of sexual orientation, and regardless of the type of childhood maltreatment (CM) they had suffered. Looking back, I realize the significance of first hearing the voices of the socially obscured, multiply marginalized, in order to approach "majority" women critically. A survey would not have been attractive to any of these women in exposing their marginalization, addiction and violent victimization. When the idea the participant wants to express is not in the instrument, a message is delivered that one's experience is "not on the map." This invalidation leads to mistrust and avoidance not only of research, but of health care. In personal stories, socio-political-cultural context and subjective uniqueness resonate. Additionally, the use of narrative can detail the intersections of gender, race, sexual orientation, gender identity and other sources of marginalization (Anderson & McCormack, 2010; Delgado & Stephancic, 2001; Mintz, California State University San Marcos College of Education, & Services, 2011).

Illuminating the edges of experience

Former research on women survivors of abuse had questioned the veracity of abuse memories, referring instead to a "false memory syndrome" (Bremner, Shobe, & Kihlstrom, 2000; Loftus, 1996; Perlman, 1996). From a feminist perspective, in my research, and through a paper I did with Dr. Lori Kondora, there was much to refute in this assertion and invalidation of women survivors. In the data women did not describe "dissociating," but rather, they said, "I always knew the memories were there, I just put it to the back of my mind," and "Why even think about those things? They just make me unhappy." Thus, we critiqued "dissociation" and "false memories" as infantilizing and invalidating (Hall, 1996a, 2003a; Hall & Kondora, 1997; Hall & Powell, 2000).

For qualitative researchers to expand on their work in a defined area, it makes sense to do supplemental scholarship in the form of reviews that draw in other research, using different methods, as well as explore relevant theories.

A caveat, however, is that merely using a narrative or phenomenological approach does not guarantee experiential validation. Interview questions may insidiously *invalidate* experience if they are not carefully constructed, guided by cultural experts (Kvale, 1996). For example, the question "What is it like to be an abuse survivor?" might invalidate many Appalachian women, who do not use the terms "abuse" or "survivor." "How have you become successful?" may alienate those who do not feel successful. Qualitative research involves creativity in the design of an interview guide, which is not simply a reiteration of the research questions, but language and sequence that will encourage the participant to talk about the "edges" of experience. Thus, in approaching the topic obliquely, versus head on, we asked, "What made it hard for you growing up?" (Hall et al., 2009). Furthermore, creative approaches abound in qualitative research, exposing "erased" and languageless aspects of experience, through photovoice, observation, video, artwork, and film (Plunkett, Leipert, & Ray, 2012; Rich, Lamola, & Woods, 2006; Walia & Leipert, 2012; Warson, 2012).

Powerful paradigm shifts

From the perspective of post-positivist science, usual "next questions" have to do with refinements of established theories. Kuhn held that scientific revolutions shatter normative quantitative paradigms. A completely new set of questions arises (Kuhn, 1970; Kuhn & Hacking, 2012). On the other hand, qualitative research has bigger aims. Because of the complexity and openness of qualitative research, as in thick description, researcher immersion, theoretical sampling, etc., marginal questions can be raised: "What are immediate responses to being told one has cancer?" "How do children describe being short of breath?" "How do persons with severe and persistent mental illness relay their perceptual experiences, in their own words?"

At the turn of the decade, I encountered a statistic that perhaps as many as 22% of survivors of CM become very successful in adulthood (McGloin & Widom, 2001). This was unheard of; the literature was rife with evidence of severe, multiple, negative sequelae of CM (Banyard, Williams, & Siegel, 2001; Briere, 1992; Browne & Finkelor, 1986; Cicchetti & Toth, 1997; Classen, Field, Koopman, Nevill-Manning, & Spiegel, 2001; Duncan, Saunders, Kilpatrick, Hanson, & Resnick, 1996; Kinzl & Biebl, 1992; Rorty, Yager, & Rossotto, 1994; Schetky, 1990; Weiss, Longhurst, & Mazure, 1999).

Trust in the participant's credibility and the tenet that people are experts on their own experience allow a new research paradigm to emerge: "How does this happen? How does a survivor become successful despite an abuse history?" "What does PTG [posttraumatic growth], or thriving, look like in this population?" (Carver, 1998; Casaccio, 1999; Finfgeld, 1999; Ickovics & Clark, 1998; O'Leary, 1998; Poorman, 2002; Saakvitne, Tennen, & Affleck, 1998; Tedeschi, Park, & Calhoun, 1998; Wuest & Merritt-Gray, 2001). Apparently this was innovative and comprehensive enough: our R01 proposal was funded by the National Institute for Nursing Research (NINR).

Our interdisciplinary team began with avoidance of pathologizing participants, use of multiple interviews, a large sample (n = 44) and an emphasis on PTG to discover how women were able to succeed despite their history of CM. We sought practical information, in everyday language, about what worked, and what didn't work for them over time; what they considered their strengths; how they strategized as problems arose; and who helped or not in their healing (Hall et al., 2009). But how far can we go with our findings?

Generalizability? You have to be kidding

How many qualitative studies have reported that "a limitation is that findings are not generalizable beyond the participants in the study"? Every set of findings, whether experimental or exploratory, is generalizable to some segment, but not the whole of a population, *regardless of method*. Generalizable knowledge is that which (a) can be applied to individuals and events beyond those sampled; and (b) is meant for dissemination, as in publication and presentation. Rigor in qualitative research has been viewed with suspicion and misunderstanding (Myers, 2000). And one cannot use the same criteria to judge all qualitative studies (Sandelowski, Trimble, Woodard, & Barroso, 2006). Because post-positivism has had hegemony on "research," that diminishes qualitative research, the term "transferability" has become widely used. Truthfully, the concept is closely related to generalizability; both frameworks are limited, albeit in different ways. Generalizability erodes with time, because phenomena are always changing. Even in biological research, each person's physiology is genetically and environmentally unique, so that findings on specific responses have limited generalizability and usability. Using analytic generalization, precise descriptions of similar contexts, locales and time frames, enhances and particularizes generalizability (Collingridge & Gantt, 2008). This is especially applicable to questions of human choices, responses, perceptions, interpretations and behaviors. Combining phenomenology and ethnography (Maggs-Rapport, 2001), especially in large studies, increases thoroughness and supports greater claims to generalizability. This is also amenable to funding. Thus, qualitative researchers should explain specifically the *segment* of the population, the type of context, and the *realm of experience* to which findings are generalizable and usable.

In my program of research, I have strained at the limits placed on generalizability. For example, in a secondary analysis of data from women of color recovering cocaine misusers surviving childhood maltreatment, I explored working, managing money, and parenting. Traumatic stress and economic necessity resulting from lack of family support, cultural impoverishment, limited formal education and, for some, illiteracy, led survivors to engage in high-risk sex work (Hall, 2000b). The narratives revealed ubiquitousness about these elements in the small sample. There was little reason to think that similarly situated low-income, substance-using women of color elsewhere were not experiencing these outcomes. If I had to do it over, I would have written more definitively about generalization, by referencing health disparities in HIV risk for precisely this aggregate; and that sex work and needle sharing are key in this chain of events.

Quantitative research also has limits to its generalizability. Because of the aforementioned issues with exclusion and invalidation, a quantitative study is often not generalizable to the marginalized segment. Homogeneity is assumed, and is often found in the dominant majority group, but diversity also needs to be captured. Rather than reject generalizability out of hand, qualitative studies can be treated as is any research: it will be critiqued, subjected to logical argument, or studied again to refute its generalizability. Replication will produce different themes, based on researcher perspective, but the *core* of the qualitative findings will likely remain stable.

Prediction

Random and representative samples meeting statistical standards should allow prediction for the population *not* in the sample. However, participants in a trial should correspond with actual patients seen in practice. This is the problem of ecological validity, e.g., studies of neurocognition and mental illness need to take place in real-world settings (Gioa, 2009; Vaskinn, Sergi, & Green, 2009; Yantz, Johnson-Greene, Higginson, & Emmerson, 2010). And reviews showed that more research is needed on cancer patients' attitudes, affecting their responses in randomized controlled trials (RCT) (Roy, 2012; Todd et al, 2009). Lovato lamented RCT threats to rigor: physician attitudes, patient cultural and confidentiality concerns, mistrust of research, HIV issues, language, expense, and difficulties in getting a diverse sample (Lovato, Hill, Hertert, Hunninghake, & Probstfield, 1997). Qualitative methods lend themselves to illuminating these crevices in the knowledge base, which may seem "small" but are structurally essential.

Statistical experts have moved from certainty of statistical procedures to valuing the practical significance of them, concluding that external validity is only attenuated assurance. Rules of interpretation are needed to judge the *usability* of findings (Horton, 2000). Qualitative samples that reflect group heterogeneity; that have a logical, adequate number of participants so that data saturation occurs; and that reflect marginalized experiences, are usable in that they are informative of the needs of the target group.

Finally, it is a conundrum that in the fine grain of deeply subjectively unique experience, in a multivocal, multiauthoritative paradigm, an emergent qualitative thematic can have "universal" implications. This is not without gender, race or other diversities, but represents a grounded unity about common human experiences, such as suffering and hope, in which we *recognize* each other (Levinas, 1947/1978). Each insight that illuminates this ground increases its clarity, contributing to *generalized roots of basic experiences*, expressed diversely. My own program of research has pointed to some basic experiences of women suffering trauma; their stories are unique *and* recognizable, and have implications for other types of trauma-related suffering.

Causality in qualitative research

Qualitative analyses can reveal specific elements of causality not reachable by other means. This is a somewhat heretical statement from the standpoints of post-positivism as well as postmodernism. Yet in knowledge development, attributions are regularly made surmising what is "behind" a given piece of evidence. In the 1990s (and even now), a common technique for substance-related treatment was confrontation and diminishment of the sufferer as merely an "addict," and withholding of treatment until the person is "truly ready." I posed a real case. A substance-misusing woman who was treated dismissively and harshly by a counselor, and sent home to feel ashamed and hopeless, was nurtured by a friend through a suicidal period. The woman later returned to the counselor in a more humbled and "ready" disposition. The counselor concluded that his confrontation had been effective. A single case study detailing the nurturing approach behind the scenes disrupted a faulty "causal" assumption about women in recovery, and "what really worked" in entry to treatment (Hall, 1993b).

Qualitative researchers can engage those in the scientific community who use discourses of internal and external validity, especially in the context of evidence-based practice. Many criteria have been developed to judge the solidity of critical, naturalistic findings as having context-bound applicability. Debate continues about issues of rigor in qualitative research circles (Tobin & Begley, 2004). Post-positivistic researchers argue that without conditions of experimental control and probability-based procedures, as in RCTs, causality cannot be established. Arguably, as an example, case study is a thorough, systematic method that can document chains of events, as in organizational transitions (Yin, 2012), which contribute to the establishment of causality. And qualitative insights can be prescient; implications of findings may be *actualized* long after the study is published (De Witt & Ploeg, 2006; Sandelowski et al., 2006).

In critical realist theory, reality is seen as a complex open system. Phenomena are assumed to be multiply caused, and traceable to generative mechanisms that can be inductively identified and described, based on observable consequences (Bhaskar, 1989). Constructivist research can establish *patterns* of how and why things happen, and related power dynamics (Bergin, Wells, & Owen, 2008; Cruikshank, 2012; Porter & Ryan, 1996).

Valuing complexity, qualitative researchers have maintained that the perspectival assumptions underlying qualitative inquiry would be violated if causality is asserted. This has justified qualitative inquiry and differentiated it from quantitative research, but veritably throws the baby out with the bathwater. Elevating description without implications of origins, the roots of phenomena, researchers may diminish the power of qualitative data to reveal who and what are behind human experiences and sociocultural patterning. No methodology escapes the fact that historical certainty is out of reach. However, narratives provide retrospective self-analyses and environmental analyses, along temporal lines (Hall, 2011; Ricoeur, 1984). A causal factor is antecedent to the outcome or effect, a criterion partially met by narrative research. The temporal order of events is discernible, within the limits of the accuracy, recall and positionality of the teller. Details might be inaccurate in retrospective narratives, but recall is also problematic in surveys (Rodgers &Herzog, 1987; Yorkston, Turner, Schluter, & McClure, 2005).

Even when multiply arranged, independent variables in experimental research fall short of "establishing" causality beyond a reasonable doubt. Additionally, quantitative researchers often report types, relative strengths and directions of non-significant *trends* in findings, with speculation that, e.g., a larger sample size might have increased significance. Hence, non-significant results are contributory to causal understanding. We should not deter the qualitative researcher from writing about findings in such a way that what *can* be said about causality *is*, in fact, said as clearly as is possible. From trends we see in qualitative data, certain outcomes logically follow. A phenomenological description or set of narratives may be enhanced by extrapolation of outcomes. In my research, for example, it is not clear what "causes" the process of "becoming resolute" for survivors of interpersonal violence. We can say, however, that the process is among the causative factors that "lead to" success, thriving and empowerment for women survivors of CM. Valuing our findings as contributory to causality is useful in putting together puzzles about human experience and behavior, and in solving clinical and societal health problems.

The social environment as the field

Qualitative research informs about the social environment. The most typical vehicle for this is ethnography, including autoethnography, cultural ethnography, urban ethnography and critical ethnography. I dealt with the question of experiential environments in "The Geography of Child Sexual Abuse." I examined narratives for evidence of subsequent social environmental impact on abuse-related family of origin dynamics (Hall, 1996b). The stories revealed that survivors' childhood experiences and perceptions of school, and then the larger community, reflected perceived "unsafeness." In growing up, survivors *expected* that abuse would continue in new environments, even after the original abuse had ended and faded in memory, and the survivor was no longer in that environment. Qualitative research can integrate and connect the intrapersonal subjective experiences, such as trauma, to social interaction in larger environments. This can be combined with multiple theorizations about what really happens in these environments. The abused, neglected child is identifiable in both overt and subtle ways, often becomes the black sheep, and is then targeted for harassment at school. Although my study could not document the actual bullying, there is now a whole body of knowledge on the reality of bullying and cyberbullying in schools, and their devastating consequences (Cooper, Clements, & Holt, 2012; Idsoe, Dyregrov, & Idsoe, 2012; Jones, Waite, & Thomas Clements, 2012; Lemstra, Nielsen, Rogers, Thompson, & Moraros, 2012; Radliff, Wheaton, Robinson, & Morris, 2012). Combining the qualitative findings with this body of knowledge, it is clear that the real, and not only perceived, abusive dynamics persist in social geographic environments outside the family. The analysis suggested a "universal precautions" approach might be used, in which it is assumed that any child might be an abused child. Safe spaces should be created in the environment where bullying, derogatory speech and sexual contact could not occur. This tactic would interrupt the abused child's global perception of being in an unsafe world. Thus, the qualities of environments and their subjective effects can be located through qualitative research, cast against a background of extant findings, and new interventions or policies can be assessed for socio-cultural-political effectiveness (Hall, 1996b).

Clinical relevance

Qualitative research can, and should, be directly *usable* in the clinical field, whether that is a clinic, hospital or the community. It need not always be a stepping stone toward instrument development, followed by experimentation which then has relevance in the "real world." In a participatory critical ethnography about breastfeeding, accessing the cultural voice, the researchers validated experiences of stigma; and findings were used to achieve a specific policy intervention that mandated shopping centers to provide space for breastfeeding (Groleau, Zelkowitz, & Cabral, 2009).

Qualitative research needs to be untangled from a web of criticism about vagueness and nebulousness that has prevented the full force of qualitative findings to enhance or change practices. The narratives of qualitative inquiry should not be labeled "anecdotal." Anecdotes reveal isolated instances, brought into a dialogue to suggest that there is further evidence. Qualitative research is organized, analytical, critical and iterative in its processes. Rigorous systematic inquiry adds more clinical credibility to findings than that of mere anecdotes. And as qualitative researchers in particular areas, we ought to make criteria specific as we do for feminist research, expressed as *scientific adequacy* (Hall & Stevens, 1991). Description, knowledge about perceptions and beliefs and interpretation are all clinically usable.

In illustration, a nurse practitioner had a copy of the article on thriving among women survivors of CM. His patient was a cancer survivor who had battled many recurrences and had outlived medical expectations for her length of life. The nurse gave the article to the patient, stating that it was not exactly about her experiences, but might be helpful. At the next appointment, woman was clearly excited about how relevant the article was to her experiences as a cancer thriver. Thus, even a "scientifically" written account of the process of "becoming resolute" was immediately meaningful. This suggests a potential benefit for patients traumatized in ways besides CM. Qualitatively based knowledge spans a range from basic descriptive to more definitive practice-applicable findings and should be included under the rubric of evidence-based practice.

Medication side effects can be quantified in clinical trials. Yet many of the reasons for non-adherence in drug therapies are embedded in negative subjective experiences, or skeptical beliefs about particular drugs. Qualitative researchers can interpret such subjective data. This is as valuable as is evidence of physiologic effectiveness, because a drug will not be used by patients if their subjective beliefs and concerns toward it are not addressed. Dulling of emotions, anticipated sexual dysfunction or fears of addiction are subjective motivations best understood phenomenologically. While not interventional, this contributes to "comparative effectiveness."

The reluctance of researchers in authoritatively tying qualitative findings to relevant clinical contexts is perhaps a reflection of timidity in the face of criticism from proponents of "harder science." If descriptive and interpretive claims prove not to be clinically relevant, one might question the trustworthiness of the particular study's findings, versus crumpling under a critique of qualitative research as a whole. In short, if a given qualitative study is not relevant to clinical practice, then why conduct it?

Costs and funding

It is a myth that qualitative research is inexpensive. Costs include payment of interdisciplinary team members, consultation, transcription, coding and the sheer time involved in analytic procedures. Despite impressions that it is unlikely, qualitative researchers can obtain adequate funding. How? Characteristics of funded projects include innovation, comparison, large-scale, clinical relevance, and generation of new knowledge. Funded studies target poorly understood, intractable, costly health problems, such as depression, end-of-life care, cancer, substance misuse, HIV, pain, anxiety, and traumatic stress. Health problems of neglected populations such as transgendered persons (Grant et al., 2011; Morgan & Stevens, 2008; Stevens & Morgan, 2001), or veterans and their families, including traumatic brain injury, PTSD, intimate partner violence, and suicide are current major concerns (Brenner, Homaifar, Adler, Wolfman, & Kemp, 2009). Many such problems lend themselves to grounded theory, and ethnographic, narrative and phenomenological study can provide subjective and critical analysis of these problems, identifying barriers to treatment acceptance and adherence. However, funders are not impressed with sole description, and sample sizes that cannot capture group diversity, or cannot achieve the study aims. With access to adequate numbers, a probability sample might be considered in qualitative research (Morse & Neihaus, 2009).

Establishing clarity on an obscured aspect of a problem (e.g., why behaviors don't change despite intervention) can lead to reduction of care costs; this is attractive. Research that is *pragmatic* is fundable. Capturing the nature of experiences like problem-solving or rehabilitation can lead to short cuts in healing processes that decrease human and monetary costs. In my early studies I focused on how lesbians actually *constructed* their substance abuse as a problem; one has to recognize the problem, in its context, before one will try to solve it (Hall, 1994b), supporting earlier appropriate intervention.

The study needs a substantive goal, i.e., that societal burden is decreased. Statistical findings provide only part of the story when the "how" is not visible. How did this result occur? What are the experiential processes that led to a statistically significant result? What is it about intervention A that makes it efficacious, yet unpopular with patients (ineffective)? How do we lay the groundwork for measurement of an emergent human experience, such as thriving in transgender persons?

In many proposals, a quantitative researcher has added open-ended questions to a survey and plans content or thematic analysis on these responses in order to augment the design, when what is really needed is a full qualitative arm of the study using mixed or multiple methods. Mixed methods and interprofessional and interdisciplinary teams have evolved to resolve these dilemmas. Qualitative researchers need to step into their rightful place in this research environment. Quantitative and qualitative methods are joined in much mixed methods research because either method alone is insufficient to answer the research question(s). The two sets of data come together at a point of interface that varies by design (Morse & Neihaus, 2009). Complex mixed methods designs reflect pluralistic frameworks. These studies are increasingly funded. Mixed methods researchers need qualitative expertise. Thus, qualitative researchers should conceptualize what we do as a valuable resource in the whole knowledge development enterprise.

Advocacy and social justice

Qualitative research can attest to human experiences of suffering. By this I mean that we become witnesses, advocates, as we closely read participants' stories. Most participatory action research (PAR) or community action research has a qualitative component and depends on social justice values and the political openness of the qualitative team. Critical race theory, postcolonialism, feminism and queer theory underscore the use of narratives and/or focus groups from the marginalized group or the engaged community. Such narratives are stories around which members can collectivize in group dialogue, thus developing *counternarratives* (Campesino, Ruiz, Glover, & Koithan, 2009; Shapiro, 2011) to the dominant cultural position. The audiences for these counternarratives are powerful others, including health care providers (HCPs), and more importantly, fellow marginalized others. The data themselves are empowering, not the researchers. Advocacy research often constitutes a crucial part of a change or liberation process, and thus the qualitative contribution to the change is its documentation, a means of *praxis* (action-reflection) (Holmes & Warelow, 1997) and part of its legacy.

A difficult aspect of engaging in this kind of research is the initiation of rapport with, e.g., communities of color, women, sexual minorities, economically repressed groups, and immigrants; and it takes courage to step out politically in our research trajectories. Yet it is often the next step when oppression is evident. White, middle-class academic researchers often expect automatic *distrust* or reticence from these communities that need exposure and resolution of disparities, through research. In my experience with marginalized groups, however, most are open to sharing their stories, often because until that point no one has actually sat down and listened. In a recent interview I had in a pilot study about subtle racism with an African American man, his opening statement was, "The first thing I want to say is that I am honored to be able to give this interview." There is empowerment in "going on the record." Thus qualitative research heightens in value, and in fact can be essential to the social change needed. Collaboration with community leaders is often welcomed; they recognize the power of "having data."

Qualitative research can be harmful

Problems emergent from past research in general include false or inequitable comparisons, exclusion, poor interviewing, culturally biased tools, exoticism, and assumptions of intragroup homogeneity. Qualitative researchers should astutely prioritize the interests of those whose experiences we are making visible, plan how the study will proceed, and assure that questions are framed in nonpathologizing ways (Rothblu, 1994; Sue, Bucceri, Lin, Nadal, & Torino, 2007). For me, a delicate study was a secondary analysis of the core internalized messages or discourses revealed in narratives of women suffering from addiction and violence (Hall, 2000a). The point was to "boil down" negative self-images, within the life course, to their most basic themes. The negativity took two invalidating forms: "I do not exist" and "I am bad or wrong." Analysis revealed differentiation between the two core messages: negation of existence versus vilification of identity and action. I wrote up this study so as not to pathologize the women who held these painfully negative core beliefs. The prevailing societal notions about survivors as "permanent victims" who can never overcome these powerful, negative core beliefs was carefully avoided; it simply did not hold empirically.

In any study of marginalized groups, stigmatization and pathologization are dangers, but these can be avoided if decisions are made early in the research process. These include decisions about inclusion/exclusion criteria, the framing of the study in consultation with group members, for example, in flyers, the informed consent document and the choice and careful wording of interview questions. Some harm cannot be controlled. Studying lesbians' alcohol problems (Hall, 1994c), I documented past drug use in a group of *recovering* lesbians. The information was "twisted" in the Family Research Council website; the study "proved" that all lesbians are drug abusers. I asked that the citation be removed, to no avail. Similar research was also "misinterpreted."

Qualitative research as language-focused

Qualitative researchers examine language as multidimensional, complex, and inexhaustible in meaning. Much of what people say can be linguistically be seen to have multiple "layers" of meaning. Power-laden messages are embedded in "talk" even about mundane events and participants' self-interpretations of experience (Bourdieu & Thompson, 1991). Media statements and images are also laden with these messages that exert social control and perpetuate stigmatization and stereotyping. I examined the discourse, the construction, of lesbianism, by medicine, in a historical investigation, which exposed the inevitably heterosexist, heteronormative and privileged speech that could be gleaned from medical texts pre-gay activism (Hall. 1993a; Stevens & Hall, 1991).

These *discourses* or *ideologies* are in often in cohesion with constantly constructed and reinforced beliefs, serving the interests of the dominant majority. For example, in a narrative about help-seeking, a person with CA said that they felt "iced out" by a provider when the provider stated in an offhand remark that, "Chemotherapy patients are very brave." This innocuous-sounding statement contains embedded ideologies reflecting Euroamerican values, such as rugged individualism, and negativity of death at all costs. The ideology is "Good cancer patients express courage in the face of death, which is an adversary." This ideology "protects" the dominant majority, perhaps especially HCPs, from having to face the inevitability of death, and the intense suffering that chemotherapy causes. It further marginalizes the patient who perceives chemotherapy as unacceptable and unwanted. Qualitative analysis that identifies oppressive discourses and ideologies can give voice to the marginalized CA sufferer, who may hold that death is inevitable and not to be avoided "at all costs." It is also important to identify non-oppressive discourses or ideologies that can be validating and liberating. For example, the above-mentioned client might say, "I am quitting this chemotherapy and going home. I have had enough." The underlying discourse is that human beings have basic rights over their bodies, and that people have options outside of the majority cultural norms. Counterideologies are often embedded in counternarratives (Reissman, 2008). In my current research, at the pilot stage, my colleague and I are investigating the experience of subtle racism, or microaggressions (Hall & Fields, 2012; Sue et al., 2007; Sue, Lin, Torino, Capodilupo, & Rivera, 2009; Sue et al., 2011), that occur between African Americans and Euroamericans in daily, even mundane interactions (Hall & Fields, 2012). This investigation stemmed from a realization that racism is a form of interpersonal trauma. Discourses of white privilege and white domination are evident. For a Euroamerican to say, "Excuse me, where are the handbags?" to an African American who happens to be shopping in a department store delivers the message, "You must be a service worker because you are a person of color." For a Euroamerican to say that we live in a postracial society, or that they are "colorblind," indicates the message, "You can no longer complain of, or perhaps even talk of, racism." These discourses/ ideologies are exposed in qualitative data, through narrative discourse analysis. This, then, is another powerful thing that qualitative research can do.

The power of a program of qualitative research

Listening to hidden, marginalized populations, I gained a critical perspective that guided future studies. I explored complex interrelated experiences such as interpersonal violence, racism and substance misuse in the life course of traumatized women. I identified the core ideologies experienced at depth by them. The environmental breadth of post-abuse experiences became clearer as these women spoke of the worlds of family, school and community. My studies became more inclusive by inviting as many subgroups of participants as possible. In the context of an interdisciplinary team I devised a complex narrative method to study success or thriving in women survivors of childhood abusive trauma. Realizing that racism is traumatic, I have set out on a new path of narrative research, still connected to the original thread of my first study. On the whole, then, I have cultivated a field of related kinds of qualitative views that provide a window on trauma in marginalized populations.

Issues requiring qualitative exploration are ever-emerging, and flexibility of perspectives, questions and methods is needed. Qualitative methods have been developed and proliferated through the creativity of investigators. With the development of the Internet, qualitative research is taking new methodological turns, with new dilemmas, ethical procedures and means of interpretation. The doors are open. Indeed, qualitative inquiry is powerful and can do more than we think, and more than we can imagine.

Conclusion

I will purposefully avoid citations in my conclusions. For too long nursing has labored under a framework that does not legitimate original scholarship. There must be room in scholarship and research for independent speech and non-traditional viewpoints, and creative approaches to study complex problems.

It is controversial to claim that qualitative research should be critical, is generalizable, adds to causality, and should be clinically usable. I have intentionally pushed these envelopes because I sense that our rhetoric as qualitative researchers is often defensive, overly cautious, apologetic, and lukewarm.

Many nurse researchers have begun with a single qualitative study, and continue doing serial qualitative studies relatively in isolation. We have not reached out into interdisciplinary teams, funding resources and the opportunities of mixed methods research. Why? Qualitative research itself is marginalized. In nursing education, the business model demands securing extramural funding. Much of qualitative nursing research has been funded via small grants or internal monies. Investigators feel the increased pressure for federal funding, even as funds dwindle in the current economy, and in an anti-intellectual climate in the US.

A hopeful note is that federal agencies do realize the value of qualitative research in tailoring interventions, making procedures culturally appropriate, and reaching marginalized, high-risk groups. A mandate has been issued for studying the health and health problems of LGBTQ populations (NIH, 2011), people of color, women, children and older persons. Often treatments are developed and tested without understanding the temporal contexts, social environments, beliefs, constraints, trust and hopes of the target groups. Patients are navigating a system fraught with short-staffing, profit motives, ruthless insurance practices, fragmentation, confusion and frustration; they fear the reality of a catastrophic health event which would change their lives forever. Patients are marginalized.

The soul of nursing is invested in the subjective, as well as objective, experience of one's health and illness, and these issues are inextricably linked in an intersectionality of racialized, gendered sociopolitical environments (Hall, 1998; Van Herk, Smith, & Andrew, 2011). Moreover, one cannot know about these phenomena without asking, without documenting the experience of those affected.

Nurses are marginalized; thus we are exploring exclusionary practices and bullying within nursing education and practice. Many qualitative studies are used to discover what motivates nurses to stay in their jobs, and why they leave. And so, without saying that we are behind the eight ball, it does seem that nurses need to take a stance as different from many other professions, and valuing of nontraditional types of knowledge (Chinn & Kramer, 2008; Meleis, 2012). As the most knowledgeable advocates of those marginalized in US health care (uninsured, under-insured, people of color, women, children, immigrants, substance misusers, prison inmates, etc.), who better than qualitative nurse researchers can capture the stories, the words, in their specificity, of persons and cultural groups?

There is a great deal of explanatory power in qualitative methods when attempting to understand complex phenomena and deriving implications for policy and situational context. More emphasis in the direction of context will add, not detract, from the power of qualitative research, and this will prove essential in comparative effectiveness and critical patient outcomes research. Qualitative researchers should influence NIH research priorities and be adamant that there be qualitative funding opportunities through the NINR, as well as equal opportunity to publish in all nursing research journals.

Qualitative research is, first and foremost, scholarship. Exceptional scholarship is a powerful influence in scientific, educational and policy circles. The writing of qualitative research and related theory is thus the linchpin of what can be achieved. We need, above all, to be able to say clearly, authoritatively and persuasively what we have explored and described, and what is clinically usable knowledge. If we are mislabeled as journalists, so be it. High profile positive health legislative changes, for example, have been fostered, not only by statistical evidence, but by the persuasive power and pathos of patients' stories. They are gripping, undeniably significant, moving and pointed. Qualitative research is the most powerful scholarly means by which to carry these stories into the social and political arena.

I have spoken here from the perspective of the research I have done, and growing awareness I have had about the importance of qualitative research to nursing. I have taken a pluralistic standpoint in order to span the breadth of qualitative inquiry and advocate for the significance of qualitative methods. I did not define the specific boundaries of given approaches, but rather worked to expand the boundaries of the whole enterprise of qualitative research. Nursing is at the forefront in using qualitative methods and is the discipline most aware of the need for them in understanding persons, environments, health and transitions. Qualitative nurse researchers should move on to the next steps in creative and critical knowledge development, confident in the power of qualitative inquiry to describe, interpret, and change inequitable health situations and diminish suffering in the US as well as globally.

References

Anderson, E., & McCormack, M. (2010). Intersectionality, critical race theory, and American sporting oppression: Examining black and gay male athletes. *Journal of Homosexuality*, *57*(8), 949–967.

Banyard, V. L., Williams, L. M., & Siegel, J. A. (2001). Understanding links among childhood trauma, dissociation and women's mental health. *American Journal of Orthopsychiatry*, *71*(3), 311–321.

Bergin, M., Wells, J. S. G., & Owen, S. (2008). Critical realism: A philosophical framework for the study of gender and mental health. *Nursing Philosophy*, *9*(3), 169–179.

Bhaskar, R. (1989). *Reclaiming reality: A critical introduction to contemporary philosophy*. London: Verso.

Borreani, C., Miccinesi, G., Brunelli, C., & Lina, M. (2004). An increasing number of qualitative research papers in oncology and palliative care: Does it mean a thorough development of the methodology of research? *Health and Quality of Life Outcomes*, *2*, 7.

Bourdieu, P., & Thompson, J. B. (1991). *Language and symbolic power*. Cambridge: Polity/Basil Blackwell.

Bremner, J. D., Shobe, K. K., & Kihlstrom, J. F. (2000). False memories in women with self-reported childhood sexual abuse: An empirical study. *Psychological Science*, *11*(4), 333–337.

Brenner, L. A., Homaifar, B. Y., Adler, L. E., Wolfman, J. H., & Kemp, J. (2009). Suicidality and veterans with a history of traumatic brain injury: Precipitant events, protective factors, and prevention strategies. *Rehabilitation Psychology*, *54*(4), 390–397.

Briere, J. (1992). *Child abuse trauma: Theory and treatment of the lasting effects*. Newbury Park, CA: Sage.

Browne, A., & Finkelor, D. (1986). The impact of childhood sexual abuse: A review of the research. *Psychological Bulletin*, *99*, 66–77.

Campesino, M., Ruiz, E., Glover, J. U., & Koithan, M. (2009). Counternarratives of Mexican-origin women with breast cancer [Research Support, NIH, Extramural]. *Advances in Nursing Science*, *32*(2), E57–67.

Carver, C. S. (1998). Resilience and thriving: Issues, models and linkages. *Journal of Social Issues*, *54*(2), 245–266.

Casaccio, E. M. (1999). From surviving to thriving: A mind, body, spirit perspective in treating adults who have experienced childhood sexual abuse. Unpublished PsyD dissertation, Institute for Graduate Clinical Psychology, Philadelphia, PA.

Chinn, P. L., & Kramer, M. K. (2008). *Integrated theory and knowledge development in nursing* (7th ed.). St. Louis, MO: Mosby/Elsevier.

Cicchetti, D., & Toth, S. L. (1997). Transactional ecological systems in developmental psychopathology. In S. S. Luthar, J. A. Burack, D. Cicchetti, & J. R. Weisz (Eds.), *Developmental psychopathology: Perspectives on adjustment, risk and disorder* (pp. 317–349). New York: Cambridge University Press.

Classen, C., Field, N. P., Koopman, C., Nevill-Manning, K., & Spiegel, D. (2001). Interpersonal problems and their relationship to sexual revictimization among women sexually abused in childhood. *Journal of Interpersonal Violence*, *16*(6), 495–509.

Collingridge, D. S., & Gantt, E. E. (2008). The quality of qualitative research. *American Journal of Medical Quality: The Official Journal of the American College of Medical Quality*, *23*(5), 389–395.

Cooper, G. D., Clements, P. T., & Holt, K. E. (2012). Examining childhood bullying and adolescent suicide: Implications for school nurses. *Journal of School Nursing: The Official Publication of the National Association of School Nurses*, *28*(4), 275–283.

Cruikshank, J. (2012). Positioning positivism, critical realism, and social constructivism in the health sciences: A philosophical orientation. *Nursing Inquiry*, *19*, 71–82.

De Witt, L., & Ploeg, J. (2006). Critical appraisal of rigor in interpretive phenomenological nursing research. *Journal of Advanced Nursing*, *55*(2), 215–229.

Delgado, R., & Stephancic, J. (2001). *Critical race theory: An introduction*. Albany, NY: New York University Press.

Duncan, R. D., Saunders, B. E., Kilpatrick, D. G., Hanson, R. F., & Resnick, H. S. (1996). Childhood physical assault as a risk factor for PTSD, depression and substances abuse: Findings from a survey. *American Journal of Orthopsychiatry, 66*(3), 437–448.

Finfgeld, D. L. (1999). Courage as a process of pushing beyond the struggle. *Qualitative Health Research, 9*(6), 803–814.

Gioia, D. (2009). Understanding the ecological validity of neuropsychological testing using an ethnographic approach [Research Support, N.I.H., Extramural]. *Qualitative Health Research, 19*(10), 1495–1503.

Grant, J. M., Mottet, J. D., Tanis, J., Harrison, J., Herman, J. L., & Keisling, M. (2011). *Injustice at every turn: A report of the National Transgender Discrimination Survey*. Washington, DC: National Center for Transgender Equality.

Groleau, D., Zelkowitz, P., & Cabral, I. E. (2009). Enhancing generalizability: Moving from an intimate to a political voice. *Qualitative Health Research, 19*(3), 416–426.

Hall, J. M. (1990). Alcoholism recovery in lesbian women: A theory in development. [Case Reports]. *Scholarly Inquiry for Nursing Practice, 4*(2), 109–122; discussion 123–105.

Hall, J. M. (1992). An exploration of lesbians' images of recovery from alcohol problems. *Health Care for Women International, 13*(2), 181–198.

Hall, J. M. (1993a). Lesbians and alcohol: Patterns and paradoxes in medical notions and lesbians' beliefs [Research Support, Non-US Government Review]. *Journal of Psychoactive Drugs, 25*(2), 109–119.

Hall, J. M. (1993b). What really worked? A case analysis and discussion of confrontational intervention for substance abuse in marginalized women [Case Reports Research Support, Non-US Government Research Support, US Government, PHS]. *Archives of Psychiatric Nursing, 7*(6), 322–327.

Hall, J. M. (1994a). The experiences of lesbians in Alcoholics Anonymous. *Western Journal of Nursing Research, 16*(5), 556–576.

Hall, J. M. (1994b). How lesbians recognize and respond to alcohol problems: A theoretical model of problematization. *Advances in Nursing Science, 16*(3), 46–63.

Hall, J. M. (1994c). Lesbians recovering from alcohol problems: An ethnographic study of health care experiences. *Nursing Research, 43*(4), 238–244.

Hall, J. M. (1996a). Delayed recall of childhood abuse: Psychiatric nursing's responsibilities to clients. *Archives of Psychiatric Nursing, 10*(6), 342–346.

Hall, J. M. (1996b). Geography of childhood sexual abuse: Women's narratives of their childhood environments. [Research Support, U.S. Gov't, P.H.S.]. *Advances in Nursing Science, 18*(4), 29–47.

Hall, J. M. (1996c). Pervasive effects of childhood sexual abuse in lesbians' recovery from alcohol problems [Research Support, Non-US Government Research Support, US Government, PHS]. *Substance Use & Misuse, 31*(2), 225–239.

Hall, J. M. (1998). Lesbians surviving childhood sexual abuse: Pivotal experiences related to sexual orientation, gender, and race. *Journal of Lesbian Studies, 2*(1), 7–28.

Hall, J. M. (1999a). Lesbians in alcohol recovery surviving childhood sexual abuse and parental substance misuse [Research Support, US Government, PHS]. *International Journal of Psychiatric Nursing Research, 5*(1), 507–515.

Hall, J. M. (1999b). Marginalization revisited: Critical, postmodern and liberation perspectives. *Advances in Nursing Science, 22*(2), 88–102.

Hall, J. M. (2000a). Core issues for women child abuse survivors in recovery from substance misuse. *Qualitative Health Research, 10*(5), 612–631.

Hall, J. M. (2000b). Women survivors of childhood abuse: The impact of traumatic stress on education and work [Research Support, Non-US Government]. *Issues in Mental Health Nursing, 21*(5), 443–471.

Hall, J. M. (2003a). Dissociative experiences of women child abuse survivors: A selective constructivist review. *Trauma, Violence & Abuse, 4*(4), 283–308.

Hall, J. M. (2003b). Positive self-transitions in women child abuse survivors [Research Support, Non-US Government]. *Issues in Mental Health Nursing, 24*(6–7), 647–666.

Hall, J. M. (2011). Narrative methods in a study of trauma recovery. *Qualitative Health Research, 21*(1), 3–13.

Hall, J. M., & Fields, B. (2012). Race and microaggression in nursing knowledge development. *Advances in Nursing Science, 35*(1), 25–38.

Hall, J. M., & Kondora, L. L. (1997). Beyond "true" and "false" memories: Remembering and recovery in the survival of childhood sexual abuse [Historical Article Research Support, US Government, PHS Review]. *Advances in Nursing Science, 19*(4), 37–54.

Hall, J. M., & Powell, J. (2000). Dissociative experiences as described by women survivors of childhood abuse. *Journal of Interpersonal Violence, 15*(4), 184–203.

Hall, J. M., Roman, M. W., Thomas, S. P., Travis, C. B., Powell, J., Tennison, C. R., et al. (2009). Thriving as becoming resolute in narratives of women surviving childhood maltreatment. [Research Support, NIH, Extramural]. *American Journal of Orthopsychiatry, 79*(3), 375–386.

Hall, J. M., & Stevens, P. E. (1991). Rigor in feminist research. *Advances in Nursing Science, 13*(3), 16–29.

Hall, J. M., & Stevens, P. E. (1992). A nursing view of the US-Iraq war: Psychosocial health consequences. *Nursing Outlook, 40*(3), 113–120.

Hall, J. M., Stevens, P. E., & Meleis, A. I. (1992). Experiences of women clerical workers in patient care areas. *Journal of Nursing Administration, 22*(5), 11–17.

Hall, J. M., Stevens, P. E., & Meleis, A. I. (1994). Marginalization: A guiding concept for valuing diversity in nursing knowledge development. *Advances in Nursing Science, 16*(4), 23–41.

Holmes, C. A., & Warelow, P. J. (1997). Culture, needs and nursing: A critical theory approach. *Journal of Advanced Nursing, 25*(3), 463–470.

Horton, R. (2000). Common sense and figures: The rhetoric of validity in medicine (Bradford Hill Memorial Lecture 1999). *Statistics in Medicine, 19*(23), 3149–3164.

Ickovics, J. R., & Clark, C. L. (1998). Paradigm shift: Why a focus on health is important. *Journal of Social Issues, 54*(2), 237–244.

Idsoe, T., Dyregrov, A., & Idsoe, E. C. (2012). Bullying and PTSD symptoms. *Journal of Abnormal Child Psychology, 40*(6), 901–911.

Jones, S. N., Waite, R., & Thomas Clements, P. (2012). An evolutionary concept analysis of school violence: From bullying to death. *Journal of Forensic Nursing, 8*(1), 4–12.

Kinzl, J., & Biebl, W. (1992). Long-term effects of incest: Life events triggering mental disorders in female patients with sexual abuse in childhood. *Child Abuse & Neglect, 16*(4), 567–573.

Kuhn, T. S. (1970). *The structure of scientific revolutions* (2nd ed.). Chicago: University of Chicago Press.

Kuhn, T. S., & Hacking, I. (2012). *The structure of scientific revolutions* (4th ed.). Chicago: University of Chicago Press.

Kvale, S. (1996). *InterViews: An introduction to qualitative research interviewing*. Thousand Oaks, CA: Sage.

Lemstra, M. E., Nielsen, G., Rogers, M. R., Thompson, A. T., & Moraros, J. S. (2012). Risk indicators and outcomes associated with bullying in youth aged 9–15 years [Research Support, Non-US Government]. *Canadian Journal of Public Health/Revue Canadienne de Santé Publique, 103*(1), 9–13.

Levinas, E. (1947/1978). *Existence and its existents*. The Hague: Nijhoff.

Loftus, E. F. (1996). Memory distortion and false memory creation. *Bulletin of American Academy of Psychiatry Law, 24*(3), 281–295.

Lovato, L. C., Hill, K., Hertert, S., Hunninghake, D. B., & Probstfield, J. L. (1997). Recruitment for controlled clinical trials: Literature summary and annotated bibliography. *Controlled Clinical Trials, 18*(4), 328–352.

Maggs-Rapport, F. (2001). "Best research practice": In pursuit of methodological rigour. *Journal of Advanced Nursing, 35*(3), 373–383.

McGloin, J. M., & Widom, C. S. (2001). Resilience among abused and neglected children grown up. *Developmental Psychopathology, 13*(4), 1021–1038.

Meleis, A. I. (2012). *Theoretical nursing: Development and progress*. New York: Lippincott, Williams and Wilkins.

Mintz, L. M., California State University San Marcos College of Education, & Services (2011). *Gender variance on campus: A critical analysis of transgender voices*. San Diego, CA: California State University San Marcos and University of California, San Diego.

Morgan, S. W., & Stevens, P. E. (2008). Transgender identity development as represented by a group of female-to-male transgendered adults. *Issues in Mental Health Nursing, 29*(6), 585–599.

Morse, J. M., & Neihaus, L. (2009). *Mixed method design: Principles and procedures* (Vol. 4). Walnut Creek, CA: Left Coast Press.

Myers, M. (2000). Qualitative research and the generalizability question: Standing firm with Proteus. *Qualitative Report, 4*(3/4).

NIH. (2011) *The health of lesbian, gay, bisexual, and transgender people: Building a foundation for better understanding*. Washington, DC: NIH.

O'Leary, V. E. (1998). Strength in the face of adversity: Individual and social thriving. *Journal of Social Issues, 54*(2), 425–446.

Perlman, S. D. (1996). "Reality" and countertransference in the treatment of sexual abuse patients: The false memory controversy. *Journal of American Academy of Psychoanalysis, 24*(1), 115–135.

Plunkett, R., Leipert, B. D., & Ray, S. L. (2012). Unspoken phenomena: Using the photovoice method to enrich phenomenological inquiry. *Nursing Inquiry.* doi: 10.1111/j.1440-1800.2012.00594.x.

Poorman, P. B. (2002). Perceptions of thriving by women who have experienced abuse or status-related oppression. *Psychology of Women Quarterly, 26*, 51–62.

Porter, S., & Ryan, S. (1996). Breaking the boundaries between nursing and sociology: A critical realist ethnography of the theory–practice gap. *Journal of Advanced Nursing, 24*(2), 413–420.

Radliff, K. M., Wheaton, J. E., Robinson, K., & Morris, J. (2012). Illuminating the relationship between bullying and substance use among middle and high school youth. *Addictive Behaviors, 37*(4), 569–572.

Reissman, C. K. (2008). *Narrative methods for the human sciences.* Thousand Oaks, CA: Sage.

Rich, M., Lamola, S., & Woods, E. R. (2006). Effects of creating visual illness narratives on quality of life with asthma: A pilot intervention study [Clinical Trial Research Support, NIH, Extramural Research Support, Non-US Government]. *Journal of Adolescent Health: Official Publication of the Society for Adolescent Medicine, 38*(6), 748–752.

Ricoeur, P. (1984). *Time and narrative* (Vol. 1). Chicago: University of Chicago Press.

Rodgers, W. L., & Herzog, A. R. (1987). Interviewing older adults: The accuracy of factual information [Research Support, US Government, PHS]. *Journal of Gerontology, 42*(4), 387–394.

Rorty, M., Yager, J., & Rossotto, M. A. (1994). Child sexual, physical, and psychological abuse in bulimia nervosa. *American Journal of Psychiatry, 151*, 1122–1126.

Rothblum, E. D. (1994). "I only read about myself on bathroom walls": The need for research on the mental health of lesbians and gay men. *Journal of Consulting and Clinical Psychology, 62*(2), 213–220.

Roy, J. (2012). Randomized treatment-belief trials. *Contemporary Clinical Trials, 33*(1), 172–177.

Saakvitne, K. W., Tennen, H., & Affleck, G. (1998). Exploring thriving in the context of clinical trauma theory: Constructivist self-developmental theory. *Journal of Social Issues, 54*(2), 279–299.

Sandelowski, M., Trimble, F., Woodard, E. K., & Barroso, J. (2006). From synthesis to script: Transforming qualitative research findings for use in practice [Research Support, NIH, Extramural Research Support, Non-US Government]. *Qualitative Health Research, 16*(10), 1350–1370.

Schetky, D. H. (1990). A review of the literature on the long-term effects of childhood sexual abuse. In R. P. Kluft (Ed.), *Incest-related syndromes of adult psychopathology* (pp. 35–44). Washington, DC: American Psychiatric Press.

Shapiro, J. (2011). Illness narratives: Reliability, authenticity and the empathic witness. *Medical Humanities, 37*(2), 68–72.

Stevens, P. E., & Hall, J. M. (1991). A critical historical analysis of the medical construction of lesbianism. *International Journal of Health Services: Planning, Administration, Evaluation, 21*(2), 291–307.

Stevens, P. E., & Hall, J. M. (2001). Sexuality and safer sex: The issues for lesbians and bisexual women [Research Support, Non-US Government Research Support, US Government, PHS Review]. *Journal of Obstetric, Gynecologic, and Neonatal Nursing: JOGNN / NAACOG, 30*(4), 439–447.

Stevens, P. E., & Morgan, S. (2001). Health of lesbian, gay, bisexual, and transgender youth. *Journal of Pediatric Health Care 15*(1), 24–34.

Sue, D. W., Bucceri, J., Lin, A. I., Nadal, K. L., & Torino, G. C. (2007). Racial microaggressions and the Asian American experience. *Cultural Diversity & Ethnic Minority Psychology, 13*(1), 72–81.

Sue, D. W., Capodilupo, C. M., Torino, G. C., Bucceri, J. M., Holder, A. M., Nadal, K. L., et al. (2007). Racial microaggressions in everyday life: Implications for clinical practice. *American Psychologist, 62*(4), 271–286.

Sue, D. W., Lin, A. I., Torino, G. C., Capodilupo, C. M., & Rivera, D. P. (2009). Racial microaggressions and difficult dialogues on race in the classroom. *Cultural Diversity & Ethnic Minority Psychology, 15*(2), 183–190.

Sue, D. W., Rivera, D. P., Watkins, N. L., Kim, R. H., Kim, S., & Williams, C. D. (2011). Racial dialogues: challenges faculty of color face in the classroom. *Cultural Diversity & Ethnic Minority Psychology, 17*(3), 331–340.

Tedeschi, R. G., Park, C. L., & Calhoun, L. G. (Eds.). (1998). *Posttraumatic growth: Positive changes in the aftermath of crisis.* Mahwah, NJ: Lawrence Erlbaum Associates.

Thomas, S. P., & Hall, J. M. (2008). Life trajectories of female child abuse survivors thriving in adulthood. [Research Support, NIH, Extramural]. *Qualitative Health Research, 18*(2), 149–166.

Tobin, G. A., & Begley, C. M. (2004). Methodological rigour within a qualitative framework [Research Support, Non-US Government Review]. *Journal of Advanced Nursing, 48*(4), 388–396.

Todd, A. M., Laird, B. J., Boyle, D., Boyd, A. C., Colvin, L. A., & Fallon, M. T. (2009). A systematic review examining the literature on attitudes of patients with advanced cancer toward research. *Journal of Pain and Symptom Management, 37*(6), 1078–1085.

Van Herk, K. A., Smith, D., & Andrew, C. (2011). Examining our privileges and oppressions: Incorporating an intersectionality paradigm into nursing. *Nursing Inquiry, 18*(1), 29–39.

Vaskinn, A., Sergi, M. J., & Green, M. F. (2009). The challenges of ecological validity in the measurement of social perception in schizophrenia [Comparative Study Research Support, NIH, Extramural Research Support, Non-US Government]. *Journal of Nervous and Mental Disease, 197*(9), 700–702.

Walia, S., & Leipert, B. (2012). Perceived facilitators and barriers to physical activity for rural youth: An exploratory study using photovoice. *Rural and Remote Health, 12*, 1842.

Warson, E. (2012). Healing pathways: Art therapy for American Indian cancer survivors. *Journal of Cancer Education: The Official Journal of the American Association for Cancer Education, 27*(Suppl. 1), 47–56.

Weiss, E. L., Longhurst, J. G., & Mazure, C. M. (1999). Childhood sexual abuse as a risk factor for depression in women: Psychosocial and neurobiological correlates. *American Journal of Psychiatry, 156*(6), 816–828.

Wuest, J., & Merritt-Gray, M. (2001). Beyond survival: Reclaiming self after leaving an abusive male partner. *Canadian Journal of Nursing Research, 32*(4), 79–94.

Yantz, C. L., Johnson-Greene, D., Higginson, C., & Emmerson, L. (2010). Functional cooking skills and neuropsychological functioning in patients with stroke: An ecological validity study. [Research Support, NIH, Extramural]. *Neuropsychological Rehabilitation, 20*(5), 725–738.

Yin, R. K. (2012). *Applications of case study research* (3rd ed.). Thousand Oaks, CA: Sage.

Yorkston, E., Turner, C., Schluter, P., & McClure, R. (2005). Validity and reliability of responses to a self-report home safety survey designed for use in a community-based child injury prevention programme [Research Support, Non-US Government Validation Studies]. *International Journal of Injury Control and Safety Promotion, 12*(3), 193–196.

5

Learning about the nature of fatigue

Karin Olson

Introduction

My interest in fatigue grew out of discussions with the oncology nurses with whom I worked in the early 1990s. The nurses had become increasingly concerned about the frequency and severity of fatigue in their patients, and had questions about what nurses could do to support these individuals and their families. In this chapter I will trace our journey from their clinical observations to where we are today and show how we used qualitative research to learn about the nature of fatigue. I will begin with a description of the clinical observations that caught our interest and our identification of behavioral patterns that distinguished those with fatigue from those without fatigue. I will then provide a brief review of the literature as it was at the time I began studying fatigue and describe how we used this work to reconceptualize fatigue. In the third section I present the conceptual framework for the prevention and management of fatigue that we developed based on our qualitative studies. I also describe several new areas of inquiry that grew out of our conceptual work, including our work related to symptom clusters and the social construction of fatigue. Finally, I discuss some of the implications of our work for clinical practice, education and research.

Clinical observations

My interest in fatigue began when I was the coordinator of nursing research at a large cancer center in western Canada. One of the nurses in our outpatient department told me about an individual in her clinic who had colorectal cancer and who had withdrawn from a potentially curative protocol because he was "too tired." He attributed his lack of energy to his treatment, and although he understood that his disease was potentially curable, he decided to withdraw from treatment because he found the lack of energy unbearable.

My colleagues and I decided that a good next step was for me to spend some time observing in the outpatient clinics so that I could meet other patients with fatigue. I was surprised to find that while many patients had varying degrees of fatigue, there were also some individuals with advanced disease who were receiving aggressive treatment but who did not report fatigue. We were surprised. Were they just ignoring their fatigue? Did they feel reluctant to report their fatigue for some reason? Did they really not have fatigue? If not, why not?

Individuals with and without fatigue

We decided to explore the experience of fatigue further. We were interested in learning more about why some individuals reported fatigue while others with the same treatment and disease profile did not report fatigue. Although there were many descriptive studies of fatigue in the literature, we could not find any studies describing the absence of fatigue in individuals who would be expected to have significant fatigue. Given the lack of research in this area, we began with a qualitative study. We chose to design our study using grounded theory because our clinical observations suggested that social interactions heavily influenced the ways individuals approached the management of their cancer experience. Grounded theory was the most appropriate design choice, given this observation, because its assumptions are rooted in symbolic interactions, and thus its analytic structures help the researcher closely examine social processes.

Our starting point was a question about whether social interaction could explain why some people with advanced cancer experienced fatigue while others did not experience fatigue. In an early grant, I restated this question as a statement and called it my central thesis. Some readers may disagree with this approach, but in my view it is important for qualitative researchers to be explicit about their starting points for two reasons. First, the starting point, often framed as a research question, helps the researcher decide which design should be used. The choice of a research design that is not well suited to the starting point of the study will seriously limit the ability of the researcher to answer the research question. The starting point also needs to be stated so that the researcher can show that it has been included in but has not constrained the data collection process. To limit the data collection to the ideas posed in the starting point implies that the key concepts related to the study are already known and prevents the researcher from discovering potentially important information related to the overall topic of the study that may lie beyond the ideas that framed the starting point. For these reasons, the failure to locate one's starting point may threaten the validity of a qualitative study.

The first step in our study was a focus group with individuals who had already completed treatment for lung or colorectal cancer. The aim of the focus group discussion was to learn more about the best way to describe our study to participants so that they would understand its focus. One of the problems we anticipated was that because the word "fatigue" is not part of everyday vocabulary in English, interview participants would not understand the purpose of the study. Participants in the focus group said that we should use the word "tiredness" rather than "fatigue" in our study, but should tell participants that we wanted them to focus on the kind of tiredness, if any, that was different from the tiredness that came at the end of a busy week. We used these descriptions about the focus of our study with participants. In our research group meetings and our analysis, we labeled the tiredness that came at the end of a busy week *ordinary tiredness* and labeled the tiredness that was different from ordinary tiredness *fatigue*.

The general interest in our study began to grow at our cancer center. The members of the ethics committee thought the study was very interesting and gave approval but suggested that we also collect information about hemoglobin level, transfusion history, and weight to describe our sample. They also noted that some authors (Oliff et al., 1987) had proposed relationships between fatigue and cytokines, such as TNF alpha, IL-2, and IL-6 based on animal studies, and so suggested that we also analyze blood samples for these markers as well. Our colleagues understood that our sample would be small, but thought we would have enough cases to analyze the biomarker data using non-parametric approaches. In retrospect we now know that these biological data were very important because they helped us interpret our qualitative findings. In the paper reporting the result of this study (Olson et al., 2002) we said we used a grounded theory design, but given the methodological work on mixed methods approaches since this study was

65

conducted, it would have been more appropriate to say that we used a mixed methods design with a qualitative drive (Morse, 2003).

Participants were interviewed pre-treatment, mid-treatment, and post-treatment and evaluable data were obtained for 18 individuals (n = 10 gastrointestinal cancer patients; n = 8 lung cancer patients). Participants did not complete a fatigue instrument but were simply asked to compare their tiredness, if any, to the tiredness one might experience at the end of a busy week. We considered individuals fatigued if they said their tiredness was different from the tiredness they had at the end of a busy week. Participants were asked to describe experiences that would help our team understand what their tiredness was like. Data were analyzed using a standard constant comparative approach. Four participants reported only the type of tiredness that comes at the end of a busy week at all three data collection points while five participants reported fatigue at all three time points. The remaining participants reported no fatigue at time 1, but did report fatigue at time 2 and/or time 3.

We identified a distinct behavioral pattern that distinguished individuals with fatigue from those without fatigue, and labeled this pattern *gliding*. Gliders were able to do three things:

*   find order in the midst of the chaos of a cancer diagnosis;
*   restructure their daily routine so that it included only those activities that were either personally meaningful or were required in order to manage their disease and treatment;
*   monitor their energy level, making adjustments to their activities as needed so that they always had some energy in reserve in case it was needed.

Gliders noted that their abilities to undertake these tasks were partly rooted in the strong supportive networks within which they lived, but were also related to skills learned previous to their cancer experience. The individuals who reported fatigue, on the other hand, reported difficulty finding order in chaos, were unsure about how to restructure their daily routines, and described a limited ability to accurately ascertain energy level.

There was no relationship between fatigue and any of the cytokines or weight loss, but low hemoglobin was associated with fatigue during and after treatment in the lung cancer group only. Low hemoglobin was not associated with fatigue in the gastrointestinal cancer group, despite the fact that the majority of participants were slightly anemic by conventional standards, but we did find an association between increased absolute neutrophil count and fatigue pre-treatment in this group, probably due to recent surgery. Although the relationship between hemoglobin and fatigue was different for the two tumor groups in this study, the behavioral patterns were the same across both tumor groups.

Revisiting the conceptual definition of fatigue

The results of the above study increased our curiosity about the nature of fatigue. In a broad search of the literature, we found that people had been writing about fatigue for many years. The earliest reference we could find was to work completed by Galvani in 1786 (as cited in Rasch & Burke, 1967), in which he discussed fatigue in relation to electrical potentials in the muscles of the legs of frogs. One hundred years later, Beard (1869) described fatigue as a psychological response to the demands of daily life associated with urbanization and increasing competitiveness in the business world, which he said led to chemical changes in the central nervous system and a buildup of related byproducts in peripheral muscles. Cowles (1893) distinguished two types of fatigue—one that could be considered a normal part of daily life, and one that was pathological; he advocated treating pathological fatigue with rest followed by mild exercise, arguing that exercise would increase appetite and promote the excretion of the waste products that had accumulated in the muscles.

Writers in the first half of the twentieth century continued to view fatigue in relation to energy expenditure. Bartley and Chute (1947) published the first analysis of fatigue as a concept and portrayed it as an early warning system that indicated an impending shortage of physiological resources for ongoing function, given current demands. This work was used as the foundation for definitions of fatigue developed by others such as Grandjean (1968), who focused on functional status and alertness.

At the time that I started working on fatigue, the definition of fatigue proposed by Grandjean (1968) was used as the foundation for most nursing research in this field. From my observations of patients and my discussions with them, this definition seemed incomplete. In addition to changes in functional status and alertness, our patients' descriptions of fatigue included difficulties with thinking clearly, marked changes in memory, and increases in anxiety. In addition, the definition proposed by Grandjean could not help us explain why some patients with advanced disease who were receiving aggressive treatment did not report fatigue. As a result, I began to think about ways to expand the conceptual definition of fatigue.

One day I came across a paper published by Bartlett (1953). This paper was interesting for two reasons. First, Bartlett said that fatigue could develop quickly if the energy demand was much greater than the energy available, and second, he pointing out that because the sensations associated with fatigue arose in response to excessive energy expenditure, they arrived too late to be useful as an "early warning system." It seemed to me that the work of Bartlett was consistent with the ideas about the stress response developed by Selye (1952, 1956, 1971). Selye (1952) said that stressors, whether good or bad, could give rise to the general adaptation syndrome (GAS), which he described as a physiologic response comprised of an alarm reaction, resistance, and exhaustion. He noted that during the resistance phase, the energy required for adaptation was high, and that once this energy was depleted, exhaustion followed; if unchecked, exhaustion would result in death.

At this time (the late 1990s), I was able to find four authors who had explored fatigue in the context of stress theory. Cameron (1973) labeled the factors that lead to fatigue as stressors and proposed that exposure to these stressors over time would lead to fatigue. Rhoten (1982) studied fatigue in the context of surgery and described the preoperative state, the surgical intervention, anesthesia, pain, and pain medication as stressors. Aistars (1987) was the first author to explore links between stress and fatigue in individuals with cancer. She said that fatigue was a function of the sources of the stress, perceptions of stress, coping mechanisms, and the duration of the stress. Unfortunately, her model has not been formally tested. Glaus (1993, 1998) later proposed that the stressors associated with fatigue in individuals with cancer could be modified by factors rooted in culture and reflected in language, but did not test these ideas.

Reconceptualizing fatigue using a pragmatic utility approach

Based on this review, I decided to see if I could find a core set of characteristics of fatigue that were common across populations who experienced it for different reasons such as illness, work, and recreation. The ill populations I selected included individuals with a diagnosis of chronic fatigue syndrome, a major depressive disorder, and cancer. The work population I selected was shift workers, and the recreational population I selected was recreational athletes. These five populations were selected because fatigue was commonly reported in the literature about these groups.

There are many approaches to concept development, but I chose to use the pragmatic utility approach developed by Morse (2000) because I wanted to build my conceptualization based on published data. I developed a set of search terms used to describe fatigue in our previous study (Olson et al., 2002) and then used these terms to conduct a search of CINAHL, Medline, PubMed, Psych INFO, SPORTDiscus, and CancerLit for the years from 1995 to 2001. Studies were selected for inclusion if the authors discussed the conceptual nature of fatigue in shift workers, athletes, or individuals with CFS, depression, or cancer, based on qualitative data. Our team identified six characteristics of fatigue were common across all five study populations. These characteristics included muscular changes, cognitive changes, sleep disruption, emotional changes, changes in body sensation, and social disruption (Olson & Morse, 2005).

We learned four important things from our examination of the fatigue literature. First, we learned that contrary to current thinking, tiredness, fatigue, and exhaustion seemed to be distinguishable from each other by rate of onset, recovery, and energy expenditure. Tiredness and fatigue generally developed over time. Tiredness was generally proportional to energy expended, but fatigue seemed out of proportion to the energy expended. Individuals with fatigue generally were surprised that they were "so tired" given their level of activity. Exhaustion occurred suddenly, sometimes without any obvious energy expenditure, and was unexpected. Second, we learned that tiredness seemed to be a precondition for fatigue. If individuals adapted to/recovered from tiredness, they did not develop fatigue. If they were unable to adapt to tiredness for some reason, however, they eventually developed fatigue. Adaptation to/recovery from fatigue was possible but took longer than adaptation to/recovery from tiredness. Individuals who did not adapt to/recover from fatigue progressed to exhaustion. Third, we learned that the onset of fatigue could be prevented or at least delayed if individuals acknowledged tiredness and attended to its underlying causes. The final and most important point stemming from the concept analysis project was the realization that the manifestations of tiredness, fatigue, and exhaustion were the same in all five study populations.

In order to further validate the findings of the concept analysis, we undertook a series of five studies, one in each of the study populations described above (Olson, 2007; Olson, Krawchuk, & Quddusi, 2007; Porr, Olson, & Hegadoren, 2010). In these studies we used both ethnoscience and grounded theory, alone or in combination, to learn more about the manifestations of tiredness, fatigue, and exhaustion. In each case we began by using ethnoscience and recruited between 15 and 30 individuals from each population. We chose to use ethnoscience because it provides a systematic analytic strategy for studying the language people use to describe experience (Leininger, 1985). Although the use of ethnoscience is relatively new in nursing, it has been used by ethnographers for many years to build classification systems based on language. The goal in ethnoscience is to locate underlying beliefs and values that shape behavior. The primary analytic strategy here is to identify the main words used to describe some experience, and then construct a set of taxonomies that show how these words are related to each other. We used this approach to look for patterns in the language individuals used to describe fatigue, and then compared our findings across our five study populations. The results of these studies were consistent with the findings of our concept analysis, and helped us construct the following definitions for tiredness, fatigue, and exhaustion:

- tiredness: forgetfulness and impatience but no changes in muscle function, sleep, or social interactions,
- fatigue: difficulty concentrating, worry, loss of stamina greater than expected given energy expenditure, decreased sleep quality, heightened sensitivity to stimuli, and decreased social interaction,

• exhaustion: confusion, no expressed emotion, unexpected and sudden loss of energy, difficulty with both staying awake and sleeping, unable to control body process such as temperature, no social interaction (Olson, 2007).

In the study of fatigue in depression we used grounded theory in addition to ethnoscience, because we also wanted to learn more about the social interactions that shaped the ways study participants managed fatigue. Morse (2003) describes this type of design as a multi-method design. The results from both the ethnoscience and the grounded theory portions were complete and could have been published separately. We chose to publish them in one paper because they used the same dataset and we thought it would be easier to integrate the results from the two studies.

An interesting part of this study was our finding regarding the wearing of masks (Porr et al., 2010). Participants reported that they wore masks when out in public to help them "fit in" with society's expectations. On occasion, but only when absolutely necessary, they went out without their masks. These occasions were often unexpected and were usually related to care for one's children or family members. At home, the participants were able to remove their masks, but they restricted those who were allowed to see them at this time. Home was generally a safe place where participants could rebuild the energy needed to put their masks back on and head out into public spaces.

Construction of a conceptual framework

Now that we had solid conceptual definitions of fatigue and related concepts, the next step was to construct a conceptual framework that showed the relationships among these concepts and that could be used to guide the development of interventions. The main strategies here were additional literature review and discussion within our research team. Based on this work we combined bodily sensation and muscular changes into muscle endurance, and added nutrition, other symptoms, and key demographic variables (sex, age, diagnostic stage) as stressors contributing to adaptive capacity. We also proposed that adaptive capacity and allostatic overload (McEwen, 1998, 2007) were positively correlated, and added explicit recognition of the contribution of the social context. The current configuration of our conceptual framework, the Revised Edmonton Fatigue Framework, is shown in Figure 5.1.

Our research team considers this framework to be an initial etiological model. The main propositions depicted in our framework are:

1 Adaptive capacity is a function of nutrition, cognition, muscle endurance, sleep, social interaction, emotional reactivity, demographic factors (disease stage, age, and gender), other symptoms, and the social contexts within which these elements occur.
2 Adaptive capacity is inversely related to allostatic overload and fatigue.
3 As adaptive capacity increases, allostatic overload and fatigue decline.

The development of the Revised Edmonton Fatigue Framework was a very exciting phase of our work, but was also a little unnerving for a couple of reasons. First, since adaptive capacity was a relatively new concept, we needed to operationalize it, which we eventually did by constructing an instrument called the Adaptive Capacity Index (Olson et al., 2011). The construction of this instrument was necessary so that we could test hypotheses related to adaptive capacity and allostatic overload. Second, I realized that I was opening up whole areas of research based in the biological sciences for which I had absolutely no background. In order to proceed I needed to find colleagues in these areas who could help me find ways to link the biological

Karin Olson

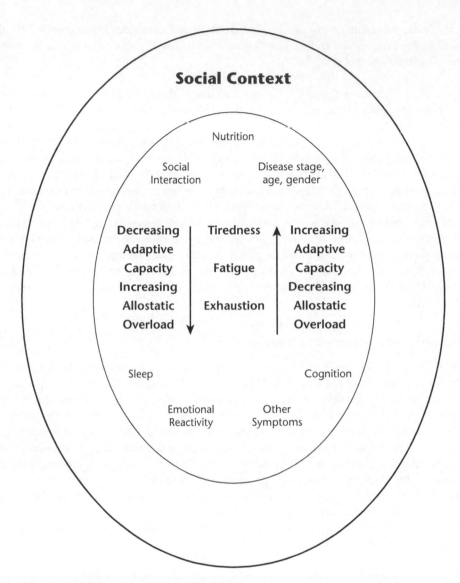

Figure 5.1 Revised Edmonton Fatigue Framework

and psychosocial components of the framework. My research team has grown to include physicians and individuals with PhDs in immunology, psychology, physiology, and biochemistry. We are currently planning a large study using a mixed methods design to test the Revised Edmonton Fatigue Framework shown in Figure 5.1.

Fatigue in the context of symptom clusters

Our concept analysis work required our research group to think more about symptom clusters. This point is now represented in our model as *Other Symptoms*. Fatigue is usually experienced along with other symptoms, and we became increasingly interested in the idea that the collective impact of symptoms could be viewed as one of the stressors contributing to a reduction in adaptive

70

capacity. All of the studies I could find about symptom clusters used a factor analysis approach. One of the problems with this approach is that a symptom is only allowed to be part of one factor. Our qualitative results suggested that fatigue was related to many other symptoms and that the relationships among the symptoms changed over time. When tested using structural equation modeling, these results of our qualitative studies were supported (Hayduk, Olson, Quan, Cree, & Cui, 2010; Olson et al., 2008). We are currently working on a third paper in which we are comparing the results from factor analysis and from structural equation modeling to see which approach fits our data set better.

The social construction of symptom experience

Another outcome of our conceptual work on fatigue was that we began to think more about the social construction of symptom experience. Beginning from the assumption that language is the primary symbol system through which meaning is conveyed, we were interested in learning more about the relationship between the meaning of experience and the context within which it occurs. For example, from the participants in our study of fatigue among recreational athletes, we learned that fatigue was a normal part of a training protocol and that, once participants demonstrated fatigue, their training protocols required that they switch to less vigorous activities so that their bodies could recover. The failure to incorporate this recovery phase adversely influenced the ability of the athlete to improve his/her level of performance. Thus fatigue was viewed as normal and expected. Among individuals with cancer, however, fatigue was associated with uncertainty and concerns that one's disease had become more advanced.

Based on these findings, we started to think about all the different contexts that could influence the meaning of fatigue. Up to this point we had only studied fatigue among Canadians, and we began to wonder about the influence of beliefs and values related to geography. The outside circle in our model, shown in Figure 5.1, represents this point. Our curiosity about social context led to our current study of cancer-related fatigue in five countries (Canada, Thailand, Italy, England, and Sweden). These countries were explicitly chosen to include one additional English-speaking country, and several other countries where the predominant language was not English but where I could find PhD-prepared researchers with expertise in qualitative research and cancer care. The three papers from this phase of our work have been published or are in press (Olson et al., 2007; Pongthavornkamol et al., 2012; Kirshbaum et al., in press), and one additional article is under review.

We used the ethnoscience study of fatigue in Canada from our earlier concept analysis work as the starting point for this project. Each of the lead researchers in the remaining four countries used our Canadian proposal to write a proposal for her work. Graffigna, the principal investigator of our Italian project, also led the preparation of a paper describing the processes used in ethnoscience and discussed its utility for work of this nature (Graffigna, Vegni, Barelo, Olson, & Bosio, 2011).

This set of studies provided us with an opportunity to think more about the Theory of Technique, a problem we first identified in an unrelated project (Graffigna, Bosio, & Olson, 2009; Graffigna, Olson, & Bosio, 2010). The Theory of Technique highlights ways in which local conventions related to the production of research results, such as ethics and recruitment procedures, may influence the study findings and complicate comparisons across contexts. In our studies of fatigue in individuals in Canada, Thailand, Italy, England, and Sweden, we have carefully tracked local conventions regarding research techniques and in our comparative analysis will be including a discussion of the ways in which we think variations in these research techniques influenced our study findings.

Implications for clinical practice, education, and research

The test of our conceptual framework is not yet completed, but we have proposed some initial implications that are consistent with our findings so far. For individuals experiencing tiredness the primary focus should be on teaching these individuals to acknowledge tiredness and then to implement strategies that address the problems contributing to tiredness. This process may be more difficult than expected because tiredness is a familiar part of everyday life and most adults have years of experience ignoring tiredness in order to meet deadlines and various obligations. In addition, the sensations of tiredness are subtle. As noted above, the primary characteristics of tiredness are increased forgetfulness and impatience, with no change in muscle endurance, sleep, or social interaction (Olson, 2007).

The first step in helping a person acknowledge tiredness and attend to underlying causes is to conduct an assessment of the stressors identified in the Revised Edmonton Fatigue Framework. Cognition, muscle endurance, social interaction, and emotional reactivity are already included in the Adaptive Capacity Index, so the only additional components initially required are a symptom assessment, a nutrition assessment, and a brief interview. The interview should focus on learning more about the individual's social context and the extent to which they are able to explicitly practice the three steps of the gliding process noted above—finding order in chaos, creating a new routine, and monitoring energy level. The intervention would be tailored for each person, based on the results of this assessment. Over the long term, our goal is to develop a bank of evidence-based interventions from which one could draw, depending on assessment results.

The clinical implications for someone who already has fatigue or exhaustion would begin with the same assessments noted above, but a key aspect of the interview would be to learn more about barriers to gliding. The interventions would likely become more complex because the scope of the problem would be larger but the available energy would become increasingly limited.

When considering the care of individuals with any chronic illness, the first assessment should be undertaken prior to treatment, as early intervention would be expected to reduce progression to fatigue and delays/modifications to treatment. The intervention should also be family-based rather than individual in focus. This approach would provide an opportunity to incorporate family members who would like to participate and to support families as they work through issues related to having a family member diagnosed with a serious illness.

Implications for education

The primary implication of our work for the education of nurses at the undergraduate and graduate levels is the importance of including a solid foundation in the biological and psychosocial content that underpins health. Nursing students need to be able to discuss core biological and psychosocial processes and be skilled at finding and building relationships with experts in these fields, particularly if they are planning to do graduate work in nursing. It is also critical that students have a solid grounding in both quantitative and qualitative research designs, understand how to move between designs, and how to incorporate both designs in a single study where necessary.

Implications for research

The development of interventions for fatigue has been limited by the lack of an etiological model. The Revised Edmonton Fatigue Framework was developed to address this gap. The primary implication for research arising from our work is the importance of continuing to refine our framework. Our current work is focused on identifying the best biomarkers for assessing the stressors included in the framework. We are particularly interested in understanding the impact of inflammation on these stressors and on the development of fatigue. As the framework is tested and refined, our ability to develop focused interventions for fatigue will increase.

Conclusion

My goal in this chapter has been to show how we used qualitative research, either by itself or in conjunction with quantitative approaches, to learn more about the nature of fatigue. I have traced the work of our research group from early clinical observations to the development of the Revised Edmonton Fatigue Framework, and an exploration of the social construction of fatigue. The qualitative designs we used allowed us to tap into information that we could not have obtained any other way. I have described some initial ways in which we could use this information to improve clinical practice, expand education, and inform future research. In the long term, my sincere hope is that this work will influence the care provided for individuals with fatigue and will improve their quality of life.

References

Aistars, J. (1987). Fatigue in the cancer patient: A conceptual approach to a clinical problem. *Oncology Nursing Forum, 14*, 25–30.

Bartlett, F. (1953). Psychological criteria of fatigue. In W. Floyd & A. Welford (Eds.), *Symposium on fatigue* (pp. 1–5). London: H. K. Lewis.

Bartley, S., & Chute, E. (1947). *Fatigue and impairment in man*. New York: McGraw-Hill.

Beard, G. (1869). Neurasthenia, or nervous exhaustion. *Boston Medical and Surgical Journal, 3*, 217–221.

Cameron, C. (1973). A theory of fatigue. *Ergonomics, 16*, 633–648.

Cowles, E. (1893). The mental symptoms of fatigue. *New York Medical Journal, 58*, 345–352.

Glaus, A. (1993). Assessment of fatigue in cancer and noncancer patients and in healthy individuals. *Supportive Care in Cancer, 1*, 305–315.

Glaus, A. (1998). *Fatigue in patients with cancer*. Heidelberg: Springer-Verlag.

Graffigna, G., Bosio, A.C., & Olson, K. (2009). Face-to-face vs. online focus groups in two different countries: Do qualitative data collection strategies work the same way in different cultural contexts? In P. Liamputtong (Ed.), *Doing cross-cultural research: Ethical and methodological perspectives* (pp. 265–286). New York: Springer.

Graffigna, G., Olson, K., & Bosio, C. (2010). How do ethics assessments frame the results of qualitative research? A theory of technique approach. *International Journal of Social Research Methodology, 13*(4), 341–355.

Graffigna, G., Vegni, E., Barelo, S., Olson, K., & Bosio, C. (2011). Studying the social construction of cancer-related fatigue experience: The heuristic value of ethnoscience. *Patient Education and Counseling, 82*(3), 402–409.

Grandjean, E. (1968). Fatigue: Its physiological and psychological significance. *Ergonomics, 11*, 427–436.

Hayduk, L., Olson, K., Quan, H., Cree, M., & Cui, Y. (2010). Evidence confirming and clarifying the changing causal foundations of palliative care symptom restructuring. *Quality of Life Research, 19*(3), 299–306.

Kirshbaum, M., Olson, K., Pongthavornkamol, K., & Graffigna, G. (in press). Understanding the meaning of fatigue at the end of life. *European Journal of Oncology Nursing*.

Leininger, M. (1985). Ethnoscience method and componential analysis. In M. Leininger, *Qualitative research methods in nursing* (pp. 237–249), Orlando, FL: Grune & Stratton.

McEwen, B. (1998). Protective and damaging effects of stress mediators. *New England Journal of Medicine, 338*(3), 171–179.

McEwen, B. (2007). Physiology and neurobiology of stress and adaptation: Central role of the brain. *Physiological Reviews, 87*, 873–904.

Morse, J. M. (2000). Exploring pragmatic utility: Concept analysis by critically appraising the literature. In

B. Rodgers, & K. Knaffle (Eds.), *Concept development in nursing* (2nd ed.) (pp. 333–352). Philadelphia, PA: W. B. Saunders.

Morse, J. M. (2003). Principles of mixed and multi-method research design. In A. Tashakkori & C. Teddlie (Eds.), *Handbook of mixed methods in social and behavioral research* (pp. 189–208). Thousand Oaks, CA: Sage.

Oliff, A., Defeo-Jones, D., Boyer, M., Marinez, D., Kiefer, D., Vuocolo, G., Wolfe, A., & Socher, S. (1987). Tumors secreting human TNF/Cachectin induced cachexia in mice. *Cell, 50,* 555–563.

Olson, K. (2007). A new way of thinking about fatigue: A reconceptualization. *Oncology Nursing Forum, 34*(1), 93–99.

Olson, K., Hayduk, L., Cree, M., Cui, Y., Quan, H., Hanson, J., Lawlor, P., & Strasser, F. (2008). The causal foundations of variations in cancer-related symptom clusters during the final weeks of palliative care. *BMC Medical Research Methodology, 8,* 36.

Olson, K., Krawchuk, A., & Quddusi, T. (2007). Fatigue in individuals with advanced cancer in active treatment and palliative settings. *Cancer Nursing, 30*(4), E1–E10.

Olson, K., & Morse, J. M. (2005). Delineating the concept of fatigue using a pragmatic utility approach. In J. Cutcliffe & H. McKenna (Eds.), *The essential concepts of nursing* (pp. 141–159). Edinburgh: Elsevier.

Olson, K., Rogers, W. T., Cui, Y., Cree, M., Baracos, V., Rust, T., et al. (2011). Measuring fatigue in advanced cancer patients by assessing adaptive capacity: An instrument development study. *International Journal of Nursing Studies, 48*(8), 986–994.

Olson, K., Tom, B., Hewitt, J., Whittingham, J., Buchanan, L., & Ganton, G. (2002). Evolving routines: Preventing fatigue associated with lung and colorectal cancer. *Qualitative Health Research, 12*(5), 655–670.

Pongthavornkamol, K., Olson, K., Soparatanapaisarn, N., Chatchaisucha, S., Kamkhon, A., Potaros, D., Krishbaum, M., & Graffigna, G. (2012). Comparing the meanings of fatigue in individuals with cancer in Thailand and Canada. *Cancer Nursing, 35*(5), E1–E9.

Porr, C., Olson, K., & Hegadoren, K. (2010). Tiredness, fatigue, and exhaustion in the context of a major depressive disorder. *Qualitative Health Research, 20*(10), 1315–1326.

Rasch, P., & Burke, R. (1967). The history of kinesiology. In P. Rasch & R. Burke (Eds.), *Kinesiology and applied anatomy: The science of human movements* (3rd ed.) (pp. 1–17). Philadelphia, PA: Lea and Febiger.

Rhoten, D. (1982). Fatigue and the postsurgical patient. In C. Norris (Ed.), *Concept clarification in nursing* (pp. 277–300). Rockville, MD: Aspen.

Selye, H. (1952). *The story of the adaptation syndrome.* Montreal: Acta.

Selye, H. (1956). *The stress of life.* New York: McGraw-Hill.

Selye, H. (1971). *Hormones and resistance* (Vol. 1). New York: Springer.

6

Using a qualitative method to describe the experiences of living with chronic pain syndrome

Siv Söderberg

Introduction

This chapter focuses on describing how qualitative methods have been used in nursing research in order to develop knowledge about people's experiences of living with chronic pain syndrome. The qualitative methods that are presented for describing and understanding the needs of people living with a chronic pain condition are qualitative content analysis and phenomenological hermeneutic interpretation. During the past decade, my research has mainly focused on the experience of living with chronic illness. The research data have first and foremost been obtained from personal narrative interviews, as is the research presented in this chapter.

Personal narrative interviews can be described as conversations rather than interviews. The word "conversation" as opposed to the word "interview" implies a discussion and best captures the attitude toward this interaction. A conversation has a central focus and it is not one-sided (Bergum, 1991). The purpose of the narrative interviews or "conversations" was to get the participants in the different studies to speak as specifically as possible about their own experience in order to clarify their meanings. The interviews focused on the experiences of living with the illness, and the participants were guided by questions to talk about their lives involving chronic pain syndrome. This is in agreement with Kvale (1997, pp. 25, 32) who describes the qualitative research interviews as a specific form of conversation aimed at understanding dimensions from the interviewees' life world. The interviews were guided by questions, i.e., a framework stemming from and mirroring the aims of the studies. This means that the interviewer is free to build a conversation within a particular subject area, but the participants are also encouraged to tell their story (cf. Patton, 2002). The strength of interviewing starting from a guide is that the outline increases the comprehensiveness of the data and makes data collection to some extent systematic for the participants. Anticipated logic gaps in the data can be closed. The weakness of this approach is that important and salient areas may be inadvertently omitted. This was probably avoided as the question guides were general and the questions had a narrative approach.

The participants in the different studies were chosen by a purposive sampling, i.e., the researcher selected the participants who fulfilled the needs of the study (Polit & Beck, 2012). Morse (1991) argues that:

> a small randomly selected sample violates both the quantitative principle that requires an adequate sample size in order to ensure representativeness and the qualitative principle of

appropriateness that requires purposeful sampling (i.e., selecting the informants best able to meet the informational needs of the study).

(p. 127)

According to Morse (1991), the major criticism of this type of sampling is that the sample is biased by the selection process, i.e., these methods encourage a certain type of informants with a certain type of knowledge. This criticism, however, does not take into account that this is the intent in using these methods. In qualitative research "bias" is used in a positive way, as a tool to facilitate the research, to provide a theoretical richness in seeking to elucidate the experiences as richly and accurately as possible. The sample size in qualitative methods cannot be predetermined, because it is dependent on the nature of data collected and where that data takes the researcher (Sandelowski, 1986).

Research from an insider view

The experience of illness can be viewed from the perspective of an outsider and an insider. The outsider perspective implies minimizing or ignoring the subjective reality of the ill person. The insider perspective focuses directly and explicitly on the experience of existing in their illness (Conrad, 1987). People who live with illness have relevant stories to tell and common-sense wisdom to share about what to do and how to cope. Listening to the voices of people with illness is central to gaining an insight into their world. It is important to know how people experience and manage their illness and how it influences their everyday lives. One way to obtain knowledge about the illness experience of living with a chronic pain syndrome is to use qualitative methods.

Living with a chronic condition

Illness is one of several stressful events that can occur in a person's life. People can experience illness that may or may not be based on a disease; there can be illness without disease or disease without illness. Illness is the experience of loss or dysfunction and has more to do with perception, experiences and behavior than with physiological processes (Conrad, 1987; Morse & Johnson, 1991). People do not see their illness primarily as a disease process; they experience the illness in terms of symptoms and their effects on daily living (Olsson, 2010; Söderberg, 1999; Toombs, 1992, 1995). The loss of strength, energy and vitality becomes evident when people are struck by illness. Illness means a threat to the person's experience of being in the world. The ill person becomes a person wounded in a specific way (Frank, 1995; Pellegrino, 1982).

Fibromyalgia (FM) is a common pain syndrome characterized by diffuse musculoskeletal pain and fatigue; it is a common condition that can be found all over the world. The prevalence of the syndrome has been estimated at 2% of the general population, with a difference between women (3.4%) and men (0.5%) (Saxena & Solitar, 2010). The majority of people with FM are women between the ages of 20 and 50, but FM has been described both in children and in the elderly. The syndrome is determined by the presence of pain and musculoskeletal tender points on physical examination. Other common symptoms that people with FM experience are fatigue, morning stiffness, poor sleep, headaches and irritable colon. Since the cause of the syndrome is not yet fully understood, the diagnosis is established by using diagnostic criteria (Bennett et al., 2010). The criteria for the diagnosis of FM available today were established in 1990 by the American College of Rheumatology (ACR) (Wolfe et al., 1990).

Transition in chronic illness

Living with a chronic pain syndrome means living a life strongly influenced by changes. This can be regarded as an ongoing process of transition. There is no universal agreement on a definition of transitions (Murphy, 1990), but the common thread in all transition experiences is change (Shaul, 1997). Schumacher and Meleis (1994) described the universal properties of transitions as processes, directions, and changes in fundamental life patterns. Different types of transitions have been recognized that are relevant to nursing, for example, developmental, situational, health-illness, and organizational. Transition can be described as the movement from one life phase, status or condition to another (Engström & Söderberg, 2011). Meleis and Trangenstein (1994) described transitions as a change "in health status, in role relations, in expectations, or in abilities."

In order to describe the process of transition for women with FM an interview study (Söderberg & Lundman, 2001) was performed. A purposive sample of 25 women with FM was interviewed with narrative interviews (Mishler, 1986; Sandelowski, 1991) and these interviews were analyzed using a thematic content analysis (Downe-Wamboldt, 1992). The women were asked to narrate their daily life with FM. The interviews were then transcribed verbatim. The analysis started with a reading where textual units were identified (cf. Krippendorff, 1980), textual units describing the process of transition, i.e., changes related to living with FM. The textual units were then sorted out and categorized. A list of categories was created for each interview and compared to identify those commonly occurred in all interviews. The analysis revealed five categories of transitions: in daily life patterns, in working life, in family life, in social life, and in learning to live with FM. After identifying the categories, a theme, the latent message, which appears in category after category, was identified (cf. Baxter, 1994). The theme identified was "Fibromyalgia as the choreographer of activity and relationships to others."

The findings from this study showed that living a life with FM means disruptions and changes in life and in relation to other people. Paradoxically, the women were feeling ill, but they experienced that other people, because of the invisibility of the illness, considered them to be healthy. The illness started either gradually or with a more acute onset. They delineated changes in daily life, family life, working life and social life related to the illness. The imbalance between the women's will to do things and their lack of strength was salient. In order to manage, the women highlighted the importance of learning to live with the changes. Learning to live was regarded as a way of gaining control over their altered lives; it meant adjusting and accepting the disruption to life. The women expressed emotional reactions such as anger and irritation about being prevented from having one's life as it once was. The women sometimes attempted to transcend the illness; they went dancing or skiing despite the knowledge that they would became worse afterwards. They needed to do something that they enjoyed and felt that they could accomplish; this was important to maintain self-esteem for the women with FM. Changes in everyday life related to FM were caused first and foremost by pain, fatigue, and lack of strength. An imbalance between the women's will to perform and their strength to accomplish was found.

Women with FM experienced an "interfering obstacle," labeled in the theme "choreographer of activity and relationships." As a consequence, their social lives became more restricted, affecting their relationships with other people. The women stated that they were better able to understand people with illness based on their own experiences of living with FM. Changes in their working lives were also obvious, both in the housework and at their paid employment. At home they had to ask other family members to help. In their working lives some of the women received a pension, were sick-listed or had changed their job in some way which influenced their financial situation. Some of the women had problems at work; they did not have the strength to carry out their work and they felt alienated and that they were sometimes treated badly.

This research showed that the women were of the opinion that there is a lack of knowledge in society about FM and emphasized the importance of spreading knowledge aimed at working against prejudice. How they were received by other people influenced the experience of living with FM. Understanding the transition process facilitates the support of people with chronic illness and can guide health care providers in supporting people so that they can manage their lives with chronic illness.

A core story (Polkinghorne, 1988, pp. 164–165; Riessman, 1993, pp. 35, 60) was then formulated based on the categories and the theme in order to illuminate the process of transitions experienced by the women with FM. The core story is presented below:

> To be a woman with FM means leading a life marked by radical changes caused by the illness. FM is the choreographer of activity and relationships. The alterations start gradually or with a more acute onset and change the woman's daily life pattern, her relations to other people and her working life. This radical change has meant a change from an active life to a more passive one. Although the woman has the desire to do things as before, she does not have the power and lives more in the present, i.e., one day at a time. Learning to live with the illness is a way of managing. It is also important to do things which are pleasant. Sometimes the woman tries to transcend the illness and go dancing, skiing or riding. Despite the fact that FM creates a significant change in one's life, these changes are invisible to almost everyone except the woman who actually experiences them. The woman's role in the family changes in one way but not in another. The woman needs more help to manage the housework than before, but she still takes main responsibility for the housework. The husband and the children must help more. The relationship with the husband is influenced by the illness. The experience of being affected by FM gives the woman an increased understanding of other people living with illness. Despite this change in her life and anger and irritation there is also hope for improvement in the future.
>
> *(Söderberg & Lundman, 2001, p. 6251)*

Impact on daily living and relationships

In two studies a phenomenological hermeneutic method of interpretation was used to elucidate meanings of living with FM (Söderberg, Lundman, & Norberg, 1999) and meanings of pain for women with FM (Juuso, Skär, Olsson, & Söderberg, 2011). The phenomenological hermeneutic interpretation was inspired by the French philosopher Paul Ricoeur (1976) and described by Lindseth and Norberg (2004). The process of interpretation consists of three phases. The process starts with a naïve understanding, followed by a structural analysis aimed at explaining the text and finally an interpretation of the text as a whole, leading to a comprehensive understanding. There is an ongoing dialectic movement between the whole and the parts of the text, between understanding and explanation. According to Ricoeur (1976, p. 72),

> We explain something to someone else in order that he can understand. And what he has understood, he can in turn explain to a third part. Thus, understanding and explanation tend to overlap and to pass over into each other.

In explanation, we explicate the meaning, while in understanding we comprehend or grasp as a whole the chain of partial meanings in one act of synthesis (Ricoeur, 1976, p. 72). The aim of the naïve understanding is to achieve a grasp of the immediately experienced meaning and to elicit a first interpretation about the meaning of the text as a whole (Ricoeur, 1976, pp. 74–75).

The aim of the structural analysis (i.e., de-contextualization of the text) is to explain the text in order to gain an understanding. The final phase is an interpretation of the text as a whole, where the naïve understanding and the structural analysis together with the authors' pre-understanding are brought together into a new comprehensive understanding (i.e., re-contextualizing of text). To understand a text is to follow its movement from what it says to what it talks about (Ricoeur, 1976, pp. 87–88). The interpretation process is not as linear as this description may suggest. During the interpretation there is a back and forth movement between the whole and the parts of the data.

A purposive sample of 14 women with FM was interviewed using a narrative approach (Söderberg, Lundman, & Norberg, 1999). The women were asked to narrate their experiences of living with FM, guided by questions about symptoms, daily living, relations with other people, and thoughts and feelings. Meanings of living with FM were interpreted as a struggle to achieve relief from the bodily experiences of FM, the consequences in everyday life, and the threat to the self. The findings were presented in three interlaced themes: loss of freedom, threat to integrity, and a struggle to achieve understanding and relief. Freedom in life was influenced by bodily changes, changes in everyday life, and changes in financial circumstances. A life with FM means first and foremost living with pain and fatigue. The women experienced pain almost permanently and had not found any treatment that afforded more than passing relief. Changes in everyday life related to FM were caused primarily by pain, fatigue and lack of strength. An imbalance between the women's will to act and their strength to accomplish was found. They experienced pain and fatigue as an "interfering obstacle," and as a consequence, their social life became more restricted, affecting their relationships with other people.

Women with FM described a threat to their integrity and human dignity. They struggled against the illness, against not being believed and they struggled for relief. The women expressed the feeling that they were not regarded as a credible person and felt that they were not respected. This was related to the fact that FM is invisible and has an obscure etiology. This threatens the women's integrity and was seen as a struggle for dignity. To be credible was to be given a diagnosis, to be examined, to be offered the opportunity to take part in a research group, to be taken seriously and not to be ridiculed. A good encounter was described as one in which they were not mistrusted, were listened to and were allowed time to tell their stories. The women struggled for understanding and relief. To obtain relief was to get a diagnosis, because this meant that the illness existed and to be given the information that the syndrome is not fatal. Knowledge about FM made it easier to accept the situation and contributed to living a life with dignity. Meeting other women in the same situation and having the feeling of being understood by other people brought relief and a sense of not being alone. Another way to get relief was to plan daily life in accordance with the illness. The women with FM emphasized that in struggling for relief they turned to alternative care. They tried every option to get relief.

In a phenomenological hermeneutic study by Juuso, Skär, Olsson, and Söderberg (2011) a purposive sample of 15 women with FM were asked to talk as freely as possible about their experience of pain related to FM. The findings showed that FM pain invaded the whole body; it was always present, unpredictable and fluctuating. Meanings of pain were presented in two interlaced themes: experiencing an unwilling body, and experiencing a good life despite it all. The women described how their body was in pain the whole time, but it was an invisible body feeling, something that made them feel questioned. One woman said: "Others can't understand what they can't see." Health care personnel had repeatedly disbelieved them. They avoided asking for help related to other people's judgmental attitudes and expressed a fear of being seen as silly, lazy and stupid, feelings that made them reluctant to talk about their pain. The women with FM described how they experienced that their body did not function as when it was healthy. They had to plan their everyday life and had to wait for their body to catch up with their ideas. The pain was described in two ways: a pain that was always present and a more intense pain. These different pains could be described as an everyday pain and pain on pain.

Ways of normalizing their daily lives included walking outdoors, gardening and doing handiwork. These activities enabled them to overcome the pain and distracted their thoughts. Being with friends enabled them to focus on issues other than pain and was important for their self-esteem; additionally, it promoted the strength to keep control and never give up. As one woman said, "The only way to survive is actually to be optimistic and try to make the best of everything." They also described that they did not accept the pain but had learned to live with it. Despite the always present pain, the women with FM said that they were living a good life. For a long time they had hoped for a recovery and had wished that life would return to normal, but ultimately, they realized that pain was a part of their daily life and they became reconciled to this.

The findings from this study are in line with a study with women with a whiplash injury (Juuso & Söderberg, manuscript). A purposive sample of eight women with a whiplash injury were interviewed with a narrative approach. The women described great changes in everyday life quite similar to those women with FM.

It was difficult for women with FM to explicitly describe the pain experience. In a study (Söderberg & Norberg, 1995) women with FM were asked to discuss their experiences of pain. The interviews were analyzed with a focus on the content in their pain descriptions. Several of the women became emotionally affected and used metaphorical expressions to describe their pain. One woman said, "It feels as if my upper arms have been cut off" and another woman said, "It feels as if it is burning, almost the same feeling as when you put your feet in warm water, boiling, as if it was too warm; it gets really hot, it burns so fiercely." This was interpreted as being a way in which the women could disclose tacit knowledge. The expression was seen as an "as if" meaning, a figure of speech, meant to convey some property of the total pain experience. In using metaphorical pain language, women with FM described their pain in ways that were interpreted as having experiences comparable to being tortured. The women experienced pain almost permanently and had not found any treatment that afforded more than passing relief. Metaphorical expressions were also used to describe the meaning of the lived experience of pain and fatigue. The pain and fatigue were found to be intertwined (Söderberg & Lundman, 2001; Söderberg, Lundman, & Norberg, 1999, 2002). Study of the use of language, especially metaphors, is a valuable approach to an understanding of the lived world of people with illnesses. The metaphors used by women with FM are vital to an understanding of their experiences of pain and fatigue. Metaphors do not add facts to a description; they add depth of meaning of the nature of a phenomenon, as expressed through its relationship to something else (Czechmeister, 1994). This means that the metaphorical expressions used by the women with FM add to their descriptions the deep meaning of the phenomena of pain and fatigue.

A phenomenological hermeneutic study by Paulson, Norberg, and Söderberg (2002) shows that men with fibromyalgia-type pain experience a difference to some extent as compared to the experiences of women with FM. A purposive sample of 14 men with fibromyalgia-type pain was interviewed concerning their experiences of living with chronic pain. The participants in the study fulfilled the ACR criteria of FM (Wolfe et al., 1990). The interviews focused on the men's symptoms, daily life, working life, family life and social life. The findings showed that the men strived to endure the changes in daily life related to their pain. The analysis of the interviews revealed three interlaced themes: experiencing the body as an obstruction, being a different man, and striving to endure. The body was experienced as being sluggish with constantly aching muscles. The men had greater difficulty working as compared to when they were healthy; these problems were related to experiencing their bodies as obstructive. The bodily pain fluctuated, and as a consequence, it was impossible to make plans. The men described feelings of not being a whole person as they could not live as they did before the illness. They felt that family and employers believed that they really were in pain, but this was not the same as true understanding. It was especially hard for their children to understand why their father could not participate in games with them. It was important for the men to live as normally as possible, and they were reluctant to show people in their surroundings that they felt ill. The men feared being looked upon as whiners. Despite a pessimistic view of the future, they retained different wishes and goals in life.

To conclude, striving to live life when not feeling well requires balancing life during the calm and difficult phases of the illness. It involves struggling for a tolerable existence, a process that takes a long time. The findings from this study could provide guidelines for health care staff members to give empathic and supportive care to men living with a long-term illness.

Pain causes fatigue and fatigue causes pain

Pain and fatigue were the symptoms that dominated the women with FM in the different studies that are presented in this chapter. Understanding the meaning of symptoms is pivotal to curing and healing and increases the possibility of supporting and empowering women with FM. Therefore, to achieve a deeper understanding of the meaning of the lived experience of fatigue among women with FM, we found it important to compare their experiences with those of healthy women. Therefore, the aim of this phenomenological hermeneutic study (Söderberg, Lundman, & Norberg, 2002) was to elucidate the meaning of fatigue as narrated by women with FM and healthy women. A purposive sample of 25 women with FM and 25 aged-matched (within three years) healthy women were interviewed using a narrative approach. The healthy women served as a reference group. The healthy women were students, office employees and health care personnel. They regarded themselves as healthy and were not suffering from any known chronic illness.

The women with FM described fatigue as equally severe and sometimes even more severe than the pain; it was experienced as an all-pervading problem. The fatigue was described as a whole body experience; using metaphorical speech, the body felt as if it were "carrying a heavy bag" and the body was jaded, losing energy. The meaning of the lived experience of fatigue was captured in four themes: (1) the body as a burden; (2) an absent presence; (3) an interfering obstacle; and (4) the hope of possible relief. Another theme of fatigue was a feeling of being "absently present," the feeling of being present but simultaneously being absent; it was a feeling of being enveloped in wool. The fatigue was depicted as uncontrollable and a feeling of being constantly sleepy; to rest at night did not help. Fatigue colored the experience of the lived body; when people are healthy, the body paradoxically is present by being absent, in fatigue the body becomes present urgently or in an alien way, thus a new relationship to the body is established. The lived body became objectified, an "it" that influenced one's power to be involved with the world in the same way as before the illness. The women with FM narrated fatigue differently than the healthy women. Fatigue among the women with FM was not caused by work; rather, it appears regardless of activity or inactivity. It exists in and of itself, and it is hard to relieve.

The healthy women did not talk about "fatigue" but "tiredness," which is something natural. They needed recovery and rest. The women with FM expressed hope of a possibility of relief in their altered situation. The findings illuminated that in illness the surrounding world looks and feels different than it does in health, because the relation between the lived body and the environment is altered.

Pain and well-being

In a phenomenological hermeneutic study (Juuso, Skär, Olsson, & Söderberg, 2012) a purposive sample of 13 women diagnosed with FM participated. The women were asked to talk about when they felt well despite living with FM. The findings showed that meanings of feeling well for women with FM could be understood as having the power to maintain strength, a possibility of managing daily life independently and being able to find their own pace and to have willpower. The women with FM said that they felt well when they had the strength to be independent during the day. It gave them a feeling of inner calm and happiness. In the summer the women described that they had more strength and felt lighter. Although they were not pain-free, they felt more alert and healthier, a feeling they attributed to the light and the warm weather in the summer. The women described how being acknowledged and listened to was important for them to feel well. Additionally, friends and good social relations also contributed to a feeling of well-being. In conclusion, the study showed that it was possible for women with FM to feel well despite their severe pain and fatigue.

The experiences of close relatives to people living with a chronic pain syndrome

The article "Living with a woman with fibromyalgia from the perspective of the husband' (Söderberg, Strand, Haapala, & Lundman, 2003) presents five men's experiences of living with a woman with the diagnosis of FM. Personal audio-taped interviews with a narrative approach were conducted (Mishler, 1986; Sandelowski, 1991). The interviews were guided by the following question: "Please tell me about your wife, and about your life together. Tell me also about how your daily life has been affected by your wife's illness, about how FM has affected relationships with your children, and how relationships to others have been influenced by FM." Clarifying questions were used, e.g., "What do you mean now?" or "Can you give me an example?" A qualitative thematic content analysis was used to analyze the interview text. Thematic content analysis can be described as a process of identifying, coding and categorizing the primary pattern of the data (i.e., the content) (Downe-Wamboldt, 1992; Patton, 2002). The data analysis began with reading each interview several times to get a sense of the whole (Sandelowski, 1995). Guided by the aim of the study, a reading followed to identify meaning units. The meaning units were condensed and sorted into 38 categories. The categories were related to each other and subsumed into seven themes, i.e., threads of meaning that appeared in category after category (Baxter, 1994). This study showed that the whole family was influenced and limited when a family member was affected by illness; in this case, a women affected by FM. The husbands experienced greater responsibility and participation in the children's upbringing. Central to the findings was the need of information for the whole family, a responsibility that the men felt was the duty of the health care personnel. Given information, the husbands believed that they would be able to better understand the women's illness.

A purposive sample of 14 female partners living with a man with FM participated in a phenomenological hermeneutic study by Paulson, Norberg, and Söderberg (2003). The aim of the study was to elucidate meanings of being a female partner to a man with FM pain. The women were asked to speak freely about their experiences. The women were asked the following open-ended question: "Please tell me about your experiences of living with a man affected by long-term pain." The findings were presented in three interlaced themes: (1) struggling to give support and comfort; (2) struggling to keep going; and (3) experiencing lack of understanding and support. The findings showed that living with a man with fibromyalgic pain meant living a life in the shadow of the man's pain.

Daily life was strongly influenced by the man's illness, and it was no longer possible to take daily life for granted. The social life was restricted for the family, and it was frustrating for the partners that the men did not want to communicate their pain. The partners felt excluded from the men's emotions. The women described how they felt drained by the long duration of the men's illness, and they had responsibility day in and day out, which led to a feeling of an almost constant fatigue. They felt alone although they were a couple. The study also showed that the female partners lacked support from the health care system. In conclusion, the study showed that meanings of female partners' experiences of living with a man with fibromyalgic pain meant living with an unwelcome family member with whom they had to struggle. The study also emphasized the importance of partners being acknowledged by the health care system.

Conclusion: impact on nursing care and suggestions for improvement

There is no such thing as illness; only people with illness (Cassell, 2004). People with illness only spend a small part of their lives in the role of a patient. The individual as a whole is the basis of every contact in health care. Every illness can be seen as a threat to the self and to one's sense of human dignity (Cassell, 2004; Morse, 1997). A prerequisite for the protection of human dignity in health care is an awareness of the vulnerability of people with illness and their dependency on the power of the health care personnel to answer individual needs (Söderberg, 1999, 2009; Söderberg, Olsson, & Skär, 2012).

Conclusions that can be drawn based on these findings are the need for communication based on shared understanding between people with chronic illness and health care personnel in order to give support. This seems to be applicable and important for the participants in the research presented in this chapter.

Implications for clinical practice

This knowledge has to be taken into consideration by health care personnel in care planning. This research shows the need for information about chronic pain syndrome. Health care personnel have a great responsibility to provide information about the illness to enable people with chronic pain and their close relatives to better understand and thus increase opportunities to support and help achieve a better life with the illness. Care, support and acknowledgment from health care personnel and public authorities are of significant importance, especially in cases of illnesses such as FM, a poorly understood disorder. It is particularly important to understand how people with chronic illness and their relatives experience the illness. To preserve people's dignity within the health care system, the staff must pay attention to individual human needs (Söderberg, 1999). Kuyper and Wester (1998) emphasized that a key factor for support to people with chronic illness and their families is the attitude and communication skills of the health care personnel. This seems to be applicable and important for all participants in the research presented in this chapter.

According to Drew (1986), the essence of health care, apart from all the complexities of a scientifically and technologically advanced system of care, is something that happens between people. To care refers to a way of relating to another person; it is a relationship that develops with changes in both the one who cares and the one who is cared for. Listening to people with illness means acquiring knowledge that will bring with it a greater understanding of the people's experiences of their lives with illness (Söderberg, 1999, 2009). If health care workers want to understand what people experience, a dialogue must be initiated with the person, a dialogue that allows the person to provide a first-person narrative of the illness.

References

Baxter, L. A. (1994). Content analysis. In R. M. Montgomery & S. Duck (Eds.), *Studying interpersonal interaction* (pp. 239–254). New York: Guilford Press.

Bennett, R. M., Russell, J., Cappelleri, J. C., Bushmakin, A. G., Zlateva, G., & Sadosky, A. (2010). Identification of symptom and functional domains that fibromyalgia patients would like to see improved: A cluster analysis. *BMC Musculoskeletal Disorders*, *11*, 134. Advance online publication.

Bergum, V. (1991). Being a phenomenological researcher. In J. M. Morse (Ed.), *Qualitative nursing research: A contemporary dialogue* (pp. 55–71). London: Sage.

Cassell, E. J. (2004). *The nature of suffering and the goals of medicine*. Oxford: Oxford University Press.

Conrad, P. (1987). The experience of illness: Recent and new directions. *Research in the Sociology of Health Care*, *6*, 1–31.

Czechmeister, C. A. (1994). Metaphor in illness and nursing: A two-edged sword. A discussion of the social use of metaphor in everyday language, and implications of nursing and nursing education. *Journal of Advanced Nursing*, *19*, 1226–1233.

Downe-Wamboldt, B. (1992). Content analysis: Method, applications, and issues. *Health Care for Women International*, *13*, 313–321.

Drew, N. (1986). Exclusion and confirmation: A phenomenology of patients' experiences with caregivers. *IMAGE: Journal of Nursing Scholarship*, *18*, 39–43.

Engström, Å., & Söderberg, S. (2011). Transitions as experienced by close relatives of people with traumatic brain injury. *Journal of Neuroscience Nursing*, *43*, 253–260.

Frank, A. W. (1995). *The wounded storyteller*. Chicago: University of Chicago Press.

Juuso, P., Skär, L., Olsson, M., & Söderberg, S. (2011). Living with a double burden: Meanings of pain for women with fibromyalgia. *International Journal of Qualitative Studies on Health and Well-being*, *6*, 7184. doi: 10.3402/v6i3.7184.

Juuso, P., Skär, L., Olsson, M., & Söderberg, S. (2012). Meanings of feeling well for women with fibromyalgia. *Health Care for Women International*. DOI: 10.1080/07399332.2012.736573.

Juuso, P., & Söderberg, S. (manuscript). Women's narrations about living with a whiplash injury.

Krippendorff, K. (1980). *Content analysis: An introduction to its methodology*. Beverly Hills, CA: Sage.

Kvale, S. (1997). *Den kvalitativa forskningsintervjun* [Interviews]. Lund: Studentlitteratur (in Swedish, English translation).

Kuyper, M. B., & Wester, F. (1998). In the shadow: The impact of chronic illness on the patient's partner. *Qualitative Health Research*, *8*, 237–253.

Lindseth, A., & Norberg, A. (2004). A phenomenological hermeneutical method for researching lived experience. *Scandinavian Journal of Caring Sciences*, *18*, 145–153.

Meleis, A. I., & Trangenstein, P. A. (1994). Facilitation transitions: Redefinition of the nursing mission. *Nursing Outlook*, *42*, 255–259.

Mishler, E. G. (1986). *Research interviewing: Context and narrative*. Cambridge, MA: Harvard University Press.

Morse, J. M. (1991). *Qualitative nursing research*. London: Sage.

Morse, J. M. (1997). Responding to threats to integrity of self. *Advances in Nursing Science*, *19*, 21–36.

Morse, J. M., & Johnson, J. L. (1991). Understanding the illness experience. In J. M. Morse & J. L. Johnson (Eds.), *The illness experience: Dimensions of suffering* (pp. 1–12). London: Sage.

Murphy, S. A. (1990). Human responses to transitions: A holistic nursing perspective. *Holistic Nursing Practice*, *4*, 1–7.

Olsson, M. (2010). Meanings of women's experiences of living with multiple sclerosis. Doctoral dissertation. Luleå University of Technology, Luleå, Sweden.

Patton, M. Q. (2002). *Qualitative research and evaluation methods*. Thousand Oaks, CA: Sage.

Paulson, M., Danielsson, E., & Söderberg, S. (2002). Struggling for a tolerable existence: The meaning of men's lived experiences of living with pain of fibromyalgia type. *Qualitative Health Research*, *12*, 239–251.

Paulson, M., Norberg, A., & Söderberg, S. (2003). Living in the shadow of fibromyalgic pain: The meaning of female partners' experiences. *Journal of Clinical Nursing*, *12*, 235–243.

Pellegrino, E. D. (1982). Being ill and being healed: Some reflections on the grounding of medical morality. In V. Kestenbaum (Ed.), *The humanity of the ill* (pp. 157–166). Knoxville: University of Tennessee Press.

Polit, D. F., & Beck, C. T. (2012). *Nursing research: Generating and assessing evidence for nursing practice* (9th ed.). Philadelphia, PA: Lippincott, Williams & Wilkins.

Polkinghorne, D. E. (1988). *Narrative knowing and the human sciences*. Albany, NY: State University of New York Press.

Ricoeur, P. (1976). *Interpretation theory: Discourse and the surplus of meaning.* Fort Worth, TX: Christian University Press.

Riessman, C.K (1993). *Narrative analysis: Qualitative research methods series 30.* London: Sage.

Sandelowski, M. (1986). The problems of rigor in qualitative research. *Advances in Nursing Science, 8,* 27–37.

Sandelowski, M. (1991). Telling stories: Narrative approaches in qualitative research. *IMAGE: Journal of Nursing Scholarship, 23,* 161–166.

Sandelowski, M. (1995). Qualitative analysis: What it is and how to begin. *Research in Nursing and Health, 18,* 371–375.

Saxena, A., & Solitar, B.M. (2010). Fibromyalgia: Knowns, unknowns and current treatment. *Bulletin of the NYU Hospital for Joint Diseases, 68,* 157–161.

Schumacher, K. L., & Meleis, A. J. (1994). Transitions: A central concept in nursing. *IMAGE: Journal of Nursing Scholarship, 26,* 119–127.

Shaul, M. P. (1997). Transitions in chronic illness: Rheumatoid arthritis in women. *Rehabilitation Nursing, 22,* 199–205.

Söderberg, S. (1999). Women's experiences of living with fibromyalgia: Struggling for dignity. Medical dissertation, Umeå University, Umeå, Sweden.

Söderberg, S. (Ed.). (2009). *Att leva med sjukdom* [Living with illness]. Stockholm: Norstedts Akademiska Förslag (in Swedish).

Söderberg, S., & Lundman, B. (2001). Transitions experienced by women with fibromyalgia. *Health Care for Women International, 22,* 617–631.

Söderberg, S., Lundman, B., & Norberg, A. (1999). Struggling for dignity: Women's experiences of living with fibromyalgia. *Qualitative Health Research, 9,* 575–587.

Söderberg, S., Lundman, B., & Norberg, A. (2002). The meaning of fatigue and tiredness for women with fibromyalgia and healthy women. *Journal of Clinical Nursing, 11,* 247–255.

Söderberg, S., & Norberg, A. (1995). Metaphorical pain language among fibromyalgia patients. *Scandinavian Journal of Caring Sciences, 9,* 55–59.

Söderberg, S., Olsson, M., & Skär, L. (2012). A hidden kind of suffering: Female patients' complaints to Patient's Advisory Committee. *Scandinavian Journal of Caring Sciences, 26,* 144–150.

Söderberg, S., Strand, M., Haapala, M., & Lundman, B. (2003). Living with a woman with fibromyalgia from the perspective of the husband. *Journal of Advanced Nursing, 42,* 143–150.

Toombs, S. K (1992). The meaning of illness: A phenomenological account of the different perspectives of physician and patient. In H. T. Engelhardt Jr. & S. F. Spicker (Eds.), *Philosophy and medicine* (Vol. 42, pp. 1–16l). Dordrecht: Kluwer Academic Publishers.

Toombs, S. K. (1995). Sufficient unto the day. In S. K Toombs, D. Barnard, & R. A. Carson (Eds.), *Chronic illness: From experience to policy* (pp. 3–24). Bloomington: Indiana University Press.

Wolfe, F., Smythe, H. A., Yunus, M. B., Bennett, R. M., Bombardier, C., Goldenberg, D. L., et al. (1990). The American College of Rheumatology 1990 criteria for the classification of fibromyalgia. *Arthritis and Rheumatism, 33,* 160–172.

7

Qualitative research program in the care of ventilator-dependent ICU patients

Mary Beth Happ

Introduction

Critical illness and its treatment in the technologically complex setting of the intensive care unit involve multifaceted physiological, psychosocial, and technological processes and human–technology interactions. Qualitative research can provide insights into understanding the experience of critical illness from the perspectives of patients, their family members, and clinician care providers. Qualitative research can also explicate the social and cultural context and processes of interaction during critical care treatment. This chapter illustrates the sequential use of a variety of qualitative research approaches to address questions about patient care and patient–caregiver interaction during critical illness. My program of research has been concerned with the condition or circumstance of prolonged mechanical ventilation (MV). This line of inquiry originated with questions about human–technology interaction among critically ill older adults (Happ, 1998a, 1998b, 2000a, 2000b, 2002), proceeded to investigation of the processes of care and communication during weaning from prolonged mechanical ventilation (Broyles, Colbert, Tate, Swigart, & Happ, 2008; Crighton, Coyne, Tate, Swigart, & Happ, 2008b; Happ et al., 2007a; Happ, Swigart, Tate, Hoffman, & Arnold, 2007b; Happ, Tate, Swigart, Divirgilio-Thomas, & Hoffman, 2010; Hoffman et al., 2004; Sereika et al., 2011; Tate & Happ, 2011; Tate, Devito Dabbs, Hoffman, Milbrandt, & Happ, 2012) and progressed to a mixed methods research program focused on understanding and improving communication among patients who were unable to speak during respiratory support and treatment.

The problem of ventilator dependence serves as a focal point. While my research questions drove the selection of research method, the process of conducting qualitative, exploratory research with ventilator-dependent patients, clinicians and family members in the ICU was iterative and took topical and methodological directions that were not initially anticipated. Thus, I have used a variety of qualitative research methods and techniques and have addressed topics ranging from device disruption (a.k.a. "treatment interference") to nurse–patient communication. In addition to journal publications of study results, case exemplars and methods explication hopefully contributed to advancing nursing science and education.

Grounded theory study of treatment interference in the ICU

Acute and critical care nurses frequently confront the dilemma of how to care for patients who pull at or attempt to remove the technologic devices, such as monitoring leads, endotracheal tubes, and intravenous lines, that are necessary for their immediate care and recovery. This phenomenon, termed "treatment interference" by gerontological researchers and "device disruption" by those in acute-critical care, can have life-threatening consequences, particularly for critically ill older adults (Happ, 1998a). Although prior descriptive correlation studies suggested that agitation, anxiety, confusion, and discomfort were possible factors contributing to treatment interference, a complete description or explanation of treatment interference was lacking. There was a gap in knowledge about the way nurses respond to treatment interference among hospitalized older adults. I sought to examine the behavioral cues, patient attributes, and circumstances surrounding treatment interference in critically ill older adults and nurses' responses to this clinical problem. The study addressed the following research question: "What is the interactional process of treatment interference in critically ill older adults?"

Methods summary

The study was conducted in a medical intensive care unit and the adjoining intermediate intensive care unit of a large metropolitan teaching hospital. Data were collected using interactive unstructured informal interviews, participant observation, open-ended formal interviews, and document (patient clinical records and policies/procedures) analysis during a 28-week period. Older adults were followed longitudinally throughout their ICU stay using "event analysis" as a guide to data collection (Happ, Swigart, Tate, & Crighton, 2004b; Pelto & Pelto, 1978). Observations and observational (informal) interviews focused on medical devices and device disruption events, patient behaviors, clinician responses and circumstances leading to or viewed as preventative of device disruption.

Sample

Critically ill patients, aged 65 and over, and the nurses who cared for them were the primary study participants. Family members (significant family or friend support persons) and physicians were included in interviews as "secondary" informants. Purposive sampling was used initially to ensure diverse representation of informants recognizing that the process of interfering with treatment devices may differ by patient age, cognitive status, severity of illness, technologic device, and nurse preparation or unit tenure. Additional informants were selected according to theoretical needs of the research as data analysis progressed (Glaser, 1978). Elderly patients who did not attempt to pull at or disrupt devices were sought as alternative cases. Midway through data collection, theoretical sampling of elderly patients who were expected to survive became necessary as death and responses to invasive technology at the end of life became a recurrent pattern. Nurses who were particularly familiar with a study case were interviewed first about their impressions of the particular case, and then regarding larger issues of older adults' responses to technologic devices. Second, nurses and physicians who were considered to be experts in the care of older adult patients were approached for interviews.

The final sample consisted of 16 critically ill adults, aged 64–87 years, followed longitudinally through the course of their ICU and post-ICU stays. Eleven of the 16 patients died in hospital, most in the ICU or step-down ICU. All except two patients required the use of mechanical ventilation at some time during hospitalization. Clearly, this was a seriously ill group with several study patients characteristic of the "chronically" critically ill (Daly et al., 1991).

Four patients were interviewed and two cognitively impaired patients provided informal interview data. Most of the 65 registered nurses employed in the two adjacent units were interviewed at least informally about older patient responses to technologic devices. Nine nurses, four nurses from each unit plus the clinical nurse specialist, participated in formal interviews; three were interviewed twice. Four family members of elderly study participants were interviewed and were representative in terms of age, gender, relationship, and ethnicity. Three physicians (two men and one woman) were interviewed formally. They were identified for interviews by their involvement with specific patients or clinical interest. In addition, informal discussions with three experienced attending physicians (all male) about their perceptions of responses of older adults to technologic devices and the phenomenon of device self-removal were included in the data.

Results

Technological access

Three major conditional categories were explicated within this BSP: *voicelessness, awareness, limitations and possibilities*. Technological access was the basic social-psychological process (BSP) identified in the data. Technological access is the core process in which invasive lines and tubes (such as the pulmonary artery catheter, intravenous lines, and endotracheal tubes) and noninvasive devices (such as cardiac or oxygen saturation monitors) are employed to visualize bodily functions or systems for diagnostic or monitoring information, or to administer treatment. Information gained through technological access is used continuously for diagnostic and treatment decision-making.

The use of technological devices in this setting involved a dynamic interplay between limitations and possibilities, benefits and burdens, healing and harm. During critical illness, practitioners, patients, and family members became intimately entwined in initiating, maintaining, and discontinuing technological access. Although physicians were primarily responsible for initiating technological access, particularly access involving invasive devices, critical care nurses maintained technological access and, in many cases, began the process of discontinuation (Happ, 1998b) (see Figure 7.1).

Technological access enabled fully aggressive critical care, including advanced cardiopulmonary resuscitation, monitoring, and life support. Inability to access a patient through necessary technology severely restricted treatment options. In such instances, grim prognoses and determinations of medical futility were achieved relatively quickly. At the other end of the spectrum, fully accessed was a condition in which a maximum number of bodily functions and processes were visible or physically accessible for information or intervention. One nurse described fully accessed as "a catheter in every orifice." Full access provided information about system deterioration or dysfunction which, at least implicitly, obligated treatment (Happ, 1998b).

Maintaining technological access

Nurses bore the primary responsibility for maintaining technological devices in the ICU (Happ, 2000b). Maintaining technological access involved the nurse's skillful assessment of patient "awareness" and "trustworthiness" with regard to the medical devices and the nurse's interpretation of the patient's behaviors. Critical care nurses were most protective of those devices for which accidental removal was perceived as "dangerous" or life-threatening (e.g., endotracheal tubes, arterial catheters, and central venous catheters). In circumstances of dangerous access, prevention of treatment interference was a significant component of maintaining the device and nurses' tolerance of patient behaviors perceived as having the potential to dislodge a device was low. In addition to assessing patient factors (e.g., cognitive status, mobility, strength, trustworthiness), nurses considered device factors such as replacement difficulty and the necessity of the

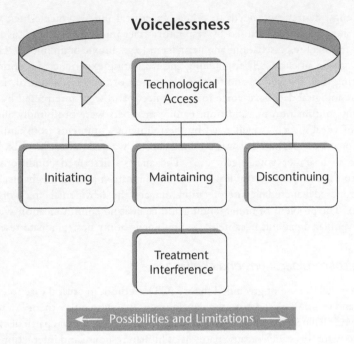

Figure 7.1 Model of technological access during critical illness

Source: Happ et al. (1998b).

device with regard to maintaining the device. Nurses used verbal strategies (e.g., explaining, threatening), distraction, deception, comfort measures, watchful family members, physical restraints, and sedation to prevent treatment interference.

Discontinuing technological access

Discontinuing technological access occurred when physiological conditions improved, alternative accesses were employed, or decisions were made to limit or withdraw treatment. In some instances, discontinuing access was routine and governed by protocol. For instance, after a specified period, an intravascular device poses a risk of serious infection and is removed or replaced. Because many study patients died during their critical illness, discontinuing access was primarily related to the limitation or withdrawal of life support technologies. In cases of terminal critical illness, adult patients sometimes expressed their wish and/or readiness to die by willful removal of one or more devices. At least three of the patients in this study exhibited this response to the devices, particularly endotracheal or tracheal intubation. Each of these patients had a terminal malignant illness and/or end-stage organ failure with no hope of recovery. The exemplar case for this dimension of discontinuing access was published in *Palliative and End of Life Pearls* (Happ, 2002) and illustrated the importance of understanding the meaning of the patient's treatment interference behavior.

Voicelessness

All behavior has meaning to the social interactionist. Thus, I began to understand treatment interference behaviors as communicative behaviors within the context of the patients' profound communication barriers. *Voicelessness* was developed as a contextual condition representing the gamut of communication barriers that limit critically ill patients' abilities to fully represent their thoughts, feelings, desires, and needs to others. In critical illness, voicelessness encompasses mechanically impaired speech caused by respiratory tract intubation, as well as mental status changes, both transient (e.g., sedation) and permanent (e.g., anoxic brain injury) (Happ, 2000a). Voicelessness can be an extremely frightening and frustrating experience for critically ill older adults, rendering them powerless and forcing abdication of decisional control. I noticed that alarms and physiological data gave voice to patient needs and were interpreted by nurses often without patient confirmation or validation. Family members were profoundly affected by the patient's loss of vocal speech as evidenced by the following comments from family members: "She's [still] not able to talk and that was our big goal." "I wanted to hear her talk. I thought I'd never be able to hear her voice again . . ." The analysis described conditions and factors contributing to the interpretation of nonvocal communication among mechanically ventilated patients and proposed that credible interpretation mitigates the detrimental effects of voicelessness (Happ, 2000a). The problem of understanding and facilitating communication with nonvocal, mechanically ventilated patients became the central focus of my post-graduate research.

Methodological considerations and challenges

This study extended the use of grounded theory (GT) methods in critical care to consider both physiological and technological data in the development of a substantive theory of technological access during critical illness (Happ & Kagan, 2001). Grounded theory was particularly well suited as a methodology for this study because patterns of human response and interaction were clearly the focus. Second, the literature showed a need for full description of the phenomenon of treatment interference, including alternative cases and patient/family perspectives. Grounded theory methods afforded techniques of purposive and theoretical sampling and comparison among multiple data sources. Event analysis provided a focus to data collection in that physiological (vital signs, electrolyte abnormalities, etc.) and clinical data (sedation use, physical restraint use, rationale for device placement/re-placement) as well as behavioral responses and participants' perspectives about devices before, during and after device disruption events were reviewed and analyzed.

The biggest challenge to conducting GT in this environment is observer distraction and fatigue. Observations can be difficult to conduct in the technologically complex, fast-paced and dynamic setting of the ICU because there is so much visual, behavioral, and auditory data for the observer to "take in" or "record." Event analysis of actual or potential device disruption events and longitudinal case analysis provided boundaries and filters for data collection and analysis (Happ & Kagan, 2001; Happ et al., 2004b). Data collection with family members and clinicians focused on the case and/or "events" of interest. Longitudinal data collection afforded prolonged engagement and a rich set of data for each study participant; however, protracted ICU stays led to decisions to limit data collection in a "selective" style of data collection or sampling.

Because patients are unable to speak during MV and have fluctuating states of consciousness, ascertaining the patient's perspective can be challenging. A few patients in my study were able to participate in interviews shortly after the breathing tube was removed. For those who were unable to be interviewed (a large number died), the patient's experience was only available through the eyes of the observer, family and clinicians. In later studies, we applied the practical guidelines offered by Higgins and Daly (Higgins & Daly, 1999) for determining decisional capacity for research participation and for collecting interview data with this vulnerable population. We also refined our communication skills with nonspeaking ICU patients to ascertain their experience more directly in a prospective approach; however, this problem remains an obstacle in conducting qualitative research in this setting.

Ethnographic study of care and communication in weaning patients from prolonged mechanical ventilation

Event analysis and longitudinal case analysis techniques were further exploited in an ethnographic study of care and communication during ventilator weaning in the ICU (R01-NR07973). This study addressed the clinical problem of weaning patients from prolonged mechanical ventilation. The study was conceived and conducted as a companion study to an existing clinical trial which compared care for patients weaning from prolonged mechanical ventilation managed by an acute care nurse practitioner to "usual" care led by pulmonary and critical care medicine fellows (Hoffman, Tasota, Zullo, Scharfenberg, & Donahoe, 2005). Our aim was not to compare advanced practice nurses and physicians, but to understand the processes of care common to successful (or unsuccessful) patterns of ventilator weaning for patients who experienced difficult and prolonged trajectories of mechanical ventilation. Prolonged mechanical ventilation (PMV) was defined as four or more days of mechanical ventilation and at least two unsuccessful weaning attempts. We purposively selected 30 patients for variability on age, gender, race, admitting diagnosis, neurocognitive status (Glasgow Coma Score) (Teasdale & Jennett, 1974) severity of illness (APACHE III score) (Knaus et al., 1991) and clinician predictions of likelihood of weaning success. These criteria were derived from the literature on weaning from PMV, the companion clinical trial (Hoffman et al., 2005) and our ongoing analysis.

Methods summary

The study was a focused ethnography (Fetterman, 1998) conducted in the 20-bed medical intensive care unit (MICU) of a tertiary care medical center from November 2001 to July 2003. Most PMV patients were transferred to the step-down ICU for weaning trials. Patient care was managed by critical care/pulmonary fellows or an acute care nurse practitioner under the direction of an attending physician. Nurses and respiratory therapists rotated between the more acute MICU and the step-down ICU. We followed patients longitudinally throughout the period of weaning from MV in the ICU.

Data collection techniques included field observations of weaning events conducted by one of two researchers (myself and trained project coordinator) in the clinical setting 4–5 days a week including evenings and weekends (Happ et al., 2004b; Happ, Dabbs, Tate, Hricik, & Erlen, 2006). Observations followed a semi-structured guide, adapted from previous work (Happ, Roesch, & Garrett, 2004a; Happ, Roesch, & Kagan, 2005) that included description of patient activities and care activities during weaning. Observations focused primarily on weaning trials and the weaning process and were recorded by handwritten and dictated field notes. Informal interviews were conducted during fieldwork. Formal, semi-structured, audiotaped interviews were conducted with selected patients (n = 18), clinicians (n = 31), and family members (n = 31). Clinicians (11 physicians, 10 nurses, 7 respiratory therapists, 3 others) were selected to participate in interviews based on their involvement in the care of study patients. The patient interview guide included questions about their experience and feelings during weaning, actions by others that they perceived as helpful and/or unhelpful during weaning from PMV. Clinicians and family members were asked similar questions about actions that they perceived to be helpful or unhelpful to patients during weaning. We followed the sample for 655 days; of those, weaning events occurred on 439 days. We observed 89 weaning events (approximately 20% of all possible events) averaging 5.6 observed events/patient. The remaining weaning events were followed via clinical record documentation and in follow-up interviews with clinicians (Happ et al., 2007a; Happ, Swigart, Tate, Hoffman, & Arnold, 2007b).

Results

Weaning progress

The process of weaning from PMV was composed of a series of interrelated weaning events that followed a relapsing, variable, and unsteady course. Weaning progress was the primary theme describing the purpose and overarching clinical goal for the care and communication for these patients. The language used to describe the initiation of weaning from PMV reflected forward movement and improvement in health status. This was also signified by the relocation of the PMV patient from the "acute" wing of the MICU to the step-down or "chronic" wing. Weaning progress was measured in daily time off MV and reduction of ventilator settings. Event analysis revealed the sequence of respiratory therapist behaviors and interactions between respiratory therapist, nurse, and patient in the initiation of ventilator weaning trials (Happ et al., 2004b, p. 245) (Figure 7.2).

Unfortunately, weaning rarely progressed in a predictable and positive direction for these patients on PMV. Only four of the 30 patients showed a steadily progressive weaning pattern. These patients were mostly young (< 60 years old), recovering from acute respiratory distress syndrome, and had few complications or comorbidities affecting other organ systems. Participants, particularly clinicians and families, described the weaning process as long, slow and fraught with "setbacks." Setbacks were recognized as common occurrences, and avoiding setbacks was a major goal in the care of PMV patients.

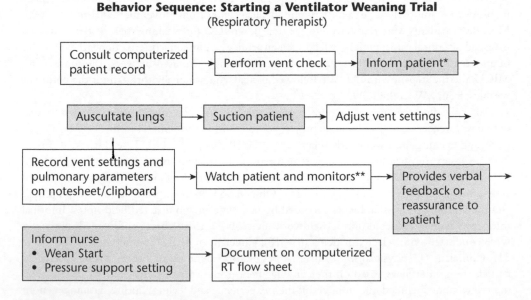

Behavior Sequence: Starting a Ventilator Weaning Trial
(Respiratory Therapist)

Figure 7.2 Ventilator weaning event sequence

Notes:
RT = Respiratory Therapist
Shaded boxes indicate actions that are variable.
*If patient is anxious, RT does not inform, but may ask nurse to administer anxiolytic medication.
**Surveillance time varies depending on patient response.

Source: Happ et al. (2004b).

Ventilator weaning provided a window on to other critical care events and processes of social interaction that potentially influenced the weaning process and trajectory of care and communication during weaning. We followed a variety of analytic lines in understanding the weaning process and potential factors related to weaning progress and setbacks.

Patient involvement in treatment decisions

Communication about treatment decisions was a common, recurrent pattern that occurred amid ventilator weaning progress and setbacks. We noticed that patients were included in decisions about a variety of health care issues and so, we sought to describe and analyze this pattern of communication in more detail. This analytic line was of interest as part of the processes of communication during PMV weaning *and* because this phenomenon was not well described in the ICU treatment decision-making literature.

We defined patient involvement in treatment decisions as "active inclusion of the patient by speaking directly to the patient about the choice, advising the family to speak to the patients, and/or receiving written or nonverbal communication from the patient to clinicians or family members about the choice" (Happ et al., 2007b, p. 363). In addition to data from observations and interviews, transcripts and field notes from observations of 11 family meetings for six patients from this group were included in this analysis. From this dataset, we identified 31 health-related decision-making events involving 12 patients, with nearly 20% (6/31) of the conversations initiated by the patient. Despite clinician and family attempts to involve patients in health-related decisions, much of the patients' input was confirmation or validation of decisions made by others on their behalf. This analysis revealed a practice, by clinicians and family members, of including patients' health-related decision-making during prolonged critical illness. It provided evidence that a larger portion of MV patients may be participating in decisions than has been previously reported. The findings raised clinical ethical questions about the extent to which seriously ill patients with cognitive and communication impairments should be engaged in decision-making about life-sustaining treatments and the preparation or support that clinicians should receive to best engage these vulnerable patients in these decisions (Happ et al., 2007b). This led to a new line in my program of research that is a current mixed methods study of patient involvement in treatment decisions before and after an intervention to improve patient communication in the ICU (Happ, 2010–2012).

Family visitation

Family bedside visitation was another recurrent pattern of communication and psychosocial interaction in the data. We noticed that family members were often present at the bedside during weaning events and that they engaged in some common behaviors and communication during bedside visitation (Happ et al., 2007a). Clinicians alternately described families as helpful and hindering weaning progress. They described family members who became anxious or made the patient anxious by hovering over the patient which resulted in premature discontinuation of the weaning trial. On the other hand, nurses praised individual family members who encouraged or distracted the patient during a weaning trial with "normalizing" talk, reading or hand holding. This raised the question, "What is the effect of family visitation on duration of weaning trials?"

We turned to the clinical record for documentation of family visits and ventilator weaning trial duration. Fortunately, nurses in this setting had meticulously documented family visitation and respiratory therapists had documented ventilator weaning trial start and end times. We created a dichotomous variable for "family visitation during the weaning trial" and applied it to each day of ventilator weaning. Because we did not have granular information about arrival and departure times for family visitation, we used the gross dichotomous categorization of present/absent to characterize family presence at any time during a weaning trial. Descriptive statistics and random coefficient modeling were employed.

Families were present during 46% of weaning trials (when more than one trial occurred in a single day, these were collapsed). Daily weaning trials were significantly longer in duration when families were present (mean = 9.80 hours) than when patients endured ventilator weaning without family visitation (mean = 7.62 hours) ($p < .0001$). On the whole, it appeared that families were more help than hindrance. Certainly, there are several limitations, alternative explanations, and unanswered questions in this analysis. These retrospective data are valid only to the extent that nurses accurately documented family visitation. There were likely errors and omissions in documentation. Nurses may have been effective gatekeepers of visitation by those families whom they assessed as "hindrances" to weaning. Duration and characterization (positive/negative) of family visits may be important variables as well. The significance of these findings rests in the empirical challenge to common clinical notions about the "stress" of family bedside visitation. In addition, the qualitative analysis of observation and interview data provided a schema and behavioral sequence of family bedside behaviors during weaning from PMV that could be applied to future intervention development and research (Happ et al., 2007a).

Bathing and weaning

Bathing during ventilator weaning was another recurrent theme in which clinical wisdom was contradictory and unsupported by evidence. Bathing and hygiene care were conducted within the context of strong personal and social values and beliefs about bathing and cleanliness. Nurses identified hygiene care as central to what they did for PMV patients to ready them for weaning. Family members equated hygiene care with nursing care quality, "a nurse who is more attentive is going to keep her patient clean" (Happ, Tate, Swigart, Divirgilio-Thomas, & Hoffman, 2010, p. S51). However, clinicians, family members, and patients expressed concern that bathing was too tiring for the patient during ventilator weaning trials. Clinicians' opinions of conducting baths during weaning trials were ambiguous and characterized by contradiction. Respiratory therapists often worked around the patient's bath which was scheduled and implemented by the nurse, sometimes delaying the initiation of a ventilator weaning trial until after the bath was completed. Both respiratory therapists and nurses recognized individual variation in patients' responses and tolerance to bathing during PMV weaning trials (Happ et al., 2010).

The ambiguity and contradiction in the qualitative data about the effect of bathing on weaning led us to return to the clinical record documentation with a quantitative question: "What is the association between baths and duration of the ventilator weaning trial?" We also explored the association between patient demographic and clinical characteristics (age, severity of illness, number of hospital days before weaning trials) and the initiation of bathing during the weaning trial. Because nurses were meticulous about documenting baths, we collected data from the clinical record on baths according to three timing categories: baths conducted (1) during weaning trials; (2) one hour before initiation of a weaning trial; and (3) during nocturnal hours (2:00a.m.–5:00a.m.) for each weaning day. Hierarchical linear regression (i.e., random coefficient) modeling was applied (Sereika et al., 2011).

There were 306 bathing events recorded during the time periods of interest; half of these (n = 155) occurred during the nocturnal period and 44% (n = 135) occurred during weaning trials. Considering that 439 weaning days were examined, baths during weaning trials occurred at a rate of 30.7%. Weaning trials in which baths occurred during the trial were of significantly longer duration (11.14 ± 0.82 hours) than those in which bathing did not occur (8.40 ± 0.77 hours) (b = 2.74, SE = .47, t = 5.78, $p < .0001$). Bathing one hour before the weaning trial or during the nighttime hours was not significantly associated with weaning trial duration (Sereika et al., 2011).

Our statistician wondered about a practice pattern in which baths during weaning trials occur later in the weaning trajectory and whether patient characteristics influenced this practice. However, the data showed no clear pattern regarding when the first bath during a weaning trial occurred. In fact, some patients were bathed during their first recorded trial. None of the patient factors hypothesized to influence the initiation of bathing during ventilator weaning trial was significantly associated with time to the first occurrence of a bath during weaning trials. The findings may reflect nurses' clinical judgment about when and if patients could tolerate baths during ventilator weaning trials. Alternatively, decisions may be influenced by clinical convenience and the bath and/or the nurses' presence may have provided comfort, relaxation, and reassurance to patients during weaning from PMV (Sereika et al., 2011).

Secondary analysis

Research trainees with our team followed and expanded additional themes/lines in the analysis. For example, as the longitudinal case analysis developed narratives of individual cases, doctoral student Lauren Broyles noted that several patients had prior mental health (e.g., depression, anxiety), substance abuse, or chronic pain conditions that complicated their care and recovery from dependence on MV. She led an exploration of clinicians' evaluation and management of mental health, substance abuse, and chronic pain conditions in 12 patients with prolonged critical illness from the parent study sample (Broyles et al., 2008). The evaluation and management of mental health, substance abuse, and chronic pain conditions were highly variable and inconsistent across cases. Factors facilitating the evaluation and management of these conditions included family members acting as history keepers, subspecialty consultations, and anticipating alcohol withdrawal. Limited history taking and the use of "cognitive short cuts" were barriers to the evaluation and management of mental health, substance abuse, and chronic pain conditions in the ICU (Broyles et al., 2008).

A single longitudinal case narrative provided data for exploring the transition to palliative care at end of life in the ICU (Crighton et al., 2008b), using dimensional analysis in a single qualitative case study design. Multiple perspectives (clinician, family, patient) and data sources (interviews, observation, family meeting, and clinical record review), including a follow-up contact with the patient's spouse after discharge were included. The case illustrated the process of unifying divergent goals of care, turning points in care and decisional communication, and rationale for the shift from fully aggressive life-sustaining treatment to palliative end-of-life care in the ICU.

Anxiety and agitation were frequently exhibited by patients on PMV and were considered to be barriers to weaning progress; however, events of anxiety and agitation were not limited to ventilator weaning trials. Doctoral student Judith Tate used qualitative secondary analysis to explore events of anxiety and agitation during and outside of ventilator weaning trials. Data were abstracted from a set of uncoded study documents using keywords derived from the literature and clinical experts as indicators of anxiety or agitation. Each event of anxiety or agitation was analyzed using dimensional analysis techniques to identify properties, conditions, context and consequence (Kools, McCarthy, Durham, & Robrecht, 1996). A model of anxiety and agitation in mechanical ventilation was produced from this analysis (Tate, Devito Dabbs, Hoffman, Milbrandt, & Happ. 2012). A case exemplar illustrated the importance of a patient's history and good history-taking in understanding and effectively treating anxiety, agitation and delirium in the ICU setting (Tate & Happ, 2011).

Methodological considerations and challenges

There are several methodological considerations and challenges in conducting ethnography in the ICU setting. Observers in the ICU must establish credibility and rapport with a variety of clinicians, patients and family members. Sensitivity to clinical events, tension, communication styles, and workflow was an essential characteristic. We anticipated and managed patient and family confusion about our role. For example, when patients or family members asked our opinion about a patient's progress or treatment choice, we carefully deflected or turned it around using techniques such as agreement and refocusing: "Yes, I saw that. Tell me what you have been thinking about that."

Ethnographic methods permitted an iterative process of qualitative data collection and analysis, hypothesis (or research question) generation, and additional data collection. This was a powerful and creative process. This method generated an enormous database of over 1100 textual documents and more than eight different spreadsheets (or matrices) (Miles & Huberman, 1994) of combined quantitative and qualitative data. Choosing which analytic lines to follow, who from the team would lead each analytic effort, and the timing (and additional funding) of such analyses were particularly challenging. We had not originally planned quantitative questions or analysis and had not funded the statistical support or micro-analytic data collection and management regarding bathing and family visitation. From this project, we learned to think differently and more proactively when planning this type of study in the future. We recommend including a statistician on the team from the planning stages of an ethnography to analysis.

Reporting and publication of iterative analyses can also be challenging. In the case of the bathing inquiry, reviewers and the journal editor required us to label the work as "secondary analysis" rather than as a mixed methods study and to divide the report into two complementary (qualitative and quantitative) papers. Although we complied with this request to insure publication of the study findings without additional delays, the compromise left an unsatisfactory, altered portrayal of the research approach. On the other hand, dividing the report into two articles provided room to expand the findings sections in ways that would not be possible in a single article.

Qualitative description in intervention development and testing

This section describes the use of qualitative methods in the development and testing of a multi-level intervention to facilitate communication with ventilator-dependent ICU patients. In these studies focused on understanding and improving communication with nonvocal ICU patients, we employed qualitative description for problem description, intervention development, measurement development, and evaluation.

The first study established that seriously ill MV patients had the capacity to communicate with clinician caregivers and family visitors despite the barriers of intubation, MV and life-threatening illness. We used qualitative content analysis of clinical records (document review) of 50 randomly selected MV patients who died in the ICU for topic and method of communication (Happ et al., 2004c). Additional patient characteristics hypothesized to influence communication were collected as well, such as physical restraint and sedation/analgesia use. Most patients (75%) communicated at some time during MV, primarily about pain, other symptoms, feelings or physical needs. They used head nods and mouthing words most often to communicate.

In pilot studies exploring the feasibility of the use of electronic communication devices with MV patients, we used semi-structured observation and conducted semi-formal and debriefing interviews with family members, patients and clinicians about their experience using the electronic speech generating devices (Happ et al., 2004a, 2005). Qualitative content analysis was employed to categorize barriers and facilitators of device use from the interviews and observations. Communication devices were used most often to communicate with family visitors. Poor device positioning, deterioration in patient condition, staff time constraints, staff unfamiliarity with device, and complex message screens were primary barriers to device use.

These pilot studies led to the development and testing of an intervention to improve communication with nonvocal patients during MV treatment in the ICU. The intervention consists of communication skills training for nurses, the provision of augmentative and alternative communication tools and individualized speech language pathologist support. The intervention was tested in a quasi-experimental sequential cohort Study of Patient–nurse Effectiveness with Assisted Communication Strategies (SPEACS) (Happ et al., 2008).

Qualitative methods were employed in several ways in this arm of my research program. We used a quantitative observational approach to measure video-recorded nurse–patient interaction to test the impact of the intervention on nurse–patient communication. This "new" quantitative measure of communication frequency, quality and success was developed and refined using qualitative techniques. For example, communication topic codes and ratings of communication success and level of partner assistance with the communication were refined after coding several sample or "pilot" video recordings. The video recordings, observational field notes, enrollment notes, and intervention logs provided data for case exemplars describing individualized speech language pathologist consultation and intervention during the intervention phase of the SPEACS study (Radtke, Baumann, Garrett, & Happ, 2011). We conducted qualitative analysis of SPEACS study enrollment notes, observation notes, and intervention logs to describe family involvement in the use of augmentative and alternative communication tools (Broyles et al., 2012). We conducted qualitative focus groups to understand the experience and nurse perceptions of communication using the SPEACS intervention program (Radtke, Tate, & Happ, 2012). After receiving the SPEACS training, which they evaluated as generally helpful, nurses still prioritized communication about physical needs with nonvocal patients as most important; however, they recognized the complexity and potential importance of other patient messages. Primary barriers to integrating the SPEACS program into practice included patients' mental status and time constraints. The participants recommended training more or all of the ICU staff in basic communication skills with nonvocal patients.

Secondary analysis was applied to patient–caregiver communication interactions in the video recordings and clinical record documentation for a more granular description and analysis of symptom identification and treatment during MV (Campbell & Happ, 2010). We started with an existing symptom checklist instrument, and used an iterative process of adding symptom definitions and qualitative content identifying new symptoms to develop an instrument that could be reliably applied to video-recorded observations and clinical record documentation (Happ et al., 2011). We have also applied qualitative analysis to a subsample of the video recordings to explore nurse gaze in the interaction between nurses and nonvocal patients, explicating three types of nurse gaze: hearing, assessing, and technical doing (Crighton et al., 2008a). Students continue to use the SPEACS dataset for additional analyses to describe nurse–patient interaction behaviors (Nilsen, 2011–2013) and to examine the progression of electronic communication device use over time (Nock & Happ, 2011).

Our team continues to use qualitative techniques in translational intervention studies. For example, we recently conducted focus groups with 33 nurses who participated in the SPEACS-2 project, which implemented a one-hour online nurse training program, provision of communication materials, and speech language pathologist consultation in six ICUs in two University of Pittsburgh Medical Center hospitals. These results may help explain variation among ICUs in intervention enactment. We also use qualitative description in a complementary mode in intervention fidelity monitoring (Song et al., 2010a) and to analyze survey comments.

Methodological considerations and challenges

Qualitative research either nested within or as a follow-up to an intervention study can provide insights into components of the intervention that work and those that require refinement. The researcher must carefully determine timing of qualitative data collection to avoid interfering with or affecting the intervention or outcome measurement (Song et al., 2010b). Data collection options include interviews, focus groups, responses to open-ended questions or comments on surveys, or recording comments and feedback from clinicians, patients and families (i.e., constituents).

Conclusion

This chapter has illustrated a qualitative and mixed methods program of research in the care of ventilator-dependent adults. The program moved from descriptive, theory-building research to intervention development and testing in an iterative process that includes qualitative feedback and program evaluation. Research, practice and educational impact of the program are intertwined.

Research impact

This line of inquiry has been sustained with external funding for more than 15 years. Research in this topical area is growing and is spawning studies of augmentative and alternative communication devices for the voiceless hospitalized patient (Rodriguez, Rowe, & Koeppel, 2012). It is important to note that in addition to the work presented from my program of research, there is a large body of qualitative studies and personal accounts of the experience of mechanical ventilation during critical illness (Bergbom et al., 1999; Bergbom & Askwall, 2000; Bergbom-Engberg & Haljamäe, 1989; Bergbom-Engberg & Haljamäe, 1993; Carroll, 2004, 2007; Eriksson et al., 2011; Fitch, 1989; Frace, 1982; Granberg et al., 1998; Gries & Fernsler, 1988; Hallenberg et al., 1990; Happ, 2000a; Hupcey, 2000; Jablonski, 1994; Jenny & Logan, 1994, 1996; Karlsson et al., 2012; Logan & Jenny, 1997; Menzel, 1998; Patak et al., 2004; Pennock et al., 1994; Rier, 2000; Riggio et al., 1982; Ringdal et al., 2006; Robillard, 1994). The list includes nurse researchers and social scientists, particularly from Europe, who have programs of research centered on the experience of patients and family members during critical illness and MV. The problem of voicelessness has been embedded in these studies but is recently becoming more visible as a central and problematic feature of the MV experience (Carroll, 2007; Karlsson et al., 2012). The quantity of studies suggests that a qualitative metasynthesis may be needed (Sandelowski & Barroso, 2007).

Clinical practice impact

The clinical practice impact of this work is closely linked to the educational and research impact. The SPEACS and SPEACS-2 studies provided education to ICU nurses and communication tools for patient use in eight different intensive care units each over periods as long as two years. Nurses were introduced to speech language pathologist consultation and support for patient communication in the ICU setting. We are currently working with the UPMC Health System to sustain and expand these resources for care and communication in the ICUs.

Qualitative research in combination with evidence on the incidence and long-term effects of psychological and physical symptoms during prolonged acute MV, termed post-intensive care syndrome (Davidson et al., 2012) has finally mobilized the critical care scientific community regarding the need to improve the experience of patients and families (Bienvenu & Neufeld, 2011; Society for Critical Care Medicine, 2011).

Educational impact

The educational impact of this work has been in both the methodological and practice arenas. We have published several papers describing methods used in this program of research (Broyles et al., 2008; Haidet et al., 2009; Happ & Kagan, 2001; Happ et al., 2004b). More than 350 critical care nurses have received Basic Communication Skills Training through the SPEACS and SPEACS-2 continuing education courses. The SPEACS training course and case exemplars from the SPEACS study were used to develop a training module for the AACN online continuing education program, *Best Practices for Elder Care Course* (Radtke et al., 2009). Our communication assessment and intervention tips were included in the Geriatric Nursing Education Consortium module on Assessment and Management of Older Adults with Complex Illness in the Critical Care Unit (Balas et al., 2007–2009) and in a podcast of that program (Aselage et al., 2010). Future educational plans include incorporating the SPEACS training program into undergraduate and graduate curricula locally and nationally and providing the SPEACS-2 training program as an online continuing education offering available to nurses nationally and internationally.

References

Aselage, M., Balas, M. C., Casey, C. M. & Happ, M. B. (2010). Assessment and management of older adults with complex illness in the critical care unit. *GNEC Geriatric Nurse Podcast.* Available at: http:/consultgerim.org/resources/media/?vid_id=10957786#player_container.

Balas, M. C., Casey, C., & Happ, M. B. (2007–2009). Assessment and management of older adults with complex illness in the critical care unit. Paper presented at the AACN/John A. Hartford Foundation Geriatric Nursing Education Consortium (GNEC) Faculty Development Conference.

Bergbom, I., & Askwall, A. (2000). The nearest and dearest: A lifeline for ICU patients. *Intensive & Critical Care Nursing, 16,* 384–395.

Bergbom, I., Svensson, C., Berggren, E., & Kamsula, M. (1999). Patients' and relatives' opinions and feelings about diaries kept by nurses in an intensive care unit: Pilot study. *Intensive & Critical Care Nursing, 15,* 185–191.

Bergbom-Engberg, I., & Haliamäe, H. (1989). Assessment of patients' experience of discomforts during respirator therapy. *Critical Care Medicine, 17,* 1068–1072.

Bergbom-Engberg, I., & Haliamäe, H. (1993). The communication process with ventilator patients in the ICU as perceived by the nursing staff. *Intensive & Critical Care Nursing, 9,* 40–47.

Bienvenu, O. J., & Neufeld, K. J. (2011). Post-traumatic stress disorder in medical settings: Focus on the critically ill. *Current Psychiatry Reports, 13,* 3–9.

Broyles, L. M., Colbert, A. M., Tate, J. A., Swigart, V. A., & Happ, M. B. (2008). Clinicians' evaluation and management of mental health, substance abuse, and chronic pain conditions in the intensive care unit. *Critical Care Medicine, 36,* 87–93.

Broyles, L. M., Tate, J. A., & Happ, M. B. (2012). Use of augmentative and alternative communication by family members in the ICU. *American Journal of Critical Care, 21,* e21–e32.

Campbell, G. B., & Happ, M. B. (2010). Symptom identification in the chronically critically ill. *AACN Advanced Critical Care, 21,* 64–79.

Carroll, S. (2004). Nonvocal ventilated patients' perceptions of being understood. *Western Journal of Nursing Research 26,* 85–103.

Carroll, S. (2007). Silent, slow lifeworld: The communication experience of nonvocal ventilated patients. *Qualitative Health Research, 17,* 1165–1177.

Crighton, M. H., Coyne, B. M., Tate, J., Swigart, V., & Happ, M. B. (2008b). Transitioning to end-of-life care in the intensive care unit: a case of unifying divergent desires. *Cancer Nursing, 31*, 478–484.

Crighton, M., Swigart, V., & Happ, M. B. (2008a). The role of gaze in nurse–patient interactions in the ICU. Paper presented at CANS 2008 State of the Science Congress, Washington, DC.

Daly, B. J., Rudy, E. B., Thompson, K. S., & Happ, M. B. (1991). Development of a special care unit for chronically critically ill patients. *Heart & Lung, 20*, 45–51.

Davidson, J. E., Jones, C., & Bienvenu, O. J. (2012). Family response to critical illness: Postintensive care syndrome-family. *Critical Care Medicine, 40*, 618–624.

Eriksson, T., Bergbom, I., & Lindahl, B. (2011). The experiences of patients and their families of visiting whilst in an intensive care unit: A hermeneutic interview study. *Intensive & Critical Care Nursing, 27*, 60–6.

Fetterman, D. (1998). *Ethnography: Step-by-step*, Thousand Oaks, CA: Sage Publishing.

Fitch, M. (1989). The patient's reaction to ventilation. *Canadian Critical Care Nursing Journal, 6*, 13–16.

Frace, R. M. (1982). Mechanical ventilation: The patient's viewpoint. *Today's OR Nurse, 4*, 16–21.

Glaser, B. G. (1978). *Theoretical sensitivity*. Mill Valley, CA: The Sociological Press.

Granberg, A., Bergbom-Engberg, I., & Lundberg, D. (1998). Patients' experience of being critically ill or severely injured and cared for in an intensive care unit in relation to the ICU syndrome. Part I. *Intensive & Critical Care Nursing, 14*, 294–307.

Gries, M. L., & Fernsler, J. (1988). Patient perceptions of the mechanical ventilation experience. *Focus on Critical Care, 15*, 52–59.

Haidet, K. K., Tate, J., Divirgilio-Thomas, D., Kolanowski, A., & Happ, M. B. (2009). Methods to improve reliability of video-recorded behavioral data. *Research in Nursing & Health, 32*, 465–474.

Hallenberg, B., Bergbom-Engberg, I., & Haljamäe, H. (1990). Patients' experiences of postoperative respirator treatment: Influence of anaesthetic and pain treatment regimens. *Acta Anaesthesiologica Scandinavica, 34*, 557–562.

Happ, M. B. (1998a). Treatment interference in acutely and critically ill adults. *American Journal of Critical Care, 7*, 224–235.

Happ, M. (1998b). Treatment interference in critically ill older adults. PhD doctoral dissertation, University of Pennsylvania. Paper AAI9829911. http://repository.upenn.edu/dissertations/AAI9829911.

Happ, M. B. (2000a). Interpretation of nonvocal behavior and the meaning of voicelessness in critical care. *Social Science & Medicine, 50*, 1247–1255.

Happ, M. B. (2000b). Preventing treatment interference: The nurse's role in maintaining technologic devices. *Heart & Lung, 29*, 60–69.

Happ, M. B. (2002). Patient 67: An 80 year-old man in respiratory failure who repeatedly removes catheters and tubes. In J. Heffner, & I. Byock (Eds.), *Palliative and end of life pearls*. Philadelphia, PA: Hanley & Belfus, Inc.

Happ, M. B. (2010–2012). Patient participation in treatment decisions before and after a program to facilitate patient communication in the ICU. University of Pittsburgh School of Nursing: Greenwall Foundation Kornfeld Program on Bioethics and Patient Care.

Happ, M. B., Dabbs, A. D., Tate, J., Hricik, A., & Erlen, J. (2006). Exemplars of mixed methods data combination and analysis. *Nursing Research, 55*, S43–S49.

Happ, M. B., & Kagan, S. H. (2001). Methodological considerations for grounded theory research in critical care settings. *Nursing Research, 50*, 188–192.

Happ, M. B., Radtke, J., Campbell, G., Houze, M., & Sereika, S. (2011). Observational measurement of symptom identification and treatment in ICU. Poster presented at Symptom Mechanisms, Measurement, and Management NINR/NIH-CC Joint Conference, Bethesda, MD.

Happ, M. B., Roesch. K., & Garrett, K. (2004a). Electronic voice-output communication aids for temporarily nonspeaking patients in a medical intensive care unit: A feasibility study. *Heart & Lung, 33*, 92–101.

Happ, M. B., Roesch, T. K., & Kagan, S. H. (2005). Patient communication following head and neck cancer surgery: A pilot study using electronic speech-generating devices. *Oncology Nursing Forum, 32*, 1179–1187.

Happ, M. B., Sereika, S., Garrett, K., & Tate, J. (2008). Use of the quasi–experimental sequential cohort design in the Study of Patient–Nurse Effectiveness with Assisted Communication Strategies (SPEACS). *Contemporary Clinical Trials, 29*, 801–808.

Happ, M. B., Swigart, V. A., Tate, J. A., Arnold, R. M., Sereika, S. M., & Hoffman, L. A. (2007a). Family presence and surveillance during weaning from prolonged mechanical ventilation. *Heart & Lung, 36*, 47–57.

Happ, M. B., Swigart, V., Tate, J., & Crighton, M. H. (2004b). Event analysis techniques. *Advances in Nursing Science*, *27*, 239–248.

Happ, M. B., Tate, J. A., Swigart, V. A., Divirgilio-Thomas, D., & Hoffman, L. A. (2010). Wash and wean: Bathing patients undergoing weaning trials during prolonged mechanical ventilation. *Heart & Lung*, *39*, S47–S56.

Happ, M. B., Swigart, V. A., Tate, J. A., Hoffman, L. A., & Arnold, R. M. (2007b). Patient involvement in health-related decisions during prolonged critical illness. *Research in Nursing & Health*, *30*, 361–372.

Happ, M. B., Tuite, P., Dobbin, K., Divirgilio-Thomas, D., & Kitutu, J. (2004c). Communication ability, method, and content among nonspeaking nonsurviving patients treated with mechanical ventilation in the intensive care unit. *American Journal of Critical Care*, *13*, 210–218; quiz 219–220.

Higgins, P. A., & Daly, B. J. (1999). Research methodology issues related to interviewing the mechanically ventilated patient. *Western Journal of Nursing Research*, *21*, 773–784.

Hoffman, L. A., Happ, M. B., Scharfenberg, C., Divirgilio-Thomas, D., & Tasota, F. J. (2004). Perceptions of physicians, nurses, and respiratory therapists about the role of acute care nurse practitioners. *American Journal of Critical Care*, *13*, 480–488.

Hoffman, L. A., Tasota, F. J., Zullo, T. G., Scharfenberg, C., & Donahoe, M. P. (2005). Outcomes of care managed by an acute care nurse practitioner/attending physician team in a subacute medical intensive care unit. *American Journal of Critical Care*, *14*, 121–130; quiz 131–132.

Hupcey, J. E. (2000). Feeling safe: The psychosocial needs of ICU patients. *Journal of Nursing Scholarship*, *32*, 361–367.

Jablonski, R. (1994). The experience of being mechanically ventilated. *Qualitative Health Research*, *4*, 186–207.

Jenny, J., & Logan, J. (1994). Promoting ventilator independence: A grounded theory perspective. *Dimensions of Critical Care Nursing*, *13*, 29–37.

Jenny, J., & Logan, J. (1996). Caring and comfort metaphors used by patients in critical care. *Image, the Journal of Nursing Scholarship*, *28*, 349–352.

Karlsson, V., Bergbom, I., & Forsberg, A. (2012). The lived experiences of adult intensive care patients who were conscious during mechanical ventilation: A phenomenological-hermeneutic study. *Intensive & Critical Care Nursing*, *28*, 6–15.

Knaus, W. A., Wagner, D. P., Draper, E. A., Zimmerman, J. E., Bergner, M., Bastos, P. G., et al. (1991). The APACHE III prognostic system: Risk prediction of hospital mortality for critically ill hospitalized adults. *Chest*, *100*, 1619–1636.

Kools, S., McCarthy, M., Durham, R., & Robrecht, L. (1996). Dimensional analysis: Broadening the conception of grounded theory. *Qualitative Health Research*, *6*, 312–330.

Logan, J., & Jenny, J. (1997). Qualitative analysis of patients' work during mechanical ventilation and weaning. *Heart & Lung*, *26*, 140–147.

Menzel, L. K. (1998). Factors related to the emotional responses of intubated patients to being unable to speak. *Heart & Lung*, *27*, 245–252.

Miles, M., & Huberman, A. (1994). *Qualitative data analysis: An expanded source book*. Thousand Oaks, CA: Sage.

Nilsen, M. L. (2011–2013). *Interaction behaviors effect on nursing care quality of older adults in the ICU*. Pittsburgh: University of Pittsburgh School of Nursing, National Institute of Nursing Research. F31 NR012856.

Nock, R., & Happ, M. B. (2011). AAC use in nonvocal patients in the ICU setting. Poster presented at Eastern Nursing Research Society 23rd Annual Scientific Sessions, Philadelphia, PA.

Patak, L., Gawlinski, A., Fung, N. I., Doering, L., & Berg, J. (2004). Patients' reports of health care practitioner interventions that are related to communication during mechanical ventilation. *Heart & Lung*, *33*, 308–320.

Pelto, P., & Pelto, G. (1978). *Anthropologic research: The structure of inquiry*. London: Cambridge University Press.

Pennock, B., Crawshaw, L., Maher, T., Price, T., & Kaplan, P. (1994). Distressful events in the ICU as perceived by patients recovering from coronary artery bypass surgery. *Heart & Lung*, *23*, 323–327.

Radtke, J. V., Baumann, B. M., Garrett, K. L., & Happ, M. B. (2011). Listening to the voiceless patient: Case reports in assisted communication in the intensive care unit. *Journal of Palliative Medicine*, *14*, 791–795.

Radtke, J. V., Nilsen, M., & Happ, M. B. (2009). Case study: Mrs. Moore – module 7. *Best Practices for Elder Care Course* American Association of Critical Care Nurses online (updated 2011).

Radtke, J. V., Tate, J. A., & Happ, M. B. (2012). Nurses' perceptions of communication training in the ICU. *Intensive & Critical Care Nursing*, *28*, 16–25.

Rier, D. (2000). The missing voice of the critically ill: A medical sociologist's first-hand account. *Sociology of Health and Illness*, *22*, 68–93.

Riggio, R. E., Singer, R. D., Hartman, K., & Sneider, R. (1982). Psychological issues in the care of critically-ill respirator patients: Differential perceptions of patients, relatives, and staff. *Psychological Reports*, *51*, 363–369.

Ringdal, M., Johansson, L., Lundberg, D., & Bergbom, I. (2006). Delusional memories from the intensive care unit: Experienced by patients with physical trauma. *Intensive & Critical Care Nursing*, *22*, 346–354.

Robillard, A. (1994). Communication problems in the intensive care unit. *Qualitative Sociology*, *17*, 383–395.

Rodriguez, C. S., Rowe, M., & Koeppel, B. (2012). Sudden speechlessness: Representing the needs of hospitalized patients. *Journal of Medical Speech-Language Pathology*, *20*(2), 44–53.

Sandelowski, M., & Barroso, J. (2007). *Handbook for synthesizing qualitative research*. New York: Springer.

Sereika, S. M., Tate, J. A., Divirgilio-Thomas, D., Hoffman, L. A., Swigart, V. A., Broyles, L., Roesch, T., & Happ, M. B. (2011). The association between bathing and weaning trial duration. *Heart & Lung*, *40*, 41–48.

Society for Critical Care Medicine (2011). Post intensive care syndrome (webcast).

Song, M.-K., Happ, M. B., & Sandelowski, M. (2010a). Development of a tool to assess fidelity to a psycho-educational intervention. *Journal of Advanced Nursing*, *66*, 673–682.

Song, M.-K., Sandelowski, M., & Happ, M. B. (2010b). Current practices and emerging trends in conducting mixed-methods intervention studies in the health sciences. In A. Tashakkori, & C. Teddlie (Eds.), *Handbook of mixed methods research* (2nd ed.). Thousand Oaks, CA: Sage.

Tate, J. A., Devito Dabbs, A., Hoffman, L. A., Milbrandt, E., & Happ, M. B. (2012). Anxiety and agitation in mechanically ventilated patients. *Qualitative Health Research*, *22*, 157–173.

Tate, J. A., & Happ, M. B. (2011). Neurocognitive problems in critically ill older adults: The importance of history. *Geriatric Nursing*, *32*, 285–287.

Teasdale, G., & Jennett, B. (1974). Assessment of coma and impaired consciousness. A practical scale. *Lancet*, *2*, 81–84.

8

Cultural aspects of Latino early childhood obesity

Lauren Clark, Susan L. Johnson,
Mary E. O'Connor, and Jane Lassetter

Introduction

The problem of Latino childhood obesity[1] is well known, and experts agree that the sooner it is addressed in a child's life, the better. Strong evidence from nationwide studies suggests that obesity begins in infancy for Mexican Americans. National data demonstrate the dramatic increase in weight-for-recumbent length above the 95th percentile (using the NCHS growth chart) among Mexican American children between National Health and Nutrition Examination Survey (NHANES) and the Third National Health and Nutrition Examination Survey (NHANES III) (Ogden et al., 2006). High rates of childhood obesity affect the long-term health potential of children, since childhood obesity tracks into adulthood—the older the obese child, the greater the chance he or she will become an obese adult (Guo, Roche, Chumlea, Gardner, & Siervogel, 1994; Whitaker, 1997). Despite the well-documented problem of Latino early childhood obesity (Ogden, Flegal, Carroll, & Johnson, 2002), less is known about Latino family and community cultural understandings of early childhood obesity and preferred approaches to support healthy early childhood feeding, nutrition, and weight status.

For clinicians, the challenge of caring for overweight children begins at diagnosis. Standards for body mass index (BMI) to classify overweight and obesity are clear (Ogden, Carroll, Kit, & Flegal, 2012). Once diagnosed, clinicians can access a variety of evidence-based resources to guide their treatment plans and enlist the cooperation of families (e.g., Annesi, Pierce, Bonaparte, & Smith, 2009; Foster et al., 2008; Holt, Wooldridge, Story, & Sofka, 2011; National Association of Pediatric Nurse Practitioners, 2006). Although diagnosis and treatment initiation are challenging and complex processes for clinicians, prevention of childhood obesity is arguably more difficult. Helping families to understand the changes in lifestyles that would prevent obesity and incorporating such a discussion during a short office visit remain a challenge for pediatric clinicians. Effective childhood obesity prevention will depend on qualitative research to fill gaps of understanding about Latino families' cultural values and patterns of infant feeding that produce obese children. Qualitative knowledge about how Latino families rear children who are of normal weight would be more useful, as the strengths identified in those families and their social networks could be a basis for helping other at-risk families.

The purpose of our research was to explore the criteria used by Latino mothers, fathers, and grandparents to identify children from birth to 18 months of age who are normal weight, overweight, or obese; their descriptions of those children; and their preferred approaches for reinforcing childcare and feeding to achieve an "ideal" or healthy infant body shape. Specifically, we framed our research questions to address the kinds of behaviors, foods, and feeding patterns identified by parents and grandparents as contributing to early childhood obesity in their communities. We also investigated what Latino parents and grandparents consider to be appropriate interventions for infants or children who would be considered "obese" or "overweight" in their community. To accomplish this, we developed a methodology to help parents describe their children's weight and their attributions of parenting skills in caring for overweight, normal and underweight infants.

Background

We use the term "Latino" to refer to Mexican American and Mexican immigrant families who participated in our research. We identified a community, which we call Los Alamos Verdes, known to have a mixture of Mexican immigrants and older, established Mexican American families. One of our key informants referred to the area by its local name of "Little Mexico." The typical pattern of settlement in the area is characterized by single young adults and young families immigrating from Mexico to live with extended lateral kin. Families and friends from the same town in Mexico tend to reside together, especially during the early months after their arrival. Few of these young families have access to local grandparents, although they telephone Mexico occasionally and send remittances regularly. A major Catholic church is headquartered in Los Alamos Verdes, and offers a familiar focal point for new immigrants. Community life is characterized by busy schedules of lower-income young families settling into a routine of work and family life. New residents find work nearby, have children, and use the community health center for low-cost primary care. Eventually young families mature and some move to more established communities nearby.

Of the patients using the low-income urban community health center clinic where we recruited many study participants, more than 90% of immigrant families were Mexican (Young & O'Connor, 2005). Even so, the clinical population demonstrated intracultural variation related to an urban or rural upbringing in Mexico, the length of residence in the US, processes of acculturation experienced in the US, and the specific kinds of syncretism they create as they merge and adapt their cultural lifeways over time. This kind of intracultural variation does not overshadow core cultural values about parenting and generations of cultural knowledge about feeding infants. Each family had a somewhat unique approach to child feeding, but an identifiable set of common cultural beliefs and values about child growth and infant feeding is also identifiable. Our clinical experience and a history of ethnographies on Latino child and family health suggest that Mexican Americans share historically rooted expectations for health care and early childhood growth and feeding (Alexander, Sherman, & Clark, 1991; Clark, 2002; Clark & Redman, 2007; Kay, 1977).

Los Alamos Verdes has experienced patterns of health disparity common in Latino communities such as higher rates of obesity, diabetes, and complications from diabetes in comparison to the national average (Vega, Rodriguez, & Gruskin, 2009). Type II diabetes among adults, which is associated with obesity, affects nearly every family. Complications of diabetes (such as amputations and kidney failure) were common, according to our informants who readily linked obesity to these outcomes. Even with high levels of need, there are few community-level, culturally competent interventions available. Clinical care of individuals already affected with diabetic complications is most common, rather than community-wide prevention efforts geared toward those who are at risk but not yet overweight, obese, or diabetic. Our overall goal was to provide a background of ethnographic data that could inform the development of new clinical and community practices specific to the cultural needs of the local Latino population.

Methodology

As a team of clinician-researchers, we were familiar with a community we will call "Los Alamos Verdes," a geographically identifiable area in the Denver, Colorado, metropolitan area. We had worked with families in the area for about two decades each as a nurse-anthropologist (LC), pediatric nutritionist (SJ), and pediatrician (MO). Another team member joined us near the end of our work (JL), extending some of our methods in her research. Our ethnographic work reported here spanned several studies and took place over 15 years. For many nurse-anthropologists, funded research is a slice in a long trajectory of ethnographic fieldwork conducted over time and across several initiatives. All of our research was conducted with the approval of the appropriate human subjects review boards.

Design

The purpose of our focused ethnography was to describe the cultural constructions of inter-generational Latino parents and grandparents in Los Alamos Verdes about food, feeding, child growth, and childrearing, and how they acted on those understandings.

Our focused ethnography incorporated a combination of participant observation in the community, focus groups, and semi-structured individual interviews with mothers, fathers, grandmothers, and grandfathers. Another aspect of the ethnography described elsewhere included interviews with biomedical pediatric health care providers about their views of the cultural aspects of Latino child health and obesity prevention in Los Alamos Verdes (Johnson, Clark, Goree, O'Connor, & Zimmer, 2008). We also conducted a related study with *curanderos* who were knowledgeable about Latino family health and nutrition (Clark, Bunik, & Johnson, 2010).

Sampling

To understand Los Alamos Verdes, we sampled social situations and clinical care settings over time. For the focused ethnography with parents and grandparents, we set our inclusion criteria such that parent/grandparent participants all had a child/grandchild 18 months of age or younger. They all lived in or near Los Alamos Verdes. Acculturation of participants was measured on the five-point Short Acculturation Scale for Hispanics (SASH) (Marín, Sabogal, Marín, Otero-Sabogal, & Perez-Stable, 1987). By definition, cultural knowledge is widely shared among parents and grandparents, regardless of parents' own or their children's weight status, so inclusion criteria did not select for an overweight sample. To recruit parents and grandparents, we worked with health care providers at two clinics and two affiliated Women, Infants, and Children Supplemental Nutrition Program (WIC) programs. Providers briefly explained the study purpose and encouraged prospective participants to meet us in the waiting room for more information. We also attended weekly public health immunization clinics where we described our study in English and Spanish to waiting parents and encouraged waiting parents/grandparents to approach us if they were interested in learning more about the study.

Methods

A cornerstone of ethnography is fieldwork, characterized by participant observation and formal and informal interviews recorded in fieldnotes and transcripts (Spradley, 1980; Angrosino, 2007). Informal conversations were easily guided toward our topic of interest, and these interviews included conversations with the nuns at the Catholic church, visits with neighborhood women in their homes, and discussions with *curanderos* about their views of local health concerns. Formal interviews followed an interview guide designed for a focus group or individual interview.

Participant observation led us to attend mass, baptisms, and community fiestas at the local Catholic church. We subscribed to the local Spanish-language newspaper, listened to Spanish radio stations, and periodically visited *botanicas* and *tiendas* (local herb shops and stores) to identify key informants in the community (such as the *curanderos*) and to observe the range of child health products and parents' shopping behaviors. We attended neighborhood meetings to observe how people collectively identified and addressed neighborhood concerns. *Fieldnotes* about our experiences recorded how people in Los Alamos Verdes talked about childhood obesity, in particular, and other health issues. Our fieldnotes also contained reflections about how behaviors we observed differed from or expanded on what participants said were their usual behaviors. Our fieldwork and participant observation provided complementary background data, offered a wider context to frame our results, and provided a means of informal member-checking findings from focus groups and interviews in successive conversations.

Focus groups were constituted to explore specific questions about shared cultural knowledge informing early childhood feeding practices and child body shape and size preferences. Focus groups are well suited for investigating complex behaviors and motivations when variation among group members is likely high (Morgan & Krueger, 1993). Participant observation and clinical experience primed us to develop questions to explore specific cultural aspects of childhood obesity (see Table 8.1).

Participants included 60 parents and grandparents and 38 health care providers across 14 focus groups. We gave each parent a $25 gift certificate to a local grocery store chain. Providers were offered lunch before the focus groups. Gender-specific focus groups were arranged for parents and grandparents. These consisted of mothers/grandmothers and fathers/grandfathers. These groups explored gendered knowledge in households and avoided the gender-based dominance possible in mixed-gender focus groups. Generation-specific groups were hosted with mothers only to explore tensions between genders and generations. Focus groups were hosted at libraries and clinics located on bus routes, and participants were invited to join either English or Spanish groups.

A series of six *silhouettes* of a Latino child approximately 9 months of age and of increasing adiposity were commissioned (Figure 8.1). In the silhouettes, the first child depicted appears considerably underweight and the sixth child depicted appears very overweight. We used the silhouettes in focus groups to open discussion about the topic of linguistic indicators of childhood health and the social value of different body sizes and levels of adiposity. We also asked projective questions about the kind of family the infant of each body size might have, and how the lightest and heaviest infants were cared for in their families. Fetterman (1989) refers to visual images as "can openers" that increase familiarity among focus group members and elicit projective responses from them.

Our silhouettes maintained key features of earlier silhouettes developed by Kramer and colleagues (1983). All silhouettes used the same infant face, size, shape, and posture. The boys had a blue diaper, and the girls had a pink diaper and a pink hair bow. We modified the original string of silhouettes by providing colored shading to represent Mexican American infants' skin

Table 8.1 Basic outline of focus group questions for parents/grandparents about childhood feeding and weight

Topic	Specific questions and prompts
Introductions, consent process, ground rules of focus group	
What characteristics do parents and grandparents identify as indicators of obesity and overweight?	Show the infant silhouettes Start with the smallest baby • What **words** would you apply to this baby? How would you describe this baby? (probe for both physical descriptors and for behavioral or personality descriptors) • If this were your baby's body how would you describe your baby? • How would your doctor or nurse talk about your baby? • How would you prefer that they talk about your baby's weight status? • What would you think of a mother who has a baby that looks like this? Repeat the questions with the largest baby Looking at all the baby drawings, at what point is a baby too big to be healthy? Which picture would represent that? Show the growth chart. Have you seen this kind of a chart before? Explain what it tracks with basic information. Show the obese child growth chart. Explain that it shows the child gaining weight at a rate faster than the child's growth in height • If a doctor or nurse showed you this growth chart, what would you think?
What kinds of behaviors, foods and feeding patterns or other environmental situations are identified by parents as contributing to early childhood obesity in the community?	Why do you think some children are overweight and others are not? How has your world changed since you were a child (in terms of food and activity?) How do you think this affects children? Do you think your child might become overweight one day? Is there anything you can do to keep your child from becoming overweight? How do you know when babies are hungry? How do you know when babies are full? Scenario: Let me tell you at story about a very nice family. There was a mother, Maria, a father, Jose, and three little girls. They lived with Maria's mother. The grandmother watched the girls during the day while Maria worked cleaning houses. The father played with the little girls every night after work, and took them outside on their tricycles. They got together on the weekends with their family for barbecues and birthday parties, but during the week the family ate together in the morning and the evening. The youngest girl, Claudia, turned 1 year old and weighed 32 pounds. The doctor was very concerned, and asked the mother what was causing this incredible weight gain for the baby.

Table 8.1 Continued

Topic	Specific questions and prompts
	Was the doctor right to be worried about Claudia's weight?
	What do you think was going on with the family that Claudia was gaining so much weight?
	How did the grandmother and the dad fit in? In what ways were they involved in managing children's feeding and weight?
	What advice would you give to Maria about the baby?
Clarification and Summary	

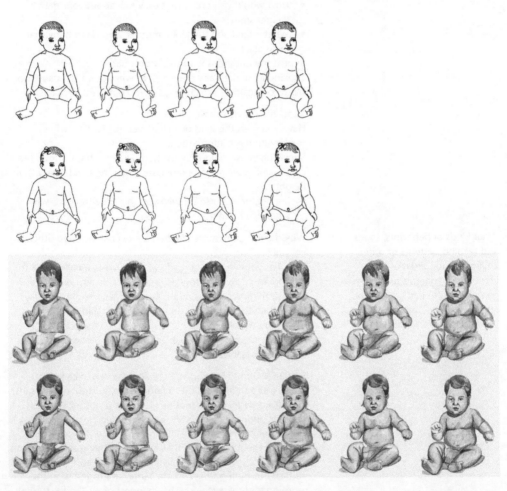

Figure 8.1 Infant silhouettes developed by Kramer, Barr, Leduc Boisjoly, and Pless (1983, p. 331) (above) and those commissioned for this research study

Source: Reprinted with permission from Elsevier Limited.

pigment and suggest curvature and form. After the first focus group we learned that the heaviest infant depicted was not viewed as very large at all. As a result, we added two new drawings at the heavier end of the weight continuum. These heaviest infants facilitated discussions about the value and meaning of very large infant bodies, eliciting parents' and grandparents' linguistic indicators and attributions about infants and caregiving relationships. The silhouettes sparked participants to share stories of the kinds of families, particularly the kinds of mothers, who reared children at the weight extremes.

Semi-structured interviews included the technique of *freelisting* (Weller & Romney, 1988). The rationale underlying freelisting is that cultural knowledge is, by definition, shared. Another assumption is that cultural knowledge is not equivalent to scientific knowledge, and parents and professionals can have different (but not "wrong") knowledge structures. Freelisting suited our research purpose by systematically eliciting emic knowledge of Latino early childhood obesity risk factors and protective factors. Freelisting matched the needs of a clinic-based interview setting. Lengthy, private individual interviews were impractical given parents'/grandparents' time constraints and the clinics' space constraints. Freelisting can be done in a short period of time and without a tape recorder. We conducted the interviews ourselves, and also hired trained, bilingual, bicultural women of childbearing or middle age who were familiar with Los Alamos Verdes to collect freelists.

The freelisting interview began by asking the parent or grandparent their thoughts about why Mexican or Mexican American children are overweight. This could be a confrontational question. To diffuse any reference to their own children, we framed the question as a general one, and asked for their expert opinion about Mexican children in their acquaintance generally. The participant would consider this question then begin talking about the contributors to overweight among local children. The researcher would transcribe each answer verbatim (in either or both English and Spanish), paying careful attention to the exact words and the order of the reasons listed. After the participant stopped listing answers, the researcher would provide a prompt, such as "Can you think of any more reasons?" Other elicitation techniques included nonspecific prompting, reading back the list of items and asking if there are more, and using listed items as semantic cues for other, similar items (Brewer, 2002). If the participant continued freelisting, the researcher would continue to transcribe the answers as before. The probes for more responses would continue until the participant said that his/her list was complete and he/she had nothing more to add.

The second freelisting interview question was "What are some behaviors that protect Mexican and Mexican American children from becoming overweight?" Again, the researcher would listen, transcribe verbatim, and probe until the participant said the list was complete. Then the participant would add stories or information she or he considered pertinent. This part of the conversation was tape-recorded. After the interviews, participants were given a small gift ($10 long-distance telephone card or grocery store gift card) and thanked for their time.

Data analysis

Interviews and focus groups were transcribed. Fieldnotes were also entered into the dataset, either appended to the transcripts or as separate documents. The silhouettes were used in focus groups to elicit discussion, and those data were also part of the focus group transcript submitted for analysis. Analysis of discourse and narrative was managed with a qualitative data management program, AtlasTi (Scientific Software 6.2, 2010) in the original language (English or Spanish) of the interview. A different software program, Anthropac (Analytic Technologies, 1996), was used to analyze freelisting. One of us (LC) inductively developed a coding dictionary to index segments of text that referred directly or more obliquely to our interest in the cultural and family context of childhood feeding, growth, and the development of overweight. By indexing each segment of data on the same topic with the same codeword in the AtlasTi software, we identified hierarchies of meaning and categories of analysis. Focus group transcripts, interviews, and fieldnotes were analyzed for themes and patterns to build evidence across the different aspects of the study (Carey, 1994; Morse, 2001).

Analysis of freelists was handled in a separate analysis based on two ideas. First, "things most familiar or most important to people will be mentioned before things that are less familiar or less important." Also, "people who know a lot about a subject [in this case early childhood feeding and obesity] will have more to say (longer freelists) about it than people who know less" (Fleisher & Harrington, 1998, p. 79). The first step in the analysis of freelists was to code the data. Often, lists will contain a phrase or sentence that can be reduced to a codeword encapsulating meaning. Other phrases on other participants' lists may share the same meaning, and would be assigned the same codeword, consistent with the coding process used in other kinds of qualitative research. Analysis of freelists results in frequency of mention of each idea or codeword (a percentage of respondents who listed that idea), an average rank of each codeword (meaning rank order among the codewords), and a salience score for the codewords. The salience score is based on two other scores: frequency and rank. As a result, salience is a measure of how much knowledge informants share and how important that knowledge is in the cultural domain. To generate these various frequencies, rankings, and scores, Anthropac software was used. Even without the software, salience is easy to calculate. It involves dividing the rank order of a codeword by the number of items in an individual's freelist. After that, the researcher sums the salience scores for each item across respondents and divides by the number of respondents to arrive at a composite salience value. Codewords that were most salient in the composite analysis were viewed as culturally agreed-upon indicators of early childhood obesity risk, and those that were not salient were considered idiosyncratic beliefs.

Results

A total of 160 parents and grandparents participated in the interviews (83 mothers, 48 fathers, 21 grandmothers, and 8 grandfathers). Participants in the interviews were not invited to participate in focus groups. In general, participants in the focused ethnography were Spanish speakers oriented toward traditional values and behaviors. The language of the interviews was predominantly Spanish (75% of the interviews). Acculturation was measured on the five-point Short Acculturation Scale for Hispanics, with a lower score indicating lower acculturation (SASH mean = 1.9, range 1.2–4.8). Parents and grandparents had a mean body mass index (BMI) of 28 (range: 19–38), indicating they were in the overweight category (a BMI of 25–30 is indicative of overweight). Cultural themes, freelists of obesity-producing and obesity-preventive behaviors for young children, and data from silhouettes about the language of childhood obesity comprise the ethnographic results.

Themes

Themes describe the cultural knowledge of Latino parents and grandparents in Los Alamos Verdes about food, feeding, child growth, and childrearing, and how this knowledge informs their behaviors. Each theme was identified across data sources and expresses central cultural beliefs (DeSantis & Ugarriza, 2000).

A Mexican way of feeding babies

Child feeding displayed and embodied ethnic identity. Literally, feeding is an act of embodiment of food given to sustain a child's body and shape it to fit cultural values about infant body type. The Mexican way of feeding babies is how the community viewed their child feeding practices.

Complementary feeding

Weaning foods or first foods are known as complementary foods, specifically because they complement breast milk or infant formula. Adhering to a Mexican way of feeding babies is a dismissal of physician and nurse recommendations, specifically the recommendation for exclusive breastfeeding or infant formula until 6 months of age. "We go against what the doctors say," said one mother. "Like when her, the doctor, said don't feed her until she's 7 months. I started her at one month." Another mother said, "What we do that most Americans don't do, is feed them food right away." The evidence-based knowledge that guides health care recommendations about what and how soon to feed infants non-milk foods differs from the emic knowledge of how to feed a Mexican baby. Early infant feeding is part of the social value placed on mealtimes in Mexican families. "When you're sitting at the table, everyone should be eating." Because babies are curious and reach for food and utensils, some mothers identified this as readiness to join in eating regular food with the family.

Types of complementary foods varied, but were often introduced to infants in their first few months of life. "I mean, my son at 6 months was eating a tortilla with frijoles. Dip it, give it to him," said one mother. Traditional complementary foods included *caldo* (soup) or *probaditas* or "tastes" of beans, eggs, potato, or tortillas. Smoothies or *liquados*, candy, or "anything" were answers given as we probed about common complementary foods.

Ubiquity of the bottle

Bottle feeding is another aspect of the Mexican way of feeding babies. Our participant observation identified bottle feeding as beginning early, usually shortly after birth, and continuing until ages 2 or 3. Long-term bottle-feeding with high-calorie strawberry milk or chocolate milk was common. When asked why flavored milk instead of regular formula or low-fat cow's milk, parents said they doubted their children would "like" anything else. Guidelines from the medical community about milk-only fluids in the bottle and weaning from the bottle shortly after the first birthday may have been offered, but local practice deviates from those recommendations. Our photographic research emphasized the ubiquity of the bottle in daily life of children 12–18 months of age, and the early pairing of child feeding with television viewing (Clark & Zimmer, 2001).

Indulging the baby

Giving babies flavored milks with extra calories and no additional nutritional value is one way of indulging babies, giving them what they want, and demonstrating the parenting value of attentiveness to a baby's desires. Participants believed a baby should not be restricted, but shown love by a responsive parent. A mother of an overweight 1-year-old son was encouraged by the child's health care provider to monitor and restrict unnecessary caloric intake. She responded, "At a year, I wouldn't get my son into a diet. I would just rather let him stick to being fat for a little while." Being fat was presumably the baby's chosen and preferred way of being, or at a minimum, the way that babies "should be." Another mother, when speaking of a sweet treat offered to her overweight nephew, said, "His parents knew the baby would like it, so they gave it to him. Of course, any kid would like it." The focus group developed this theme further, with an exchange between mothers:

> *Mother 1*: I want to give the baby what he wants.
> *Mother 2*: They want anything that's sweet.
> *Mother 3*: My kid loves chocolate.
> *Mother 1*: Sometimes I let 'em taste suckers, so I know he's gonna like it, so I give him a little bit, a taste of it. His daddy gets mad at me though. "Quit giving him that, you'll give him a stomach ache."

These are examples of how childrearing beliefs translate into child feeding behaviors and aligned with Mexican self-identity. The same nurturing environment and parenting behaviors that are associated with sensitivity to children's needs and their self-directed development are also linked to parental indulgence in child-directed feeding behaviors driven by flavor and sweetness that contribute to over-feeding and under-nutrition.

When weight is a problem

According to parents and grandparents, children being overweight is not always a problem, even when a child's weight-for-length meets clinical definitions of obesity. In Los Alamos Verdes, weight is a problem when it is a social liability, a functional or developmental hindrance, or a gendered issue. It is through these social and cultural evaluations, rather than by knowing weight on a scale, that parents and grandparents come to know that a child's weight is a problem.

Social age-related problems

The negative social consequences of children's obesity are clear to parents, who say "When they go to preschool, or when they're about three years old, then they start to be teased by their friends. Then they won't invite them to play because they're fat." Other parents say the social consequences arrive most profoundly at a later stage. "Don't worry until kindergarten. Let them be as fat as they want until kindergarten. Kindergarten is a problem, they might get teased." Others saw the problem occurring even later for boys: "It's a problem when boys are adolescents. Because then they're interested in girls."

Functional health and development problems

Not only is excess body weight a social problem, but a functional and developmental problem as well. Parents and grandparents noted that some babies were too big for their car seat, too big for diapers, and so fat they were "having problems with walking" or moving ("tienen problemas para caminar" or "para movimientos"). Overweight babies "can't breathe" and develop both health and developmental problems. An overweight child is not a problem until weight becomes a functional issue for the parent or child.

Gendered aspects of obesity

The gendered nature of body weight, particularly at adolescence, identifies young men as more "like their Dads" and manly if they are large, and young women less attractive and less desirable if they are overweight. "Girls should be nice and pretty, skinnier" than boys as they get older. "The girl can be fat until the quinceañera," or 15th-year coming-out celebration. Then they should be "nice and pretty, skinnier." For these individuals there was little realization that being overweight early in childhood could make it more difficult to be "skinnier" as adolescents.

To illustrate the family pressures to socialize boys into men through food, a woman told of her brother-in-law, who was overweight and had an overweight son. The story illustrates how the child was taught to eat like a man, a Mexican man, and became overweight like his father.

I asked him, "Why are you feeding your son so much? Especially if you are having a hard time losing the weight?" I'm not too sure they are really thinking about the whole outcome later on. Hispanic people eat a lot of fattening things, pork, and he doesn't have a problem sitting down with a big ol' thing of grease, *chicharrones* (fried pork skins), and it's like "Here, son." So it's hard for my nephew to lose weight with his Dad doing that. It's mostly the boys that have the problems, so whatever the Dad eats, the boy has to eat.

Mexican foods and celebrations inscribe ethnic and gender identities. Eating particular foods and food quantities forges community bonds. Baptisms, birthdays, and communions were formal occasions to prepare food and spend the day eating, as were weekend barbecues where children learned how to eat and enjoy ethnic foods.

Freelists

Parents and grandparents freelisted practices they believed to be responsible for the development of childhood overweight (Table 8.2). All of the most salient responses were food-related rather than activity-related. None addressed the feeding interaction between parents and children (such as authoritarian feeding styles) or feeding practices (like "topping off" each feeding by encouraging intake beyond satiety cues). Most common in the freelists were food items such as sweets, junk food, greasy food, or breads/flours/tortillas. Few participants noted that bottle feeding or too many bottles could contribute to children's obesity (n = 2), or that flavored milks (n = 1) might be adding too many calories to the diet. Two parents thought that breastfeeding may contribute to children becoming overweight.

Parents and grandparents also free-listed practices that protected against overweight: Eating vegetables and fruits, and (to a lesser degree) engaging in physical activity formed a discernible core of belief. The remainder of the protective factors were a combination of food prohibitions mirroring the risk factors (greasy foods, sweets, junk foods) and popular-culture ideas about water, white meats, and juice. For infants, juice is not considered a protective factor among health care providers, but rather a risk factor for unnecessary calories, especially when added to the calories obtained from formula or milk. The perception that juice is healthy and promotes a healthy weight could be registering the influence of WIC-provided food coupons for juice given to

Table 8.2 Parents' and grandparents' freelisted responses to the question, "Why are Mexican or Mexican-American children overweight?"

Item	Frequency	Smith's S (Salience Score)
Tortillas	29	0.310
Fast food	33	0.268
Eating too much	27	0.264
Sweets	33	0.213
Soda	28	0.208
Junk food	26	0.188
No activity	23	0.111
Grease	21	0.211
Bread	19	0.180
Red meat	16	0.131
Flour	14	0.154
No los cuida (not taking care of them)	13	0.096

Table 8.3 Parents' and grandparents' freelisted responses to the question, "What are some behaviors that protect Mexican and Mexican-American children from becoming overweight?"

Item	Frequency	Smith's S (Salience Score)
Eat vegetables	39	0.373
Engage in physical activity	44	0.358
Eat fruits	33	0.304
Don't allow grease	24	0.214
Eat healthier foods	17	0.179
Don't allow sweets	19	0.157
Don't eat too much	14	0.145
Have scheduled feedings	13	0.133
Drink water	17	0.124
Don't allow soda	18	0.122
Eat white meat	14	0.107
Eat soup or *caldo*	11	0.101
Drink juice	13	0.098
Don't allow junk food	13	0.085

breastfeeding women and infants. With a few exceptions, beliefs elicited by the freelisting procedure were congruent with evidence-based medicine (Table 8.3). It seems that lack of knowledge was not the underlying root cause of infant obesity in this group.

Silhouettes and the language of childhood obesity

On the continuum from very thin to very overweight infants, parents used anchor terms for the larger children such as *gordo/a* or *gordito/a*. The three largest infants were considered in the category of *gordo*. *Gordo* literally means "fat." *Gordito* is a euphemistic diminutive literally translated as "little fatty." *Gordito* may be considered flattering or even a term of endearment in a family, and does not convey a clear message from a health care provider to a parent about body weight when used in a clinical encounter. *Bien gordo* was the term used for the two drawings in the middle of the weight continuum, with the term referring to a well-formed, robust child who is appropriately proportioned. *Sobre peso* means "overweight," and is a clear way of discussing a child's overweight status without accidentally lapsing into *gordito* and confusing the message. *El peso que debiera* means a child who weighs what he should, even if that weight appears to a parent to be too thin or *flaco*.

Focus groups spent quite a bit of time discussing how children who were of the appropriate weight were sometimes viewed as too thin, often because overweight siblings and cousins were used as the reference group. *El peso que debiera* (the weight they should be) was suggested as a way of referring to appropriately sized infants to reassure parents that they are not too thin. *Más Gordito* is, literally, "more fat," as is *pasadito de peso*, and both are probably too colloquial to get a clear weight message across, although you will hear parents use these words. Parents and grandparents perceive the infants in the middle of the spectrum to be "normal" or "ideal." They also view the slightly slimmer infants as more likely to be breastfed, and the fattest infants more shockingly obese when they discuss the girl silhouettes than the boy silhouettes. When asked at what point an infant was "too fat" or "obese," parents indicated the heaviest two infants in the pictorial series, but also referred to the thematic elements describing when health is a problem. In those instances, the body weight was considered "obesity" if the child was a girl, was being teased, or was "too big to fit" into diapers or the car seat.

The context of healthcare in the urban immigrant community

Cultural themes and freelists are contextualized by a political economy that embeds differential power in relationships between health care providers, health care agencies, immigrants, and other residents in Los Alamos Verdes. The community health center pediatric/teen clinic does serve as a medical home for children and teenagers in the community. It provides well-child care and care for chronic problems and acute illnesses and attempts to match families with a regular provider. It is also the site of a WIC clinic. However, many Latino families rely on a patchwork of health care services. They may seek immunizations from public health clinics, illness care from free clinics or emergency departments, and well-child care from a school-based health center, or they may forego child health services altogether until an emergency looms. Health care providers are uncertain how to broach a conversation about a child weight issue if they fear the family might sever their tenuous contact with the health care setting over a linguistic error or misunderstanding. Providers' challenges communicating in Spanish to parents with variable levels of health literacy require thoughtfulness and time that may be at odds with the busy pace of the community health center environment.

In the worst case, parents given hasty assessment results about child weight status could launch an over-zealous campaign to slim their child. Relying on cultural beliefs that tortillas or greasy food or red meat are responsible for overweight, they may decide to alter the infant's diet significantly. Without a thoughtful coordinated plan for weight monitoring and family-level behavioral feeding changes, providers are justifiably concerned that parents could launch an inadvisable child slimming effort that could threaten healthy growth and development. Without continuous follow-up or contact with the clinic, the results could be disastrous. As one public health nurse said, "I think we [at the immunization clinic] see that child on such a limited basis, I would be reluctant to encourage a parent to decrease the feedings of a baby less than twelve months, because I'm not going to have any follow-up with that child."

Discussion

Applying focused ethnographic results in community outpatient clinics can improve the health care experience for families and health outcomes for children. Because many parents ask how their baby is growing during well child checkups, health care providers can use cultural knowledge and community preferences about child body size to start a conversation. Health care providers identify the protective effects of breastfeeding and associate childhood obesity with prolonged bottle feeding, calorically dense flavored milks, over-feeding, and a host of other issues that map approximately, but not completely, on the cultural knowledge of parents and grandparents (Johnson et al., 2008).

Intergenerational disagreements about how to best feed a baby can be tense. Clinicians can prepare parents to introduce current biomedical recommendations at home with other family members. Such recommendations would value traditional feeding practices like breastfeeding and appropriately timed, high-fiber and low-fat complementary foods (like pinto beans and corn tortillas) typical of traditional Mexican cuisine. Reinforcing parents' cultural knowledge that fruits, vegetables, and physical activity prevent obesity is relatively easy for clinicians, since most families report that children like fruits and playing outside.

The cultural belief that a boy should be big like his father may partially explain the increased obesity rates in school-age Hispanic boys. The results from NHANES 2007–2008 show the highest rates of obesity for all race and ethnic groups to be among Mexican-American boys aged 2–19 years when compared to non-Hispanic white or black boys and Mexican-American girls.

In infancy and toddler years, Mexican-American boys surpass Mexican-American girls as twice as likely to be overweight (weight/length ≥ 95% for children <2 years of age) (Ogden, Carroll, Curtin, Lamb, & Flegal, 2010). Intergenerational involvement in feeding, the role of the grandparents and extended kin in multi-generational households, and cultural expectations for body size are topics worthy of additional research.

The cultural aspects of Latino childhood obesity are part of the broader topic of the social determinants of health. Latino families throughout the US encounter structural determinants of physical activity and healthy eating, from living quarters without backyards to lack of transportation during the daytime for women at home with children. Neighborhoods viewed as unsafe and lacking sidewalks and streetlights are a persistent reason for lack of outdoor playtime for children, and the relatively high cost of organized youth sports programs further discourages physical activity. Daily walks for mothers and their toddlers set a pattern of family physical activity. Walking groups for urban Latinas are a culturally congruent health promotion intervention with promise for further development (Clarke et al., 2007; Keller & Cantue, 2008). Food deserts, or neighborhoods without access to affordable full-service grocery stores, could be addressed through public policy to benefit many urban communities.

Conclusion

Despite widespread media attention and scientific information about childhood obesity, health care providers encounter in practice a common refrain from parents of overweight children: "What do you mean, my child is overweight?" The mismatch between parents and health care providers in the cultural construction of childhood obesity is a classic example of how to apply a focused ethnography to improve cross-cultural clinical interactions. We know that *how* parents define childhood weight status in their own families and within their local socio-cultural environments is as culturally specific as providers' clinical definitions of childhood obesity. By asking, "What do you mean, my child is overweight?" the parent also presents a challenge to the provider to explain the scientific definitional characteristics of obesity in a sensitive, culturally competent manner and enlist parental involvement in establishing a "normal" weight for the child in biomedical as well as social and functional terms. Improving the health care of young children who are already overweight or at risk for overweight depends on structuring a dialogue with parents based on evidence about obesity prevention integrated with an understanding of cultural norms and feeding practices specific to the family.

Note

1   We use obesity in this article to identify the children who are overweight with a BMI >85th percentile or above the 95th percentile and officially categorized as "obese" (Ogden, Carroll, Kit, & Flegal, 2012).

References

Alexander, M. A., Sherman, J. B., & Clark, L. (1991). Obesity in Mexican-American preschool children: A population group at risk. *Public Health Nursing, 8*, 53–58.

Angrosino, M.V. (2007). *Naturalistic observation*. Walnut Creek, CA: Left Coast Press.

Annesi, J. J., Pierce, L. L., Bonaparte, W. A., & Smith, A. E. (2009). Preliminary effects of the Youth Fit for Life protocol on body mass index in Mexican American children in YMCA before- and after-school care programs. *Hispanic Health Care International, 7*(3), 123–129.

Brewer, D. D. (2002). Supplementary interviewing techniques to maximize output in free listing tasks. *Field Methods, 14*(1),108–118.

Carey M.A (1994). The group effect in focus groups: Planning, implementing, and interpreting focus group research. In J. M. Morse (Ed.), *Critical issues in qualitative research methods* (pp. 225–241). Thousand Oaks, CA: Sage.

Clark, L. (2002). Mexican-origin mothers' experiences using children's health care services. *Western Journal of Nursing Research, 24*, 159–179.

Clark, L., Bunik, M., & Johnson, S. L. (2010). Research opportunities with curanderos to address childhood overweight in Latino families. *Qualitative Health Research, 20*(1), 4–14.

Clark, L., & Redman, R. W. (2007). Mexican immigrant mothers' expectations for children's health services. *Western Journal of Nursing Research, 29*, 670–690.

Clark, L., & Zimmer, L. (2001). What more we learned about Mexican-origin children's health from a photographic research component. *Field Methods, 13*(4), 303–328.

Clarke, K. K., Freeland-Graves, J., Klohe-Lehman, D. M., Milani, T. J., Nuss, H. J., & Laffrey, S. (2007). Promotion of physical activity in low-income mothers using pedometers. *Journal of the American Dietetic Association, 107*, 962–967.

DeSantis, L., & Ugarriza, D. N. (2000). The concept of theme as used in qualitative nursing research. *Western Journal of Nursing Research, 22*(3), 351–372. doi: 10.1177/01939459 0002200308.

Fetterman, D. M. (1989). *Ethnography step by step.* Newbury Park, CA: Sage.

Fleisher, M. S., & Harrington J. A. (1998). Freelisting: Management at a women's federal prison camp. In V. C. de Munck & E. J. Sobo (Eds.), *Using methods in the field: A practical introduction and casebook* (pp. 69–84). Walnut Creek, CA: Altamira.

Foster, G. D., Sherman, S., Borradaile, K. E., Grundy, K. M., Vander Veur, S. S., Nachmani, J., & Shults, J. (2008). A policy-based school intervention to prevent overweight and obesity. *Pediatrics, 121*(4), e794–802.

Guo, S. S., Roche, A. F., Chumlea, W. C., Gardner, J. D., & Siervogel, R. M. (1994). The predictive value of childhood body mass index values for overweight at age 35 y. *American Journal of Clinical Nutrition, 59*, 995–999.

Holt, K., Wooldridge, N., Story, M., & Sofka, D. (Eds.). (2011). *Bright futures: Nutrition* (3rd ed.). Elk Grove Village, IL: American Academy of Pediatrics.

Johnson, S. L., Clark, L., Goree, K., O'Connor, M., & Zimmer, L. M. (2008). Healthcare providers' perceptions of the factors contributing to infant obesity in a low-income Mexican American community. *Journal for Specialists in Pediatric Nursing, 13*(3), 180–190.

Kay, M. (1977). Health and illness in a Mexican American barrio. In E. H. Spicer (Ed.), *Ethnic medicine in the Southwest* (pp. 99–166). Tucson: University of Arizona Press.

Keller, C. S. & Cantue, A. (2008). Camina por salud: Walking in Mexican-American women. *Applied Nursing Research, 21*, 110–113.

Kramer, M. S., Barr, R. G., Leduc, D. G., Boisjoly, C., & Pless, I. B. (1983). Maternal psychological determinants of infant obesity: Development and testing of two new instruments. *Journal of Chronic Disease, 36*, 329–335.

Marín, G., Sabogal, F., Marín, B., Otero-Sabogal, R., & Perez-Stable, E. (1987). Development of a short acculturation scale for Hispanics. *Hispanic Journal of Behavioral Sciences, 9*(183), 183–205.

Morgan, D. L., & Krueger, R. A. (1993). When to use focus groups and why. In D. L. Morgan (Ed.), *Successful focus groups: Advancing the state of the art* (pp. 3–19). Newbury Park, CA: Sage.

Morse, J. M. (2001). Qualitative verification: Building evidence by extending basic findings. In J. M. Morse, J. M. Swanon, & A. J. Kuzel, *The nature of qualitative evidence* (pp. 203–220). Thousand Oaks, CA: Sage.

National Association of Pediatric Nurse Practitioners (NAPNAP). (2006). *Healthy eating and activity together (HEAT™) clinical practice guideline: Identifying and preventing overweight in childhood.* Cherry Hill, NJ: NAPNAP.

Ogden, C. L., Carroll, M. D., Curtin, L. R., Lamb, M. M., & Flegal, K. M. (2010). Prevalence of high body mass index in US children and adolescents, 2007–2008. *JAMA, 303*, 242–249.

Ogden, C. L., Carroll, M. D., Curtin, L. R., McDowell, M. A., Tabak, C. J., & Flegal, K. M. (2006). Prevalence of overweight and obesity in the United States, 1999–2004. *JAMA, 295*, 1549–1555.

Ogden, C. L., Carroll, M. D., Kit, B. K., & Flegal, K. M. (2012). NCHS data brief: Prevalence of obesity in the United States, 2009–2010. Retrieved from: http://www.cdc.gov/nchs/data/databriefs/db82.pdf.

Ogden, C. L., Flegal, K. M., Carroll, M. D., & Johnson, C. I. (2002). Prevalence and trends in overweight among US children and adolescents, 1999–2000. *JAMA, 288*, 1728–1732.

Spradley, J. P. (1980). *Participant observation.* New York: Holt, Rinehart & Winston.

Vega, W. A., Rodriguez, M. A., & Gruskin, E. (2009). Health disparities in the Latino population. *Epidemiologic Reviews, 31*, 99–112.

Weller, S., & Romney, A. K. (1988). *Systematic data collection*. Newbury Park, CA: Sage.

Whitaker, R. (1997). Predicting obesity in young adulthood from childhood and parental obesity. *New England Journal of Medicine, 337*, 869–873.

Young, J., & O'Connor, M. E. (2005). Risk factors associated with latent tuberculosis infection in Mexican-American children. *Pediatrics 115*(5), e647–653.

9

Bringing visibility to an invisible phenomenon

A postpartum depression research program

Cheryl Tatano Beck

"Qualitative research can put flesh on the bones of quantitative results, bringing the results to life through in-depth case elaboration" (Patton, 1990, p. 123). As Selikoff (1991) noted "statistics are human beings with the tears wiped away" (p. 126). Qualitative research can allow nurses a privileged insider's view of what it is like to walk a mile in the shoes of our patients so that we can develop appropriate and effective interventions. Qualitative research can provide the best data to develop items for instrument development. The items can be derived from patients' own words which will resonate with persons completing the instrument. Substantive, grounded theory developed from qualitative research is an extremely valuable approach to midrange theory. As Lasiuk and Ferguson (2005) stated, "Midrange theory has the potential to address the theory–practice gap that continues to plague nursing and to develop the substantive practice knowledge needed to advance nursing as a discipline" (p. 134).

In this chapter I will illustrate the impact, the "so what?", that qualitative research can have on clinical practice through my research program on postpartum depression. In the late 1980s when I began my research trajectory there were no qualitative studies published on postpartum depression. In nursing and medical obstetric textbooks only a few sentences about postpartum depression were devoted to this disorder. From my clinical practice I knew how devastating postpartum depression was to new mothers but their voices describing the crippling impact of this mood disorder were missing from the literature. It was at this juncture in time that I began my research program with a qualitative study.

This initial study was a descriptive phenomenological study of the lived experience of postpartum depression (Beck, 1992). Using Colaizzi's (1978) method of data analysis, 11 themes emerged from the in-depth descriptions provided by seven mothers of their experiences of postpartum depression. These 11 themes can be found in the left column in Table 9.1. Together, these 11 themes described the essence of postpartum depression.

Building on that phenomenological study, next I wanted to investigate the process mothers went through to recover from the depths of their depression. I also wanted to discover the basic problem or central concern women experienced with this devastating mood disorder. Grounded theory was the perfect match to help answer these questions. Data collection took place over an 18-month period (Beck, 1993). Data were obtained by means of participant observation in a postpartum depression support group and also from 12 in-depth interviews. Using Glaser and Strauss' (1967) constant comparative method, loss of control emerged as the basic problem

Table 9.1 Comparison of phenomenological and grounded theory studies on postpartum depression

Phenomenological study	*Grounded theory study*
Theme 1. Enveloped in unbearable loneliness, the mother is uncomfortable with others and believes that no one understands what she is experiencing.	**Stage 2.** Dying of self: Isolating oneself
Theme 2. Contemplating death provides a glimmer of hope for the end of her living nightmare.	**Stage 2.** Dying of self: Contemplating and attempting self-destruction
Theme 3. Obsessive thoughts of being a bad mother and questioning what is happening consume the mother's waking hours.	**Stage 1** Encountering terror: Relentless obsessive thinking
Theme 4. Haunted by the fear that any normalcy in her life is irretrievable, the mother grieves her loss of self.	**Stage 2** Dying of self: Alarming unrealness
Theme 5. Life is empty of all previous interests and goals.	**Stage 2.** Dying of self: Isolating oneself
Theme 6. The mother carries a suffocating burden of fear and guilt at the thought of harming her infant	**Stage 2.** Dying of self: Contemplating and attempting self-destruction
Theme 7. Shrouded in fogginess, the mother's ability to concentrate is diminished.	**Stage 1.** Encountering terror: Enveloping fogginess
Theme 8. The mother envisions herself as a robot stripped of all positive feelings and just going through motions.	**Stage 2** Dying of self: Alarming unrealness
Theme 9. Experiencing uncontrollable anxiety attacks leads to a feeling of being on the edge of insanity.	**Stage 1** Encountering terror: Horrifying anxiety
Theme 10. Loss of control of her emotions is alarming and difficult to accept.	**Basic social psychological problem:** Loss of control
Theme 11. Besieged with insecurities, the mother needs to be mothered herself.	**Basic social psychological problem:** Loss of control

Source: Reprinted with permission from Beck (1993), p. 46.

mothers had to contend with; loss of control both of their emotions and thought processes. Mothers suffering from postpartum depression attempted to cope with this loss of control through a four-stage process called teetering on the edge (Figure 9.1). These four stages consisted of: (1) encountering terror; (2) dying of self; (3) struggling to survive; and (4) regaining control.

Comparing the results of my phenomenological study (Beck, 1992) with my grounded theory study (Beck, 1993) provided a triangulation of two qualitative methods which allowed the illumination of clinical realities that escape alternative approaches (Wilson & Hutchinson, 1991). In the right column of Table 9.1 can be seen how the grounded theory study confirmed and extended the findings of the phenomenological study. The first two stages of teetering on the edge substantive theory confirmed the first nine themes from the phenomenological study. In

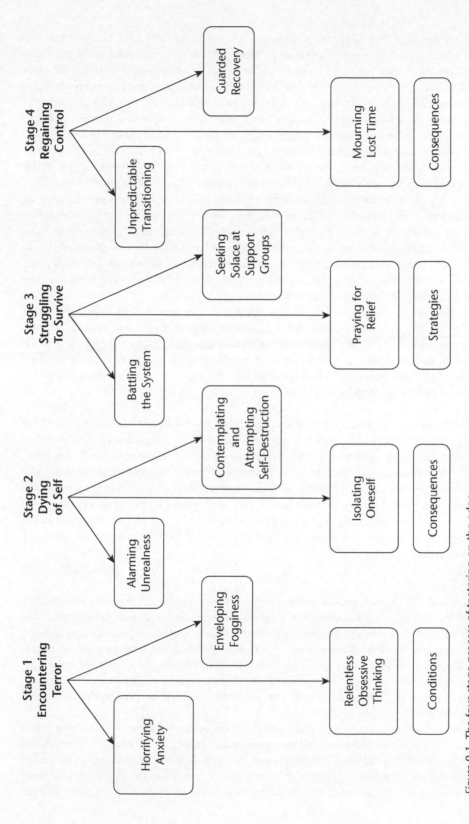

Figure 9.1 The four-stage process of teetering on the edge

Source: Reprinted with permission from Beck (1993), p. 43.

teetering on the edge, loss of control, which was a component in themes 10 and 11 in the phenomenological study, emerged as the basic problem mothers contended with. Since grounded theory focuses on process, strategies mothers used to regain control of their lives and the consequences of these strategies were revealed. In the grounded theory study mothers admitted contemplating ending their own lives. Contributing to their dangerous thoughts of death was the consuming guilt women bore due to their perceptions of being failures as mothers and also, for some women, due to uncontrollable thoughts of harming their infants. As one woman shared, "I would go into my baby's room and think, put the blanket over his head. He's nothing. Then I'd start crying hysterically. I felt like the worst person in the world, the worst mother in the world. I felt tremendous guilt and just wanted to hurt myself" (Beck, 1993, pp. 45–46).

Next in my program of research I wanted to focus more on this most serious issue of postpartum depression and mother–infant relationships. To get an idea how great a problem this was I conducted a meta-analysis of 19 quantitative studies in which the effects of postpartum depression on maternal–infant interaction during the first year of life had been examined (Beck, 1995). The glimpse of this problem from my grounded theory study led me down this path. Results of the meta-analysis indicated that this postpartum mood disorder had a moderate to large negative effect on maternal–infant interactions.

Now came my best example of qualitative research putting the flesh on the bones of quantitative findings. I conducted a descriptive phenomenological study concentrating this time on postpartum depressed mothers' experiences interacting with their children in order to provide a voice for women to explain just what they were experiencing (Beck, 1996). Twelve mothers participated in in-depth interviews. The following quote from the first mother interviewed added the tears to my quantitative meta-analysis findings:

> My husband and son got back from the store. I think my 3-year-old son wanted to tell me about something that had happened. It was physically so hard to listen that I really remember just trying to put up some kind of wall so that I wouldn't be battered to death. At this point I was really sitting on the couch trying to figure out whether I could ever move again, and I started to cry. My son started hitting me with his fists, and he said, "Where are you mom?" It was really painful because I didn't have a clue as to where I was either. He was really trying to wake something up, but it was just too far gone. There was no way that I could retrieve the mom that he remembered and hoped he would find, let alone the mother I wanted to be for my new baby.
>
> *(Beck, 1996, p. 98)*

Using Colaizzi's (1978) data analysis method in this phenomenological research, nine themes were revealed that captured the essence of mothers' experiences interacting with their infants (Beck, 1996). In their day-to-day interactions with their infants, mothers experienced guilt, anger, loss, and irrational thinking. Women were completely overwhelmed with their role as a new mother. Women shared that when caring for their infants they felt like robots just going through the motions. In order to survive their postpartum depression, women erected "a wall" to separate themselves emotionally from their infants. This emotional wall led to some mothers failing to respond to their infants' clues.

Phenomenological studies have helped throughout my research trajectory to discover subtle differences among postpartum mood and anxiety disorders (Beck, 2011). Some mothers shared in the earlier qualitative studies I had conducted that they had been misdiagnosed as having postpartum depression when in actuality they were suffering from some other crippling postpartum mood or anxiety disorder, such as postpartum onset of panic disorder. Due to their misdiagnoses women suffered unnecessarily due to incorrect treatment. Using phenomenology as the research method permitted mothers' vivid, detailed descriptions to identify for clinicians subtle differences in symptom patterns. Through phenomenology, nuances in the diagnostic profiles of postpartum depression versus postpartum panic disorder and posttraumatic stress disorder (PTSD) due to birth trauma emerged as I was able "to walk a mile" in the shoes of women suffering from these disorders.

The themes that emerged from three of my phenomenological studies helped identify discrete differences from women with these postpartum mood and anxiety disorders in regards to loneliness/isolation, cognitive impairment, guilt, and loss of control. These three phenomenological studies focused on: (1) postpartum depression (Beck, 1992); (2) postpartum onset of panic disorder (Beck, 1998); and (3) PTSD due to traumatic childbirth (Beck, 2004). In postpartum depression, mothers experienced loneliness because of their belief that neither their family, friends, nor health care professionals really understood the depths of their despair. With postpartum onset of panic disorder, mothers isolated themselves and experienced loneliness for a different reason. Because women feared the onset of another terrifying panic attack, they isolated themselves and curtailed daily activities that would take them outside of their home. Women preferred to be in the safety of their home if another panic attack occurred. Mothers with PTSD due to childbirth also experienced isolation. These women isolated themselves by attempting to avoid triggers to their traumatic birth. For example, women would isolate themselves from other mothers with infants and, at times, from their own infants.

In regards to cognitive impairment, women explained that with postpartum depression they felt like fog was rolling into their brains and their mental acuity was diminished. With postpartum onset of panic disorder, mothers' cognitive functioning was drastically reduced during a panic attack. Some women described experiencing irrational thinking during panic attacks, such as catastrophic misinterpretations of the physical symptoms they experienced. Between panic attacks women's diminished cognitive functioning was more of a chronic problem as the fear of another panic attack distracted women due to their being consumed with worry. PTSD following traumatic childbirth also affected women's cognitive functioning. When mothers had flashbacks to their traumatic births, their mental acuity decreased.

When considering guilt, postpartum depressed mothers experienced this distressing emotion due to their belief that they were not able to love their infants the way they should and also at times due to horrific thoughts of harming their infants. On the other hand, women with postpartum onset of panic disorder bore the heavy burden of guilt but for a different reason. Their guilt focused on their belief that they repeatedly disappointed their infants as they drastically curtailed their everyday activities. Some women who were experiencing PTSD due to their traumatic childbirth experienced suffocating guilt as a consequence of their distancing themselves from their infants who were a constant reminder of their birth trauma.

Loss of control was a key component in all three postpartum mood and anxiety disorders. In panic disorder mothers had no control regarding when their next panic attack would strike. During a panic attack mothers felt like they were totally out of control, while in postpartum depression, women shared that they could not control any aspect of their lives; neither their emotions nor their thoughts. Women with PTSD due to childbirth shared that they could not control the videotape of their birth trauma that kept running in their minds. Mothers described that their minds were on automatic replay leaving them feeling like there were loop tracks in their brain. Mothers suffering with PTSD also described loss of control in relation to their anger. Women lashed out their anger at the health care professionals who were present during their traumatic labor and delivery for betraying their trust, at their partners who did not stand up for them during their childbirth, and at themselves for letting this birth trauma happen.

By this time in my research trajectory a number of qualitative studies on postpartum depression had been published by other researchers. Even though the number of qualitative studies had increased, knowledge development would have been hindered unless the powerful results from these studies were synthesized. Therefore, I conducted a metasynthesis (Beck, 2002). A thorough review of the literature revealed 18 qualitative studies that had been published between 1990 and 1999. Using Noblit and Hare's (1988) method for synthesizing qualitative studies, four overarching themes were identified (Figure 9.2): (1) incongruity between expectations and reality of motherhood; (2) spiraling downward; (3) pervasive loss; and (4) making gains.

At this point in my research program I was considering testing an intervention for postpartum depression that I would design based on the findings from my series of qualitative studies. I would need to use a screening scale as the first step in selecting a sample for this intervention study. The Edinburgh Postnatal Depression Scale (EPDS; Cox, Holden, & Sagovsky, 1987) was the only scale available at that time. When I assessed the EPDS' content validity I discovered that it was not assessing the gamut of postpartum depressive symptoms mothers had repeatedly shared with me in my qualitative research. The EPDS did not have items measuring cognitive impairment, loss of self, guilt/shame, and eating disturbances. I had never planned on developing an instrument as part of my research trajectory but it became clear to me that this would indeed be my next project. My series of qualitative studies on postpartum depression (Beck, 1992, 1993, 1996) provided the conceptual basis for the development of my instrument, the Postpartum Depression

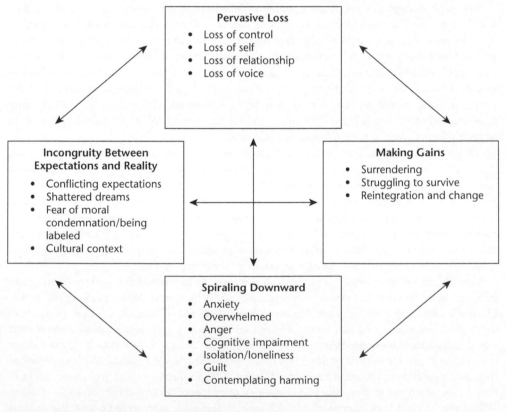

Figure 9.2 Four perspectives involved with postpartum depression

Source: Reprinted with permission from Beck (2002), p. 461.

Screening Scale (PDSS; Beck & Gable, 2002). The conceptual and operational definitions were all based on my qualitative findings. Seven dimensions of the PDSS were decided upon: Sleeping/Eating Disturbances, Anxiety/Insecurity, Emotional Lability, Cognitive Impairment, Loss of Self, Guilt/Shame, and Contemplating Harming Oneself. Each dimension had five items for a total of 35 items on the PDSS.

When qualitative findings are available, it is critical that these be used to develop items to preserve the meaning of the qualitative data. Both the language and expressions of postpartum depressed women in my qualitative studies were used to develop meaningful instrument items. The items on the PDSS were created from actual quotes from the interviews I had conducted with the women. Table 9.2 provides examples of the generation of selected items (Beck & Gable, 2001a). Content validity of the PDSS was assessed by a panel of four experts in postpartum depression. The content experts were given the theoretical definitions of each dimension of the PDSS and then they rated how well the items fit with the dimension. Figure 9.3 illustrates this step for the Emotional Lability dimension (Beck & Gable, 2001a).

The psychometrics of the PDSS were assessed and compared with the EPDS (Cox et al., 1987) and also with the Beck Depression Inventory-II (BDI-II; Beck, Steer, & Brown, 1996) which is a general depression scale that was used frequently by researchers to screen for postpartum depression. The community sample of 150 mothers completed these three instruments in random order and then immediately were interviewed by a nurse psychotherapist using the Structured Clinical Interview for DSM-IV mood disorder diagnoses (First, Spitzer, Gibbon, & Williams, 1997). When screening for major postpartum depression, the PDSS achieved sensitivity of 94% and specificity of 98%. The EPDS had a sensitivity of 78% and specificity of 99% while the BDI-II's sensitivity was 56% and specificity was 100%. Why I believe the PDSS was the instrument that screened most effectively had to do with its qualitative roots. The PDSS displayed higher

Table 9.2 Development of selected PDSS items from qualitative data

Quote	Item
I was extremely obsessive with my thoughts. They would never stop. I could not control them.	I could not control the thoughts that kept coming into my mind.
I felt like a robot. I went through the motions of my life taking care of the baby without any joy.	I felt like a robot just going through the motions of taking care of my baby.
Sometimes inside me was just exploding and there was no way for me to exhibit it other than anger.	I felt full of anger ready to explode.
I felt tremendous guilt and the fact that I couldn't love my baby like I should made it even worse.	I felt guilty because I could not feel as much love for my baby as I should.
It was like I was in a fog. The fogginess would set in.	I felt like I was in a fog.
I couldn't fall asleep even when my baby was sleeping. I had a difficult time getting to sleep even though I was exhausted.	I had trouble sleeping even when my baby was asleep.
I had such a hard time even making a simple decision like what to cook for dinner. I couldn't control my emotions. One minute I'd be fine. The next minute I'd be crying. It was like my emotions were on a roller coaster.	I had a difficult time making even a simple decision. I felt like my emotions were on a roller coaster.

Source: Reprinted with permission from Beck & Gable (2001a), p. 208.

Emotional Lability

A mother's feeling that she is living a joyless existence just going through the motions. Joy is not experienced even when caring for her baby. Interest in doing many activities that used to bring her enjoyment is lost. The mother cannot control her emotions. Uncontrolled crying can occur. She may feel irritable and full of anger ready to explode.

Items	This item fits in this dimension very well[1]				
Over the last 2 weeks, I					
1. Felt like a robot just going through the motions taking care of my baby	SD	D	U	(A)	(SA)
2. Was scared that I would never be happy again	SD	D	U	A	(SA)
3. Did not enjoy taking care of my baby	SD	D	U	(A)	SA
4. Cried a lot for no real reason	SD	D	U	A	(SA)
5. Lost interest in doing anything that I used to enjoy	SD	D	U	(A)	SA
6. Had no control over my emotions	SD	D	U	A	(SA)
7. Did not feel any love toward my baby	SD	D	(U)	A	SA
8. Felt like every little thing got on my nerves	SD	D	U	A	(SA)

[1]Rating Scale: SD Strongly Disagree
D Disagree
U Neither Disagree or Agree
A Agree
SA Strongly Agree

Figure 9.3 Example of a completed content validity rating form
Source: Reprinted with permission from Beck and Gable (2001a), p. 213.

sensitivity especially in the symptom profiles of sleeping disturbances, cognitive impairment, and anxiety (Beck & Gable, 2001b). The PDSS was the only scale out of the three that situated its items in the context of new motherhood, using mothers' own phrases from my qualitative research.

The PDSS' popularity is increasing around the globe. For example, psychometric studies have been published for the Portuguese version of the PDSS (Pereira et al., 2010; Zubaran et al., 2009; Zubaran et al., 2010), the Chinese version of the PDSS (Li, Liu, Zhang, Wang, & Chen, 2011), and its Spanish version (Beck, Bernal, & Froman, 2003; Beck & Gable 2003, 2005; Quelopana & Champion, 2010). Using the PDSS Spanish Version, Quelopana, Champion, and Reyes-Rubilar (2011) reported that 45% of the Chilean sample of women reported elevated depressive symptoms including suicidal thoughts, sleeping/eating disturbances, and emotional lability. In the US, the PDSS-Short Form was recently used in the Listening to Mothers II national survey to assess postpartum depressive symptoms (Beck, Gable, Sakala, & Declercq, 2011). Out of the sample of 1573 women who participated in this national survey, 63% screened positive for elevated postpartum depressive symptomatology. In Portugal, Pereira et al. (2011) successfully used the Portuguese PDSS as a screening instrument for prenatal depression. This is the first time any language version of the PDSS was used to assess prenatal depression.

In grounded theory, modification should never stop (Glaser, 2001). As new data become available, the substantive theory should be modified to accommodate the varying conditions in order to increase the theory's power and completeness. Glaser (2001, p. 15) stressed that "all is data" in grounded theory. As new studies are published, their findings are compared as additional data. A grounded theory is modified as the new data-literature is woven into it.

Maximizing differences among comparative groups is one approach Glaser described as a powerful method to extend a grounded theory.

I have modified my teetering on the edge grounded theory of postpartum (Beck, 1993) in 2007 and again in 2012. The original grounded theory was based on data from only Caucasian, middle-class women suffering with postpartum depression. In 2007 I first modified my grounded theory to increase its scope to include data from postpartum depressed mothers from other cultures than just Caucasian women in the United States. In this first modification I used data from ten transcultural qualitative studies on women's experiences of postpartum depression that had been published by other researchers since 1993 when teetering on the edge was developed. Five years later I modified my grounded theory of postpartum depression a second time (Beck, 2012). Seventeen new transcultural studies of postpartum depressed women had been published since my 2007 modification and their data were used in this second modification. The countries where the qualitative studies were conducted included the United Kingdom, Australia, New Zealand, Canada, Indonesia, Sweden, Taiwan, United Arab Emirates, Ethiopia, and the Democratic Republic of Congo. Qualitative data from these cross-cultural experiences were used for the continuing modifications to each of the four stages of teetering on the edge substantive theory. Figure 9.4 provides an illustration of this modification for Stage 1, encountering

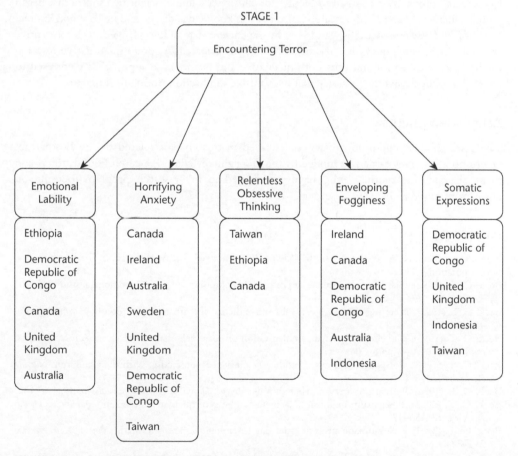

Figure 9.4 Second modification of teetering on the edge: Stage 1

Source: Reprinted with permission from Beck (2012), p. 265.

terror. A similar process was used for Stages 2–4 but due to space limitations in this chapter only one stage is presented. Under each category in Figure 9.4 are listed the countries other than the United States where the qualitative studies took place and mothers from those countries had endorsed the categories. These lists include countries from both my first and second modifications.

This second modification of my grounded theory has wider applicability since its categories have now been expanded from data from all these different cultural orientations regarding mothers' experiences of postpartum depression. In some cultures the women used somatic expressions to describe their postpartum depression which have important implications for screening for this devastating mood disorder in mothers from those cultures.

My most recent study in my program of research on postpartum depression was a double blind randomized control trial testing the effect of a diet enriched in DHA during pregnancy on postpartum depressive symptoms. Mothers were assessed three times during the postpartum period using my PDSS. The experimental group had significantly lower scores on the PDSS than the control group (Judge, Beck, et al., under review).

Conclusion

My research program on postpartum depression illustrates a line of scientific inquiry that began with qualitative research. This research trajectory was knowledge driven and not method limited. My choice of research methods was driven by the current state of knowledge in this substantive area and the research questions that needed to be investigated. At times quantitative research methods were called for and thus both qualitative and quantitative approaches were used to develop a productive line of inquiry that has valuable implications for clinical practice.

Acknowledgments

The research that supported the work described in this chapter related to the Postpartum Depression Screening Scale was funded by the Donaghue Medical Research Foundation. I also thank the amazing mothers who have participated in my research program focusing on postpartum mood and anxiety disorders.

References

Beck, A. T., Steer, R. A., & Brown, G. K. (1996). *BDI-II Manual*, San Antonio, TX: The Psychological Corporation.

Beck, C. T. (1992). The lived experience of postpartum depression: A phenomenological study. *Nursing Research, 41*, 166–170.

Beck, C. T. (1993). Teetering on the edge: A substantive theory of postpartum depression. *Nursing Research, 42*, 42–48.

Beck, C. T. (1995). The effect of postpartum depression on maternal–infant interaction: A meta-analysis. *Nursing Research, 44*, 298–304.

Beck, C. T. (1996). Postpartum depressed mothers' experiences interacting with their children. *Nursing Research, 45*, 98–104.

Beck, C. T. (1998). Postpartum onset of panic disorder. *Image: Journal of Nursing Scholarship, 30*, 131–135.

Beck, C. T. (2002). Postpartum depression: A meta-synthesis of qualitative research. *Qualitative Health Research, 12*, 453–472.

Beck, C. T. (2004). Posttraumatic stress disorder due to childbirth: The aftermath. *Nursing Research, 53*, 216–224.

Beck, C. T. (2007). Exemplar: Teetering on the edge: A continually emerging theory of postpartum depression. In P. L. Munhall (Ed.), *Nursing research: A qualitative perspective* (pp. 273–292). Sudbury, MA: Jones & Bartlett.

Beck, C. T. (2011). Revealing the subtle differences among postpartum mood and anxiety disorders: Phenomenology holds the key. In G. Thomson, F. Dykes, & S. Downe (Eds.), *Qualitative research in midwifery and childbirth: Phenomenological approaches* (pp.193–214). New York: Routledge.

Beck, C. T. (2012). Exemplar: Teetering on the edge: A second grounded theory modification. In P. L. Munhall (Ed.), *Nursing research: A qualitative perspective* (5th ed.) (pp. 257–284). Sudbury, MA: Jones & Bartlett Publishers.

Beck, C. T., Bernal, H., & Froman, R. (2003). Methods to document the semantic equivalence of a translated scale, *Research in Nursing & Health, 26*, 64–73.

Beck, C. T. & Gable, R. K. (2001a). Ensuring content validity: An illustration of the process. *Journal of Nursing Measurement, 9*, 201–215.

Beck, C. T. & Gable, R. K. (2001b). Comparative analysis of the performance of the Postpartum Depression Screening Scale with two other depression instruments, *Nursing Research, 50*, 242–250.

Beck, C. T., & Gable, R. K. (2002). *Postpartum Depression Screening Scale manual.* Los Angeles, CA: Western Psychological Services.

Beck, C. T. & Gable, R. K. (2003). Postpartum Depression Screening Scale: Spanish version. *Nursing Research, 52*, 296–306.

Beck, C. T. & Gable, R. K. (2005). Screening performance of the Postpartum Depression Screening Scale: Spanish version. *Journal of Transcultural Nursing, 16*, 331–338.

Beck, C. T., Gable, R. K., Sakala, C., & Declercq, E. R. (2011). Postpartum depression in new mothers: Results from a two-stage U.S. national survey. *Journal of Midwifery and Women's Health, 56*, 427–435.

Colaizzi, P. (1978). Psychological research as the phenomenologist views it. In R. Valle, & M. King (Eds.), *Existential phenomenological alternative for psychology* (pp. 48–71). New York: Oxford University Press.

Cox, J. L., Holden, J. M., & Sagovsky, R. (1987). Detection of postnatal depression: Development of the 10-item Edinburgh Postnatal Depression Scale. *British Journal of Psychiatry, 150,* 782–786.

First, M. B., Spitzer, R. L., Gibbon, M., & Williams, J. B. (1977). *User's guide for the structured clinical interview for DSM-IV axis disorders*, Washington, DC: American Psychiatric Press.

Glaser, B. (2001). *The grounded theory perspective I: Conceptualization contrasted with description.* Mill Valley, CA: Sociology Press.

Glaser, B., & Strauss, A. (1967). *The discovery of grounded theory.* Chicago: Aldine.

Judge, M. P., Beck, C. T., Durham, H., McKelvey, M. M., & Lammi-Keefe, C. J. (under review). Maternal DHA consumption during pregnancy decreases postpartum depressive symptomatology.

Lasiuk, G. C., & Ferguson, L. M. (2005). From practice to midrange theory and back again: Beck's theory of postpartum depression. *Advances in Nursing Science, 28*, 127–136.

Li, L., Liu, F., Zhang, H., Wang, L., & Chen, X. (2011). Chinese version of the Postpartum Depression Screening Scale: Translation and validation. *Nursing Research, 60*, 231–239.

Noblit, G. W., & Hare, R. D. (1988), *Meta-ethnography: Synthesizing qualitative studies.* Newbury Park, CA: Sage.

Patton, M. Q. (1990). *Qualitative evaluation and research methods.* Newbury Park, CA: Sage.

Pereira, A. T., Bos, S. C., Marques, M., Maia, B. R., Soares, M. J., Valente, J., et al. (2010). The Portuguese version of the Postpartum Depression Screening Scale. *Journal of Psychosomatic Obstetrics & Gynecology, 31*, 90–100.

Pereira, A. T., Bos, S. C., Marques, M., Maia, B. R., Soares, M., Valente, J., et al. (2011). The Postpartum Depression Screening Scale: Is it valid to screen for antenatal depression? *Archives of Women's Mental Health, 14,* 227–238.

Quelopana, A. M., & Champion, J. D. (2010). Validation of the Postpartum Depression Screening Scale: Spanish version in women from Arica, Chile. *Ciencia y Enfermeria, 16*, 37–47.

Quelopana, A. M., Champion. J. D., & Reyes-Rubilar, T. (2011). Factors associated in postpartum depression in Chilean women. *Health Care for Women International, 32,* 939–949.

Selikoff, I. J. (1991). Asbestos disease, 1990–2020: The risks of asbestos risk assessment. *Toxicology and Industrial Health, 7*, 117–126.

Wilson, H., & Hutchinson, S. (1991). Triangulation of qualitative methods: Heideggerian hermeneutics and grounded theory, *Qualitative Health Research, 1,* 263–276.

Zubaran, C., Foresti, K., Schumacher, M. V., Amoretti, A. L., Muller, L. C., Thorell, M. R., et al. (2009). Validation of a screening instrument for postpartum depression in Southern Brazil. *Journal of Psychosomatic Obstetrics & Gynecology, 30*, 244–254.

Zubaran, C., Schumacher, M. V., Foresti, K., Thorell, M. R., Amoretti, A., & Muller, L. (2010). The Portuguese version of the Postpartum Depression Screening Scale-Short Form, *The Journal of Obstetrics & Gynaecology Research, 36*, 950–957.

Part II
Qualitative research methods

10

Descriptive phenomenology

Cheryl Tatano Beck

As Giorgi (1989) warned: "lack of exposure to phenomenological philosophy results in a limited understanding of the phenomenological method and its demands" (p. 71). Phenomenology is both a philosophy and a method. The philosophy of phenomenology provides the foundation for the method. This chapter on the state of the science of descriptive phenomenology in nursing research begins with a description of Husserlian philosophy which provides the underpinnings for this method. Next, the procedure used to review the literature on descriptive phenomenological studies conducted by nurse researchers for the past 20 years is detailed. The results of this extensive search are then discussed. The methods for the three most frequently used descriptive phenomenological methods by nurse researchers are identified and compared. Then the general topics of the phenomena most often studied by nurse researchers in descriptive phenomenological studies are described. Comparisons across countries are included in this section. In the last part of this chapter an illustration of the use of Colaizzi's (1978) method of descriptive phenomenology is provided. This study of the experience of subsequent childbirth following a previous traumatic birth (Beck & Watson, 2010) is one of the most recent studies in the author of this chapter's research program on traumatic childbirth and its resulting posttraumatic stress disorder.

The philosophy of phenomenology

Edmund Husserl is often called the father of phenomenology. In the beginning of his career he was a mathematician but later turned philosopher. Husserl became alarmed by what he termed a crisis in science. He believed that science was degenerating into a study of mere facts and with that came the loss of its meaning for life. He established phenomenology: "not as a science of facts, but as a science of essential Being (as eidetic science); a science which aims exclusively at establishing 'knowledge of essences' and absolutely 'no facts'" (Husserl, 1913/1962, p. 40). Husserl's philosophy of phenomenology provided a new way of looking at things: "One that contrasts at every point with the natural attitude of experience and thought; to move freely along this new way without ever reverting to the old viewpoints, to learn to see what stands before our eyes, to distinguish, to describe" (Husserl, 1913/1962, p. 39).

Critical to Husserl's philosophy of phenomenology is the concept of reduction which "discloses an entirely unsuspected, vast field of research . . . If we miss the meaning of reduction, which is the unique entrance to this new realm, everything is lost" (Husserl, 1981, p. 319). The process of phenomenological reduction entails changing one's natural or naïve attitude toward the world. Reduction involves bracketing or putting aside one's presuppositions and what one knows about a phenomenon being studied so that one can see it without imposing past knowledge or experience upon the phenomenon. Husserl was striving for the elimination of presuppositions that have not been thoroughly examined. As he explained:

> I do not turn my back on the world to retreat into an unworldly and, therefore, uninteresting special field of theoretical study. On the contrary, this alone enables me to explore the world radically. Once the inadequacy of the naïve attitude has been realized, this is the only possible way of establishing science in its genuine radicality.
>
> *(Husserl, 1981, p. 322)*

In the natural attitude the everyday world is just there for persons who naïvely view ongoing life. We need to abstain from this naïve attitude. Husserl encouraged his followers that they "are not left with a meaningless, habitual abstention; rather it is through this abstention that the gaze of the philosopher in truth first becomes fully free" (Husserl, 1954/1970, p. 151). By denying ourselves the natural life world, one is in a position above this.

The process of reduction allows one freedom to search for the essence of a phenomenon, its most invariant meaning. Free imaginative variation is one approach that can be used to discover essences. By means of free imaginative variation, a person varies descriptive features of a specific phenomenon in imagination so that the invariant or essential characteristics of the phenomenon are identified. If a change of the characteristic changes the identity of the phenomenon, then it would be considered an essential feature.

Phenomenological reduction is a source of disagreement among philosophers. Heidegger, one of Husserl's star students, turned away from his distinguished professor because of reduction. Heidegger's philosophy is addressed in Chapter 11 in this volume on interpretive phenomenology.

Literature search

Published descriptive phenomenological studies conducted by nurse researchers were located by means of electronic searches for the past 20 years using PubMed and CINAHL. Key words such as "phenomenology," "phenomenological study," and "descriptive phenomenology" were used to locate appropriate studies. As an extra added measure in order to locate as many studies as possible, the 74 journals listed in the Journal Citation Reports for the Nursing subject category in the social science edition were individually reviewed using the same keywords as used in the PubMed and CINAHL searches.

Criteria for inclusion were that: (1) the study was a descriptive phenomenological study; (2) conducted by at least one nurse researcher; (3) a specific descriptive phenomenological method was identified; and (4) the study was in English. If only a brief, general statement was included in the methodology section of an article, such as just stating that the study was a descriptive phenomenological study in which themes were identified, that study was not included in this literature review. A limitation of this review is that descriptive phenomenological studies conducted by nurse researchers that were published in languages other than English were not included.

Results

Descriptive phenomenological studies published by international nurse researchers over-whelmingly used one of the methods developed by the Duquesne School of Phenomenology. Colaizzi's (1973, 1978) method (n = 310) was by far the most frequently used approach by nurse researchers during this 20-year period (Table 10.1). Giorgi's (1985) approach was the second most frequently cited method (n = 96), followed by van Kaam's (1966) method (n = 11). In Table 10.1 can also be found a breakdown of the studies by country. The majority of studies were conducted by nurse researchers in the US. Nurse researchers in the UK ranked second, followed by Taiwan in the number of descriptive phenomenological studies published in this 20-year period.

In a small number of studies, a modification of Colaizzi's method developed by Moustakas (1994) (n = 7) was employed. Porter (1995), a nurse researcher, developed what she termed a phenomenological alternative to the activities of daily living research tradition. It was based on Husserl's phenomenology. She herself has conducted 21 studies on older widows' experiences using her method.

Colaizzi's (1978), Giorgi's (1985) and van Kaam's (1966) steps involved in their phenomeno-logical methods are summarized in Table 10.2. Even though all three of these methods were developed by researchers in the discipline of psychology at Duquesne University, disagreement prevails among them. When nurse researchers are deciding which method to use in their descriptive phenomenological study, it is essential that they read the primary sources for each method being considered. For instance, in all three methods, phenomenological reduction is addressed but there are some variations. Colaizzi calls for phenomenologists to interrogate their presuppositions about the phenomenon being studied so that they uncover their beliefs and attitudes. Colaizzi falls short of asking users of his research method to bracket their presuppositions

Table 10.1 Descriptive phenomenological methods used in 20-year period by country

Country	Colaizzi	Giorgi	van Kaam	Total
USA	204	33	3	240
Taiwan	28	3	0	31
UK	27	9	0	36
China	8	4	4	16
Sweden	4	21	1	26
Ireland	8	0	1	9
Canada	7	5	1	13
Australia	8	5	0	13
Finland	8	1	0	9
New Zealand	1	2	0	3
Norway	1	7	0	8
South Africa	0	1	0	1
The Netherlands	1	0	0	1
Korea	2	0	0	2
Turkey	2	0	0	2
Iceland	1	0	0	1
Spain	0	3	1	4
Japan	0	2	0	2
Total	310	96	11	417

Table 10.2 Comparison of three phenomenological methods

Colaizzi	Giorgi	van Kaam
Read all of the subjects' descriptions in order to acquire a feeling for them	One reads the entire description in order to get a sense of the whole	Listing and preliminary grouping of descriptive expressions which must be agreed upon by expert judges. Final listing presents percentages of these categories in that particular sample
Return to each protocol and extract significant statements	Researcher discriminates units from the participants' description of the phenomenon being studied	In reduction the researcher reduces the concrete, vague, and overlapping expressions of the participants to more precisely descriptive terms. There again, intersubjective agreement among judges is necessary
Spell out the meaning of each significant statement, known as formulating meanings	Researcher does this from within a psychological perspective and with a focus on the phenomenon under study	Elimination of these elements that are not inherent in the phenomenon being studied or which represent a blending of this phenomenon with other phenomena that most frequently accompany it
Organize the formulated meanings into clusters of themes		
Refer these clusters of themes back to the original protocols in order to validate them	Researcher expresses the psychological insight contained in each of the meaning units more directly	
At this point, discrepancies may be noted among and/or between the various clusters. Researchers must refuse temptation of ignoring data or themes which do not fit	Researcher synthesizes all of the transformed meaning units into a consistent statement regarding the participants' experiences. This is referred to as the structure of the experience and can be expressed on a specific or a general level	A hypothetical identification and description of the phenomenon being studied are written
Results so far integrated into an exhaustive description of phenomenon under study		The hypothetical description is applied to randomly selected cases of the sample. If necessary, the hypothesized description is revised. This revised description must be tested again on a new random sample of cases

Table 10.2 Continued

Colaizzi	Giorgi	van Kaam
Formulate the exhaustive description of investigated phenomenon in as unequivocal a statement of identification as possible		
A final validating step can be achieved by returning to each subject asking about the findings so far		When operations described in previous steps have been carried out successfully, the formerly hypothetical identification of the phenomenon under study may be considered to be valid identification and description

Source: Beck (1994), pp. 256–257.

but instead directs them to use their uncovered presuppositions to help formulate their research questions.

Giorgi (1985) is very upfront with the need for reduction in his method: "What is required is that the analysis and descriptive results of the researcher take place within the phenomenological reduction" (Giorgi, 2000, p. 6). He goes on to stress that reduction in itself is not a research method but one step in the method. In van Kaam's (1966) method he purports that by explication an enlightened awareness of a phenomenon is produced. In Table 10.2 are listed his steps of explication: "Explication is based on the raw data instead of the researcher's own personal experience of the phenomenon" (p. 305). Van Kaam stresses that the researcher "must restrict himself in his explication to the expression of what is given in awareness. During the process of explication, he ought not to involve himself in any implicit philosophizing" (p. 306). He went on to warn that "a scientist who begins with his own analyzed experience may be prejudiced from the very beginning" (p. 308).

Another issue where these three methods differ is in the use of the participants and judges to review the results of the data analysis. Colaizzi (1978) considered participants in a phenomeno-logical study as co-researchers. He called for dialogal research where the dialogue occurs only among persons on equal levels, negating the distinction between researcher and participant. Colaizzi stressed the need to have the co-researchers validate the fundamental structure of the phenomenon under study. Giorgi (1988), on the other hand, argued against having participants in a research study validate the results. Giorgi believed that asking participants to evaluate the findings is inappropriate since they had described their experiences from an everyday perspective. In Giorgi's method, the phenomenologist seeks the psychological meaning of participants' everyday experiences and the two perspectives do not coincide.

Van Kaam's (1966) method has a quantitative flavor to it with his terms such as "randomly selected cases." He called for the use of expert judges to review the steps of data analysis in a study in order to prevent subjectivism. What the researcher keeps is only the data analysis that the expert judges consensually validated. Giorgi (1989) opposed the use of expert judges because it emphasized facts such as whether themes listed under a category fit that category. According to Giorgi, that type of step is not appropriate in a phenomenological framework which stresses essential meaning with the help of free imaginative variation. Neither does Colaizzi (1978) call

137

for expert judges to validate the steps of data analysis as van Kaam does. Colaizzi is the only one of the three phenomenologists who has the participants themselves validate the results of data analysis. Nurse researchers need to be aware of the differences in these descriptive phenomenological methods so they can make an informed choice and stay true to the chosen method and avoid method slurring (Beck, 1994).

Moustakas (1994) developed a modification of analysis of phenomenological data based on a combination of the methods of Colaizzi (1973), Stevick (1971), and Keen (1975). The following are the steps in Moustakas' (1994, p. 122) modification:

1 Using a phenomenological approach, obtain a full description of your experience of the phenomenon.
2 From the verbatim transcript of your experience complete the following steps:
  a Consider each statement with respect to significance for description of the experience.
  b Record all relevant statements.
  c List each nonrepetitive, nonoverlapping statement. These are the invariant horizons or meaning units of the experience.
  d Relate and cluster the invariant meaning units into themes.
  e Synthesize the invariant meaning units and themes into a description of the textures of the experience. Include verbatim examples.
  f Reflect on your own textural description. Through imaginative variation, construct a description of the structures of your experience.
  g Construct a textural-structural description of the meanings and essences of your experience.
3 From the verbatim transcript of the experience of each of the other co-researchers, complete the above steps, a–g.
4 From the individual textural-structural descriptions of all co-researchers' experiences, construct a composite textural-structural description of the meanings and essences of the experience, integrating all individual textural-structural descriptions into a universal description of the experience representing the group as a whole.

Two examples of studies using Moustakas' method included a study of the experience of pregnancy complications in single older women (Mandel, 2010) and the process of acquiring practical knowledge by emergency nurses in Taiwan (Chu & Hsu, 2011).

Porter (1995) adapted a phenomenological alternative to the activities of daily living research to study older widows' lived experiences. Her analysis method was based on Husserl's phenomenology. Since individuals structure their lived experiences by means of their intentional acts, Porter called for interview and observational data to be obtained concerning persons' intentional acts and their perceptions of these acts. Based on Husserl's (1913/1962) strategies of "describing, comparing, distinguishing, and inferring" (p. 93), Porter analyzed data inductively and deductively to develop the structures of lived experiences. "Three categories of structures, ranging from specific to general, were developed: (a) intention, (b) component phenomenon, and (c) phenomenon. A taxonomy of mutually exclusive phenomena was not created because such a product is inconsistent with Husserl's ideas" (Porter, 1995, p. 32). Porter provided an example of how related structures of older widows' lived experiences were developed from data: "(a) thinking about movement, an intention; (b) exercising caution, a component phenomenon; and (c) reducing my risks, a phenomenon" (p. 32).

Using her method Porter conducted over 20 studies in her research program with older widows. Some examples of these studies included intentions of older homebound women to reduce the risk of falling again (Porter, Matsuda, & Lindbloom, 2010), and older homebound women negotiating reliance on a cane or walker (Porter, Benson, & Matsuda, 2011).

Topics of phenomena studied

The top three phenomena most frequently investigated by nurse researchers using descriptive phenomenology during this span of 20 years were: (1) experiences of nurses/nursing students (n = 103); (2) patients' experiences in childbearing (n = 41); and (3) oncology patients' experiences (n = 35).

Nurses' experiences

Examples of the descriptive phenomenological studies nurse researchers conducted with the focus on nurses' experiences are provided from the following countries: the United States, the United Kingdom, Canada, Australia, Ireland, China, the Philippines, Sweden, and Switzerland. In the US, Kindy, Petersen, and Parkhurst (2005) studied nurses' experiences in psychiatric units with high risk of assault. The perceptions of nurses in the UK of expert palliative care were investigated by Johnston and Smith (2006). In Canada, pediatric intensive care unit nurses' experiences of grief were examined (Rashotte et al., 1997). Another study focused on caring for clients with a dual diagnosis in rural communities in Australia (Deans & Soar, 2005). In Ireland, Hilliard and O'Neill (2010) concentrated on nurses' emotional experiences of caring for children with burns. Caring practices in Chinese professional contexts were described by Pang et al. (2000) and in the Philippines Arthur et al. (2006) investigated the experiences of primary health care nurses in a school of nursing. Experiences of community health nurses in Sweden regarding fathers' participation in child health care were explored (Alehagen, Hagg, Kalen-Enterlov, & Johansson, 2011). In Switzerland, Hantikainen and Kappeli (2000) explored nurses' experiences using restraints with nursing home residents.

Nursing students' experiences were also studied. Examples of these descriptive phenomenological studies carried out by nurse researchers include studies in Taiwan, the US, and Korea. In Taiwan, Jiang, Chou, and Tsai (2006) examined grief reactions of nursing students to the sudden death of a classmate. Also in Taiwan, Hung, Huang, and Lin (2009) investigated the first experiences of clinical practice of psychiatric nursing students. Love (2010) reported on the experiences of African American nursing students in a predominantly White university in the US. Also in the US, nursing students' experiences caring for dying patients (Beck, 1997) and of faculty incivility in nursing education (Clark, 2008) have been examined. So and Shin (2011) examined the experiences of Korean nursing students in a spiritual care practicum.

Childbirth experiences

Nurse researchers in the US, Sweden, Taiwan, Finland, New Zealand, and the UK have published descriptive phenomenological studies on different aspects of childbirth. Illustrations of the breadth of childbearing experiences that have been studied include the experience of pregnancy and motherhood after a diagnosis with HIV in the US (Sanders, 2008), decision-making experiences of mothers selecting waterbirth in Taiwan (Wu & Chung, 2003), women's experiences of antenatal care in Finland (Bondas, 2002), antenatal testing in the UK and subsequent birth of a child with Down's syndrome (Sooben, 2010), and first-time parents' experiences of their intimate relationship in Sweden (Ahlborg & Strandmark, 2001).

Fathers have also been the focus of descriptive phenomenological studies by nurse researchers. For example, in New Zealand, fathers' experiences of PTSD following childbirth were explored by White (2007). First-time expectant fathers' experiences of having a spouse tocolyzed in the hospital were examined in Taiwan (Hsieh, Kao, & Gau, 2006). In the US, Schachman (2010) studied first-time fatherhood in combat-deployed troops.

Oncological patients' experiences

Nurses researchers have studied patients' experiences in oncology on an international scope in the US, the UK, Canada, China, Sweden, Denmark, Taiwan, Norway, Turkey, and Ireland. In the US, Stegenga and Ward-Smith (2009) studied adolescents' perceptions of receiving the diagnosis of cancer. The experience of eating problems for patients with head and neck cancer during radiation was the focus of Larsson et al.'s. (2003) study in Sweden. In the UK, Worster and Holmes (2009) investigated the preoperative experiences of patients undergoing surgery for colorectal cancer, while, in China, Wu et al. (2010) examined the experiences of cancer-related fatigue in children with leukemia. Living with gynecologic cancer was the focus of Akyuz et al.'s (2008) study in Turkey. Chemotherapy-induced alopecia was investigated in Ireland (Power & Condon, 2008) and life attitudes in patients with nasopharyngeal carcinoma in Taiwan (Chou et al., 2007). In Norway, cancer inpatients' communication needs were the focus of Kvale's (2007) research, while the experiences of grandparents who had a grandchild with cancer were examined by Charlebois and Bouchard (2007).

Illustration of a descriptive phenomenological study

One of the studies from my research program on traumatic childbirth is now described as an example of a descriptive phenomenological study using Colaizzi's (1978) method. Subsequent childbirth after a previous traumatic birth involved an Internet study of 35 women (Beck & Watson, 2010). One of the benefits of using the Internet to recruit participants is the international sample that it yields. Out of the 35 mothers, 15 (43%) were from the US, 8 (23%), from the UK, 6 (17%) from New Zealand, 5 (14%) from Australia, and 1 (3%) from Canada. The recruitment notice for the study was placed on the website of Trauma and Birth Stress (TABS; www.tabs.org.nz) which is a charitable trust in New Zealand. Mothers who were interested in participating in this research sent their experiences of their subsequent births after a previous birth trauma as attachments to the first author via her university email address. Data collection continued for 2 years and 2 months and involved the women responding to the statement "Please describe in as much detail as you can remember your subsequent pregnancy, labor, and delivery following your previous traumatic birth."

Using Colaizzi's (1978) method, Table 10.3 illustrates how one paragraph from a participant was divided up into 10 significant statements. Analysis of the 35 written descriptions resulted in 274 significant statements. The formulated meanings for these significant statements about the phenomenon of subsequent childbirth following an earlier birth trauma were clustered into four themes: (1) riding the turbulent wave of panic during pregnancy; (2) strategizing: attempts to reclaim their body and complete the journey to motherhood; (3) bringing reverence to the birthing process and empowering women; and (4) still elusive: the longed-for healing birth experience.

Based on these four themes the fundamental structure was developed that identified the essence of the phenomenon (Table 10.4). Two mothers reviewed the themes and fundamental structure of the phenomenon under study and totally agreed with them.

Table 10.3 Example of extracting significant statements

Number	Significant statements
1	One thing that I'd noticed when I was a child was that when my parents got together with other adults, the talk eventually turned to two things: for my father (a Vietnam veteran) and the other men the talk turned to the war and interestingly, to me as a small child, for my mother and the other women the talk always turned to childbirth.
2	It was as if, from a young age, for me, the connections between the two were drawn. A man is tested through war, a women is tested through childbirth.
3	My dad, as abusive as he was, was considered a "good man" because he'd been a good soldier and so, I reasoned forward with a child's intelligence, that all that really mattered for a woman was to be strong and capable in childbirth.
4	And I failed. In the past, with the previous two births (particularly with the one that resulted in PTSD) – that's what it felt like. I failed at being a woman.
5	I don't think that I am alone in feeling. I have a sneaking suspicion that this is pretty universal.
6	Just as a man who "talks" under torture in a POW situation feels as though he's failed, a woman who can't "handle" tortuous situations during childbirth feels like she's failed. It is not true. But it feels true.
7	My dad received two Purple Hearts and a Bronze Star during Vietnam. He, by most standards, would be considered a hero. Where are my Purple Hearts? My Bronze Star? I've fought a war, no less terrifying, no less destroying but there are no accolades. At least that's what it feels like.
8	I am viewed as flawed if not downright strange that I find L & D [Labor and Delivery] so terrifying.
9	The medical establishment thinks that I am "mental" and I have no common ground on which to discuss my childbirth experiences with "normal" women.
10	I know, I've tried. And that makes me feel isolated and inferior.

Source: Beck and Watson (2010), p. 244.

Table 10.4 Fundamental structure of the phenomenon

Subsequent childbirth after a previous traumatic birth far exceeds the confines of the actual labor and delivery. During the 9 months of pregnancy women ride turbulent waves of panic, terror, and fear that the looming birth could be a repeat of the emotional and/or physical torture they had endured with their previous labor and delivery. Women strategized during pregnancy how they could reclaim their bodies that had been violated and traumatized by their previous childbirth. Women vowed to themselves that things would be different and that this time they would complete their journey to motherhood. Mothers employed strategies to try to bring a reverence to the birthing process and rectify all that had gone so wrong with their prior childbirth. The array of various strategies entailed such actions as hiring doulas for support during labor and delivery, becoming avid readers of childbirth books, writing a detailed birth plan, learning birth hypnosis, interviewing obstetricians and midwives about their philosophy of birth, doing yoga, and drawing birthing art. All these well designed strategies did not ensure that all women would experience the healing childbirth they desperately longed for. For the mothers whose subsequent childbirth was a healing experience, they reclaimed their bodies, had a strong sense of control, and their birth became an empowering experience. The role of caring supporters was crucial in their labor and delivery. Women were treated with respect, dignity, and compassion. Even though their subsequent birth was positive and empowering, women were quick to note that it could never change the past. Still elusive for some women was their longed-for healing subsequent birth.

Source: Beck and Watson (2010), p. 245.

Conclusion

In this chapter the philosophical underpinnings of descriptive phenomenology were described. Published descriptive phenomenological studies conducted by nurse researchers across the globe over the past 20 years were reviewed. Trends in the methods used by these nurse researchers and also the phenomena studied were identified. Overwhelmingly the methods developed by the Duquesne School of Phenomenology were used. Colaizzi's method was the one used most frequently followed by Giorgi's method, and then van Kaam's method. Comparison of these three methods was described with disagreements noted. The three phenomena investigated most often by international nurse researchers during this 20-year period in order of frequency were the experiences of nurses/nursing students, patients' experiences in childbirth, and oncology patients' experiences. Overwhelmingly the most descriptive phenomenological studies were conducted by nurse researchers in the US followed by the UK. A limitation of this literature review, however, is the criterion that the studies needed to be published in English. In the future hopefully we can rectify the language barriers that hinder nurse researchers from around the globe also publishing in English journals so that an increased audience can learn from the rich findings from their descriptive phenomenological studies.

References

Ahlborg, T., & Strandmark, M. (2001). The baby was the focus of attention—First-time parents' experiences of their intimate relationship. *Scandinavian Journal of Caring Sciences*, *15*, 318–325.

Akyuz, A., Guvens, G., Ustunsoz, A., & Kaya, T. (2008). Living with gynecologic cancer: Experience of women and their partners. *Journal of Nursing Scholarship*, *40*, 241–247.

Alehagen, S., Hagg, M., Kalen-Enterlov, M., & Johansson, A. K. (2011). Experiences of community health nurses regarding father participation in child health care. *Journal of Child Health Care*, *15*, 153–162.

Arthur, D., Drury, J., Sy-Sinda, T., Nakao, R., Lopez, A., Gloria, G., Turtal, R., & Luna, E. (2006). A primary health care curriculum in action: The lived experience of primary health care nurses in a school of nursing in the Philippines: A phenomenological study. *International Journal of Nursing Studies*, *43*, 107–112.

Beck, C. T. (1994). Reliability and validity issues in phenomenological research. *Western Journal of Nursing Research*, *16*, 254–262.

Beck, C. T. (1997). Nursing students' experiences caring for dying patients. *Journal of Nursing Education*, *36*, 408–415.

Beck, C. T. & Watson, S. (2008). Impact of birth trauma on breast-feeding: A tale of two pathways. *Nursing Research*, *57*, 228–236.

Beck, C. T., & Watson, S. (2010). Subsequent childbirth after a previous traumatic birth. *Nursing Research*, *59*, 241–249.

Bondas, T. (2002). Finnish women's experiences of antenatal care. *Midwifery*, *18*, 61–71.

Charlebois, S., & Bouchard, L. (2007). "The worst experience": The experience of grandparents who have a grandchild with cancer. *Canadian Oncology Nursing Journal*, *17*, 26–36.

Chou, H. L., Liaw, J. J., Yu, L. H., & Tang, W. R. (2007). An exploration of life attitudes in patients with nasopharyngeal carcinoma. *Cancer Nursing*, *30*, 317–323.

Chu, W., & Hsu, L. L. (2011). The process of acquiring practical knowledge by emergency nursing professionals in Taiwan. *Journal of Emergency Nursing*, 37, 126–131.

Clark, C. M. (2008). Student voices on faculty incivility in nursing education: A conceptual model. *Nursing Education Perspectives*, *29*, 284–289.

Colaizzi, P. (1973). *Reflection and research in psychology*. Dubuque, IA: Kendall/Hunt.

Colaizzi, P. (1978). Psychological research as the phenomenologist views it. In R. Valle & M. King (Eds.), *Existential phenomenological alternative for psychology* (pp. 48–71). New York: Oxford University Press.

Deans, C., & Soar, R. (2005). Caring for clients with dual diagnosis in rural communities in Australia: The experience of mental health professionals. *Journal of Psychiatric and Mental Health Nursing*, *12*, 268–274.

Giorgi, A. (1985). *Phenomenology and psychological research*. Pittsburgh, PA: Duquesne University Press.

Giorgi, A. (1988). Validity and reliability from a phenomenological perspective. In W. Baker, L. Mos, H. Rappard, & H. Stam (Eds.), *Recent trends in theoretical psychology* (pp. 167–176). New York: Springer-Verlag.

Giorgi, A. (1989). Some theoretical and practice issues regarding the psychological phenomenological method. *Saybrook Review*, *1*, 71–85.

Giorgi, A. (2000). The status of Husserlian phenomenology in caring research. *Scandinavian Journal of Caring Science*, *14*, 1–10.

Hantikainen, V., & Kappeli, S. (2000). Using restraint with nursing home residents: A qualitative study of nursing staff perceptions and decision-making. *Journal of Advanced Nursing*, *32*, 1196–1205.

Hilliard, C., & O"Neill, M. (2010). Nurses' emotional experience of caring for children with burns. *Journal of Clinical Nursing*, *19*, 2907–2915.

Hsieh, Y. H., Kao, C. H., & Gau, M. L. (2006). First time expectant fathers whose spouses are tocolyzed in the hospital. *Journal of Nursing Research*, *14*, 65–74.

Husserl, E. (1913/1962). *Ideas: General introduction to pure phenomenology*. New York: Macmillan.

Husserl, E. (1954/1970). *The crisis of European sciences and transcendental phenomenology*. Evanston, IL: Northwestern University Press.

Husserl, E. (1981). Phenomenology and anthropology. In P. McCormick & F. Elliston (Eds.), *Husserl: Shorter works* (pp. 315–323). Notre Dame, IN: University of Notre Dame Press.

Hung, B. J., Huang, X. Y., & Lin, M. J. (2009). The first experiences of clinical practice of psychiatric nursing students in Taiwan: A phenomenological study. *Journal of Clinical Nursing*, *18*, 3126–3135.

Jiang, R.S., Chou, C.C., & Tsai, P.L. (2006). The grief reaction of nursing students related to the sudden death of a classmate. *Journal of Nursing Research*, *14*, 279–284.

Johnston, B., & Smith, L.N. (2006). Nurses' and patients' perceptions of expert palliative nursing care. *Journal of Advanced Nursing*, *54*, 700–709.

Keen, E. (1975). Doing research phenomenologically. Unpublished manuscript, Bucknell University, Lewisburg, PA.

Kindy, D., Petersen, S., & Parkhurst, D. (2005). Perilous work: Nurses' experiences in psychiatric units with high risks of assault. *Archives of Psychiatric Nursing*, *19*, 1699–1750.

Kvale, K. (2007). Do cancer patients always want to talk about difficult emotions? A qualitative study of cancer inpatients' communication needs. *European Journal of Oncology Nursing*, *11*, 320–327.

Larsson, M., Hedelin, B., & Athlin, E. (2003). Lived experiences of eating problems for patients with head and neck cancer during radiotherapy. *Journal of Clinical Nursing*, *12*, 562–570.

Love, K.L. (2010). The lived experience of socialization among African American nursing students in a predominantly White university. *Journal of Transcultural Nursing*, *21*, 342–350.

Mandel, D. (2010). The lived experience of pregnancy complications in single older women. *MCN: The American Journal of Maternal/Child Nursing*, *35*, 336–340.

Moustakas, C. (1994). *Phenomenological research methods*. Thousand Oaks, CA: Sage.

Pang, S. M., Arthur, D. G., & Wong, T. K. (2000). Drawing a qualitative distinction of caring practices in a professional context: The case of Chinese nursing. *Holistic Nursing Practice*, *15*, 22–31.

Porter, E. J. (1995). A phenomenological alternative to the "ADL research tradition." *Journal of Aging and Health*, *7*, 24–45.

Porter, E. J., Benson, J. J., & Matsuda, S. (2011). Older homebound women: Negotiating reliance on a cane or walker. *Qualitative Health Research*, *21*, 534–548.

Porter, E. J., Matsuda, S., & Lindbloom, E. J. (2010). Intentions of older homebound women to reduce the risk of falling again. *Journal of Nursing Scholarship*, *42*, 101–109.

Power, S., & Condon, C. (2008). Chemotherapy-induced alopecia: A phenomenological study. *Cancer Nursing Practice*, *7*, 44–47.

Rashotte, J., Fothergill-Bourbonnais, F., & Chamberlain, M. (1997). Pediatric intensive care nurses and their grief experiences: A phenomenological study. *Heart & Lung*, *26*, 372–386.

Sanders, L. B. (2008). Women's voices: The lived experience of pregnancy and motherhood after diagnosis with HIV. *Journal of the Association of Nurses in AIDS Care*, *19*, 47–57.

Schachman, K. A. (2010). Online fathering: First time fatherhood in combat deployed troops. *Nursing Research*, *59*, 11–17.

Shin, K. Y., Kim, M. Y., & Chung, S. E. (2009). Methods and strategies utilized in published qualitative research. *Qualitative Health Research*, *19*, 850–858.

So, W. S., & Shin, H. S. (2011). Korean students' experience in a spiritual care practicum. *Journal of Christian Nursing*, *28*, 228–234.

Sooben, R.D. (2010). Antenatal testing and the subsequent birth of a child with Down syndrome: A phenomenological study of parents' experiences. *Journal of Intellectual Disabilities, 14*, 79–94.

Stegenga, K., & Ward-Smith, P. (2009). On receiving the diagnosis of cancer: The adolescent experience. *Journal of Pediatric Oncology Nursing, 26*, 75–80.

Stevick, E. L. (1971). An empirical investigation of the experience of anger. In A. Giorgi, W. Fisher, & R. Von Eckartsberg (Eds.), *Duquesne studies in phenomenological psychology*. (Vol. 1, pp. 132–148). Pittsburgh, PA: Duquesne University Press.

van Kaam, A. (1966). *Existential foundations of psychology*. Pittsburgh, PA: Duquesne University Press.

White, G. (2007). You cope by breaking down in private: Fathers and PTSD following childbirth. *British Journal of Midwifery, 15*, 39–45.

Worster, B., & Holmes, S. (2009). A phenomenological study of the postoperative experiences of patients undergoing surgery for colorectal cancer. *European Journal of Oncology Nursing, 13*, 315–322.

Wu, C. J., & Chung, U. L. (2003). The decision-making experience of mothers selecting waterbirth. *Journal of Nursing Research, 11*, 261–267.

Wu, M., Hsu, L., Zhang, B., Shen, N., Lu, H., & Li, S. (2010). The experiences of cancer-related fatigue among Chinese children with leukaemia: A phenomenological study. *International Journal of Nursing Studies, 47*, 49–59.

11

Interpretive phenomenology

Patricia L. Munhall

> Discussing or talking is the way in which we articulate significantly the intelligibility of
> Being-in-the-world. The way in which discourse gets expressed is Language.
>
> *(M. Heidegger, 1927/1962)*

Introduction

This chapter introduces the reader to interpretive phenomenology as not only a research method
but also as a way of being-in-the-world. We are always in the world as long as we are alive and
we are always in experience. Some individuals seem to go blithely about their life without much
reflection as to meaning or understanding. Others, though, seek meaning as in the meaning of
being human and what experience means in different contexts. We might say those individuals
are assuming a phenomenological perspective in their life as a way of being in the world in
interaction with self and others.

I believe it is essential to become phenomenological in your own being if you are to embark
on phenomenological research and, in particular, interpretive phenomenology. Therefore, in this
chapter I am going to discuss the philosophical tenets of interpretive phenomenology, how we
become unknowing so that we can listen with the third ear[1] to hear new and different interpretations
of reality, search for meaning in experience for self and others and become more understanding,
empathic, authentic and compassionate. These characteristics are essential to attunement with
another, to hear their language through their distinctive voice and their distinctive narratives.

Another aim of this chapter is to *inquire* how one uses an interpretive phenomenological
philosophy as a research approach. We will engage in this interpretive process in search of
understanding and meaning of experience for others who through language provide narratives
for the researcher. The respect we show these narratives, in order to understand them in an
authentic manner, calls upon us to understand the irreducibility of human beings, the postmodern
and multistoried world, intersubjectivity, the situated context of being, suspending our
assumptions, being atheoretical and becoming childlike, reflecting wonder and awe as the varied
meanings and interpretation awaken us to our taken-for-granted beliefs and knowledge that
presently structure our approach to caring for others.

The findings of interpretive phenomenological research lead us to include understanding the
meaning of experience for self and others, liberating us from our assumptions, preconceptions,

and myths, legitimizing differences among peoples, and emancipating us from outdated beliefs or stereotypes which often oppress people and cultures. From voices often silenced we attend to the fluid core of being human and our research leads to individualized care, understanding and meaning. This calls for an understanding of intersubjectivity where two subjective perspectives in a phenomenological project intersect, which will be discussed in this chapter.

The difference between descriptive and interpretive phenomenology should become apparent and will be called out for you to consider. Also in the nursing literature interpretive analysis and hermeneutic analysis seem to be used interchangeably and in this chapter I will follow this trend.

"Understanding meaning" is paramount to interpretive phenomenology. This is not a "how to do" chapter but I would like to focus on some key tenets that may assist you in carrying and understanding the interpretive project. Included then in this chapter is a brief outline of van Manen's method of doing phenomenology and then my own approach, which attempts to modify or add to his approach specifically for a practice discipline such as nursing.

To assist the reader in understanding the scope of interpretive phenomenology from an international perspective, a random sample from a literature review provides actual research projects, as illustrated in Table 11.1, entitled "International interpretive phenomenological nursing studies: a random sample." I find it so encouraging to read how worldwide interpretive phenomenology is being performed in Thailand, Sweden, England, Canada, as well as the USA. Reading these research projects, I come to appreciate in a deeper way how influential one's situated context (to be discussed) is essential in this relational way of understanding the meaning of experience. We encounter the particulars of our life-worlds and thoughtfully can address the myriad of differences in interpretation.

One caveat, and it is a critical one, is this chapter is just a brush stroke due to space restrictions. Perhaps that should be in the chapter title: "*A Brush Stroke* of Interpretive Phenomenology"! One stroke against many blank pages and there is so much more to be known and learned beyond this brief overview. References will be listed to expand your knowledge and if you do pursue this approach, with further immersion into the philosophy I assure you, you will find meaning in and understanding of interpretive phenomenology as well as a heightened consciousness to the meaning in experience.

Another more practical caveat is that there will be repetition as points made in one context will be repeated in another context, so if you have the feeling you already read that, you have! However, the meaning will be within that context.

Table 11.1 International interpretive phenomenological nursing studies: a random sample*

Title:	"The body gives way, things happen": Older women describe breast cancer with a non-supportive intimate partner
Authors:	Sawin, Erika Metzler
Affiliation:	James Madison University, 801 Carrier Dr., MSC 4305, Harrisonburg, VA 22807, USA
Source:	*European Journal of Oncology Nursing* (EUR J ONCOL NURS), 2012 Feb; 16(1): 64–70
Title:	Thai Buddhists' experiences caring for family members who died a peaceful death in intensive care
Authors:	Kongsuwan, Waraporn; Chaipetch, Orapan
Affiliation:	Assistant Professor, Medical Nursing Department, Faculty of Nursing, Prince of Songkla University, Hat Yai, Songkhla, Thailand
	Head Nurse of Surgical Ward, Nursing Department, Songklanagarind Hospital, Faculty of Medicine, Prince of Songkla University, Hat Yai, Songkhla, Thailand
Source:	*International Journal of Palliative Nursing* (INT J PALLIAT NURS), 2011 Jul; 17(7): 329–336 (36 ref)

Title: Is there a place for ontological hermeneutics in mental-health nursing research? A review of a hermeneutic study

Authors: Chang, K. H.; Horrocks, S

Affiliation: Department of Nursing, Faculty of Medicine and Health Sciences, University Malaysia Sarawak, Sarawak, Malaysia.

Source: *International Journal of Nursing Practice* (INT J NURS PRACT), 2008 Oct; 14(5): 383–390 (28 ref)

Title: Patients' lived experience of myeloma

Authors: Dowling, M.; Kelly, M.

Source: *Nursing Standard* (NURS STAND), 2011 Mar 16–22; 25(28): 38–44 (48 ref)

Title: Living with an adult family member using advanced medical technology at home

Authors: Fex, Angelika; Flensner, Gullvi; Ek, Anna-Christina; Söderhamn, Olle

Affiliation: University West, Trollhättan, Sweden
               Linköping University, Linköping, Sweden
               University West, Trollhättan, Sweden

Source: *Nursing Inquiry* (NURS INQUIRY), 2011 Dec; 18(4): 336–347 (29 ref)

Title: The meaning of breast cancer risk for African American Women

Authors: Phillips, Janice; Cohen, Marlene Z.

Affiliation: Alpha Lambda, Former Manager-Nursing Research, Research Associate, Center for Clinical Cancer Genetics and Global Health, University of Chicago Medical Center, Chicago, IL Gamma Pi at Large, Professor and Kenneth E. Morehead Endowed Chair in Nursing, Associate Dean for Research, University of Nebraska Medical Center, College of Nursing, Omaha, NE

Source: *Journal of Nursing Scholarship* (J NURS SCHOLARSH), 2011 Sept; 43(3): 239–247 (20 ref)

Title: Individual arrangements for elderly patients after hospitalization: a phenomenological-hermeneutic study based on experiences from nurse leaders in the municipality [Norwegian].

Authors: Tingvoll, Wivi-Ann; Fredriksen, Sven-Tore Dreyer

Affiliation: Førstelektor, Høgskolen i Narvik, Lodve langes gt. 2 Postboks 385, NO – 8505 Narvik

Source: *Nordic Journal of Nursing Research & Clinical Studies / Vård i Norden* (VARD I NORDEN), 2011; 31(3): 40–44 (33 ref)

Title: Improving access to government health care in rural Bangladesh: The voice of older adult women.

Authors: Hossen, Abul; Westhues, Anne

Affiliation: Faculty of Social Work, Wilfrid Laurier University, Canada
               Faculty of Social Work, Wilfrid Laurier University, Canada

Source: *Health Care for Women International* (HEALTH CARE WOMEN INT), 2011 Dec; 32(12): 1088–1110 (75 ref)

Note: * Studies like these could fill up an entire book. Just know that many search engines in your library will lead you to studies done either about your phenomenon of interest, international studies and excellent philosophical articles. I find it very "meaningful" to see how phenomenology has captured the interest of nurses all over the world.

The meaning of human understanding

Let's begin this chapter with what might be the most important rationale for the use of interpretive phenomenology as a research method in nursing and why that makes this method so compelling to the practice of nursing. Think for a minute what you yourself would like most from your family, friends, colleagues and those with whom you have either a personal or professional relationship. What is it that makes you feel "heard"?

Does being understood come to mind? Does the realization that someone understands what you *mean*, the meaning of what you might be experiencing or attempting to communicate, seem critical to you? How do you feel when someone utterly fails to understand what you are saying, as though they did not even hear you? How do you feel when someone suggests something to you that seems so opposed to who you are as a person? Moreover, that someone seems to know what is best for you when you clearly have voiced the meaning something holds for you.

Now think of our patients, the health care system, the academic setting and for a moment reflect upon the prescribed ways of *doing*, the structured assessments, evaluations, and protocols. The systems in most places where our patients, colleagues and we find ourselves are often deterministic, formula-based without consideration of individual contexts, and most importantly understanding of individuals.

This chapter on interpretive phenomenology as a research method proposes that we as nurse researchers have a means of inquiry that not only leads to understanding another individual but also to understanding the meaning that an experience has for an individual. We appreciate that for ourselves and my goal in this chapter is to have you understand the meaning this has for our patients and those we serve and interact with in different settings.

An advantage of this method is that its approach can be used as a philosophical perspective for your professional practice and also your personal life. Personally and professionally there will be fewer misunderstandings, conflicts, and complications in communication and practice when you live from a phenomenological perspective. Your life and who you are change once you begin to think in an interpretive phenomenological way and use interpretive phenomenology as a research approach. You approach others and experience from a different worldview than positivism and embrace the complexities, *ambiguities and the messiness of life situations* between and among people.

This is a challenge and if you have been reading the prior chapters you will have already an understanding of what underpins qualitative research thinking. However, since I am thinking phenomenologically I *cannot assume* that, so I might be repeating some of what has already been discussed.

Just so we understand where we are headed, we are going to become immersed in focusing on *understanding the meaning of being human in experience* of self and others. This we will do with respect for context and contingencies of individual lives, their differences and commonalities. Important to this project are the philosophical underpinnings of interpretive phenomenology, the concept of meaning, unknowing or de-centering, intersubjectivity and approaches to interpretive research method.

Interpretive phenomenology as method

Interpretive phenomenology has been defined in different ways by different researchers, so there are actually different interpretations of interpretive phenomenology. Patricia Benner (1994), whose excellent work on interpretive phenomenology deserves our attention, states:

> The goal of studying persons, events, and practices in their own term is to understand world, self and other. The interpreter moves back and forth between the foreground and back-ground, between situations and between the practical worlds of the participants.

(p. 99)

As you can see, the word "meaning" does not appear here, upon further reading you will find meaning is an important part of what Benner writes on in interpretive phenomenology. I want to use this, though as an example of different definitions. Phenomenology itself has often been defined "as the study of lived experience." Inherent in that is the voice of the individual who has lived through the experience. Though not explicitly stated but in the epigraph of this chapter is the critical emphasis on language. Language is paramount. The voices of individuals are to be heard unfiltered through our own lens of the world. Individuals narrate the meaning of their experience and include the contingencies of their life-worlds.

When we move from the world of descriptive phenomenology with its philosophical underpinnings derivative of Husserl's philosophy and the belief that there are characteristics that are common to any lived experience, which can be categorized as universal essences or eidetic structures (Natanson, 1973) to the world of interpretive phenomenology, we are able to see the vast differences in these two approaches (discussed in the next section). *It is critical for the researcher to be aware of these differences* and be able to follow the philosophical reasoning of Husserl and others for descriptive phenomenology and Heidegger and others for interpretive phenomenology.

Another definition of interpretive phenomenology using the alternative word "hermeneutics" for "interpretive" does include *meaning*:

> In relation to the study of human experience, hermeneutics goes beyond mere description of core concepts and essences to look for meanings embedded in common life practices. These meanings are not always apparent to the participants but can be gleaned from the narratives produced by them.
>
> *(Lopez & Willis, 2004, p. 728)*

My approach to the interpretive method (see p. 158) differs somewhat with this definition in that I believe we are on more authentic grounding if we explore the meaning with the participants themselves, rather than us "extracting" the meaning from narratives. If you are as a researcher going to "extract" meanings from narratives, you need to return to the individual to ascertain if you did indeed capture his or her meaning.

Adding another dimension to our understanding of what interpretive phenomenology comprises is to be found in the following quote by Caelli: "Contemporary interpretive phenomenology seeks to understand the situated meanings of phenomena in the sense that such knowledge is to be understood within the specific environment or problem domain of the participant" (Caelli, 2000, p. 371, citing Slezak, 1994). Here we see the importance of the situated context of our participants, the life-worlds of spatiality, temporality, embodiment and relational and or the contingencies of each person's being (Munhall, 2012, pp.159–162).

Heidegger's philosophy underpins the interpretive, or hermeneutic research tradition (Cohen, 1987; Lopez & Willis, 2004). The researcher is keenly interested in what Heidegger has called the "life-world" and his philosophical concept of "throwness." We are "thrown" or born into this world during a specific time of history, into a specific location, culture, economic status, in a body which may be healthy or not, male, female and further "thrown" or born into a country, nationality, family intact or not intact, we may or may not have siblings, friends, support and/or colleagues. These then are the life-worlds of temporality, spatiality, embodiment and relational; our "being-in-the-world."

Rorty (1991) emphasized how important individual contingencies are to understanding; the way individuals are embedded in their world with social, cultural, historical, relational, economic, nationality and political contingencies. Each individual occupies their own situated context, which will influence their subjective experience of what it means to be human "be-ing" in their world.

When doing any kind of phenomenology, a researcher should make clear how they are implementing and following the particular philosophy and worldviews of particular philosophers.

In other words, the method should be a reflection of the worldview in this case of Heidegger and other philosophers who have followed him, such as Merleau-Ponty (1962), Gadamer (1976), Dreyfus (1972), Rorty (1991), or van Manen (1990), among many others.

For instance, when conducting an interpretive phenomenological inquiry, the following philosophical underpinnings should be followed, and incorporated in the description of the method, which you need to describe in detail. This has the added benefit of providing a way to evaluate your inquiry while keeping you within the philosophical perspective you have adapted. In Heideggerian phenomenology, the interpretation and self-understanding are handed down through language and culture, called the "background" (Allen, Benner, & Diekelmann, 1986). The idea of the background (much like the situated context and life-world) is critical because it provides conditions for human actions and perceptions. It is where the individual is, a history to the present moment, and a view of "what can be." Other Heideggerian tenets include the following: meaning is found in the *transaction* between an individual and a situation so that the individual both constitutes and is co-constituted by the situation. I will address this in a discussion of intersubjectivity. A critical assumption of this phenomenological perspective as mentioned, is its emphasis on language, which imbues and informs experience. Language does not exist apart from thought or perception, for language reveals and conceals the human life-world of the individual (Munhall, 2012, pp. 35–38).

The meaning of the interpretive project

When we deliver care to others without understanding the individual, we are practicing based on aggregate knowledge. One size will fit all. Protocols are supposed to have the same outcome. We know this is not the case, yet in the quest for certainty, models of care have led to the blind acceptance of procedure manuals, prescriptive theory, stereotyping of care for different cultures or just plain stereotyping of care. Interpretive phenomenology used as a research method allows us entrance into life-worlds of differences, beliefs, attitudes and whole different understandings of variant meanings for individuals based on their history, temporality, embodiment, and their own subjective interpretation of meaning in an experience. This self-interpretation is atheoretical. Instead, the self interprets based on one's background, embedded in their history, cultural traditions and language.

Rather than the mechanistic view of the scientific method, which of course has many purposes of its own, it is a method of epistemology. Interpretive phenomenology moves us also to the world of ontology, the study of meaning in the world of being. What does it mean to be in this world? What does it mean to become ill? What does it mean to become an adolescent, a parent, a nurse, and a patient? What does it mean to be lonely, to be fearful, to feel happy or sad or any emotion in experience? The meanings to these questions are unique to the individual and do not lead to a title, "The Meaning of Loneliness." Instead it might lead to a title such as "The Meaning of Loneliness: Different Voices."

All the above questions are questions of significance because if we gain understanding as to the various and different meaning of these experiences we will have a *variety of directions* and possible ways to guide nursing practice and health care policy (Morse, 1996). Perhaps most importantly, we become capable of delivering the best care to an individual, instead of a prescriptive care based on an aggregate of people collapsed to a statistical mean. Interestingly enough, there may not even be one person representing the statistical mean! I wonder sometimes why we are surprised that there are so many complications when caring for people. We are actually practicing to a statistical mean and need instead, to every extent possible, practice to the individual. Perhaps this could be interpreted as utopian thinking, as in "who has the time?" but when I think of the innumerable complications in health care, I see an ethical imperative to individualize care, and time is the lesser of the ethical concerns.

Additionally, and incredibly important, are the possibilities that interpretive phenomenology offers specific groups who have been labeled, stereotyped, or have prescriptive roles because of unquestioned beliefs or assumptions and, because of these accepted factors, are oppressed groups. The search for understanding the meaning of experience for these groups has and continues to *result in the liberation and emancipation of such people.*

This approach to research then has an ethical imperative for a humanistic profession, as is nursing, one that professes caring for the individuals, families, communities and different cultures. I believe we have a moral calling to those we care for, to see them, to listen with the third ear, to know that all is not revealed and what is concealed could be of life-saving importance, and *that we are unknowing and the knower is the other individual and that an individual's perception is what constitutes their reality.* Interpretive phenomenology can assist us in uncovering and coming to know and understand the individual human being before us who is a mystery to us. How can we design care for this human being without first acknowledging that we do not know this person?

Philosophical differences between descriptive phenomenology and interpretive phenomenology

There are important philosophical differences between descriptive and interpretive phenomenology. For those readers who have read about phenomenology as a research method, you might have noticed that not all researchers distinguish which school or philosophical phenomenological method they are using when they use "the phenomenological method." This actually illustrates the time we are in (temporal world!). Thirty years ago, using the phenomenological method in nursing meant mostly using a descriptive approach as exemplified in Chapter 10. Dr. Beck refers to these methods developed by the Duquesne School of Phenomenology, which were derived from the philosophical beliefs of Edmund Husserl, sometimes called the "Father of Phenomenology." His philosophy is excellently described in that chapter.

As with many "fathers"[2] of a specific philosophy, there will be strict followers and then there will be others who diverge, taking some of the original meaning, synthesizing or integrating a new and different worldview which will then result in an emerging, in this case, a different phenomenology. The predominant philosopher whose works and worldview have influenced the development of interpretive phenomenology is Heidegger, a student of Husserl.

A major difference emerges at this point, and the phenomenological project changes focus to *what humans experience,* rather than what *they consciously know* (Lopez & Willis, 2004). Husserl's idea of reduction was challenged by Heidegger's philosophical "being-in-the-world." Heidegger (1927/1962) posited that human beings are embedded in their life-worlds, linked to social, cultural and political contexts. This concept is called situated freedom (Leonard, 1999) and has been also extolled by Rorty (1991) as to the importance of life contingencies as to where we are, our historicity, location, age, and culture, anything that contributes to our life circumstance. To Sartre (1993), this is situated freedom and contingencies or the situated context that existentially gives rise to the meaning of human experience.

The interpretive phenomenologist from this perspective, rather than seeking essences, themes, or purely descriptive categories, focuses primarily on the supremacy of meaning.

Heidegger also believed that bracketing was not achievable although making preconceptions known and held in abeyance is part of hermeneutic interpretive phenomenology (Lopez & Willis, 2004).

When I did a search for interpretive phenomenology, oftentimes "hermeneutic analysis" was the result, as though the words are interchangeable. From my perspective this emphasis on hermeneutics has been of import to interpretive phenomenology but not without some drawbacks. Hermeneutics was an ancient way of interpreting religious texts, and then applied to the interpretation of other texts. What has happened and is still practiced in some phenomenological methods is that the language of people, their voices are taped, transcribed and then researchers engage in varying ways of trying to interpret the text, rather than having the *individual interpret their own words, showing what they did mean* in their personal description of experience.

This can easily be accomplished (this will be mentioned again in the next section) by incorporating in your dialogue (interview) with an individual the question of meaning. I suggest quite simply to ask, or to say, "I am not sure what you mean by that" during the dialogue, interview or conversation where a narrative of experience is being told.

In closing this section I would like to emphasize that there must be a clear association and integration of the specific philosophical underpinnings that will be guiding and be foundational to your research study. These two distinct approaches, the descriptive and the interpretive, are based on two very different philosophical worldviews and then also on the specific methods which follow. It has become necessary not only to identify the approach that is being used but critical to follow the values and claims associated with the particular philosophy. In this chapter we are discussing interpretive phenomenology. In Chapter 10, Dr. Beck was writing about descriptive phenomenology. Whichever you choose from these two different approaches to accomplish your research goal, it is imperative as you design and carry out your study that you *have complete synchrony between the philosophy and the method.*

These two approaches yield two different types of knowledge and to arrive there you go about your research with a different philosophical lens. Both make valuable contributions to understanding. Descriptive phenomenology focuses on identifying or establishing "knowledge of essences" (Husserl, 1913/1962, p. 40), themes, essential structures of an experience, which can be considered universal. Interpretive phenomenology seeks to *understand the meaning of experience, the meaning of being human* within varying situated contexts of being, the particular and the differences and how this translates into changing practice to be more authentic to the experience.

One approach is not better than another. We can see that just by looking at Chapter 9 and Beck's (1992) descriptive phenomenological study contributing a much-needed understanding of women with postpartum depression, which resulted in screening accurately for postpartum depression. This is essential knowledge and extremely valuable. Beck has undertaken an extremely impressive research program in the area of postpartum depression (among other experiences and topics, look at Beck's references, i.e., Beck herself, and you will see what I mean) and I would like to call your attention to the idea of a "research program," starting with your first study or second study in your area of interest and then pursuing other questions that may have been stimulated for your next study. In the area of interpretive phenomenology I was interested in women's anger, where several inquiries followed and the latest was about understanding the meaning of men's anger (Munhall, 1993b, 1995a, 1995b, 2007). Sarah Lauterbach also has an interpretive research program, several studies on the phenomenon of peri-natal loss (Lauterbach, 1993, 2001, 2007). This focus enables you to gain deeper understanding of the meaning of the experience that interests you, in different contexts, from different perspectives and accrue a body of knowledge for practice.

Using interpretive phenomenology instead of questionnaires or semi-structured interviews

Often we find in research methods the way we can get to know a person is to design a question-naire or semi-structured interview (some may even advocate a structured interview). There may be good reasons for that approach with some research designs but it is antithetical to interpretive phenomenology.

Every good researcher strives to be objective when doing research, meaning not getting in the way of obtaining subjective material from an individual. However, once you decide which questions to ask, you have introduced your own knowledge, presuppositions, assumptions, stereotypes, theories you have learned. Even with a semi-structured interview, the questions have those characteristics regardless of how nebulous they may sound. These questions have a way of leading an individual rather than allowing the individual to think about experience in a spontaneous way. Here is an example: I was listening to an interview by a researcher, and the interviewer asked the question, "How did you plan this?" Thus the assumption was there was a plan which then left out the possibility of spontaneity. One could argue that the person could say they did not have a plan but often unconsciously, individuals will follow the assumption of the interviewer, in this instance perhaps thinking, I should have had a plan. This is not as serious in outcome as some leading questions.

When we do interpretive phenomenology, we listen with the third ear. This takes practice as we often find out own mental chatter interfering with a very pure listening process. What does it mean to listen with the third ear? I have used the idea of "*de-centering*" from the self or *unknowing* (Munhall, 1993a, 2012, pp. 134, 135, 139). This means acknowledging your biases, preconceptions, assumptions, hunches, theories, intuitions, motives, knowledge, and ideas that you have that might guide your understanding of the meaning of another individual's experience. De-centering is getting out of your own way, unknowing is like you are attempting a blank mind, open and receptive to hearing without noise, hearing only the language of the individual.

While we can use many sources to understand the meaning of experience of another, I hold the gold standard to be the dialogue between you and the other/participant. And even "dialogue" is not the best word, though I prefer it to "interview." Dialogue often implies that there are two people in discussion, where an interpretive phenomenological dialogue is one where the researcher attempts to listen, listen, listen. Prompting may be needed. However, prompts should not be leading, they should be neutral. "Please, go on, I am not sure I understand," and if there is silence, "What are you thinking?"

Additionally, we attend to the affective domain of the individual, what is being conveyed without language through facial expressions, demeanor, emotions, and we in turn should adjust our own demeanor to mirror their emotions, communicating empathy, that the person is understood. When writing a chapter it is easy to be a purist since the demands of the world are not part of the discussion, so this is an example of a pure approach. The optimum study, I believe, is where the same researcher does the interviews and no one else. *It is essential because people do not listen in the same way and intuit intonations, nor do people respond to different people in the same way.* For the best authentic understanding to be found of an individual, there should always be one interviewer (unless the study has some variant reasons not to). Also from a purist perspective, the interpretation, as mentioned, is done by the individual not the researcher and it is the same researcher who probes for the interpretation and meaning from the individual. That researcher *then* interprets what he or she found for the larger picture, for the world of nursing and health care. Essentially there are two levels of interpretation: the participant's interpretation of meaning of experience; and the researcher's interpretation of what that interpretation means to nursing practice, health care or society.

I would like to return briefly now to this "unknowing" component of listening as a goal to strive for when doing interpretive phenomenology. Remember it also helps communication in all your endeavors of attempting understanding, personally and in practice. It is a valuable communication skill.

The researcher as the "unknower"

Because we don't know, do we? *Everyone knows* . . . How what happens the way it does? What underlies the anarchy of the train of events, the uncertainties, the mishaps, the disunity, the shocking irregularities that define human affairs? Nobody knows, Professor Roux. "Everyone knows" is the invocation of the cliché and the beginning of the banalization of experience, and it's the solemnity that's so insufferable. What we know is that, in an unclichéd way, nobody knows anything. You *can't* know anything. The things you *know* you don't know. Intention? Motive? Consequence? Meaning? All that we don't know is astonishing. Even more astonishing is what passes for knowing.

(Philip Roth, The Human Stain, *2001, pp. 208–209)*

I love this passage. I think it is elegantly written but for the purpose of this chapter, it shouts out that we really don't know at the very least another individual whom we have just met, even if we have received prior information about that person. The danger of thinking we know is that of premature closure to new information, new understanding and new meaning.

As a researcher knows, their main interest, goal and passion is to explore knowing ("but we really don't know," their main interest may be to complete their dissertation!). In this quotation Roth demonstrates how this phrase, "Everyone knows" is the banalization of experience and then later on goes on to how astonishing it is when contemplating what passes for knowing. One word in this quote that is particularly critical to interpretive phenomenology as a research method is "meaning." I would venture to guess that in this hyperactive society we live in, with instant communication and multi-tasking, the search for meaning is sadly suffering in our lives. And this search is what makes life meaningful. Roth dramatically tells us there is so much unknowing so that all attempts at "knowing" are critical to understanding who we are. Most important though, Roth acknowledges that what we think we know, all that passes as knowledge is questionable. He then asks, how could we know, when we don't know intention, motive, consequence, and meaning so all that we don't know is astonishing! Good rationale for all qualitative research methods, but for the purpose of this chapter, especially interpretive phenomenology!

As Roth implies, there is a need to question what we think we know. As a step in doing interpretive phenomenology, we examine our own "knowing." We do this so we do not have clutter or noise when we listen to others speak of their experience. We do this so what we hear is not simultaneously being collaborated with what we think we know from theory, assumptions, as with my own mind filled with presuppositions, biases and theories; all this "knowing" noise must be held in abeyance to allow the individual to speak of their experience in their own "knowing" way within their individual situated context. Cayne and Loewenthal (2011) consider this the post-existential/post-phenomenological view of the relational. The relational involves individuals who are separate yet in dialogue, and the researcher does not reduce the other to their own worldview. This is the de-centering process, which also focuses on this intersubjectivity (Munhall, 2012, p. 134).

Heidegger (1927/1962) emphasized that there is no justification to understanding a specific individual's experience with pre-existing structures such as theories or other criteria without contextualizing aspects of being and time. Here we acknowledge temporality, contingencies, and the specific situated context that each individual brings to an experience and are all components of how the experience will be individually interpreted. So interpretive phenomenology is atheoretical, without theory. Practically speaking, if you find yourself conducting such a study and the proposal outline for a study calls for a literature review, in this approach this is the place where your philosophical body of knowledge, that which is guiding your study (as with literature that guides other kinds of research) is articulated.

Intersubjectivity and the relational

Merleau-Ponty (1962) also emphasizes the relational, the perception of the particular individual, as one worldview bumps up against perhaps another worldview. When doing interpretive phenomenology, I have found such wonder at how different and in great variety others interpret a similar experience. Merleau-Ponty expresses it this way: "Here there is nothing comparable to the solution of a problem, where we discover an unknown quantity through its relation with known ones" (Merleau-Ponty, 1962, p. 178). This furthers our discussion on "unknowing" when we come to understand that it is the *in-between of two people* that is the mystery. I have come to revere this intersubjective space where my perception of reality meets with another's individual's perception of reality. Imagine, if you will, your worldview within one circle, and another individual's worldview within another circle. In normal discourse these two circles interconnect, say, halfway forming an intersubjective space and two individuals can agree, disagree or come up with a consensus.

In interpretive phenomenology, when these two circles of subjectivity or worldviews interconnect, the researcher has already de-centered his or her own worldview and is listening with "the third ear" to the subjective experience solely of the other individual.

The "unknower" so to speak, allows and in fact welcomes hearing the experience with all its relational content and meaning for that individual which will eventually be part of the answer to the research question. Interpretive phenomenology in this way gives voice to the individual and provides a method for continuous discovering within the context of the temporal, and the variety of contingencies of each individual, the meaning of experience for that individual. We have a means to authentic human understanding of another if we do not impose our own knowing. We then have found what Roth says is missing, the intention, motive, consequence and most important the meaning. We begin to know what it is like for another individual and what meaning the experience holds for that individual.

The particular and differences

Whereas many researchers attempt to understand individuals with the goal of establishing probabilities, the interpretive phenomenological researcher is investigating the vast potentials of possibilities that may differ from what is thought or known, to unveil the "unknown." To reiterate, interpretive phenomenology is not about validating theories, or making generalizations. It includes differences and the particular. Commonalities, among and between individuals, are also important to your project but not necessarily as "themes" or "essences."

If you are comfortable as a researcher approaching in dialogue with others, free of theories and predictions and are able to enter into the unknowing position, if this is for you, interpretive phenomenology offers to you a world rich in human meaning, based not on your interpretation but on the interpretation of experience of those experiencing the phenomenon. Mysteries will indeed unfold for you.

Meaning of meaning

This leads to an important consideration and that is, who is doing the interpretation of meaning? Authenticity is best accomplished when the particular individual interprets their own experience; they are the one who through dialogue searches and finds individual meaning of their experience. They come to understand their own meaning. We might prompt them along the way but not with structured or semi-structured interviews. Some prompts I have found helpful to individuals, which do not guide them to my own preconceived notions or perhaps what I thought they meant, are:

- "I am not sure what you *meant* by that"—(if more is needed) perhaps you could help me understand better.
- "What are you thinking?"—best prompt for when there is silence, and you will often be surprised as to where their mind has wandered, and you allow them to go there. There is a reason people often stop during an interview or dialogue: their mind has wandered somewhere and where it wandered is important.
- "Go ahead, tell me more"—another prompt for silence or if you are not sure of what was said.

You can see that these prompts are not leading in any way. You are only maximizing possibilities.

What to do with the material

In descriptive phenomenology listing of themes often collapses the material into a word which the researcher neatly labels in that section of the material. Here we can see the entry of the researcher. He or she listens to a section of the dialogue and interprets what the person is saying. Or the researcher might paraphrase longer periods of discussion to shorten the amount of the material; again we see the entry of the researcher. The researcher in essence is deleting material to get to something he or she believes to be the core meaning of what the person is talking about.

This often comes about because of the sheer volume of material and also the different purpose of descriptive phenomenology. *So an important question emerges as to what to do with all material you have gathered*. Again, I mention this is not a "how to do" chapter, so consulting qualitative research method books is essential. However, I have found the "what to do" question is an important one that requires a short offering to insure meaning be understood. I believe it is critical when doing interpretive phenomenology not to reduce material to themes or categories. It is interesting to note that we have many responses available to us to describe experience and that is perhaps best for descriptive phenomenology. Many experiences result in the similar responses: fear, loneliness, frustration, anger, powerlessness, hopefulness, denial, acceptance and loss are among some themes one reads.

The meaning of responses

With interpretive phenomenology we want to understand what those responses mean, so from my perspective each person's narrative and therefore meaning remain uniquely theirs and are interpreted through the lens of the person's background, situated context, history and temporality. These are all different for individuals, though of course there may be similarities. Depending on how you will be writing the results of your research, for whom and for what purpose will greatly influence how you describe your results. For example, if there were ten individuals in your study, there would be ten sections, with ten narratives, with the meaning of the experience embedded in the narrative and the interpretation of that meaning coming from the individual or, as in some instances, if the researcher has done the interpretation, it is agreed upon with the particular person. If you are sharing the results of your research in an article, then a certain amount of material will be reduced but if you had ten (not a magical number) dialogues, then you would have at least ten shortened narratives if it was an article, or complete narratives if it was a book, complete with the interpretation of meaning.

The similarities, the differences, the contingencies, or background would all be a part of the interpretation. Again the interpretation is agreed upon. "Yes, that is what I meant," "you captured it right," and "yes, that is my meaning" are what you want to hear from your research participant. This requires returning to the particular individual who should read what you have written, unless you have reason to think it would be harmful. So much more could be said, but again I must refer you to a methods book!

Exemplars of interpretive phenomenological method

Van Manen's phenomenological method

Max van Manen's phenomenological method (1990) has been for most U.S. and Canadian nurse researchers the predominant method for interpretive phenomenology although van Manen did not label it as such. Rather, he used the term "hermeneutics" and also included in the word *description* to include both the *interpretive and the descriptive*. He has influenced me and countless nurse researchers, as well as other human science researchers, to adopt a phenomenology that emphasizes pure description, which includes interpretation of lived experience.

Earle (2010, p. 289) outlines van Manen's method as follows:

i   Turning to the phenomenon to the researcher's particular interest.
ii   Investigating experience as lived rather than as conceptualized.
iii Reflecting on essential themes that characterize the phenomenon.
iv   Describing the phenomenon through writing and rewriting.
v   Maintaining a strong relation to the phenomenon.
vi   Moving back and forth in balancing the research context by considering parts and whole.

The above outline is just that: an outline of what is a rigorous process with detailed explanations and descriptions in van Manen's writings (1990). Van Manen has been extremely influential in phenomenological nursing research and I have used his method for my own classroom teaching, guiding doctoral students and inviting van Manen to do phenomenological research workshops at the annual International Institute for Human Understanding annual meetings during the years from 1996 to 1999. He was always very generous, motivating, and scholarly in his approach.

During my years of teaching, doing and guiding research I began to think about some additional steps I thought might enhance van Manen's method for nursing as a practice discipline. His predominant focus had been on pedagogy and he encourages his method to advance pedagogy in a very practical way.

Through the back and forth of students' work and research and to answer students' focus on nursing practice, I began suggesting additional steps to van Manen's method, always keeping at the forefront the philosophy of interpretive phenomenology. I also thought (in contrast to van Manen) that phenomenology could be problem-solving, in that it could illuminate needed changes in many areas, whether policy or practice (Munhall, 2007, p. 149). What I think I was doing was attempting to make van Manen's method more interpretive and at the same time more aligned with the pragmatic concerns of nursing practice and health care policy.

I suppose this was also stimulated by the simple yet profound question that can be asked after doing a research study and reading the results and asking that question, "SO WHAT?" That was when I moved to the idea of significance as a step of "What does this study mean and to who, to what and why?" So you will see in Munhall's approach to interpretive phenomenology (below), always under revision and welcoming of suggestions, there are some additional steps.

There is the step of writing: what does the meaning/s that the researcher has uncovered *mean to nursing practice or policy*? There is also the step of critique, where the interpretation is to be articulated in the form of implications and recommendations for nursing, political, cultural, health care, family and other social systems. This is an attempt to go beyond interpretation and meaning of the experience to the meaning and interpretation for practice and policy.

I have in this chapter decided to call it "Munhall's approach" to interpretive phenomenology as almost a return to my roots where I often said (1994) phenomenology was "a philosophy, a perspective, and an approach to practice and research" (p. 14). You will see these additional steps in the following outline, and this outline is fully explained in Munhall (2012, Chapter 5).

Munhall's approach to interpretive phenomenological inquiry

i Coming to the phenomenological aim of the inquiry:
   a Articulate the aim of your study in the form of a phenomenological question.
   b Distinguish the experience that is part of your study.
   c De-center yourself and come to "unknow."
ii Review of philosophical literature: immersion:
   a Describe in detail the philosophical underpinnings of interpretive phenomenology.
   b Articulate the perspectives and assumptions of the philosopher/s whose works will be illustrated in your phenomenological project.
iii Phenomenological inquiry:
   a Interviewing within the framework of intersubjectivity and "unknowing."
   b Each person as subject describes and interprets their own meaning given to an experience.
   c Integrate contingencies or life-worlds of each subject.
   d Interpretive inquiry includes existential investigation of literature on the experience (post interviewing), artistic expressions found in art, film, photography, etc.
iv Analysis of interpretive interaction:
   a Integrate existential investigation within the phenomenological context. Include situated context, expressions of subject, feelings, metaphors, as well as appearances and conceal-ments.
   b Follow-up interviews for insuring each individual's narrative captures the meaning.
v Writing the interpretive phenomenological narrative for each subject: the meaning of the experience.
   a Write inclusively of all meanings, the "general" and the "particular." Include participant's interpretation of meaning within situated context and contingencies of the participant's world.
vi Writing a narrative on the meaning of your study: what does this interpretation mean to individuals, nursing practice, health care?
vii Critique this interpretation with implications and recommendations for political, social, cultural, health care, family, and other social systems.

This approach is spelled out fully and with specific suggestions in Munhall (2012, Chapter 5). There it is referred to as Method which was an editorial decision, not mine, and also please be prepared if you do research it, that it is very detailed so as to assist a first-time researcher.

Also it is important to note that the method in this chapter has not been called "interpretive." In that chapter I do write that this goes beyond descriptive phenomenology to the interpretive but neither the chapter title nor other headings articulate it as such.

I also hope it is apparent that the additional steps added answers for questioners or critics, to the question of the "SO WHAT?" of your study.

The second level of interpretation comes from the researcher who then after studying the interpretation of the meaning of the experience for the individual is now able to interpret how this new knowledge, the commonalities and the particularities provide knowledge for nursing practice, health care policy, future direction in research, or suggestions for change. This is the step where the researcher presents the significance of the interpretive phenomenological study. Here you might find the researcher critiquing current practices and policies as a direct result of new understandings of meaning in experience. The critique yields the significance of study through implications for nursing practice and health care policy.

Conclusion

Reading the international interpretive research studies gives us in nursing reason to celebrate our common values, ethics and goals. There is in nursing worldwide interest in understanding what it means to be human in this world of experience. Imagine if we understood each other within the dyad, family, and on local, national and international stages (some might be very pleased with understanding themselves!). Imagine if through this understanding, not only tolerance but also celebration of differences evolved. Imagine if we understood the power of different meanings to individuals and to people. Meaning creates entire worldviews, some similar and others completely differing and even paradoxical.

Nursing is a profession that has an ethic of care. Inherent in that ethic is respect for the individual. Interpretive phenomenology is not only a research method but a nursing worldview, which opens windows and doors, lets possibilities, various meanings and particular perspectives, breeze through back and forth, embraced and understood. This does not always mean agreement but this in fact opens perhaps the backdoor to change for the better. This is a task of no small consequence. In my view, however, it is more than worth the effort and we as nurse researchers *care* to rise to the challenge.

Notes

1 The third ear is one that is unknowing, opened and uncluttered.
2 This idea of "father" demonstrates temporality and situated context since few women at the time were knowingly given recognition of their intellect.

References

Allen, D., Benner, P., & Diekelmann, N. (1986). Three paradigms for nursing research: Methodological implications. In P. Chinn (Ed.), *Nursing research methodology issues and implementation*. Rockville, MD: Aspen.

Beck, C. T. (1992). The lived experience of postpartum depression: A phenomenological study. *Nursing Research*, *41*(3), 166–170.

Benner, P. (Ed.). (1994). *Interpretive phenomenology: Embodiment, caring, and ethics in health and illness*. Thousand Oaks, CA: Sage.

Caelli, K. (2000). The changing face of phenomenological research: Traditional and American phenomenology in nursing. *Qualitative Health Research, 10*, 366–367.

Cayne, J., & Loewenthal, D. (2011). Post phenomenology and the between as unknown. In D. Loewenthal (Ed.), *Post existentialism and the psychological therapies*. London: Karnac.

Cohen, M. Z. (1987). A historical overview of the phenomenological movement. *Image: Journal of Nursing Scholarship, 19*(1), 31–34.

Dreyfus, H. (1972), *What computers can't do: A critique of artificial reason*. New York: Harper & Row.

Earle, V. (2010). Phenomenology as research method or substantive metaphysics? An overview of phenomenology's uses in nursing. *Nursing Philosophy, 11*, 286–296.

Gademer, H. G. (1976). *Philosophical hermeneutics*. Berkeley: University of California Press.

Heidegger, M. (1927/1962). *Being and time*. San Francisco: Harper & Row.

Husserl, E. (1913/1962). *Ideas: General introduction to pure phenomenology*. New York: Macmillan.

Lauterbach, S.S. (1993). In another world: A phenomenological perspective and discovery of meaning in mothers' experience with death of a wished-for baby: Doing phenomenology. In P. Munhall, & C. Oiler Boyd (Eds.), *Nursing research: A qualitative perspective* (pp. 133–179). New York: National League for Nursing.

Lauterbach, S. S. (2001). Longitudinal phenomenology: An example of "doing" phenomenology over time: Phenomenology of maternal mourning: Being-a-mother in another world (1992) and five years later (1997). In P. Munhall, *Nursing research: A qualitative perspective* (pp. 185–208). New York: National League for Nursing.

Lauterbach, S. S. (2007). Exemplar: meanings in mothers' experience with infant death: Three phenomenological inquiries: In another world; Five years later; What forever means. In P. Munhall, *Nursing research: A qualitative perspective* (pp. 211–237). Sudbury, MA: Jones and Bartlett.

Leonard, V. W. (1999). A Heideggerian phenomenological perspective on the concept of the person. In E. C. Polifroni & M. Welch (Eds.), *Perspectives on philosophy in nursing: An historical and contemporary anthology* (pp. 315–327). Philadelphia, PA: Lippincott.

Lopez, K. A., & Willis, D. G. (2004). Descriptive versus interpretive phenomenology: Their contributions to nursing knowledge. *Qualitative Health Research, 14*(5), 726–735.

Merleau-Ponty, M. (1962). *Phenomenology and perception*. (trans. C. Smith). New York: Humanities Press.

Morse, J. (1996). What is a method? *Qualitative Health Research, 6*(4), 468.

Munhall, P. (1993a). Unknowing: Toward another pattern of knowing. *Nursing Outlook, 41*, 125–128.

Munhall, P. (1993b). Women's anger and its meanings: A phenomenological perspective. *Health Care for Women International, 14*(6), 481–491.

Munhall, P. L. (1994). *Revisioning phenomenology: Nursing and health science research*. New York: National League for Nursing.

Munhall, P. L. (1995a). The transformation of anger into pathology. In P. Munhall, *In women's experience* (Vol. 1, pp. 295–322). New York: National League for Nursing.

Munhall, P. (1995b). Cancer of violence: Power differentials and family values. In P. Munhall & V. Fitzsimons (Eds.), *The emergence of women into the 21st century* (pp. 109–114). Sudbury, MA: Jones & Bartlett.

Munhall, P. (2002). Transformation of anger by men. In P. Munhall, E. Madden, & V. Fitzsimons (Eds.) *The emergence of men into the 21st century* (pp. 342–359). Sudbury, MA: Jones & Bartlett.

Munhall, P. (2012). *Nursing research: A qualitative perspective*. Sudbury, MA: Jones & Bartlett.

Munhall, P., & Boyd, C. (1993). *Nursing research: A qualitative perspective*. New York: National League for Nursing.

Natanson, M. (1973). *Edmund Husserl: Philosophy of infinite tasks*. Evanston, IL: Northwestern University Press.

Rorty, R. (1991). *Essays on Heidegger and others*. New York: Cambridge University Press.

Roth, P. (2001). *The human stain*. New York: Houghton Mifflin Harcourt.

Sartre, J.-P. (1993). Freedom and responsibility. In W. Baskin (Ed.), *Essays in existentialism*. New York: Kensington.

Slezak, P. (1994). Situated cognition: Empirical issue, "paradigm shift" or conceptual confusion? In A. Ram, & K. Eiselt (Eds.), *Proceedings of the 16th annual conference of the Cognitive Science Society* (pp. 806–811). Hillsdale, NJ: Lawrence Erlbaum.

Spielgelberg, H. (1976). *Doing phenomenology*. The Hague: Martinus Nijhoff.

van Manen, M. (1990). *Researching the lived experience*. Albany, NY: SUNY Press.

Recommended readings

Allen, D. G. (1995). Hermeneutics: Philosophical traditions and nursing practice research. *Nursing Science Quarterly, 8*(4), 174–182.

Anderson, W. (Ed.). (1995). *The truth about the truth: De-confusing and re-constructing the post-modern world.* New York: Tarcher/Putnam.

Annells, M. (1999). Phenomenology revisited. Evaluating phenomenology: Usefulness quality and philosophical foundations. *Nurse Researcher, 6*(3), 5–19.

Asp, M., & Fagerberg, I. (2005). Developing concepts in caring science based on a lifeworld perspective. *International Journal of Qualitative Methods, 4*(2), article 4.

Atwood, G., & Stolorow, R. (2001). *Faces in a cloud: Intersubjectivity in personality theory.* Northvale, NJ: Jason Aronson.

Bruner, J. (1992). *The acts of meaning: Four lectures on mind and culture* (Harvard-Jerusalem Lectures). Cambridge, MA: Harvard University Press.

Cerbone, D.R. (2006). *Understanding phenomenology.* Montreal: McGill-Queen's University Press.

Conroy, S. (2003). A pathway for interpretive phenomenology. *International Journal of Qualitative Methods, 2*(3), article 4.

Corben, V. (1999). Phenomenology revisited. Misusing phenomenology in nursing research: Identifying the issues. *Nurse Researcher, 6*(3), 52–56.

Flood, A. (2010). Understanding phenomenology. *Nursing Research, 17*(2), 7–15.

Frankl, V. E. (2006). *Man's search for meaning.* Boston, MA: Beacon Press.

Gademer, H. G., Weinsheimer, J., & Marshall, D. G. (2005). *Truth and method* (2nd rev. ed.). New York: Continuum.

Koch, T. (1995). Interpretive approaches in nursing research: The influence of Husserl and Heidegger. *Journal of Advanced Nursing, 21*(5), 827–836.

Koch, T. (1999). Phenomenology revisited. An interpretive research process: Revisiting phenomenological and hermeneutical approaches. *Nurse Researcher, 6*(3), 20–34.

Locke, J. (1975). *An essay concerning human understanding.* Oxford: Oxford University Press.

Morse, J. M. (Ed.) (1994). *Critical issues in qualitative research.* Menlo Park, CA: Sage.

Paterson, M., & Higgs, J. (2005). Using hermeneutics as a qualitative research approach in professional practice. *Qualitative Report, 10*(2), 339–357.

Power, E. (2004). Toward understanding in postmodern interview analysis: Interpreting the contradictory remarks of a research participant. *Qualitative Health Research, 14*(6), 858–865.

Sandelowski, M. (2002). Re-embodying qualitative inquiry. *Qualitative Health Research, 12*(1), 104–115.

Thorne, S. E., Kirkham, S. R., & Henderson, A. (1999). Ideological implications of paradigm discourse. *Nursing Inquiry, 6*(2), 123–131.

12

Glaserian grounded theory
The enduring method
Phyllis Noerager Stern

Grounded theory

You may be under the impression that a given researcher uses grounded theory (GT) method to analyze data or, conversely, does not. I believed that too, but respected researchers have restructured the original form of the method while stating that they too used "grounded theory." In this chapter I try to describe what the original method is, a bit about the histories that led to its development, a sketch of how the method is done, and finally some examples of grounded theories that have stood the test of time.

Glaserian?

"Glaserian" (Stern, 1994) is the label I gave the original method as developed by Glaser and Strauss (1967a), and which Glaser still practices, but from which Strauss departed when he found a new partner in Juliet Corbin (Strauss & Corbin, 1990). Jan Morse had asked me to discuss the conflict that ensued between Glaser and Strauss for a book she was editing (Morse, 1994). So I labeled the two versions of the method "Glaserian" and "Straussian" after each of the collaborators. Corbin suggests that just as humans mature and change so does a method (Corbin & Strauss, 2008). Doing grounded theory gives rise to deep thought, and it's not surprising that researchers keep trying to make it easier to understand, more workable. But from my point of view, the original form works just fine. Really deep thinkers like Morse (2012) and Thorne (2008) suggest that as qualitative researchers, we need to examine and re-examine the methods we use to analyze data. I believe they are correct, and I have at times tinkered with the method myself, but in the end I go back to the original.

Origins of grounded theory

Anselm, a well-known medical sociologist, was recruited to the University of California at San Francisco School of Nursing (UCSF) by then Dean Helen Nahm to strengthen the fledging doctoral program in nursing. Strauss recruited a number of sociologists to the school, among them the newly graduated Barney Glaser. Strauss' background was the sociology of the Chicago School, where his mentor was Herbert Blumer, a proponent of symbolic interactionism (1969), who in turn had been mentored by George Herbert Mead. Mead first introduced the concept of symbolic interactionism (Strauss, 1956). Symbolic interactionism (SI) is a sociological concept that gives direction to the researcher on how to collect and analyze data. According to this concept, people act and react on the basis of symbols; for example, style of dress, physical appearance, facial expression, gestures, and race. Even words are symbols. Words are not the real thing, they represent the real thing. This explains in part the reason intimate partners have trouble communicating; one partner uses what I call "family language," which the other partner misinterprets, and the fight is on.

When Strauss accepted a position at UCSF, he looked forward to teaching nurses SI, as he thought they would welcome the insights the concept allows. At the time, most sociologists were using statistical methods to prove or disprove theory.

Glaser is a graduate of Columbia, where he was a student of Paul Lazarfield (called the father of modern sociology) and Robert K. Merton. Glaser returned to his home state of California and he and Strauss met "at a gathering" (Barney Glaser, pers. comm.). Glaser had tired of disproving theory—he wanted to develop theory. For his part, Strauss had been awarded grant money to study dying patients in California hospitals, and the more the two discussed how the study might proceed, it became clear that Glaser had found the mentor he was looking for, and Strauss had found the bright young recruit he sought. In hindsight, exploding fireworks would have been an appropriate means to mark this meeting; such was their eventual impact on sociological and nursing research. Before Glaser and Strauss developed grounded theory, nursing research generally followed the medical model, using the scientific method.

The first publication from the dying study was *The Nurse and the Dying Patient*, authored by the first graduate of the Doctor of Nursing Science (DNS) program, Jean Quint (1967), closely followed by *Awareness of Dying* (Glaser & Strauss, 1967b) and two additional books on dying patients and their families (Glaser & Strauss, 1970, 1974) and a formal theory, *Status Passage*, 1971). Other sociologists were curious about the methods they used to elicit their findings, and it was then that they realized that they had merged their training—the theory-building techniques of the Chicago School with the constant comparison common in statistical research from Columbia.

Housed as they were in the School of Nursing,[1] Glaser and Strauss attracted a number of doctoral students in nursing, along with PhD students in medical sociology—a fortunate mix, providing an opportunity to learn something about one another's discipline. Morse (2012) tells us that early nursing qualitative researchers turned to anthropology for their terminal degrees. As graduates of the DNS program began to publish, nurse scholars recognized grounded theory as a method that had value for the things they cared about. Holly Wilson, who earned her PhD across the bay at Berkeley, crossed the bridge to learn grounded theory from Glaser and Strauss. Wilson published the first ever qualitative study in *Nursing Research*, a journal known for running medical model research *only* (Wilson, 1977). I believe that I owe Holly a debt of gratitude for leading the way, and showing me that it's OK to submit to high-toned journals.

Doing grounded theory

How to do it

Trust in emergence is the cardinal rule in doing grounded theory. Never go in with a theory in mind, let the data tell you what theory is hidden there. The method is so upside-down from the methods you learned about in undergraduate school that it's a task getting your head around it. Paul Wishart says it's like pulling the cork out of a wine bottle (pers. comm., 2010). Instead of beginning a project with a conceptual framework, you create one from the data. It's not an easy principle to grasp. You select an area of research because it holds your interest, and you think you know something about it. You don't. To go back to the beginning, when I did the stepfather family research, I thought I knew all about it because I lived in such a family group (Stern, 1978), but once again, it turned out that I had a lot to learn. More of that later.

Porr and I have a somewhat different impression about the so-called "worldview" of the researcher (Stern & Porr, 2011). Porr (Porr, Drummond, & Olson, 2012) began her research by looking at the symbolic interaction (SI) in the scene. SI is but one of the dozens of theoretical codes used to upgrade substantially coded data to become theoretical. Deciding which theoretical code to use beforehand is a Glaserian no-no. However, I do have trouble imagining why a nurse would attempt research without considering the SI in the scene—isn't that what we're all about? *Paying attention to what's going on will get you further into theory than sorting out your worldview.*

Doing grounded theory is similar to a detective show on TV: a crime happens, and detectives search for clues in order to solve the puzzle. They record their hunches on a whiteboard, making diagrams, and linking clues together until they have a theory of what happened, why, and by whom. That's pretty much what goes on in grounded theory. Data are coded as they are collected, categories are formed as data codes relate to one another, and then collapsed to form a more inclusive category. Theoretical codes come from sociology, but they are useful for us as we all live in a society. They can be found in Glaser (1978) and Stern and Porr (2011) and online. Theoretical codes help you think about data theoretically. Then finally it happens: you've discovered a *theory*! Early on, Glaser taught his students that they were looking for *a basic social process*, and/or for *a basic social structural process*. Now he writes that he has decided that grounded theory is a method that can be used with any kind of data, and was never meant to be used only inductively (Glaser, 2008). Recently Glaser complained that his intellectual property has been absconded (Glaser, 2009), because the vocabulary he used when describing grounded theory has been used by other authors when the methods they describe are not grounded theory at all.

Briefly, the steps in grounded theory are those below, thought of as a matrix rather than linearly: What I mean is, these are horses on a merry-go-round (you pick the one you like) instead of a ladder where your choice is to go up or down—no sideways please.

1 *Gathering data.* Data usually consists of interviews, observations, literature, but each data bit must be coded prior to the gathering of more data.
2 *Constant comparison.* Compare each data bit with all the other bits.
3 *Categorizing.* People form categories all the time. You may organize your spices in alphabetical order, or by groups of sweet or savory; you're categorizing.
4 *Overarching categories.* Through constant comparison, you break down the categories to find relationships between and among them.
5 *Memoing.* Through the entire process write memos about the data while trying to think theoretically.
6 *Theoretical coding.* Consult a table of theoretical codes and find where your data fit.
7 *Theoretical sorting.* More constant comparison as you see how your puzzle comes together.
8 *Theoretical writing.* Further analysis goes on as you write the research report.

I urge you to explore the many resources we have for learning how to do grounded theory. Glaser has continued to publish books on the method, the most important of which is *Theoretical Sensitivity* (1978). It may be rough going at first if you don't have a sociology background (it's a different language). All of Glaser's books are available through Sociology Press. Artinian, Giske, and Cone produced an excellent text in 2009. Artinian is an expert in "conceptual mapping" and each chapter has a helpful diagram illustrating how the findings were conceived. Caroline Porr and I (Stern & Porr, 2011) wrote what we hope is an easy-to-understand text on the method. Morse, Stern, Corbin, Bowers, Charmaz, and Clarke (2009) gives you a range of authors, from old school to deep thinkers' view of grounded theory.

A grounded theory deconstructed

In 1980, I published a deconstruction of my stepfather study, which people found helpful in understanding how a grounded theory is done (Stern, 1980). With that in mind, I decided to give you a glimpse into how we discovered the GT of a home fire (Stern & Kerry, 1996).

In the late 1980s, the house we lived in just outside Halifax, Nova Scotia, was destroyed by arsonists. We lived in a hotel for six weeks, then moved to an unfurnished apartment for another six while our home was being rebuilt. When I moved to Canada to accept the Directorship of Dalhousie School of Nursing, my husband having become legally blind, retired. During the time of rebuilding, I tried to carry on with directing, plus making what seemed like endless lists for the insurance company of property that needed to be replaced. Trying to carry out the activities of daily living under these circumstances seemed like a terrible burden for both of us. Due to the arson, we both felt paranoid, and frankly, we were both mentally unwell; from the loss, the disruption, the unmet need for social support, and replacement work—what's destroyed needs to be replaced, and somebody has to shop for it. All this work and the work *space* no longer existed—even my computer burned. My woman cave went up in flames. I had to do something to divert my attention from this crisis.

It has long been my belief that when all else fails—do a study about it.

Following the usual permissions, I did some interviews, and it was clear that losing one's home to fire causes varying degrees of suffering, but I wasn't getting past the descriptive stage to theory. At the time I was teaching a graduate course in grounded theory. As is usual, one of the learning exercises is sharing one another's project information with one's classmates—analysis by group— so I added my fire data to the pile. This group of graduate students made suggestions about why recovering from a home fire is so depleting: the lack of social support, the lack of understanding. Finally, Deborah Thoun and I said almost at once, "There's no ritual!" At a conference later, Jan Morse said, "There's always a ritual!" True of course: the ritual following fire loss consists of questions about injury and insurance coverage, followed by comments like, "Oh, you can get all new stuff!" You don't want new stuff, you want people to understand what you're going through, how crazy you feel. As Bolin (1985) tells us, "persons who are exposed to life-threatening events, who witness the loss of family, or who survive the catastrophic destruction of a home are the most likely to exhibit emotional distress" (p. 6). It's *comforting* ritual that's missing. After diagramming my coded data, I was able to determine where comforting ritual exists (in rural isolated places), where it's absent (in cities), and where it's purposely withheld (in slum populations where outsiders assume the fire was due to carelessness). Kerry was able to interview the French-speaking people of Eastern Canada, and this comparative data confirmed the theoretical implications of the study.

At the time of this writing, there's a massive wild fire in the state of Colorado in the Western United States. So far, 350 homes have been destroyed. In a disaster such as this first responders rush to the area, and counselors follow—it's only in single-family homes where survivors have to go it alone.

Ways of going astray

As a reviewer, I find that the most serious problem writers—nurses and others—have is that they fail to go beyond description to theory. Thinking theoretically can be scary—nurses are taught that they need to stick to the facts. In using grounded theory you need to allow yourself to dwell in the land of the unproven. I believe that everyone can be creative: you just have to learn to let it out. The table of theoretical codes can help you. Your mentor can be invaluable. On a number of campuses students have formed grounded theory clubs; student seminars where colleagues are kept on track.

I'd like to see more authors relate their findings to the larger society. What happens when one house burns doesn't help us much in understanding how the world works, unless the author helps us out. In this process you need to use your imagination: If the ritual following a house fire fails to be comforting, in what other situations does the "loss ritual" fall short? Divorce comes to mind. We don't have an established comforting ritual for divorce as we do for, say, death. I've observed that people say something trivial, such as, "You're probably better off," or assume that it's better not to talk about it at all. I find it interesting that we have support groups for folks who have lost their pets, but other comforting loss rituals are missing.

A figure can help you analyze your data and reach a theoretical level, but that's the purpose of drawing one. Then your job is to explain what's going on in the figure. More and more often I see beginners placing their emphasis on the figure at the expense of the narrative—this defeats the beauty of the method as theory and literature.

Beginners sometimes forget that the writing up of GT becomes literature: lyrical, well paced, readable. There's too much information swirling around us to attend to it all. You have to hook the potential reader with a catchy title, and an opening paragraph that holds the reader's attention, making her or him read on. A groundbreaking theory breaks no ground if nobody reads it. Some schools employ an editor. You're lucky if yours does. If not, pay someone in the English department to read your manuscript for clarity and flow.

Whichever form of grounded theory you use, as a reviewer I'm annoyed when a writer fails to cite Glaser and Strauss (1967a); they started all this. How about going back to the original source? Isn't that what academics are supposed to do?

Staying power of Glaserian grounded theory

Sue Pyles phoned. She was helping a doctoral student with a grounded theory dissertation and it is natural that she associated me with the method, because she learned it from me back in the early 1980s when she was a Master's student at Northwestern State University of Louisiana School of Nursing at Shreveport. For her thesis research, Sue wanted to know how nurses could spot a patient in danger before it "shows up in the numbers" as hospital jargon has it (blood gases and the like). The theory she discovered and named *nursing gestalt*, involved the learning process of a fledgling nurse, in the presence of a mentoring relationship, to put together scientific knowledge, differentiation, visual and verbal clues, and gut feelings to make decisions regarding the critical care of patients (Pyles & Stern, 1983).[2] My point is that a well-developed theory stands the test of time—nursing gestalt is as true of nursing care today as it was in 1983. Clarke argues that the validity of a theory depends on time, place and time in history (Clarke 2009), while I consider these elements conditions, which can be considered integral to the theory itself. As well, a Glaserian grounded theory is readily modifiable to fit a variety of circumstances; for example, Dangdomyouth studied how Thai families manage their relatives with schizophrenia at home, and she concluded that they do it with *tactful monitoring*, taking care not to embarrass the ill member, but still being attuned to the relative's mood (Dangdomyouth, Stern, Yunibhand, & Ountanee, 2008). This theory, developed with a Thai population, is echoed in a Canadian population of public health nurses and their study of single mothers living in low-income situations (Porr, Drummond, & Olson, 2012). Porr called the theory *developing a therapeutic relationship,* but the components of both processes are so similar that Porr could have named it tactful monitoring. In both situations, caretakers acted to protect the patients' pride while gaining their trust.

Of the research projects I've published, I'm probably best known for my work with stepfamilies (Stern, 1978, 1980, 1982a, 1982b) and with home-fire victims (Stern & Kerry, 1996). Of the properties I learned about stepfather families, particularly important was the role of the new family member. When the biological parent allowed him to "take over" the role of primary disciplinarian the child became a behavior problem, but when the stepparent practiced what I called integrative discipline (take it easy on the kid), the family tended to become integrated. These findings were poorly accepted by family experts at the time—the late 1970s—but presently, TV psychologist Dr Phil is advising stepfamilies that the stepparent must never take on the role of primary disciplinarian, because they have no history with the child (McGraw, 2005).

A theme that transcends most of my work is *showing respect.* The way one shows respect varies from culture to culture, and depends on context: The stepfather who shows respect by assuming the role of wiser older person rather than a disciplinarian, the fire victim who gains social support, and the Filipino immigrant who wants to maintain the birth ritual she learned from her mother.

I have kept to the processes of the original method because it works for me, it's systematic and the products are applicable. I advise you to do the same.

Notes

1   Glaser never admits to being part of the School of Nursing. He calls his university base either the University of California or the Medical Center at UCSF.
2   I failed in my attempt to do a literature search of Glaserian grounded theory because authors glaze over the specifics of the method they used when writing their abstracts, thereby making a computer search unavailable. My only choice, as I saw it, was to include the publications of colleagues I had worked with. I hope the reader will forgive the frequent self-citations.

References

Artinian, B. M., Giske, T., & Cone, P. H. (2009). *Glaserian grounded theory in nursing: Trusting emergence.* New York: Springer.

Blumer, H. (1969). *Symbolic interactionism: Perspective and method.* Englewood Cliffs, NJ: Prentice Hall.

Bolin, R. (1985). Disaster and social support. In B. Sowder (Ed.), *Disasters and mental health: Selected contemporary perspectives* (pp. 150–157). Rockville, MD: National Institutes of Mental Health.

Clarke, A. E. (2009). From grounded theory to situational analysis. In J. Morse, P. N. Stern, J. Corbin, B. Bowers, K. Charmaz, & A. E. Clarke (Eds.), *Developing grounded theory: The second generation* (pp.194–235). Walnut Creek, CA: Left Coast.

Corbin, J., & Strauss, A. (2008). *Basics of qualitative analysis* (3rd ed.). Thousand Oaks, CA: Sage

Dangdomyouth, P., Stern, P. N., Yunibhand, J., & Ountanee, A. (2008). Tactful monitoring: How Thai caregivers manage their relatives with schizophrenia at home. *Issues in Mental Health Nursing, 29,* 37–50.

Glaser, B. G. (1978). *Theoretical sensitivity.* Mill Valley, CA: Sociology Press.

Glaser, B. G. (2008). *Doing quantitative grounded theory.* Mill Valley, CA: Sociology Press.

Glaser, B. G. (2009). *Jargonizing: Using grounded theory vocabulary.* Mill Valley, CA: Sociology Press.

Glaser, B. G., & Strauss, A. (1967a). *Discovery of grounded theory.* Chicago: Aldine.

Glaser, B. G., & Strauss, A. (1967b). *Awareness of dying.* Chicago: Aldine.

Glaser. B. G., & Strauss, A. (1970). *Anguish.* Chicago: Aldine.

Glaser, B. G., & Strauss, A. (1971). *Status passage: A formal theory.* Mill Valley, CA: Sociology Press.

Glaser, B. G., & Strauss, A. (1974). *A time for dying*. Chicago: Aldine.

McGraw, P. (2005). *Family first*. New York: Free Press.

Morse, J. (Ed.). (1994). *Critical issues in qualitative inquiry*. Newbury Park, CA: Sage. (AJN Book of the Year Award for 1994.)

Morse, J. M. (2012). Introducing the first global congress for qualitative health research: What are we? What will we do—and why? *Qualitative Health Research, 22*, 147–156.

Morse, J. M., Stern, P. N., Corbin, J., Bowers, B., Charmaz, K., & Clarke, A. E. (2009). *Developing grounded theory: The second generation*. Walnut Creek, CA: Left Coast.

Porr, C., Drummond, J., & Olson. K. (2012). Establishing therapeutic relationships with vulnerable and potentially stigmatized clients. *Qualitative Health Research, 23*, 384–396.

Pyles, S. H., & Stern, P. N. (1983). Discovery of nursing gestalt in critical care nursing: The importance of the gray gorilla syndrome. *Image: The Journal of Nursing Scholarship, 2*, 51–57.

Quint, J. (1967). *The nurse and the dying patient*. New York: Macmillan.

Stern, P. N. (1978). Stepfather families: Integration around child discipline. *Issues in Mental Health Nursing, 1*, 50–56.

Stern, P. N. (1980). Grounded theory methodology: Its uses and processes. *Image: The Journal of Nursing Scholarship, 12*, 20–23.

Stern, P. N. (1982a). Affiliating in stepfather families: Teachable strategies leading to integration. *Western Journal of Nursing Research, 4*, 75–89.

Stern, P. N. (1982b). Conflicting family culture: An impediment to integration in stepfather families. *Journal of Psychosocial Nursing, 20*, 27–33.

Stern, P. N. (1994). Eroding grounded theory. In J. Morse (Ed.), *Critical issues in qualitative inquiry* (pp. 212–223). Newbury Park, CA: Sage.

Stern, P. N., & Kerry, J. (1996). Restricting life after home loss by fire. *Image: The Journal of Nursing Scholarship, 28*, 11–16.

Stern, P. N., & Porr, C. J. (2011). *Essentials of accessible grounded theory*. Walnut Creek, CA: Left Coast.

Strauss. A. (Ed.) (1956). *George Herbert Mead on social psychology*. Chicago: University of Chicago Press.

Strauss, A., & Corbin, J. (1990). *Basics of qualitative analysis*. Newbury Park, CA: Sage.

Thorne, S. (2008). *Interpretive description*. Walnut Creek, CA: Left Coast.

Wilson, H. (1977). Limiting intrusion: Social control of outsiders in a healing community. *Nursing Research, 26*, 103–110.

13

Strauss' grounded theory

Juliet Corbin

Anselm Strauss has been dead for over a decade. The world of qualitative research has proliferated since Dr. Strauss' death and the trend has been to replace older methods with either newer qualitative or with mixed qualitative/quantitative methods. While it is natural to want to be on the latest methodological bandwagon, there is something to be said for traditional methods. The aim of this chapter is to demonstrate that Dr. Strauss' approach to generating grounded theory is not a relic from the past but still a vibrant method that transcends time and is capable of generating relevant nursing knowledge.

The chapter begins with a short discussion of why theory construction is important to nursing. It will move on to a brief summary of the philosophy underlying Strauss' method. Next, it will list the components of the method. Fourth, the chapter will address some of the criticisms directed at grounded theory and Strauss' method. Fifth, it will present a summary of some of the research conducted over the past 20 years using Strauss' method. This will be followed by a summary and conclusion.

Why theory construction?

Nursing demands a variety of types of knowledge and skills from its members. It deals with the most intimate aspects of human lives in sickness and health and at times when people are most vulnerable. It involves teaching, advocating, counseling, managing, and referring as well as hands-on healing. It requires rapid and life-saving decisions and necessitates excellent communication and listening skills. It requires that nurses be researchers, administrators, managers, as well as caretakers.

Theory provides the concepts, insights, and understanding that educators, researchers and practitioners rely upon to carry out their practice, research, and teaching. Theory provides the foundation for knowledge and its development later to be tested through practice and further research. Except for a few well-known general nursing theories, many of the theories that nurses draw upon are borrowed from biological, social/psychological, and managerial sciences. These theories, though helpful, are not specific to the varied and complex practices of nursing. Nurses need theories developed by nurses from and for the profession.

Strauss was not one to sit back and generate theory only by means of logic and deductive reasoning. He believed that if researchers want to develop theory, they should go into the areas of concern and find out what people are saying and doing. Then, from that knowledge, they should develop what he called "grounded theories." To him, theory had a greater likelihood of being reflective of personal and professional issues if it is grounded. To quote Strauss, "Without grounding in data, that theory will be speculative, hence ineffective" (Strauss, 1987, p. 1). Or it might be added, not as effective as it could be had it been generated through research into the holistic practice of nursing.

Philosophies underlying Strauss' grounded theory

Though most researchers refer to Symbolic Interactionism as the philosophy driving grounded theory, Strauss' method is really a combination of Pragmatism as well as Symbolic Interaction (Strauss, 1987; Corbin, 1991). Action/interaction stands at the heart of Anselm's approach. Why action/interaction? The answer lies in the following. During his undergraduate days at the University of Virginia, Strauss was greatly influenced by the Pragmatist philosophers, most notably Dewey, who viewed action as central to human behavior. For Dewey (1922) and also for Strauss (1993), action did not refer only to the physical act of doing but encompassed the duality of thought and acting. Action led to consequences, making these an important part of the thinking/doing equation. As important as action is to method, so is interaction. Strauss was introduced to the sociological notion of interaction while at the University of Chicago where he did his graduate work. A major influence was Mead (1934) with his emphasis on interaction and the development of the self. One of his teachers was Blumer who coined the term "Symbolic Interaction" (1969). But as Strauss stated in a personal communication: "Blumer talked about concepts, theory, and Interaction but he never developed a method for putting these together in research." It was not until Strauss was working with Glaser on a study of death and dying (1965) that together they explicated a method that became known as grounded theory (Strauss & Glaser, 1967). Glaser, who had a doctorate from Columbia University, came to the research study with a background in comparative analysis and quantitative research, while Strauss brought his Pragmatist/Interactionist philosophies and his qualitative research background. Eventually Glaser and Strauss went their separate ways. Strauss continued to teach and do research at the University of California, San Francisco. It was during these years that his book *Qualitative Analysis for Social Scientists* (1987) and the first two editions of the *Basics of Qualitative Research* with Corbin (1990, 1998) were written.

Although it took Strauss years to put Pragmatism and Interactionism together into a formal Theory of Action (Strauss, 1993), the two orientations were part of his way of thinking and influenced his approach to research much earlier as explained in Strauss (1987, p. 5). For those who would like to read more about the philosophical assumptions underlying Strauss' approach to grounded theory, see Strauss (1991, pp. 3–32, 1993, pp. 1–46).

Overview

Put simply, the philosophy underlying Strauss' approach to method reads something like this. Persons are not passive recipients of the events, situations, and the problems they encounter in life. They give meaning to problems, events and situations and respond through some form of action/interaction (Dewey, 1922). Emotion is also part of action as stated by Strauss (1993, p. 31): "Action has emotional aspects. To conceive of emotion as distinguishable from action, as entities accompanying action, is to reify those aspects of action." Meanings are arrived through a process of self and other interaction (Mead, 1934). Reflected in self and other interaction are the contextual conditions in which the situation or problems or events occur. Among the possible contextual conditions are emotions, past experiences, culture, motivations, family dynamics and relationships, historical time, information levels, economic, political and power structures, and so on (Strauss, 1987). Action/interaction or their opposite, inaction, lead to consequences, such as a change in the situation or a shift in the problem, resulting in further self and other interaction, leading to a possible change in meaning, leading to potential alteration in action/interaction. The cycle of context/event/problem/meaning/action/interaction/consequences continues in an ongoing feedback loop until there is some resolution or management of the situation or problem.

Given the complexity and cyclical nature of events and responsive action/interaction, Strauss felt simple cause and effect explanations would not do. Any theoretical explanation constructed using his method would have to include as many as possible of the nuanced and complex factors that enter into situations. Perhaps this is why researchers think that Strauss' method is difficult to learn and carry out. It is a complex method designed to unravel complicated life situations then take those unraveled pieces and weave them together into a tapestry of understanding that captures the varied and ever-changing nature of human action, interaction, and emotion as well as the context in which these occur.

Constructing grounded theory

Grounded theory is aimed at breaking data apart, denoting concepts to stand for data, then weaving the data back together to form an explanatory theoretical framework by relating concepts around a central or core category. Though different approaches to doing grounded theory have evolved, and all claim to be the definitive method, it is interesting to note that though the philosophical orientations and approach to analysis of each might be a little different, the final products are similar. They all have concepts, the concepts are developed in terms of their properties and dimensions, concepts are located in context, there is process, and there is an overarching core concept that integrates all the lower-level concepts to form theory. Furthermore, the different approaches use the basic techniques of making comparisons, asking questions, theoretical sampling and saturation. Finally, some degree of validation of findings is built into the analytic process through theoretical sampling, looking for negative cases, and bringing findings back to participants. Since all researchers bring to their analyses different philosophical orientations, they are responding to different critics when making explanations of their method, and approach data in different ways, it is doubtful one could find any two researchers who explain the method in quite the same way. Researchers make choices among the various approaches based on which method most appeals to them, their familiarity with a method, the persons with whom they study, or the criticisms to which they are responding. Recently, researchers have adopted aspects of the different grounded theory approaches or at least combined or referenced the different approaches as discussed in their method sections. Or they are combining different qualitative approaches with grounded theory. Both leave doubt that any user of grounded theory or qualitative method is a true purist in terms of how method is carried out. (See, for example, Brink, 2009; Busby & Witucki-Brown, 2011; Tate, Dabbs, Hoffman, Milbrandt, & Happ, 2012; Zahourek, 2005.)

Also there appears to be some confusion about the various versions of grounded theory published by Strauss and Corbin (1990, 1998) and Corbin and Strauss (2008), with some readers assuming they are different books. Let me assure readers that the method presented in each edition is essentially the same. What is different is the manner of presentation, with each edition attempting to clarify some of the areas users of the method had questions about or that tended to misunderstand or misinterpret. Just because the third edition does not refer to open, axial, and selective coding does not mean that these forms of coding are not part of the method. What is important is not what one calls the different types of coding but a basic understanding of the logic that underlies coding, which is to identify different levels of concepts and achieve integration of all of these to form theory.

Components of grounded theory

Analysis

Analysis involves an interaction between the analyst and the data. Analysis begins when an analyst picks up a field note and reads through it to obtain a general sense of what the data are all about. The next step is to break the fieldnote into manageable but related sections, then examine each section in greater depth. A section may consist of a word, sentence, paragraph or even page, if the topic remains the same. While scrutinizing the data, the researcher asks probing questions to get at meaning. Questions such as "What seems to be going on here? What is being said in this work or phrase or sentence? What is the main idea that is being expressed?" Concepts are used to stand for meaning. Concepts are important because they enable researchers to combine different but conceptually similar pieces of raw data under one name, reducing the amount of data researchers have to work with. With the continued making of comparisons, more raw data are conceptualized under the same or different concepts and concepts are developed in terms of properties and dimensions. The process of denoting and developing concepts is called coding.

Concepts

Concepts are interpretations, the analyst's attempt to convey the intent or meaning contained in different bits of data. Though analysts aim for valid interpretations, there is no absolute way of guaranteeing the accuracy of interpretations. Even participants may not be fully aware of intent or meaning. All an analyst can do is try to "get it right" by bringing interpretations back to participants and by using the process of constant comparison to continually check out interpretations against incoming data. The important thing about analysis is to avoid paraphrasing because it does not take the data up to a conceptual level and limits the amount and type of data that can be grouped. Paraphrasing is different from "in vivo" codes. Paraphrasing is descriptive. It describes a situation or event and repeats perhaps using different words or a phrase from the data and has little applicability to other incidents or events. In vivo codes indicate that a word or two used by a participant to describe something is sufficiently abstract to group similar events or incidents, for example, using a term such as "stigma" to describe many different incidences in which persons feel slighted because of a disability or some way they appear or act.

Categories

Once an analyst has some concepts to work on, he or she can begin to group them into categories/themes. Questions that a researcher might ask of the data in order to group concepts are: "What is the main theme of the section I'm working with? What common idea expressed in data are all these concepts pointing to?" The concept used to denote a major idea contained in a group of lower-level concepts is called a category (sometimes referred to as a theme). A category may turn out to be one of the initial concepts that after consideration by the analyst is found to stand above the rest of the concepts. Or it might be a different concept that better captures the essence of what is being expressed in the section of data. An analyst will have many concepts but fewer categories or themes.

Again, categories are interpretations. They are analysts' understandings of a major idea contained in a section of data. To arrive at a category, analysts have to see an element common to a group of concepts. A bird, a plane, a kite sound like discrete objects until an analyst identifies that what they have in common is flight. A person can learn a lot about flight (now a category) by comparing each object for similarities and differences. The comparison is made along properties of flight as noted in the data such as height, distance, and mechanism of action. When making comparisons between the different objects such as height, distance, and mechanism of action, properties are dimensionalized because the analyst will notice the differences in how high each can fly, how far or the distance each can fly without stopping, and what it is that makes them fly. From the data the analyst will learn that height will vary from low to high, distance not very far to very far, and mechanism of action from self-propelled to mechanically propelled. As more data are collected, the researcher is able to add to the properties and dimensions of a category until the point of saturation, a term that indicates considerable variation has been built into the theory. Saturation not only increases understanding of how something works, but also allows the user of theory to apply it to different situations.

It is important to note that saturation does not indicate merely that "no new data are coming in" as is so often reported in grounded theory studies after five or six interviews. Rather saturation indicates that each category is defined, specified, and shows considerable variation in its properties. It is saturation of categories that gives specificity and density to the final theory.

A researcher does not want to fixate on naming a category/theme too early in the analysis. As insight grows through interaction with data, ideas that a researcher had in the beginning of the analysis about what these lower-level concepts are pointing to may prove to be irrelevant or wrong. It's not unusual to begin by naming a category one thing only to rename it something else later as more data are collected. Also researchers will find that categories may collapse into one another if overlap is discovered. The distinction between breaking data apart and putting it back together is artificial and made for explanatory purposes only. Even at the beginning of analysis, analysts are constantly having insights, thinking abstractly, and proposing relationships between lower- and higher-level concepts.

Core category

There is no theory until a core category is denoted by the researcher. The core category stands for what a researcher determines to be the main storyline or the research. The core category may be chosen from concepts already identified in the research or it may be a new concept that is broader and better able to capture the general story. The core concept should be broad enough to unify all concepts and categories and may even account for negative cases. Negative cases represent a dimensional extreme of a property. For many novice researchers, naming the core category and integrating the other categories around it is the most difficult aspect of the research. It requires the ability to stand back and make a judgment about the general meaning of the data and then choose a concept or phrase to denote this. To do this, a researcher has to trust in him or herself and have confidence that the analytic process has led him or her to this point.

Context and process

Strauss' version of grounded theory should include explanations of context and process. As mentioned, action/interaction are incomplete without relating them to context and showing how these evolve with changes in context. In any situation there are multiple conditions at work to set in motion, and facilitate or constrain action. Together these conditions make up what is called context. For example, a person says: "I went ahead and had cancer surgery because I didn't know about the possibility of choosing alternative treatments because I had been out of the country and out of touch with medical care in the U.S. for so long." The word "because" is a cue to the reasons persons give for doing what they do or say."Being out of the country and out of touch" is part of the explanation given by this person for choosing surgery. It is part of the context in which the decision to have surgery was made. By going through the data and looking for the reasons persons give for their decisions and subsequent action/interaction, researchers begin to get a sense of who, what, where, why and when persons act/interact the way that they do, rounding out explanations. Going back to the earlier explanation about categories and flight, even a concept like flight has reasons. One reason in that case happens to be the mechanisms of action, but there are also other factors such as amount of wind and ability to make use of that wind to facilitate, modify, or constrain the ability to fly.

Next, by examining the relationships of forms of action/interaction to the contextual conditions operating in each situation, researchers are able to arrive at patterns, the beginnings of theoretical integration. For example, a researcher might come up with a pattern of mechanically derived flight and another of self-propelled flight and denote the conditions under which each of these happened or are hindered. By now, the researcher has moved beyond the original concepts of bird, kite, plane, and instead is talking about flight, thereby increasing the level of abstraction.

Process

Process denotes changes or shifts in the action/interaction. These shifts or changes occur as a result of changes in conditions or context. To go back to the example of flight, to bring process into the theoretical explanation, the researcher would have to examine the data to determine how the various patterns of flight change in response to changes in conditions. For instance, what happens to mechanical flight when there is mechanical failure or bad weather? Then what happens to self-propelled flight when something happens like a broken wing?

However, at this point, researchers will not have completed the work of constructing theory. To complete the process, researchers must come up with a concept that synthesizes in a few words what the research is all about. This is where the final integrative concept becomes necessary. In the case of flight, it might be something like "Taking to the Sky: An explanation of why and how flight happens." The detailed framework that the researcher has constructed up to this point fits under this larger concept. The categories and all the explanations that pertain to them will explain why and how flight occurs and is maintained, using examples derived from the data such as bird, kite, and plane, bringing the research back full circle.

Analytic procedures

One of the most interesting aspects of working with Dr. Strauss was watching his mind at work during analysis. He was thoughtful, deliberate, and generative but careful to consider the range of possible meanings of data. He examined data from a variety of perspectives and though conceptual, he never strayed far from the raw data, constantly returning to it to check out interpretations. Though impressive to watch during analysis, Strauss did not arrive at his insights into data through magical thinking. He used a variety of heuristic devices, many of which are used by persons as part of their everyday life. For example, to show how meaning varies depending upon context and intent, Strauss brought objects to class and asked students to name the many possible uses to which objects might be put. For instance, he would bring a cup and ask students to name as many uses as they could come up with, such as a cup may be used to drink from but it also may be used to store pencils, as a flower vase, or as a weapon, depending upon the situation and the meaning given to it by a person. He also asked students to turn their interpretations upside down asking: "What would happen if . . .?" thus changing the set of conditions or context. For example: "What might happen if an experienced workman were replaced with a non-experienced one?" Strauss would draw upon experience to get students to become sensitive to data and to look for clues. For example, if the study was of work and how it is done, he might say: "When you are building a deck on your home, how do you go about getting the work done?" The answers would not be used as data but aimed to get students to think in terms of what goes into getting work done. Though these activities might seem like game playing to the uninitiated, doing these exercises was not a game. They were Strauss' way of helping students develop their analytic skills.

Asking questions and making comparisons

Asking questions and making comparisons are two of the most important basic processes of analysis and are used throughout the entire analytic process. However, the kinds of questions and details of the comparisons vary, depending upon the stage of the research and the analytic problem to hand. In terms of questions, early in the analysis, questions might be more general and thought-provoking, designed to "open up" the data. Later questions might be more specific and directed at developing and filling in categories. Making comparisons involves analysts comparing one piece of data against another, asking if the data are conceptually the same or different from another.

There are two other thinking strategies that bear mentioning because they are often misunderstood. These are the paradigm and the conditional-consequential matrix. As mentioned earlier, Strauss felt that actions/interactions were at the heart of analyses because they are indications of how persons give meaning to and respond to situations and to problems. But just noting meaning and response is not enough to construct a well-developed explanatory theory. Meaning and the subsequent action/interaction must be located within a framework of contextual conditions as explained above. Here is where the paradigm comes in. It consists of conditions/action/interactions/consequences. The idea behind it is not to structure the analysis but to remind analysts to look for the context in which action occurs and to look for consequences that result from action. This is very important to have in a theory because it is what makes it usable. The user knows under what conditions the theory will work and what the outcomes might be. Contextual factors can come from a variety of sources as described earlier and consequences sometimes have implications beyond the immediate situation, giving rise to what Corbin and Strauss (2008) called the Conditional/Consequential Matrix.

The matrix is another analytic tool reminding analysts of the wide range of areas from which contextual conditions might arise and the wide range over which consequences might have implications. Not every possibility contained in the matrix will be found in data and a researcher should not put something into the data that is not there. However, when conditions and/or consequences do show up in the data, the analyst can trace their paths.

Theoretical sampling and saturation

These are two additional components of a grounded theory study. Saturation was explained earlier. Theoretical sampling means gathering data based on relevant concepts in order to develop categories. It involves varying the conditions pertaining to categories in order to determine what might be the same and what might be different in under different conditions. The original concept has to come out of the data. For example, a researcher might study flight by looking at birds, and then want to sample flight under different circumstances such as with planes and kites. Or a researcher might theoretically sample by looking at flight of birds under different conditions such as on a foggy versus a clear day if the data indicate that there might be differences in the ability to fly.

Memos and diagrams

There has to be a way of recording insights, concepts, and their exploration and development. Memos serve this function. Strauss was adamant about researchers writing memos. He believed that it was because of the lack of memos that some grounded theory studies are lacking in detail, variation, and conceptualization and that was why many students have difficulty arriving at the core category. Unless analysts write memos, they have no way of recalling all of the many properties and dimensions associated with a concept. They have no way of keeping a written record of the evolving analytic story or of studying concepts to see which one stands out and might be a description of the storyline. Diagrams are also essential to doing solid grounded theory as they help analysts fill in gaps in logic, work out connections between concepts, and see the larger picture, allowing the analyst to arrive at the core category. Writing memos regarding personal reactions to data collection and analysis are a way of keeping the analyst aware and honest. Memos regarding personal reactions to data gathering and analysis can be assembled to form a diary or account of the personal journey taken through the research.

Review of the literature

The proof of the value of a method lies in the quality and relevance of the research produced using the method. Can anyone honestly say that research based on postmodern, constructivist, feminist or any other philosophical orientation produces knowledge that is any more significant, more in-depth, or more authentic than what can be produced through the proper application of Strauss' approach to grounded theory? Given the research reports using grounded theory methodology that I read in preparation for this chapter, I don't think so. Below are some examples of research using Strauss' grounded theory. Over the years the method consistently has generated a valuable body of knowledge on a variety of topics, covered a wide range of problems, has been used successfully to study various cultures, genders, and across age groups. The articles have been organized according to the following themes: experiencing and managing illness; life stage issues; family caregiving; health, healing, and spirituality; and nursing practice and professional issues.

Experiencing and managing illness

One of the primary functions of nursing is to provide care to persons and their families during health, illness, and disability. What better way to understand the meaning of health, illness, and disability than to step inside the shoes of those persons undergoing the experience as described in their own words? The following research reports provide insight into how persons experience illness and how they respond. Ching, Martinson, and Wong (2009, 2012) explored the psychological process and strategies used by Chinese women to adjust to a diagnosis of breast cancer. Hayder and Schnepp (2010) detailed the strategies used by persons suffering from incontinence to "Regain Some Control" over their lives. Huang, Lin, Yang, and Sun (2009) examined how

"Hospital-Based Home Care" helped persons and their caregivers cope with severe mental illness. Scharer and Singleton (2004) used the concept of "Hospitalization, the Last Resort" to demonstrate the ambivalence and stress parents felt when having to hospitalize a child with severe mental illness after all other management options had failed. Vandall-Walker and Clark (2011) adopted the term "Working to Get Through" to explain the strategies family members used to gain access to the ICU so that they might be at an ill relative's bedside. Zoffman and Kirkevold (2005) used the concept of "Keeping Life and Disease Apart" to explain how persons with diabetes cope with self-conflict and conflict with professionals over management of the disease.

Life stage issues

Nursing care is directed at more than just illness management. It is varied in scope reflecting the many life stage issues that persons encounter. The following articles describe some of the issues and responses. Alex, Hammarstrom, Norberg, and Lundman (2006) utilized the concept of "Balancing within Various Discourses" to explain how elderly Sami women preserved their cultural identities and accommodated to personal and cultural change over time. Children were the focus of a study by Chaiyawat and Jezewski (2006) who examined how Thai school-aged children describe and manage their fears. Another study of young children was that of Yearwood and McClowry (2006), who explored "The Process of Preparedness in Communicating with At-Risk Children." Chung-Park (2011) conducted a grounded theory study of decision-making in military women using the term "Taking Responsibility" to explain women's contraceptive strategies. Gonzales-Guarda, Ortega, Vasquez, and De Santis (2010) explored how environmental and cultural factors led to increased risks of substance abuse, partner violence, and HIV in young Hispanic males. Kim (2004) investigated "The Experiences of Young Korean Immigrants" and the strategies they used to adapt to their new country. St. John, Cameron, and McVeigh (2005) used grounded theory to explore how fathers met the challenges of parenting during the early weeks after the birth of their first child.

Family caregiving

Family members play an important role in caring for their ill parents both at home, in hospitals, and nursing homes. In order to assist families, it is important that nurses understand the issues and problems that families encounter and how they manage these. De la Cuesta (2005) and De la Cuesta and Sandelowski (2005) examined caretaking from the perspective of families caring for persons with advanced dementia in Columbia. Escadon (2006) studied Mexican American intergenerational caregiving, bringing in another cultural perspective on caring. Jacelon (2006) used the concept of "Managing Personal Integrity" to explain the strategies used by family members to preserve the integrity and dignity of hospitalized relatives. Legault and Ducharme (2009) investigated the process by which daughters become advocates for a parent with dementia living in a long-term care facility. Li and Shyu (2007) examined the coping processes used by Taiwanese families caring for elderly family members with hip fracture during the post-discharge period. Lopez (2009) used the concept of "Doing What's Best" to explain decision-making by family members of acutely ill nursing home residents. Shawler (2007) used the term "Evolution of Female Strength" to describe how mothers and daughters transited through a health crisis.

Health, healing, and spirituality

Nurses take a holistic approach to care whether they are dealing with health or illness. They reach out to persons in a variety of ways that go beyond the medical as demonstrated by the following articles that examine the relationship between spirituality, healing, and health. Hunter, Logan, Goulet, and Barton (2006) explored how Aboriginal people in Canada address health issues and the link between tradition and holism in nursing practice. Labun and Emblen (2007) investigated the interrelationships between health, illness, and spirituality in Punjabi Sikhs living in Canada. Lewis, Hankin, Reynolds, and Ogedegbe (2007) turned their attention to the US where they studied spirituality in the African American culture and its relationship to health promotion. The US was also the site of a study by Zahourek (2005) that focused on intentionality and its role in healing.

Nursing practice and professional issues

While it is important to study patients and families, there is also a need to examine and evaluate the nursing profession and its practice. Feng, Jezewki, and Hsu (2005) examined the meaning of child abuse to nurses in Taiwan. Career persistence in baccalaureate-prepared nurses working in acute care settings was the topic of investigation of a study by Hodges, Troyan, and Keeley (2010). Iran was the site of a study by Hossein, Fatemeh, Fatemeh, Katri, and Tahereh (2010) that examined teaching styles in clinical nursing education. In Taiwan, Huang, Ma, Shih, and Li (2008) conducted a study of the roles and functions of community mental health nurses caring for people with schizophrenia. Iran again was the site of a study by Lagerström, Josephson, Arsalani, and Fallahi-Khoshknab (2010) who explored how Iranian nurses balanced work with family life. Nurses' contribution to the rehabilitation process was the focus of a study conducted by Pryor, Walker, O'Connell, and Worrall-Carter (2009). Oncology patients' perception of what constitutes quality nursing care was the topic investigated by Radwin (2000). Schoot, Proot, ter Meulen, and de Witte (2005) investigated client–nurse interaction in chronically ill persons receiving home care from the clients' perspective. In a related study, Schoot, Proot, Legius, ter Meulen, and de Witte (2006) explored nurses' perceptions and descriptions of that care.

Criticisms and responses

Over the years there have been many criticisms of grounded theory. This section will list some of the criticisms and respond to them.

Quality of findings

One of the criticisms of grounded theory is that though there may be some significant findings, the "theories" produced do not always meet standards of quality and the blame is placed on the method. Grounded theory is only as good as the user of the method. In most instances when the "findings" are not theory or the theory lacks density and precision, the researcher is not experienced and as a consequence the method is used incorrectly or not to its full capacity. Safeguards are built into the method but it has to be carried out as designed.

Grounded theory doesn't address modern problems

Grounded theory does not prevent a researcher from looking at any of the latest issues and problems. Take social justice. Strauss was interested in social justice long before it became a trend.

Most of Strauss' writings are aimed at bringing about enlightened change to a health care system dominated by and blinded by its focus on "acute care" and unequal distribution of services, beginning with his early edited book *Where Medicine Fails* (Strauss, 1984) and later writings with colleagues on hospitals, *Social Organization of Medical Care* (Strauss, Fagerhaugh, Suczek, & Wiener, 1985), and chronic illness, *Shaping a New Health Care System* (Strauss & Corbin, 1988) among others.

Findings cannot be generalized

Grounded theory is a qualitative research method designed to explore issues and develop theory. Its purpose is to discover relevant variables, not to test them. However, if theoretical concepts are sufficiently abstract, they can be studied in different populations, thus extending their usefulness. The value of theory is that it can be modified with time and adapted to place and culture. Parts that no longer fit can be discarded. To increase generalizability, hypotheses derived from a theory can be tested by means of theory testing methodologies.

Early analysis is time-consuming and detailed

Though there are complaints that analysis in grounded theory is detailed and time-consuming, especially the line-by-line analysis, the truth is that analysts work with whole sections of data. However, line-by-line analysis does have its place. Early in the analysis it helps researchers to get into the data and become focused. Later it may be used to fill in categories or to break through analytic standstills. Theory that lacks density, scope, variation, and specificity is often due to a lack of detailed coding. There are no short cuts to theory building. Like all research, it's a demanding and intense process and those who want to develop theory must be prepared to do the work involved or choose to do descriptive type of research, which in its own way is just as valuable.

Writing memos is too much work

Many researchers fail to write memos or do so sparingly. But this is a mistake. When working with large amounts of data, it becomes impossible to recall all that passed throughout the analytic process. Memos are especially important for researchers working in groups. Little notes made in the margins do not make sense when researchers go back to retrieve them and often "brilliant" insights are lost because there was no memo to record them. Memos do something more: they keep the researcher honest. Writing and reviewing memos enables researchers to note inconsistencies and contradictions in analyses, uncover assumptions and biases, and discover gaps in logic.

Strauss' method is not a constructivist method

Though Strauss never used the terms "constructed" or "co-constructed" when talking about method, he did state that analysis consists of an interaction between the analyst and the data (Strauss, 1987). Both the researcher and participant, by the very implication of the term "interaction," play a part in the theory development—the participant through actions taken or the spoken or written word taking the form of data, and the researcher who builds, develops, or "constructs" theory from that data. The final theory is a combination of both participant and researcher and when viewed in that way is co-constructed. One of the problems comes from the title of the original book, *The Discovery of Grounded Theory* (1967) and an assumption by some persons that the word "discovery" implies there is one and only one possible theory in data and if the researcher works at it long and hard enough it can be "discovered." To understand the title a reader has to understand why the book was written the way that it was. Its purpose was to discredit the sociological trend at the time. It seems that theory was developed through logico-deductive means rather than "grounded" or constructed through analytic interpretation from data as explained earlier in this chapter.

Conclusion

Grounded theory as a methodology needs no defense. It remains a relevant and viable method that speaks for itself in the many contributions to knowledge it has made and continues to make to the nursing profession. This method, if carried out as suggested, leads to the construction of a well-developed and relevant theory. It does not claim to result in a set of generalizable and well-tested facts. Rather, its purpose is to generate variables and to suggest their relationships that in turn can be tested through hypothesis testing research. However, it doesn't always have to be tested before using because it is derived from actual data. Grounded theory is not suitable for studying all things in nursing such as the effectiveness of one nursing intervention over another. It is most useful for researching and explaining the contextual factors or conditions that facilitate or constrain persons' ability through evolving action and interaction to gain and maintain control over personal and professional problems. Most importantly, grounded theory provides concepts that can be used for discourse about relevant professional phenomena, and concepts upon which to build practice, carry out research, and teach, thereby extending the body of professional knowledge. Admittedly, doing grounded theory requires a certain fortitude and set of skills but these can be developed over time and with practice and are certainly not beyond the abilities of highly motivated persons.

References

Aléx, L., Hammarström, A., Norberg, A., & Lundman, B. (2006). Balancing within various discourses: The art of being old and living as a Sami woman. *Health Care for Women International, 27*, 873–892.

Blumer, H. (1969). *Symbolic interaction.* Englewood Cliffs, NJ: Prentice Hall.

Brink, E. (2009). Adaptation positions and behavior among post-myocardial infarction patients. *Clinical Nursing Research, 18*(2), 119–135.

Busby, S., & Witucki-Brown, J. (2011). Theory development for situational awareness in multi-casualty incidents. *Journal of Emergency Nursing, 37*(5), 444–452.

Chaiyawat, W., & Jezewski, M.A. (2006). Thai school-age children's perception of fear. *Journal of Transcultural Nursing, 17*(1), 74–81.

Ching, S. S. Y., Martinson, I., & Wong, T. K. S. (2009). Reframing: Psychological adjustment of Chinese women at the beginning of the breast cancer experience. *Qualitative Health Research, 19*(3), 339–351.

Ching, S. S. Y., Martinson, I., & Wong, T. K. S. (2012). Meaning making: Psychological adjustment to breast cancer by Chinese women. *Qualitative Health Research, 22*(2), 250–262.

Chung-Park, M. (2010). Contraceptive decision-making in military women. *Nursing Science Quarterly, 20*(3), 281–287.

Corbin, J. (1991). Anselm Strauss: An intellectual biography. In D. R. Maines (Ed.), *Social organization and social process: Essays in honor of Anselm Strauss* (pp. 17–42). New York: Aldine de Gruyter.

Corbin, J., & Strauss, A. L. (2008). *Basics of qualitative research* (3rd ed.). Thousand Oaks, CA: Sage.

De la Cuesta, C. (2005). The craft of care: Family care of relatives with advanced dementia. *Qualitative Health Research, 15*(7), 881–896.

De la Cuesta, C., & Sandelowski, M. (2005). Tenerlos en la casa: The material world and craft of family caregiving for relatives with dementia. *Journal of Transcultural Nursing, 16*(3), 218–225.

Dewey, J. (1922). *Human nature and conduct.* New York: Holt.

Escadón, S. (2006). Mexican American intergenerational caregiving model. *Western Journal of Nursing Research*, *28*(5), 564–585.

Feng, J.-Y. Jezewski, M. A., & Hhu, T-W. (2005). The meaning of child abuse in Taiwan. *Journal of Transcultural Nursing*, *16*(2), 142–149.

Glaser, B., & Strauss, A. L. (1965). *Awareness of dying*. Chicago: Aldine.

Glaser B., & Strauss, A. L. (1967). *The discovery of grounded theory*. Chicago: Aldine.

Gonzales-Guarda, R. M., Ortega, J., Vasquez, J., & De Santis, J. (2010). The mancha negra: Substance abuse, violence, and sexual risks among Hispanic males. *Western Journal of Nursing Research*, *32*(1), 128–148.

Hayder, D., & Schnepp, W. (2010). Experiencing and managing urinary incontinence: A qualitative study. *Western Journal of Nursing Research*, *32*(4), 480–496.

Hodges, H. F., Troyan, P. J., & Keeley, A. C. (2010). Career persistence in baccalaureate-prepared acute care nurses. *Journal of Nursing Scholarship*, *42*(1), 83–91.

Hossein, K. M., Fatemah, D., Fatemeh, O. S., Katri, V. J., & Tahereh, B. (2010). Teaching style in clinical nursing education: A qualitative study of Iranian nursing teachers' experiences. *Nurse Education in Practice*, *10*, 8–12.

Huang, X.-Y., Lin, M. J., Yang, T.-C., & Sun, F. K. (2009). Hospital-based home care or people with severe mental illness in Taiwan: A substantive grounded theory. *Journal of Clinical Nursing*, *18*, 2956–2968.

Huang, X.-Y., Ma, W.-F., Shih, H.-H., & Li, H.-F. (2008). Roles and functions of community mental health nurses caring for people with schizophrenia in Taiwan. *Journal of Clinical Nursing*, *17*, 3030–3040.

Hunter, L. M., Logan, J., Goulet, J.-G., & Barton, S. (2006). Aboriginal healing: Regaining balance and culture. *Journal of Transcultural Nursing*, *17*(1), 13–22.

Jacelon, C. S. (2006). Directive and supportive behaviors used by families of hospitalized older adults to affect the process of hospitalization. *Journal of Family Nursing*, *12*(3), 234–250.

Kim, S. S. (2004). The experiences of young Korean immigrants: A grounded theory study of negotiating social, cultural, and generational boundaries. *Issues in Mental Health Nursing*, *25*, 517–537.

Labun, E., & Emblen, J. D. (2007). Spirituality and health in Punjabi Sikh. *Journal of Holistic Nursing*, *25*(3), 141–148.

Lagerström, M., Josephson, M., Arsalani, N., & Fallahi-Khoshknab, M. (2010). Striving for balance between family and work demands among Iranian nurses. *Nursing Science Quarterly*, *23*(2), 166–172.

Legault, A., & Ducharme, F. (2009). Advocating for a parent with dementia in a long-term care facility. *Journal of Family Nursing*, *15*(2), 198–219.

Lewis, L. M., Hankin, S., Reynolds, D., & Ogedegbe, G. (2007). African American spirituality. *Journal of Holistic Nursing* *25*(1), 16–23.

Li, H.-J., & Shyu, Y.-I. (2007). Coping processes of Taiwanese families during the postdischarge period for an elderly family member with hip fracture. *Nursing Science Quarterly*, *20*(3), 273–279.

Lopez, R. P. (2009). Doing what's best: Decisions by families of acutely ill nursing home residents. *Western Journal of Nursing Research*, *31*(5), 613–626.

Mead, G. H. (1934). *Mind, self, and society*. Chicago: University of Chicago Press.

Pryor, J., Walker, A., O'Connell, B., & Worrall-Carter, L. (2009). Opting in and opting out: A grounded theory of nursing's contribution to inpatient rehabilitation. *Clinical Rehabilitation*, *23*, 1124–1135.

Radwin, L. (2000). Oncology patients' perceptions of quality nursing care. *Research in Nursing & Health*, *23*, 170–190.

Scharer, K., & Singleton Jones, D. (2004). Child psychiatric hospitalization: The last resort. *Issues in Mental Health Nursing*, *25*, 79–101.

Schoot, T., Proot, I., Legius, M., ter Meulen, R., & de Witte, L. (2006). Client-centered home care: Balancing between competing responsibilities. *Clinical Nursing Research*, *15*(4), 231–254.

Schoot, T., Proot, I., ter Meulen R., & de Witte, L. (2005). Actual interaction and client centeredness in home care. *Clinical Nursing Research*, *14*(4), 370–393.

Shawler, C. (2007). Empowerment of aging mothers and daughters in transition during a health crisis. *Qualitative Health Research*, *17*(6), 838–849.

St. John, W., Cameron, C., & McVeigh, C. (2005). Meeting the challenge of new fatherhood during the early weeks. *Journal of Obstetric, Gynecologic, and Neonatal Nursing*, *34*(2), 180–189.

Strauss, A. L. (Ed.). (1984). *Where medicine fails* (4th ed.). New Brunswick, NJ: Transaction.

Strauss, A. L. (1987). *Qualitative analysis for social scientists*. Cambridge: Cambridge University Press.

Strauss, A. L. (1991). *Creating sociological awareness*. New Brunswick, NJ: Transaction.

Strauss, A. L. (1993). *Continual permutations of action*. New York: Aldine de Gruyter.

Strauss, A. L., & Corbin, J. (1988). *Shaping a new health care system*. San Francisco: Jossey-Bass.

Strauss, A. L., & Corbin, J. (1998). *Basics of qualitative research* (2nd ed.). Thousand Oaks, CA: Sage.

Strauss, A. L., Fagerhaugh, S., Suczek, B., & Weiner, C. (1985). *Social organization of medical work*. Chicago: University of Chicago Press.

Tate, J. A., Devito Dabbs, A., Hoffman, L. A., Milbrandt, E. & Happ, M. B. (2012). Anxiety and agitation in mechanically ventilated patients. *Qualitative Health Research, 22*(2), 157–173.

Vandall Walker, V., & Clark, A. M. (2011). It starts with access! A grounded theory of family members working to get through critical illness. *Journal of Family Nursing, 17*(2), 148–181.

Yearwood, E. L., & McClowry, S. (2006). Duality in context: The process of preparedness in communicating with at-risk children. *Journal of Family Nursing, 12*(1), 38–55.

Zahourek, R.P. (2005). Intentionality: Evolutionary development in healing. *Journal of Holistic Nursing, 23*(1), 89–109.

Zoffmann, V., & Kirkevold, M. (2005). Life versus disease in difficult diabetes care: Conflicting perspectives disempower patients and professionals in problem solving. *Qualitative Health Research, 15*(6), 750–765.

14

New directions in grounded theory

Rita Sara Schreiber and Wanda Martin

Since its origins in 1967, grounded theory method (GTM) has gained a following in nursing and now holds a well-established place in the toolkit of nursing researchers. Since Benoliel completed the first nursing grounded theory dissertation on the *Social Consequences of Chronic Disease in Adolescence* in 1969, GTM has become the most popular qualitative research methodology among nursing doctoral students, with 938 grounded theories currently listed in ProQuest Dissertations and Theses. This is more than double the number identified as using phenomenology (380), nearly eight times those identified as using hermeneutics (124), and four times the number identified as using ethnography (63). The second most popular qualitative methodology identified was "qualitative research" (538). Admittedly, ProQuest is largely limited to dissertations from the US, but grounded theory seems to have earned its rightful place in nursing research.

Yet there is considerable variability in how researchers understand and take up GTM, particularly in the past decade or so, as people increasingly learn from the growing body of methodological literature and rely less often on mentors. Stern (1994) warned about the challenges of learning to do GTM adequately in the absence of appropriate mentorship, calling this "minus mentoring." Mentorship is taken seriously at the Grounded Theory Club, an ongoing advanced research seminar at the University of Victoria in Canada, where novice and experienced grounded theorists discuss GTM traditions and explore its emergence in the twenty-first century (Schreiber, 2001). At the same time, variation can be a potentially rich source for further development of the method, as researchers bring new ideas to the research process, unencumbered by dogmas of the past. A bit of stumbling in the dark can be productive, and although we strongly support the role of mentoring in the teaching/learning process when it comes to GTM, we also strongly value the scholarly explorations that happen when fresh eyes and creativity are brought to the methodology. It is in the tension between tradition and exploration, where the pragmatics of method and imaginative scholarship meet, that GTM matures. It is those fresh explorations of where GTM can go that we examine in this chapter.

Researchers have already begun exploring the relationships between GTM and several other research methodologies and philosophical traditions. For example, MacDonald (2001), and Kushner and Morrow (2003) have explained the fit between critical perspectives and GTM, identifying definite areas of compatibility and also potential tensions. Wuest and Merritt-Gray (2001), Wuest (1995), and Keddy, Sims, and Stern (1996) have explored the overlaps between GTM and feminism, and as with other critical perspectives, found the philosophical underpinnings allowed for some compatibility between the two. A few adventurous souls (Allen, 1995; Wilson & Hutchinson, 1991; Pursley-Crotteau, Bunting, & Draucker, 2001) have attempted to combine hermeneutics with GTM, with mixed results (which helps explain why some of us have despaired after many attempts to find areas of compatibility between the two). Yet new horizons always unfold. In the following pages, we present some areas where grounded theorists are currently pushing the boundaries of the method. We begin with a discussion of constructivist grounded theory, a major advancement in the method. This is followed by consideration of situational analysis, as well as the usefulness of bringing a complex adaptive systems (CAS) perspective to GTM. Finally, we briefly discuss the relationships between and among concept mapping, self-organizing mapping, and GTM.

Constructivism

GTM was born of the collaboration between Anselm Strauss and Barney Glaser, and the publication of *The Discovery of Grounded Theory* (1967) marked a milestone in establishing the credibility of qualitative research methods. Yet although Glaser and Strauss produced a substantial body of pioneering work together (Glaser & Strauss, 1965, 1967, 1968; Strauss & Glaser, 1970), it was always clear to their students that significant differences existed between their perspectives on GTM (Stern & Covan, 2001). Since Glaser's 1992 publication, various writers have attended to the foundations and consequences of these differences (see e.g., Annells, 1997; Kendall, 1999; MacDonald, 2001; McCann & Clarke, 2003; Chen & Boore, 2009; Cooney, 2010), identifying differences in ontological perspective (realism vs. relativist) and methods (e.g., role and meaning of verification; approaches to coding). Although these differences result in current arguments about GTM's ontological stance, MacDonald noted, based on Strauss' pragmatist orientation, congruence between GTM and an interpretivist ontology. It is clear to those who read his work that Strauss, at least, always leaned toward a social constructivist perspective of reality (Strauss, 1987; Birks, Chapman, & Francis, 2006). Charmaz, a student of Strauss, has been central to articulating the place of constructivism in grounded theory, in some ways taking the method where Strauss might have, had he lived longer.

Key concepts

Constructivism is centered on the notion that people actively create their own worlds of meaning based on their understandings and the actions and interactions that result (Vygotsky, 1978). The focus on meaning creation, and the behaviors that result, shows a direct line from the symbolic interactionist roots of GTM (Milliken & Schreiber, 2001) as well as its pragmatist beginnings (Strauss, 1987; MacDonald, 2001; Clarke, 2003). Based on the meanings of objects in the world, people demonstrate their agency by acting and interacting, as well as negotiating and renegotiating meanings. Aligned with this is a relativist ontology in which there is no single, objective social reality that can be discovered and described. Thus, reality is not independent of the researcher and participant, but multiple and individual, and grounded theorizing is always contextually situated.

According to Charmaz (2006), a constructivist perspective on grounded theory provides a way of bridging the realist, or critical realist (Chen & Boore, 2009) ontology noted in the original writing on GTM and "Blumer's call for the empirical study of meanings" with the philosophical demands of postmodernism. As in Glaser (1978), there is a strong value on firsthand knowledge of the empirical world of participants, yet at the same time recognition of the complexity of social interaction. The job of the grounded theorist then is to explicate participants' realities, and their beliefs and understandings, in an ongoing interactive process that honors phenomenological experience, while at the same time comparing the differing realities within the data with our own analytic insights in search of understanding. Most current qualitative research is based on a relativist ontology in some way.

Constructivism arises out of, but goes a step further than interpretivism, which is intended only to understand participants' actions and interactions within their contexts. An interpretivist understanding is achieved by attending closely to the source material, such as interviews, observations, or texts, and generating an explanation of the content of the stories provided. Constructivism, in contrast, is based on a recognition that the data, for example, an interview, are already one person's interpretation of a story or event, and that this rendering is a narrative reconstruction by the participant. Geertz, talking about field notes (1973) noted, "what we call our data are really our own constructions of other people's constructions of what they and their compatriots are up to" (p. 9). Thus, from a constructivist view, the researcher's role is to sift through the varied levels of constructions of "what is happening" in the data, and create his or her own explanation. In this way, the constructivist grounded theorist must appreciate and tease out the complex layering of understandings as she or he negotiates with participants in creating theory that will ultimately arise from a shared horizon between participants and researcher.

As the research process unfolds, grounded theorists use both inductive and deductive thinking, to which Charmaz (2006) adds abductive reasoning. The iterative process between induction (theory generating) and deduction (hypothesis testing) in GTM has been likened to the way in which a person on a bicycle shifts slightly from side to side in order to keep moving forward in a straight line. Abductive logic involves identifying all possible explanations for the actions and interactions in the data and checking them against the data to find the most feasible explanation. This could involve theoretically sampling to fill in gaps that could substantiate or refute a particular theoretical formulation. Abductive reasoning does not appear to be specific to constructivist GTM, and could arguably be another name for theoretical sensitivity (Glaser, 1978).

An important tenet of constructivism involves challenging and reformulating the power dynamic between participant and researcher, and illuminating the imbalances inherent in the two roles. The intent is toward an equalization of power to foster reciprocity, a shared horizon, and co-creation of meaning resulting in a theory that represents the shared, constructed reality of both participant and researcher (Charmaz, 2000; Mills, Bonner, & Francis, 2006; Mills, Chapman, Bonner, & Francis, 2007). This requires the grounded theorist to work toward neutralizing the power imbalance, for example, by explicating, via memo writing, how he or she is situated with regard to the phenomena of study, and being open to sharing this if asked by participants. This use of reflexivity is in line with the feminist notion that the exquisite intimacy of an interview brings with it an obligation of reciprocity (Oakley, 1981). Addressing the power imbalance through reciprocity also requires that the researcher enter the field with a non-judgmental stance, prepared to accommodate participants and truly hear what they have to teach. Other strategies to promote reciprocity include scheduling interviews at a time and place convenient for the participant, and giving over control of the interview and following participants' leads rather than closely following an interview schedule (Mills et al., 2006). This latter may be a challenge for novice researchers who, like all of us, are inclined to cling to the false security of a list of questions. With practice it becomes natural to work without an interview schedule or consult it merely to ensure nothing is overlooked. Another strategy aimed toward reciprocity involves providing individual participants with various written components of the data analysis, including their own transcripts, varied memos, and emerging conceptualizations (McCreaddie, Payne, & Froggatt, 2010). This is done to seek participants' thoughts, feelings, and inputs related to the analysis, and can lead to another interview and/or valuable written expansion of the ideas put forth by the researcher.

Constructivist GTM and nursing

Constructivist grounded theory has become popular in nursing, and there is no shortage of published work identified as constructivist (see e.g., Mills, Francis, & Bonner, 2007a; Mills, Chapman, Bonner, & Francis, 2007; Williams & Keady, 2008; McCreaddie et al., 2010; Marcellus, 2010). There are also several excellent discussions of constructivist GTM in nursing, including but certainly not limited to those by Mills et al. (2006), Ghezeljeh and Emami (2009), and Hunter, Murphy, Grealish, Casey, and Keady (2011). A recent CINAHL search using the terms "constructivist" or "constructivism" and "grounded theory" in the abstract resulted in 426 citations. At times it seems that only the bravest would select a non-constructivist approach to GTM, and there is substantial variation in how different researchers take up the notion of constructivism and where that leads them. Nursing researchers have used constructivist GTM to study the full range of health and health-related phenomena including dealing with cancer from varied perspectives (see e.g., Holtslander, Bally, & Steeves, 2011; McCreaddie, Payne, & Froggatt, 2010; Pieters & Heilemann, 2011; Sheehan & Draucker, 2011), teaching and learning (see e.g., Drury, Francis, & Chapman, 2008; Gardner, McCutcheon, & Fedoruk, 2010; Mills, Francis, & Bonner, 2007a), aging (see e.g., McGeorge, 2011), mental health and addictions (see e.g., Gardner, 2010; Kearney, 1996; McCreaddie, Lyons, et al., 2010; Snowden & Martin, 2010), and countless other health matters (see e.g., Williams & Keady, 2008; Kean, 2009, 2010; Jones, Waters, Oka, & McGhee, 2010; Marcellus, 2010).

As noted, however, there are differences in how grounded theorists take up constructivism, and in how they align their work with its principles. Many authors provide cogent explanations for how constructivism matches their own ontological and epistemological leanings, and highlight the strategies used to enact its principles. For example, Gardner (2010) highlighted mutuality in the relationship between researcher and participant as paralleling the therapeutic relationship between nurse and mental health patient in his study of therapeutic friendliness. He also noted that constructivist GTM was philosophically congruent with current nursing practice, and this made it an appropriate method to study it. Marcellus (2010), in her study of resilience in foster families caring for infants with prenatal substance exposure, identified in particular the co-creation of knowledge between participants and the researcher as a means of keeping the participants "present" throughout the study. Holtslander et al. (2011) specifically noted the role of the researcher in interpreting the data as their rationale for their choice of constructivist GTM.

Some authors simply state that they used constructivist grounded theory, and provide either no details about what this means, or provide a generic grounded theory rationale for the choice, and no explanation of how their studies are constructivist as opposed to other conceptualizations of grounded theory (see, e.g., Drury et al., 2008; McCreaddie, Lyons, Horsburgh, Miller, & Frew, 2011). Perhaps this is due to space limitations, or perhaps these authors have adopted Jan Morse's oft-stated wish for a time when qualitative researchers might simply state their methods without explanation, much as quantitative researchers do. Or perhaps these authors use the term loosely, although this may be unlikely because some of them have published excellent explications of constructivist GTM elsewhere (see e.g., McCreaddie, Payne, & Froggatt, 2010). Whatever the case, the reader is left to guess what, in particular, makes the study constructivist, which could be confusing for the novice grounded theorist.

A few authors describe their methodology sufficiently, and come to curious conclusions about the nature of constructivism, or even of grounded theory itself. For example, Snowden and Martin (2010) note what they see as the challenge of conducting a constructivist grounded theory based on written text as the primary data source. It is unclear whether these authors understood that text is legitimate data in GTM (Glaser & Strauss, 1967), and their reasoning for rejecting constructivist GTM was because Charmaz did not explicate how to use literature in this way. Instead, they offer what they describe as a new methodology, "concurrent analysis," partly in the hope of generating theory that can be widely generalized. McGeorge (2011) adopted constructivist GTM because she, citing Glaser and Strauss (1967) felt unable to "achieve the distancing (or 'bracketing' required by traditional grounded theory)." It is unclear how McGeorge came to understand bracketing as part of grounded theory when, in fact, the opposite is the case and the researcher's previous experience is explicitly memoed and examined against the data. Nonetheless, we have learned, sometimes to our embarrassment, that once something is in print, people will take up their own understandings of it.

Notwithstanding some of the unusual interpretations of constructivist GTM, it appears to represent the mainstream of current grounded theory research in nursing. In contrast to the 400+ citations found for constructivist GTM, a CINAHL search of "Glaserian grounded theory" in the text, using no date limitations, resulted in 34 hits while "Straussian grounded theory" resulted in eight. It is noticeable that constructivist GTM is well established in contemporary nursing research and has become the prevalent thread of the method, perhaps because it explicates the way many nurse researchers approach their work in the twenty-first century.

Situational analysis

While Charmaz was explicating constructivist GTM as a bridge between Glaser and Strauss and postmodernism, another student of Strauss, Adele Clarke (2005), was seeking ways to fully integrate postmodernism with GTM, developing what she's called situational analysis. Clarke describes situational analysis as an approach to research using a grounded *theorizing* methodology to frame basic social processes, by representing complexity through mapmaking (Clarke, 2005). Clarke has taken grounded theory beyond the focus on action and meaning in constructivist GTM described by Charmaz (2006) to focus on the situation itself as the basis of analysis, using a social worlds/arenas/negotiations framework. The researcher's interest is moved away from the individual experiences of participants to the often invisible or assumed social structural elements that impact the actors (Kearney, 2009). In this shift, Clarke is attempting to address one of the major criticisms of GTM, particularly as enacted in nursing, the relative obscurity of contextual factors related to the action and interaction within the data (Kearney, 2009). According to Clarke (2005), Strauss and Corbin (1990) emphasized context or situatedness through their use of the conditional matrix, where the elements in the context set the conditions for action as the analytical focus. This, however, was inadequate for Clarke as the condition for action is not merely part of the story, but *is* the story. Therefore, context is not merely something to be considered as background, but is the focus of the research. For Clarke, the term "context" is meaningless because it obscures so much:

> There is no such thing as "context." The conditional elements of the situation need to be specified in the analysis or the situation itself as *they are constitutive of it*, not merely surrounding it or framing it or contributing to it. They *are* it.
>
> *(p. 71; emphasis in original)*

Clarke (2005) writes that, because epistemology and ontology are closely related, any research methodology should be understood in terms of a "theory/methods package." Clarke's intent is that theory and method are inseparable, and that by understanding the epistemological basis, the stage is set for understanding the possible "truth" of social phenomena. To explain situational analysis, therefore, she identifies the epistemological foundations of basic grounded theory as pragmatism and symbolic interactionism, and then adds constructivism and postmodernism, to bring "grounded theory around the postmodern turn" (Clarke, 2005, p. 19). Clarke also relies heavily on the work of Foucault in relation to the ways in which power, disciplining, and discourses shape relational processes. The emphasis of situational analysis is on the relationships and interconnections that constitute a given situation, including the human and non-human actants, spatial and temporal elements, events, discourses, and other factors.

Although Wasserman, Clair, and Wilson (2009) have written of ways to simplify the analytical process through a parsimonious framework, Clarke (2005) embraces the complexity of situations, including the differences, contradictions, missing elements, and incoherencies in the data. In situational analysis, the researcher takes seriously the variations, power issues, contingencies, and multiplicities within the research process, and incorporates them within the analysis. Because situational analysis specifically instructs the grounded theorist to attend to and explore the human and non-human environmental circumstances, there is interest, particularly among public health nurse researchers, in exploring the methodology more fully. For example, one of us (WM) is currently studying the intersection between food safety and food security, where there are considerable differences in power, from the hungry person, to underpaid farm workers, to small farmers struggling to remain in business, to the food industry and its major corporations. Another nurse researcher (L. N. Tomm Bonde, pers. comm., December 1, 2010) is preparing to study the situation of women and HIV/AIDS in Mozambique, where the presence of NGOs, cultural practices, power issues, and the remnants of a bloody civil war interact with prevalent discourses in the HIV/AIDS community as well as biological issues to create a highly complex world (Collins, 2006). What situational analysis presents to the researcher is the ability to foreground more actively the social structures that are intimate aspects of the phenomenon of study.

Specifically, the methodology of situational analysis is developing substantive theory and story-telling through the use of maps, with a goal of critical analysis to produce a "truth" or "possible truths" (Clarke, 2005). Unlike Strauss' more limited tool, the conditional matrix, situational analysis provides a means to specify and visualize all the important human and non-human elements of a situation, emphasizing relationships, positions, social worlds and discursive positions through the use of three types of maps to cast light on the situation: (1) situational maps; (2) social world/arenas maps; and (3) positional maps.

Situational maps aid in articulating discursive and other elements of a situation and the relationships between and among the elements (Clarke, 2005). This begins with a "messy map" created by descriptively laying out human and non-human elements, asking who and what are in this situation, who and what matters in this situation, and what elements make a difference in this situation (Clarke). This map helps to frame the situation and consider what might be an invisible, or taken-for-granted aspect of the phenomenon of study (Clarke). In the case of food policy we would consider not only the policy-makers and people who are food insecure, but global conditions, trade negotiations, and even zoonotic diseases that can impact trade, to name a few potential elements. Some of these elements come from data that were collected, but might also come from personal experience of the researcher. The situational map is a growing and changing map that can highlight areas for further data collection. Once the elements of what matters are down on paper, they can be ordered into clusters or categories that make sense for the topic area, a process familiar to experienced grounded theorists. Reflecting on the descriptions in terms of these categories stimulates thinking in directions that may have otherwise been overlooked.

In order to make sense of the messy map, relational analysis is done to identify the key storylines in the data and to assist with further sampling strategies (Clarke, 2005). This involves a process of identifying and articulating relationships between points on the map describing the nature of the relationship and what connects them. For example, in Mozambique, the relationships between and among the AIDS virus, American health policy, the role of international development organizations and workers, and the position of women in post-colonial society could explain local health policies regarding sexually transmitted infections (STI) and the subsequent impact on women who play multiple roles in the epidemic. By articulating the various relationships, new insights can be gained into the challenges of creating and implementing effective HIV/AIDs policy.

A second type of map used to explore the situation is a *social worlds/arenas map*. This is where social action or activity at the intermediate level of a situation is noticeable and discourses are active (Clarke, 2005). The questions to ask the data in creating this map involve the patterns of collective commitment and the salient social worlds, who is participating, why or why not, as well as identifying the characteristics of the social world itself. A social worlds map of food policy could include municipal, provincial, and federal governments and various departments and ministries; food security networks; food industries; food banks and various feeding programs, to name a few. Social worlds are fluid, and there is no true boundary between them, so they can overlap because people are often in more than one social world at any given time, according to Clarke (2005).

The final type of map Clarke (2005) uses to chart data is an abstract *positional map* that shows various perspectives of the major discursive issues. This map highlights the different discourses or perspectives taken on issues, not those associated with individuals, groups or institutions, by locating the positions against an X and Y axis, as in the example in Figure 14.1.

Positional maps are an attempt to distinguish the politics of representation and identify the complexity of emerging behaviors. Clarke argues that positional maps, because they are free of associations with individuals or institutions, help the researcher to see situations better because they are representative of the larger picture, taken from a broader perspective.

The challenge in creating a positional map is to identify the basic issues and their different positions (Clarke, 2005). For example, in considering women and the HIV/AIDS epidemic in Mozambique, a basic issue may be the ability for women to enact their agency. One axis could be a scale where aid agencies provide more or less access to condoms for women and thereby decrease viral transmission to the rest of the population. The other axis could be the power of women within Mozambican society and how that influences their ability to make use of the

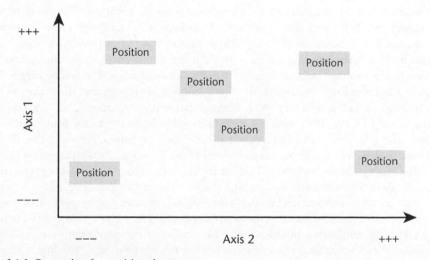

Figure 14.1 Example of a positional map

189

condoms when they have them. One position on this grid would be that women have access to condoms (high access) but are generally unable to use them in their sexual relationships because their male partners are uncooperative (low power). Another position is that women have uneven access to condoms (medium access) but are prepared and willing to take whatever other risks there are to themselves to enforce the use of condoms in their sexual relations (high power). Articulating positions on this sort of map can help the researcher identify the complexity of issues, and also to note what positions and discourses are not present in the situation.

Clarke also describes the use of project maps that do not advance analysis but bring the three types of maps together in a final visual display of the study. A project map can place a complex situation on a single page, visually representing the complexity and framing the story of the wider situation. The end result in situational analysis is not a substantive theory, as with grounded theory, but maps representing the substantive theorizing describing the story.

Situational analysis and nursing

Nurses have not been quick to adopt situational analysis as their research methodology, and we found only two dissertations based on it. A CINAHL search of the terms "situational analysis" and "Clarke" in the text returned 28 items, however, the majority were not related to Clarke's methodology. The term, "situational analysis," is commonly applied to examination of problematic situations, for example, a difficult student–patient interaction, with a view toward identifying strategies to prevent them in the future (Williams, 2001). In this way, Clarke's Situational Analysis is not the same as situational analysis making it somewhat more challenging to locate nurses' use of the method. Examples of non-Clarke situational analysis are Grigg (1997) and Turrill (2000). For the purposes of this chapter, we use the term "situational analysis" to refer to the research methodology developed by Clarke. There are a handful of situational analysis studies done by nurses, and these are each discussed briefly below, although it would be impossible to do justice here to the complexity in these studies.

Gagnon, Jacob, and Holmes (2010) used situational analysis to explore a public health campaign in Quebec, Canada, called "Condoms: They aren't a luxury," intended to prevent sexually transmitted infections in adolescents and young adults. The authors examined two of the three communication strategies of the campaign, the third having been deleted from the Ministry of Health website. The two strategies were informational posters (Zoom) and web-based messaging (What would you do for pleasure?), both with the tagline of the campaign name. Examples of messages used in the campaign include: "These panties have lived through horror," which highlights the ugly symptoms of gonorrhea (greenish vaginal discharge, dyspareunia), and "This underwear has known fear," which describes the pain and disfigurement caused by herpes. Using disorganized and organized situational maps, they identified and reorganized the major discourses of the campaign, including such messages as fatalism, moralistic, promotional, safe-sex, repression, prevention, and so forth. They were also able to identify the foundational assumptions of the campaign that risk perception influences behavior (e.g., condom use) and that fear was "considered the best way to increase the perception of risk in young adults" (Gagnon et al., 2010, p. 249), the targeted high-risk group. This led the researchers to a Foucauldian exploration of the central role of fear in the situation, finding that it is "inherently political," and is being used by the state as a bio-political technology to promote the state's objectives related to STI prevention by governing the sexual habits of young people. The authors note that this approach could backfire by reinforcing the stigma of STIs, therefore increasing transmission, because responsibility for transmission is reduced to individual, fear-based choice. The highly evocative title of the study is "Governing Through (In)security."

There are two other published studies by nurses using situational analysis techniques. Mills and colleagues (2007b, 2007c) are authors noted for their thoughtful discussions of constructivism and situational analysis in grounded theory. In one study, Mills et al. used all of the situational analysis mapping techniques within a collective action frame analysis to explore an "emerging cultural change" in Australian rural nurses, and found the combination of methods useful (2007b, p. 723). What is reported was based on their use of social worlds mapping as a stage in the data analysis that included locating themselves within the maps because of their previous and ongoing embeddedness within the situation of study. The authors paid particular attention to positions and perspectives related to stakeholder groups, and found the situation of Australian rural nurses involves difficult working conditions, anticipated staff shortages, equity issues, and ultimately fatalism regarding increased globalization. In a related study, Mills, Francis, and Bonner (2007c) used a combination of situational analysis mapping techniques and frame analysis as part of a grounded theory study of rural nurses' sense of self. They found that rural nurses "live" their work and view themselves through the lenses of culture, politics, and clinical practice. The authors also briefly reported "cultivate and grow" as the core category, and identified related conditions and properties.

Some researchers have relied on Clarke's (2005) writing, but actual use of the methodology itself is irregular, and at times unclear, often because the researcher has combined multiple related methods. For example, Lyndon (2010) used a combination of "constant comparative method, dimensional, and situational analysis" (p. 15) to study safety issues in two birthing centers in the US. Erikson (2008) primarily used constructivist grounded theory and added social worlds maps to explore how pediatric nurses in an end-of-life facility negotiate professional and personal boundaries with children and their families. She used situational analysis mapping strategies to push her analytic thinking in the course of formulating a grounded theory. Many authors cite Clarke but do not appear to have used her methodology (see, e.g., Jones et al., 2010; Leutwyler & Wallhagen, 2010).

Although nurse researchers appear to be slow to adopt situational analysis, there is some nascent interest in the methodology and a brave few have reflected on and written about it, its techniques, and what it might add to our research toolkit. These include Kearney (2009) and Mills, Chapman et al. (2007). Mills, Chapman et al. in particular provided a thoughtful and thought-provoking discussion of situational analysis in the context of the constructivist epistemological stance of the authors, illustrated though their study of rural nurses in Australia. The ontological incongruity arose when the authors considered the governing, actually constitutive role of discourse as understood in situational analysis and the nature of human agency in constructivist grounded theory. For these authors, situational analysis does not appear to provide a mechanism to appreciate, understand, and explore people's ability to influence their worlds. This contradiction, between human agency and a Foucauldian postmodernist understanding of governance is problematic and apparently irresolvable within situational analysis, at least for constructivist grounded theorists unable to find a way to hold contradictory beliefs simultaneously.

It is unclear why nurses have been so hesitant to adopt situational analysis for their research, although there might be some reluctance to remove the participant from the central role of "repository of emergent truth" (Mills, Francis, & Bonner, 2007b, p. 723). For the majority of nurses, the phenomenon of interest is the patient, who is surrounded by family, community, and so forth in an increasingly fading line of vision, a perspective that is apparently shared by practitioners and researchers alike. Benoliel (1996) and Kearney (2009) both noted the overabundance of social psychological processes, based on interview data alone, in nursing grounded theory studies, bemoaning the focus on interior experiences at the expense of the social. It seems that those nurse researchers who are exploring situational analysis have a particular interest in health from a societal perspective, as is the case with rural and public health nurses. Perhaps having the tools situational analysis provides might encourage nurse researchers to widen their gaze.

Nonetheless, situational analysis has strong roots in grounded theory, relies on the GTM process as its base, and moves beyond its positivist roots and constructivism into postmodernist thought. It also decenters the actions and interactions of individual participants as the focus to concentrate on the situation itself as the phenomenon of study, which is particularly helpful when studying complex systems. Whether situational analysis is a form of GTM or another, closely related method, is perhaps a moot question, the answer to which will depend on the perspective of the researcher.

Complex adaptive systems (CAS)

As a research method that seems adaptable to various paradigms, it was perhaps only a matter of time before grounded theorists began exploring complexity science. The links between GTM and complexity go back to the writings of Strauss (1959/1969, 1978, 1993), in which he emphasized the need to reject dualistic thinking (e.g., structure vs. process, micro vs. macro, body vs. mind) in order to advance the study of social phenomena. In his struggle to find a way to integrate micro and macro perspectives, it became clear that "the world of social phenomena was exceedingly complex" (MacDonald, 2001, p. 128), and this understanding was a large part of what resulted in the development of GTM, including coining the term "structural process" (Glaser, 1978). Thus, although use of a complexity perspective has had a long, but perhaps thin history in GTM, until recently, the connections are evident.

Brief history of complexity science

With its roots in general systems theory (Bertalanffy, 1968), complexity science is the study of adaptive, self-organizing systems that cannot be explained with the methods of traditional science (Capra, 1996). Traditional science is intentionally reductionist, and is based on the assumption that close examination of the functioning parts can explain the whole (Zimmerman, Lindberg, & Plsek, 2001). According to Kauffman (1995), the reductionist focus of traditional science has left a void in society and fostered a lost sense of our worth as humans. Complexity science fills this void through a focus on relationship patterns, how relationships are sustained, and how outcomes emerge, with an emphasis on the whole and on synergy, rather than on individual parts (Zimmerman, Lindberg, & Plsek, 2001). Viewing the world as a complex system means that "life is holistic, self-organizing, highly relational, dynamic, interconnected, nonlinear, and evolving" (Castellani & Hafferty, 2009, p. 21). Thus, complexity science involves the study of complex adaptive systems (CASs), which are systems that have an evolving structure, continuously reorganizing to adapt to changes, issues, and problems arising in their surroundings (Holland, 1992). Examples of CASs include the food industry, nursing, hospitals, and epidemics. Cilliers (2002) argues that complexity science fits within the postmodern framework because of its relationary nature and the emphasis on the continual shifting of those relationships. Complexity science, however, is not fully within the postmodern frame because complexity scientists believe in science, rigorous empirical study, theory, and synthesis, all, however, from a systems thinking perspective (Castellani & Hafferty, 2009). Traditional science is simply insufficient for researching systems, because the complexity of systems makes them unpredictable in the normal sense.

Capra (1996) describes the history of the study of systems as oscillating from mechanistic to systemic or ecological paradigms since the dawn of Western philosophy. The rise in systems thinking came from organismic biologists during the first half of the twentieth century. In contrast to traditional analytical thinking, a systems perspective involves studying the phenomenon of interest within the context of the larger whole; traditional analysis involves taking something apart to understand it. Systems thinking and cybernetics (science of organization) emerged in the 1940s, and it, along with dynamic systems theory (applied mathematics) in the late 1960s, fed into the development of complexity science in the early 1970s (Castellani & Hafferty, 2009). It is only with the introduction of modern computers that complexity scientists have been able to capture and build on the theoretical aspects developed earlier, such as general systems theory and cybernetics (Capra, 1996). No single discipline has taken up complexity science; rather, it crosses numerous disciplines, from computational science to physics, to sociology, to nursing (Zimmerman et al., 2001; Chaffee & McNeill, 2007; Castellani & Hafferty, 2009).

Key concepts

There is no single complexity theory or systematic way to study complex adaptive systems. Indeed, complexity science encompasses several perspectives. For example, the work of Prigogine and Stengers (1984) is focused on chaos theory and sensitivity to initial conditions (the butterfly effect), while the work of the Santa Fe Institute is concentrated on finding order and patterns within systems (Walby, 2007). Regardless of the approach, there are some common concepts that can offer insights when looking at a whole system including, but not limited to: agents, inter-connections, self-organization, patterns, emergence, co-evolution, and non-linearity (Anderson, Crabtree, Steele, & McDaniel, 2005; Capra, 1996; Cilliers, 1998; Holland, 1995; Kauffman, 1995).

The term *agent* is used, much like Clarke's (2005) *actant*, to avoid preconceptions in describing both human and non-human active elements that have the capacity to exchange information with their environment (Holland, 1995). Examples of agents are people, human processes such as the nursing process, discourses, and computer systems. This notion of agency, of people and processes that create activity through information exchange, expands on the constructivist view of human agency by enlarging the circle of who or what can act to include non-human forces. In doing so, it allows room for interplay between and among Foucauldian governance and individual forces within the phenomena of interest. These *interconnections* between and among agents are a key element within a CAS because they give rise to self-organization, emergence, and patterns (Anderson et al., 2005). Interconnections are created as a result of agents exchanging information, with mutual effect (Goldstein, 2008), and, along with agents, are an important feature for grounded theorists to identify as they try to make sense of what is happening in the data. For example, in studying the non-cash food economy in a region, there may be several layers of interconnection between players, who may have relationships even with food safety authorities because of other social involvements (e.g., community kitchens, school), and these interconnections may informally influence interpersonal behaviours.

Self-organization is the spontaneous process through which systems adjust to internal and external environmental changes, and is affected by the interdependent and interrelated nature of that environment (Kauffman, 1995). Capra (1996) refers to self-organization as the spontaneous emergence of order that can be identified through the recognition of patterns. What makes a system self-organizing is the lack of a centrally coordinating authority or externally imposed structure, such as planning. Examples of self-organizing systems include herd or flock behavior, spontaneous street demonstrations, the world economy, and any phenomena whose behavior cannot be readily predicted even though patterns and structures are recognizable.

Patterns are thematic recurrences, elements that repeat, and are ultimately how interactions and relationships are revealed. Patterns are the explicit focus for cybernetics, where the form and structure of organization are seen as key characteristics of life (Capra, 1996). In the grounded theory process, looking for patterns is at the core of data analysis as the researcher asks questions such as, "How is this incident similar to/different from this other incident?" "What is the pattern that holds them together?" In GTM, the researcher is continuously sifting data to identify patterns and repetitions, and comparing what appear to be emerging forms with data and embryonic concepts. In a recent study (Jantzen, 2012), the researcher identified a pattern she named "getting grounded," which involves setting high standards, being self-reflective, and focusing mindfully on patient care. Getting grounded is central to beginning a career as a nurse, and it recurs at the beginning of each shift worked, and often frequently during the day, for example, while washing hands and preparing to enter a patient's room.

Emergence is the interaction of agents and self-organization, causing properties to arise that are distinct from the properties of the individual agents themselves (Anderson et al., 2005). "Emergence" is a term used to describe system changes that were not intentionally created through traceable actions or components, and these changes arise out of what could be a series of minor, local interactions. Goldstein (1999) defined emergence as how novel and coherent structures, patterns, and properties surface in the process of self-organization of complex systems. Holland (1998) offers a simple example of emergence as a seed becoming a plant, or a fertilized egg becoming an organism; it is the notion of how something big can come from something little, given the right environment. Thus, a seed of corn can only develop into a cornstalk if properly fertilized, watered in accommodating conditions of light and temperature. Within the social world, an example of emergence is the world economy, resulting from numerous interactions at local levels, with no single leader or authority directing the course or setting the rules. From a grounded theory perspective, the concept of emergence is somewhat contested, because it is a term routinely used to describe the identification of a core concept in a study. Glaser and Strauss (1967) and Glaser (1978, 1992) contend that the core concept, or basic social process (BSP) emerges from the data, as if arising *de novo* as some sort of sacred vision. Most authors (see, e.g., Bryant, 2003; Charmaz, 2006; May, 1994; Morse, 1994) recognize the need to dwell with, and analyze data carefully, and at the same time know that, ultimately, to find the core concept, they have to "DRAG it out of the data!" (May, 1994, p. 10).

Co-evolution is the result of interaction and exchanges of energy and information that occur beyond the system boundaries, where both the CAS and the world beyond change because of the interactions (Anderson et al., 2005). A biological example of co-evolution is how the changes in a predator species can alter the adaptability of its prey (Goldstein, 2008). Depending on what is identified as the system, co-evolution can involve two closely related components of the system that evolve as a result of their mutual interactions. For example, in a small, remote community, the role of the public health nurse and that of the physician might co-evolve as a result of changes in the practice in one role. A new physician in town might feel it important to see newborns and their mothers "several times" in the first three weeks of life, making it easier for the nurse to make fewer home visits during that period, however, should something untoward happen (or the physician is replaced) that highlights the need for home visiting, nurses in that community would re-engage with that aspect of their practice. In this way, over time, the roles co-evolve in a somewhat closed system together. This highlights the need for someone researching the provision of health services in such a community to explore not just the current practices and relationships, but also historical practices and the factors that brought them into being.

Non-linearity is, literally, not a line. In mathematics, linearity means the value of a whole is equal to the sum of its parts, but in a CAS, a slight change in initial conditions might result in a large difference over time and therefore, predictability is less simple than in a linear system (Holland, 1995). Non-linearity can help explain how a single case of a new infectious disease can result in multiple incidents in one area and substantially fewer in another, even with similar public health infrastructure, such as the case of SARS in Ontario and British Columbia in Canada.

Systems thinking paradigms and nursing

Complexity science is not the only approach to whole systems thinking that is used by nurses. Ray (1998) suggests that nurses have thought in terms of systems for some time. She identifies complexity science as similar to the work of nursing theorists Rogers, Newman, Parse, Watson, Leininger, Davidson, and Reed, all of whom have recognized the importance of patterns and relationships. King's (1981) "Conceptual Framework for Nursing," based on general systems theory (Bertalanffy, 1968), defined nursing as occurring in personal, interpersonal, and social systems simultaneously and interactively. In addition, Chaffee and McNeill (2007) developed a conceptual model of nursing as a complex adaptive system. Kleffel (1996) advanced an ecocentric paradigm by linking nursing back to a systems conceptualization of the environment that includes the larger social, political, economic and global structures that affect health. In much the same light, Stevens (1989) called for a critical social reconceptualization of the environment.

Marck (2004) applied an ecological framework to understand nurses in direct patient care. Ecological restoration involves assessing the integrity or the overall health of an ecosystem by gathering information on the diversity of life forms; the process and structure for birth, growth, death, and renewal; and the context for economic development. Using tenets from ecological restoration, Marck assessed the ecological integrity of the health care system relating to nursing practice. Good restoration involves cultural, historical, social, political, moral and aesthetic considerations (Higgs, 1997).

The notion of panarchy was introduced by Gunderson, Holling, and Light (1995) and is focused on the source and role of change in systems from a socio-ecological perspective, in other words, bringing the idea of a CAS into the social arena. Panarchy refers to the dynamic interplay between and among human and other systems, such as health care or the pharmaceutical industry, as they iteratively grow, change, adapt, restructure, and sometimes renew each other. Some key concepts in panarchy are resilience, adaptive capacity, adaptive cycle, and adaptive management. Edwards, Rowan, Marck, and Grinspun (2011) worked within a panarchy framework to identify the challenges that have prevented full implementation of the nurse practitioner role in the Canadian health care system. After reviewing the relevant policy documents and other published sources as well as conducting interviews and creating complex timelines, the authors were able to construct a succinct explanation of how implementation of the role has unfolded in Canada, as well as locating pressure points for further implementation.

Grounded theory method and complex adaptive systems

There are several research methods that have been used in the study of systems, including case study (Anderson et al., 2005), concept mapping (Kane & Trochim, 2007), situational analysis (Clarke, 2005), agent-based modeling, data mining, and social network analysis, as well as grounded theory (Castellani & Hafferty, 2009). One grounded theory was produced by Turkel and Ray (2001), who created a grounded theory called "Relational Complexity: A Theory of the Nurse–Patient Relationship Within an Economic Context," using the ideas of complexity science such as relational interconnectedness, non-linearity, and creative emergence. In this study, using both qualitative and quantitative methods, the authors explored the phenomenon of nursing as an economic resource, capturing the contradiction of disorder and order produced by economics and cost containment. At the same time, they captured the unity created by the caring relationship as potentiating self-organization in the economically charged environment (Turkel & Ray, 2001). Using the concepts of non-linearity and emergence, these authors captured the paradoxes inherent in the nurse–patient relationship in a context of economic restraint, demonstrating that the value of nursing is in the relationships.

A review specifically of grounded theory research and complex adaptive systems revealed very few examples of their integration. We identified 14 articles, only two of which represented nursing (Morgan, Crossley, Stewart, et al., 2008; Swartz & Triscari, 2011); five were from health policy or administration (Atun, Kyratsis, et al., 2007; Dattee & Barlow, 2010; Hysong, Best, Pugh & Moore, 2005; Kernick & Mitchell, 2010; Lanham, McDaniel, et al., 2009); five from business management (Borzillo & Kaminska-Labbe, 2011; Chiles, Meyer, & Hench, 2004; Meyer, Gaba, & Colwell, 2005; Rhodes & Murray, 2007; Tams & Marshall, 2011); and the remainder from sustainability (Fraser, 2006) and planning (Innes & Gruber, 2005). The challenge in reviewing research reports using both grounded theory and complex adaptive systems is that there are often page limitations or other expectations from journal editors that do not allow for a sufficiently full explanation to describe highly complex ideas or methodologies. Half of the articles reviewed were extremely thin in their description of GTM, with authors making statements such as, they were inspired by Glaser and Strauss (e.g. Borzillo & Kaminska-Labbe, 2011), or they shifted from grounded theory (e.g. Chiles et al., 2004). Other authors stated that they used GTM, but how they did this was not evident and they did not cite any GTM sources (e.g. Rhodes & Murray, 2007; Lanham, McDaniel, et al., 2009; Dattee & Barlow, 2010; Kernick & Mitchell, 2010). As with GTM and constructivism, some CAS authors only mention CAS in passing, without a full exploration of the concepts of their applications of CAS as a framework for understanding the basic social process (e.g. Fraser, 2006; Morgan et al., 2008; Tams & Marshall, 2011). Thus, a researcher seeking guidance on how to use GTM to study complex adaptive systems would find little assistance in the existing body of literature on the pairing.

There are, however, some strong examples where researchers combined CAS and GTM. For example, Swartz and Triscari (2011) created a grounded theory of a collaborative learning partnership in which they describe the research process as a series of research spirals of data collection and reflections. These authors identified the research process itself as a network of open system feedback loops, resulting in transformative learning, or what can be understood as a co-evolutionary process. The non-linear, iterative process of research spirals is necessary in grounded theory to test out emerging ideas and to identify patterns that help to formulate the theory. So not only did Swartz and Triscari approach their topic area from a CAS framework, but they also applied CAS to their methodological approach. These authors demonstrate how grounded theory is a process of the researchers allowing ideas and concepts to self-organize, so the theory and understanding of the data can actually emerge. Whether it emerges as a "sacred vision" or is "dragged out of the data," there remains a distinct new understanding as a result of the way ideas and concepts self-organize within the researcher's thought process. Castellani, Castellani, and Spray (2003) compare self-organization to Strauss' concept of negotiated order, stating that:

> a self-organizing system's patterned regularity depends on and emerges out of the complex set of negotiated interactions that constitute it; conversely, these negotiated interactions depend on and are conditioned by the larger system of which they are part.
>
> *(p. 582)*

In this way, many of the concepts that are part of CAS correspond to grounded theory, making the method compatible with and appropriate for studying CASs.

There may be some distinction between studying a CAS as phenomena, and using CAS concepts within the research process. Authors such as Anderson and colleagues (2005) used a case study approach, applying complexity science concepts. Many research methodologies can be used to study a CAS, or aspects of it, but once the system is identified as a CAS, and set to be studied as one, complexity science concepts will be highlighted throughout the research process. There are varied methods to achieve this and the focus of the research will determine which methodology is best suited for the purpose.

Related/mixed methods

We have discussed some of the innovative directions researchers are taking GTM, including constructivism, situational analysis, and complexity science. In this, we have tried to confine the exploration to research in which GTM could be identified, and have highlighted some of the notable points of intersection between the methodology and the varied conceptualizations of it. It has become clear to us that GTM as a methodology allows for considerable creativity. For example, not only is it compatible with CASs, but there are other novel strategies and methods to bring to a grounded theory study that can expand or enhance traditional methods. For example, concept mapping is a participatory mixed method designed by William Trochim (1989), resulting in a structured conceptualization of participants' responses to a focused question, which are visually represented in maps (Trochim et al., 2006). In concept mapping, the participants answer the focused question, then are asked to group the entire set of responses, much as a grounded theorist might code interviews, constantly comparing each statement with the others to place similar statements in the same group. Non-metric multidimensional scaling and cluster analysis are done on the entire set of groupings to identify which statements were grouped together most often, placing them closer together on the map (Trochim, 1989). Concept mapping is similar to creation of a positional map in situational analysis, the difference being that in concept mapping the researcher asks the question(s) directly of the participants, whereas in positional mapping the researcher questions the data. In the food security/food safety study currently underway, one of the authors (WM) is using concept mapping results to enhance theoretical sensitivity in a study using situational analysis as the primary method. What this has added is a direct focus on the primary research question, allowing for the exploration of the situation to ensure that what is considered important to those working in the field is captured within the data.

Another mixed method approach to grounded theory is the self-organizing map (SOM) (Castellani et al., 2003). SOM is a modeling technique from the neural networking field of complexity theory (see Cilliers, 1998). Castellani and colleagues (2003) describe the application of SOM to grounded theory, based on the original writings of Glaser and Strauss (1967). As with concept mapping and grounded theory, SOM relies on constant comparative analysis, is a diagrammatic tool, uses theoretical sampling, and is exploratory (Castellani et al., 2003). The output for SOM is conceptual clusters, as with concept mapping. The strength of SOM is that the researcher can analyze complex quantitative data using a nonlinear clustering technique to find non-obvious patterns and relationships that can then be applied to more traditional grounded theory techniques of coding and memo writing (Castellani et al., 2003). Both concept mapping and SOM offer new directions that could be supportive of a grounded theory study, depending on the intent of the study, and exploration of mixed methods in this way may provide new tools for grounded theory research in nursing.

Conclusion

As can be seen, GTM has a long history in nursing and is well respected as a rigorous qualitative methodology, regardless of the debates that we scholars love so much. It is precisely in those tensions that grounded theorists explore the possibilities for ways of explicating and further enhancing the methodology. And as may be evident by now, GTM is not a research method that will appeal to nurse scholars whose sole mission is to elucidate the unique essence of nursing; rather, GTM has been, and continues to be strengthened from the interchange of ideas across disciplinary boundaries over time, because knowledge is always shared and research methodologies benefit from this.

In our exploration of new directions in the use of GTM, we have noted a few challenges for nursing researchers to consider as they conduct their work. First is the challenge posed by journal page limitations, which makes it difficult to explain sufficiently what is sometimes a complex methodology. It is tiring to have to choose between slimming down the findings in order to explain a methodology adequately or presenting an insufficient description of the methods, so we appreciate that some of the inconsistencies in published work may be through no fault of the authors. The second, which may be related to the first, is a tendency for researchers to say they are using grounded theory "approaches," or their study is "informed by grounded theory," when they are simply using constant comparison. Finally, is the tendency of some, particularly those new to GTM, to cite recent sources at the expense of the originals, resulting in what appears to be a thin comprehension of the methodology. The pressures of grant writing can sometimes push researchers to take their sources at face value without looking further to understand GTM in all its wondrous complexity, thus, without examining the roots of the methodology, novice researchers may come to believe, for example, that Charmaz invented memoing as part of constructivist GTM. We acknowledge that there is a significant learning curve to becoming a competent grounded theorist, particularly without a mentor. Approaching the research from a complexity science perspective, or using other emerging theoretical frameworks, makes GTM that much more challenging, thus making good mentoring especially important.

It is no longer sufficient to simply indicate a methodology used, even if it is, for example, Straussian (or Glaserian) grounded theory. Researchers must explicate their own philosophical stance related to the chosen methodology, and explain what GTM means, as well as a rationale for its use, for each particular study. This not only helps the reader better appreciate the study, but also provides sufficient guidance for novice researchers to begin formulating a rich understanding for themselves as they learn GTM. It might also enable novice grounded theorists to appreciate how much GTM, even at its most basic, requires attention to the rich, nuanced worlds of meaning that we, as nurses, are privileged to share.

Acknowledgments

The authors wish to acknowledge Lenora Marcellus for her editorial contribution to this chapter.

References

Allen, D. G. (1995). Hermeneutics: Philosophical traditions and nursing practice research. *Nursing Science Quarterly*, *8*(4), 174–182.

Anderson, R. A., Crabtree, B. F., Steele, D. J., & McDaniel, R. R., Jr. (2005). Case study research: The view from complexity science. *Qualitative Health Research*, *15*(5), 669–685.

Annells, M. (1997). Grounded theory method, part I: Within the five moments of qualitative research. *Nursing Inquiry*, *4*, 120–129.

Atun, R. A., Kyratsis, I., Jelic, G., Rados-Malicbegovic, D., & Gurol-Urganci, I. (2007). Diffusion of complex health innovations: Implementation of primary health care reforms in Bosnia and Herzegovina. *Health Policy and Planning, 22*(1), 28–39. doi: 10.1093/heapol/czl031.

Benoliel, J. Q. (1996). Grounded theory and nursing knowledge. *Qualitative Health Research, 6,* 406–428.

Bertalanffy, L. V. (1968). *General system theory: Foundations, development, applications.* New York: George Braziller.

Birks, M., Chapman, Y., & Francis, K. (2006). Moving grounded theory into the 21st Century: Part 1: An evolutionary tale. *Singapore Nursing Journal, 33*(4), 4–10.

Borzillo, S., & Kaminska-Labbe, R. (2011). Unravelling the dynamics of knowledge creation in communities of practice though complexity theory lenses. *Knowledge Management & Research Practice, 9*(4), 353–366.

Bryant, A. (2003). A constructive/ist response to Glaser. *Forum: Qualitative Social Research, 4*(1), Article 15. Available at: http://nbn-resolving.de/urn:nbn:de:0114- fqs0301155.

Capra, F. (1996). *The web of life.* New York: Anchor Books.

Castellani, B., Castellani, J., & Spray, S. L. (2003). Grounded neural networking: Modeling complex quantitative data. *Symbolic Interaction, 26*(4), 577–589.

Castellani, B., & Hafferty, F. (2009). *Sociology and complexity science: A new field of inquiry.* Berlin: Springer.

Chaffee, M. W., & McNeill, M. M. (2007). A model of nursing as a complex adaptive system. *Nursing Outlook, 55*(5), 232–241.

Charmaz, K. (2000). Grounded theory: Objectivist and constructivist methods. In N. Denzin & Y. Lincoln (Eds.), *Handbook of qualitative research* (2nd ed.) (pp. 509–535). Thousand Oaks, CA: Sage.

Charmaz, K. (2006). *Constructing grounded theory: A practical guide through qualitative analysis.* Thousand Oaks, CA: Sage.

Chen, H. Y., & Boore, J. R. (2009). Using a synthesized technique for grounded theory in nursing research. *Journal of Clinical Nursing, 18,* 2251–2260.

Chiles, T. H., Meyer, A. D., & Hench, T. J. (2004). Organizational emergence: The origin and transformation of Branson, Missouri's musical theaters. *Organization Science, 15*(5), 499–519.

Cilliers, P. (1998). *Complexity and postmodernism: Understanding complex systems.* New York: Routledge.

Cilliers, P. (2002). Why we cannot know complex things completely. *Emergence, 4*(1), 77–84.

Clarke, A. E. (2003). Situational analysis: Grounded theory mapping after the postmodern turn. *Symbolic Interactionism, 26,* 553–576.

Clarke, A. E. (2005). *Situational analysis: Grounded theory after the postmodern turn.* Thousand Oaks, CA: Sage.

Collins, J. L. (2006). *Mozambique's HIV/AIDS pandemic: Grappling with apartheid's legacy.* United Nations Research Institutes for Social Development Social Policy and Development Programme, Paper Number 24.

Cooney, A. (2010). Choosing between Glaser and Strauss: An example. *Nurse Researcher, 17*(4), 18–28.

Dattee, B., & Barlow, J. (2010). Complexity and whole-system change programmes. *Journal of Health Services Research & Policy, 15*(suppl. 2), 19–25.

Drury, V., Francis, K., & Chapman, Y. (2008). Mature learners becoming registered nurses: A grounded theory model. *Australian Journal of Advanced Nursing, 26*(2), 39–45.

Edwards, N., Rowan, M., Marck, P., & Grinspun, D. (2011). Understanding whole systems change in health care: The case of nurse practitioners in Canada. *Policy, Politics, & Nursing Practice, 12*(1), 4–17.

Erikson, A. (2008). Maintaining integrity: How nurses navigate boundaries in pediatric palliative care University of California, San Francisco, ProQuest Dissertations and Thesis (AAT 3324708).

Fraser, E. D. (2006). Crop diversification and trade liberalization: Linking global trade and local management through a regional case study. *Agriculture and Human Values, 23*(3), 271–281.

Gagnon, M., Jacob, J. D., & Holmes, D. (2010). Governing through (in)security: A critical analysis of a fear-based public health campaign. *Critical Public Health, 20*(2), 245–256.

Gardner, A. (2010). Therapeutic friendliness and the development of therapeutic leverage by mental health nurses in community rehabilitation settings. *Contemporary Nurse, 34*(2), 140–148.

Gardner, A., McCutcheon, H., & Fedoruk, M. (2010). Superficial supervision: Are we placing clinicians and clients at risk? *Contemporary Nurse, 34*(2), 258–266.

Geertz, C. (1973). *The interpretation of cultures: Selected essays.* New York: Basic Books.

Ghezeljeh, T. M., & Emami A. (2009). Grounded theory: Methodology and philosophical perspective. *Nurse Researcher, 17*(1), 15–23.

Glaser, B. G. (1978). *Theoretical sensitivity.* Mill Valley, CA: Sociology Press.

Glaser, B. G. (1992). *Basics of grounded theory analysis: Emergence vs. forcing.* Mill Valley, CA: Sociology Press.

Glaser, B. G., & Strauss, A. L. (1965). *Awareness of dying.* Chicago: Aldine.

Glaser, B. G., & Strauss, A. L. (1967). *Discovery of grounded theory*. Chicago: Aldine.

Glaser, B. G., & Strauss, A. L. (1968). *Time for dying*. Chicago: Aldine.

Goldstein, J. A. (1999). Emergence as a construct: History and issues. *Emergence: Complexity and Organization*, *1*(1), 49–72.

Goldstein, J. A. (2008). A review of *Reinventing the Sacred*: A new view of science, reason, and religion. *Emergence*, *10*(3), 117.

Grigg, E. (1997). A situational analysis of an HIV/AIDS clinical area. *Journal of Clinical Nursing*, *6*, 35–41.

Gunderson, L. H., Holling, C. S., & Light, S. S. (1995). *Barriers and bridges to the renewal of ecosystems and institutions*. New York: Columbia University Press.

Higgs, E. S. (1997). What is good ecological restoration? *Conservation Biology*, *11*(2), 338–348.

Holland, J. H. (1992). Complex adaptive systems. *Daedalus*, *121*(1), 17–30.

Holland, J. H. (1995). *Hidden order: How adaptation builds complexity*. New York: Helix Books.

Holland, J. H. (1998). *Emergence: From chaos to order*. Reading, MA: Addison-Wesley.

Holtslander, L. F, Balley, J. M., & Steeves, M. L. (2011). Walking a fine line: An exploration of the experience of finding balance for older persons bereaved after caregiving for a spouse with advanced cancer. *Journal of Oncology Nursing*, *15*(3), 254–259.

Hunter, A., Murphy, K., Grealish, A., Casey, D., & Keady, J. (2011). Navigating the grounded theory terrain. Part 1. *Nurse Researcher*, *18*(4), 6–10.

Hysong, S., Best, R., Pugh, J., & Moore, F. (2005). Not of one mind: Mental models of clinical practice guidelines in the Veterans Health Administration. *Health Services Research*, *40*(3), 829–847.

Innes, J., & Gruber, J. (2005). Planning styles in conflict: The Metropolitan Transportation Commission. *Journal of the American Planning Association*, *71*(2), 177–188.

Jantzen, D. (2012). Refining nursing practice: A grounded theory of experienced nurses' lifelong learning. Unpublished doctoral dissertation, University of Alberta, Edmonton, Alberta.

Jones, P. R., Waters, C. M., Oka, R. K., & McGhee, E. M. (2010). Increasing community capacity to reduce tobacco-related health disparities in African American communities. *Public Health Nursing*, *27*(6), 552–560.

Kane, M., & Trochim, W. M. (2007). *Concept mapping for planning and evaluation*. Thousand Oaks, CA: Sage.

Kauffman, S. (1995). *At home in the universe: The search for laws of self-organization and complexity*. New York: Oxford University Press.

Kean, S. (2009). Children's and young people's strategies to access information during a family members' critical illness. *Journal of Clinical Nursing*, *19*, 266–274.

Kean, S. (2010). The experience of ambiguous loss in families of brain injured ICU patients. *Nursing in Critical Care*, *15*(2), 66–75.

Kearney, M. (1996). Reclaiming normal life: Mothers' stages of recovery from drug use. *JOGNN: Journal of Obstetric, Gynecologic, and Neonatal Nursing*, *25*(9), 761–768.

Kearney, M. (2009). Taking grounded theory beyond psychological process. *Research in Nursing & Health*, *32*, 567–568.

Keddy, B., Sims, L., & Stern, P. N. (1996). Grounded theory as a feminist research methodology. *Journal of Advanced Nursing*, *23*, 448–453.

Kendall, J. (1999). Axial coding and the grounded theory controversy. *Western Journal of Nursing Research*, *21*, 743–757.

Kernick, D., & Mitchell, A. (2010). Working with lay people in health service research: A model of co-evolution based on complexity theory. *Journal of Interprofessional Care*, *24*(1), 31–40.

King, I. M. (1981). *A theory of nursing: Systems, concepts, process*. New York: John Wiley & Sons.

Kleffel, D. (1996). Environmental paradigms: Moving toward an ecocentric perspective. *Advances in Nursing Science*, *18*(4), 1–10.

Kushner, K. E., & Morrow, R. (2003). Grounded theory, feminist theory, critical theory: Toward theoretical triangulation. *Advances in Nursing Science*, *26*(1), 30–43.

Lanham, H. J., McDaniel, J., Crabtree, B. F., Miller, W. L., Stange, K. C., Tallia, A. F., & Nutting, P. A. (2009). How improving practice relationships among clinicians and nonclinicians can improve quality in primary care. *Joint Commission Journal of Quality Patient Safety*, *35*(9), 457–466.

Leutwyler, H. C., & Wallhagen, M. (2010). Older adults with schizophrenia finding a place to belong. *Issues in Mental Health Nursing*, *31*, 507–513.

Lyndon, A. (2010). Skillful anticipation: Maternity nurses' perspectives on maintaining safety. *Quality & Safety in Health Care*, *19*(5), e8.

MacDonald, M. A. (2001). Finding a critical perspective in grounded theory. In R. S. Schreiber & P.N. Stern (Eds.), *Using grounded theory in nursing* (pp. 113–158). Philadelphia, PA: Springer.

Marcellus, L. (2010). Supporting resilience in foster families: A model for program design that supports recruitment, retention, and satisfaction of foster families who care for infants with prenatal substance exposure. *Child Welfare, 89*(1), 7–29.

Marck, P. (2004) Ethics for practitioners: An ecological framework. In J. Storch, P. Rodney, & R. Starzomski (Eds.), *Toward a moral horizon: Nursing ethics for leadership and practice* (pp. 232–247). Toronto, ON: Pearson.

May, K. A. (1994). Abstract knowing: The case for magic in the method. In J. M. Morse (Ed.), *Critical issues in qualitative research methods* (pp. 10–21). Thousand Oaks, CA: Sage.

McCann, R., & Clarke, E. (2003). Grounded theory in nursing research: Part 1: Methodology. *Nurse Researcher, 11*(2), 7–18.

McCreaddie, M., Lyons, I., Horsburgh, D., Miller, M., & Frew, J. (2011). The insolating and insulating effects of Hepatitis C. *Gastroenterology Nursing, 34*(1), 49–59.

McCreaddie, M., Lyons, I., Watt, D., Ewing, E., Croft, J., Smith, M., & Tocher, J. (2010). Routines and rituals: A grounded theory of the pain management of drug users in acute care settings. *Journal of Clinical Nursing, 19*, 2730–2740.

McCreaddie, M., Payne, S., & Froggatt, K. (2010). Ensnared by positivity: A constructivist perspective on "being positive" in cancer care. *European Journal of Oncology Nursing, 14*, 283–290.

McGeorge, S. J. (2011). Unravelling the differences between complexity and frailty in old age: Findings from a constructivist grounded theory. *Journal of Psychiatric and Mental Health Nursing, 18*, 67–73.

Meyer, A. D., Gaba, V., & Colwell, K. A. (2005). Organizing far from equilibrium: Nonlinear change in organizational fields. *Organization Science, 16*(5), 456–473.

Milliken, P. J., & Schreiber, R. S. (2001). Can you do grounded theory without symbolic interactionism? In R. S. Schreiber & P. N. Stern (Eds.), *Using grounded theory in nursing* (pp. 177–190). Philadelphia, PA: Springer.

Mills, J., Bonner, A., & Francis, K. (2006). Adopting a constructivist approach to grounded theory: Implications for research design. *International Journal of Nursing Practice, 12*, 8–13.

Mills, J., Chapman, Y., Bonner, A., & Francis, K. (2007). Grounded theory: A methodological spiral from positivism to postmodernism. *Journal of Advanced Nursing, 58*(1), 72–79.

Mills, J., Francis, K., & Bonner, A. (2007a). The accidental mentor: Australian rural nurses developing supportive relationships in the workplace. *Rural and Remote Health, 7*, 842–852.

Mills, J., Francis, K., & Bonner, A. (2007b). The problem of workforce for the social world of Australian rural nurses: A collective action frame analysis. *Journal of Nursing Management, 15*, 721–730.

Mills, J., Francis, K., & Bonner, A. (2007c). Live my work: Rural nurses and their multiple perspectives of self. *Journal of Advanced Nursing, 59*(6), 583–590.

Morgan, D. G., Crossley, M. F., Stewart, N. J., D'Arcy, C., Forbes, D. A., Normand, S. A., & Cammer, A. L. (2008). Taking the hit: Focusing on caregiver "error" masks organizational-level risk factors for nursing aide assault. *Qualitative Health Research, 18*(3), 334–346

Morse, J. M. (1994). "Emerging from the data": The cognitive processes of analysis in qualitative inquiry. In J. M. Morse (Ed.), *Critical issues in qualitative research methods* (pp. 23–43). Thousand Oaks, CA: Sage.

Oakley, A. (1981). Interviewing women: A contradiction in terms. In H. Roberts (Ed.), *Doing feminist research* (pp. 30–74). London: Routledge & Kegan Paul.

Pieters, H. C. & Heilemann, M. V. (2011). "Once you're 82, going on 83, surviving has a different meaning": Older breast cancer survivors reflect on cancer survivorship. *Cancer Nursing, 34*(2), 124–133.

Prigogine, I., & Stengers, I. (1984). *Order out of chaos: Man's new dialogue with nature.* Boulder, CO: New Science Library.

Pursley-Crotteau, S., Bunting, S. M., & Draucker, C. B. (2001). Grounded theory and hermeneutics: Contradictory or complementary methods of nursing research. In R. S. Schreiber & P. N. Stern (Eds.), *Using grounded theory in nursing* (pp. 191–201). Philadelphia, PA: Springer.

Ray, M. (1998). Complexity and nursing science. *Nursing Science Quarterly, 11*, 91–93.

Rhodes, M. L., & Murray, J. (2007). Collaborative decision making in urban regeneration: A complex adaptive systems perspective. *International Public Management Journal, 10*(1), 79–101.

Schreiber, R. S. (2001).The grounded theory club, or who needs an expert mentor? In R. S. Schreiber & P. N. Stern (Eds.), *Using grounded theory in nursing* (pp. 97–112). Philadelphia, PA: Springer.

Sheehan, D. K., & Draucker, C. B. (2011). Interaction patterns between parents with advanced cancer and their adolescent children. *Psycho-Oncology, 20*(10), 1108–1115.

Snowden, A., & Martin, C. R. (2010). Mental health nurse prescribing: A difficult pill to swallow? *Journal of Psychiatric and Mental Health Nursing*, *17*, 543–553.

Stern, P. N. (1994). Eroding grounded theory. In J. M. Morse (Ed.), *Critical issues in qualitative research methods* (pp. 212–223). Thousand Oaks, CA: Sage.

Stern, P. N., & Covan, E. K. (2001). Early grounded theory: Its processes and products. In R. S. Schreiber & P. N. Stern (Eds.), *Using grounded theory in nursing* (pp. 17–34) Philadelphia, PA: Springer.

Stevens, P. E. (1989). A critical social reconceptualization of the environment in nursing: Implications for methodology, *Advances in Nursing Science*, *11*(4), 56–68.

Strauss, A. (1959/1969). *Mirrors and masks*. San Francisco, CA: Sociology Press.

Strauss, A. (1978). *Negotiations*. San Francisco, CA: Jossey-Bass.

Strauss, A. (1987). *Qualitative methods for social scientists*. Cambridge: Cambridge University Press.

Strauss, A. L. (1993). *Continuous permutations of action*. New York: Aldine de Gruyter.

Strauss, A., & Corbin, J. (1990). *Basics of qualitative research: Grounded theory procedures and techniques*. Newbury Park, CA: Sage.

Strauss, A. L., & Glaser, B. G. (1970). *Anguish: A case history of a dying trajectory*. Mill Valley, CA: Sociology Press.

Swartz, A. L., & Triscari, J. S. (2011). A model of transformative collaboration. *Adult Education Quarterly*, *61*(4), 324–340.

Tams, S., & Marshall, J. (2011). Responsible careers: Systemic reflexivity in shifting landscapes. *Human Relations*, *64*(1), 109–131.

Trochim, W. M. (1989). An introduction to concept mapping for planning and evaluation. *Evaluation Program Planning*, *12*, 1–16.

Trochim, W. M., Cabera, D. A., Milstein, B., Gallagher, R. S., & Leischow, S .J. (2006). Practical challenges if systems thinking and modelling in public health. *American Journal of Public Health*, *96*(3), 538–546.

Turkel, M. C., & Ray, M. A. (2001). Relational complexity: From grounded theory to instrument development and theoretical testing. *Nursing Science Quarterly*, *14*(4), 281.

Turrill, S. (2000). A situational analysis: The potential to produce evidence-based nursing practice guidelines within a regional neonatal intensive care unit. *Journal of Nursing Management*, *8*, 345–355.

Vygotsky, L. S. (1978). *Mind in society: The development of higher psychological processes*. Cambridge, MA: Harvard University Press.

Walby, S. (2007). Complexity theory, systems theory, and multiple intersecting social inequalities. *Philosophy of the Social Sciences*, *37*(4), 449–470.

Wasserman, J. A., Clair, J. M., & Wilson, K. L. (2009). Problematics of grounded theory: Innovations for developing an increasingly rigorous qualitative method. *Qualitative Research*, *9*(3), 355–381.

Williams, B. (2001). Developing critical reflection for professional practice through problem-based learning. *Journal of Advanced Nursing*, *34*(1), 27–34.

Williams, S., & Keady, J. (2008). "A stony road . . . a 19 year journey": "Bridging" through late-stage Parkinson's disease. *Journal of Research in Nursing*, *13*, 373–388.

Wilson, H. S., & Hutchinson, S. A. Triangulation of qualitative methods: Heideggerian hermeneutics and grounded theory. *Qualitative Health Research*, *1*(2), 263–272.

Wuest, J. (1995). Feminist grounded theory: An exploration of the congruency and tensions between two traditions in knowledge discovery. *Qualitative Health Research*, *5*, 125–137.

Wuest, J., & Merritt-Gray, M. (2001). Feminist grounded theory revisited: Practical issues and new understandings. In R. S. Schreiber & P. N. Stern (Eds.), *Using grounded theory in nursing* (pp. 159–175). Philadelphia, PA: Springer.

Zimmerman, B., Lindberg, C., & Plsek, P. (2001). *Edgeware: Insights from complexity science for health care leaders*. Irving: VHA Inc.

15

Traditional ethnography

Pamela J. Brink

This chapter attempts to encapsulate the history of Traditional Ethnography in both anthropology and nursing, by reviewing the development of ethnography in Anthropology, followed by a discussion of the basic requirements of a Traditional Ethnography. The third section discusses the introduction of Traditional Ethnography to nursing, while the fourth describes some of the misunderstanding found in the nursing literature about ethnography. A brief review of some of the nursing publications in the past 20 years reporting on Traditional Ethnography is followed by a comment on the future of Traditional Ethnography in nursing.

Cultural Anthropology traces its methodological roots to Malinowski's *Argonauts of the Western Pacific* (1922). From this beginning, Anthropologists came to describe their methods of data collection as field work, participant observation and eventually ethnography. The terms were used almost interchangeably. Field work, for an anthropologist, meant they were to find an isolated group of people, somewhere in the world, who had not been previously studied or written about and live with them for at least two years. This provided time for learning the language. The anthropologist generally went out alone, with visiting government officials or missionaries as their only contact with the outside world. The loneliness engendered by this isolation led to the use of field diaries as their only emotional outlet (Malinowski, 1967).

Anthropology, as a discipline, is composed of four fields: socio/cultural anthropology, linguistics, archaeology, and physical anthropology. Anthropologists were expected to qualify (pass written and oral examinations) in all four fields as a basic requirement for the degree. Field work, therefore, included data collection and analysis in all four fields. (Although graduate students in archaeology did summer "field work" on archaeological digs, field schools in cultural anthropology came much later and were not available to all students. Each anthropologist, therefore, had to learn how to do ethnography by doing it.) Knowledge of descriptive linguistics enabled the researcher to learn and document the indigenous language. Knowledge of physical anthropology provided tools for estimating the physical health and well-being of a population, including normative size, weight and development. The behavioral portion of the research included kinship charts and patterns of interaction which was often dictated by age and gender. Anthropological field research was holistic.

Initially, there was no requirement of having a "problem" to study. By living with a people for two years, some unifying theme would arise. There were general notions about how to go about collecting data, including mapping the village, collecting genealogies, counting people in every household and village, documenting who went where and who visited, writing down everything observed as soon as possible after observations. Only when the language was sufficiently learned could the researcher begin asking questions. So field work began with non-verbal observations of everything that was going on within sight, trying to get as involved as the people would allow with festivities and activities of daily living. Gaining the trust of the people being studied was of paramount importance.

Most of the information about how to "do" field work came from chance remarks in lectures and seminars, talking to returning field workers to find out what they did. The only book devoted to the collection and analysis of data in the field was geared to archaeology and was revised and updated regularly (see Committee of the Royal Anthropological Institute, 1967). Laura Bohannan, under the pseudonym Eleanor Bowen (1961), wrote a humorous account of her doctoral field work in Nigeria in *Return to Laughter* in which her major professor told her to take along "leaky tennis shoes." This was the sum of her training in field methods. For the most part, anthropology students were simply told to "read ethnographies" with the vague hope that somehow, through some kind of osmosis, they would discover how to collect and analyze the data for their own field work.

There was no text available on "how to do" ethnography until Spradley and McCurdy's (1972) popular book came out, followed by the book by Agar in 1980. Wax's (1986) book on Field Methods came even later. Many ethnographies mentioned how the researcher went about field work but it was not consistent. There was very little about methods in anthropological journals. The focus was on the findings rather than how one went about obtaining those results. Everyone "assumed" that everyone else was doing the same things, more or less. If there was an article on ethnographic field methods, it usually appeared in Sociology journals as Sociology was deeply concerned with research methods. See, for example, the article by Schwartz and Schwartz (1955) on Participant Observation. In fact, a very useful "how to" text on field work was written by Sociologists (Schatzman & Strauss, 1973).

As travel to remote peoples became more difficult, American anthropologists turned to studying indigenous peoples within the continental United States, Canada and Mexico. In addition, as few anthropologists were independently wealthy, grants were sought to support field research. Granting agencies, more familiar with the hard sciences and sociological research, required a problem focus for the research. Anthropologists found they had to narrow their ethnographies not only by geographic region or tribe but also by selecting a particular event, tradition or ritual such as childbirth, initiation rites, funerary customs, pottery making, weaving, or adolescent initiation rites. (If the culture group had not previously been studied, the researcher might find that the culture trait to be studied did not exist in that particular group although all the other surrounding groups did have the custom!)

Anthropological field work began to focus upon specific fields of study as well as geographical areas. Anthropology became more involved in urban populations, so Urban Anthropology became an area of study with its requisite form of field work. Anthropologists interested in schools and education developed field methods specifically for Educational Anthropology. Medical anthropology evolved out of an interest in health and illness issues within indigenous populations. Field work, that included data collection in all four fields of anthropology, began to disappear, focusing instead on the sub-fields.

Granting agencies not only demanded a problem focus for research grants, they required some sort of theoretical basis for the research, as well as a detailed description of the methods of data collection and analysis to be used. General methods books for Anthropologists began to appear in the 1970s but were not solely on ethnography (Pelto, 1970). Ethnographies shifted from describing a culture group to describing a particular issue within a culture group.

Ethnography is as intrinsic to Anthropology as Anatomy and Physiology are to Medicine and Nursing. To ignore the rationale behind ethnography, derived from Anthropology, is to limit an understanding of this form of research.

The basics of Traditional Ethnography

Ethnography provides a rich description of a particular social group that is well defined, naturally occurring, interacts daily in face-to-face contacts, has rules and regulations for individual as well as group behavior, and is a small, geographically defined population. Ethnographies use multiple methods of data collection, in combination, in order to obtain that rich description. No single data collection method will yield ethnography.

Early in the history of anthropology, the field worker was expected to enter the field as a stranger with no preconceived ideas as to what would be found. Culture shock was an expectation (Oberg, 1954) and part of the rites of passage (Van Gennep, Vizedon, & Caffee, 1961). Ethnographers usually entered the field alone although some husband-and-wife teams occurred (Whiting, 1963). The group needed to be small enough for the ethnographer to become familiar with everyone at least by sight. The ethnographer usually lived with the group; some ethnographers lived within a family household (Reid, 1969).

Field work began with unobtrusive observations of daily activities. Since the ethnographer was not familiar with the language, interviews (whether formal or informal) were impossible. The ethnographer could employ a member of the group as a "chief informant" or interpreter. Other individuals could be chosen to serve as informants about aspects of group customs and behaviors. Informants served for the entire term of the research project or were used briefly. Asking appropriate questions of appropriate informants is one of the hallmarks of Traditional Ethnography.

During the initial phase of field work, the researcher spent time mapping the village; noting the placement of houses, roads, and other buildings. If a village, spatial arrangements of houses, farms, gardens, markets, schools, and water sources were noted and later labels were given to these places such as the compounds of the traditional birth attendant, the traditional healer, or chief's house. As the ethnographer was invited into homes, floor plans and surrounding land are also noted. If invited to a meal in a home, foods and food rituals are noted. If each home has a garden and livestock, these too are noted. Basic census data were collected for each household with its attendant kinship systems.

If the ethnography is of a particular hospital ward or neighborhood, the same requirement for mapping spatial arrangements remains. (For example, the classic Nightingale hospital ward allowed for easy observations of all patients on the ward whereas the hospital ward of today with its enclosed single and double rooms requires the nurse to actually open a door and enter a room to see what is going on.) This observation period is a critical first step in the research. It takes time and cannot be rushed.

As the group comes to acknowledge and accept the researcher, some form of participation in the life of the group becomes possible. Participation usually begins with public rituals open to anyone to attend before moving to more intimate group rituals, as the ethnographer becomes more accepted and trusted. Any research report labeled as an ethnography that does not include participant observation is not a Traditional Ethnography. Participant observation, in all its stages, is the cornerstone of ethnography (Roper & Shapira, 1999).

Other data routinely collected by the ethnographer included any written documentation such as census data from church records or actual census data, or other historical records. Material objects in the environment (artifacts) also provided information on how the group believes and behaves. Any data that help in understanding the group being studied were collected.

Reliability and validity, as well as triangulation of data (Brink, 1991), are built into the process. Observations of events are repeated throughout the period of field work. Consistency of information is sought from a variety of informants. All information is checked and rechecked with questions asked for clarification. All conflicting information is clarified and missing data is sought. Explanations are obtained of what is observed and how it fits into the beliefs of the group. Data analysis occurs throughout field work rather than at the end.

Obtaining Ethics Review Board approvals may be problematic. Allbutt and Masters (2010) found that Ethics Review Boards do not really understand ethnography. Griffiths (2008) was concerned with the morality of obtaining individual signed consents from very ill people. Permission to study the group may come from the chief of the tribe, the tribal council, the hospital administration or whoever is responsible for the functioning of the group. The ethnographer usually explains to each person just who they are and what they are doing. The population being studied may or may not be familiar with research of any kind so accept the researcher at face value, based upon their behavior.

The general misunderstanding of ethnography and the study of indigenous culture groups arises, in this author's opinion, because of a general ignorance of Anthropology in American nursing. Although American schools of nursing routinely require an introductory course in Sociology, few also require an introductory course in Anthropology.

The introduction of ethnography to nursing

Three early papers describing participant observation as a research method appeared in *Nursing Research* (Pearsall, 1965; Byerly, 1969; and Ragucci, 1972). A fourth paper (Gale, 1973) appeared in the *American Journal of Nursing*. The first reference to ethnography (Aamodt et al., 1979) was found in the papers presented at, and subsequently published in, the annual Communicating Nursing Research Conference. Another paper by Aamodt (1982) appeared in the *Western Journal of Nursing Research*, closely followed by the widely quoted Robertson and Boyle (1984) article in the *Journal of Advanced Nursing*. A book by Munhall and Oiler included a chapter on ethnography by Germain (1986). The National League for Nursing's compilation of research methods in nursing included a chapter on ethnography by Omery and Sarter (1988).

A paper by Macgregor (1967) introduced the concept of culture and described some of the reasons behind the seemingly uncooperative behavior of certain patients. Leininger (1967) spoke to giving nursing care to a patient from another culture. About the same time, the first group of American nurses was studying for their doctoral degrees in anthropology, either under private USPHS grants or under a group grant (Gortner, 1991). Some of the dissertations by this early group of nurse anthropologists were traditional ethnographies involving field work with indigenous peoples (Brink, 1969; Gazaway, 1974; Osborne, 1968; Reid, 1969), in ethnic neighborhoods (Ragucci, 1972) or hospital wards (Germain, 1979; Kayser-Jones, 1981). Most of these doctoral dissertations never appeared in nursing journals.

Nurse-anthropologists were keenly interested in bringing their knowledge of the theory and methods of Anthropology to nursing. The first books introducing anthropology to the broader nursing community appeared in the 1970s (Bauwens, 1978; Brink, 1976; Leininger, 1971). Byerly and Brink (1979) proposed a model course introducing Anthropological principles and methods to nursing. Nursing ethnographies appeared in papers read at national and regional nursing conferences (Aamodt, 1972; Cahill, 1967; Ford, 1973). These early nursing research conferences were by invitation only, limiting both presenters and attendees.

Controversial uses of Traditional Ethnography in nursing

There appear to be two major areas of confusion in the nursing literature on what constitutes Traditional Ethnography. One area is the question of what constitutes a target population or culture group, and the other is on the methods of data collection.

Some nurses believe that when they create a focus group, and then join the group as a participant, subsequently observing the interactions of the group, they are doing ethnography. This is a distortion of the mandates for both the target group as well as participant observation. Any research report labeled an ethnography that is based solely upon a researcher-created group demonstrates an ignorance of ethnography. Focus groups are not a naturally occurring group and no longer exist after the research has been completed. A focus group may be used in conjunction with other methods of data collection but cannot stand alone as the basis for ethnography.

A study using only an interview protocol, with or without pre-set questions, does not yield ethnography. The publication of Spradley's book *Ethnographic Interviewing* (1979) created the idea that his interview technique yielded ethnography. These nurses did not read Spradley's (1980) companion volume on *Participant Observation*. Spradley's interviewing technique, when used as the only method of data collection yields Ethnoscience or Ethnographic Semantics (Kay, 1974; Kay & Evaneshko, 1982).

Interviewing, without participant observation, can lead to misunderstanding. For example, new nurses to the Canadian North are often overheard repeating the same question of an Inuit patient. What the nurses are missing is that the Inuit is in fact responding to the question by squeezing their eyes, a common non-verbal communication. The nurse misses the cues and believes the patient is not responding (Nancy Edgecombe, pers. comm.).

Traditional Ethnography looks for knowledge about a group as it currently exists. When a change is deliberately introduced, as in a field experiment, the group no longer exists as the ethnographer found it. (There are those who say that the introduction of the ethnographer into the setting will cause a change. There is always a "before and after" when introducing any change. The presence of the researcher is an inadvertent change over which the researcher has no control. In fact, the researcher has no way of knowing what the group was like before entering the group so cannot study any before-and-after scenarios.)

Some nurses equate Applied Anthropology with Traditional Ethnography. Traditional Ethnography seeks knowledge for its own sake. Applied disciplines seek knowledge for immediate applicability or for future use. Applied anthropology is the blend of the desire to know with the desire to see what will happen if something is changed. It is a field experiment that is expected to occur only after there is a knowledge base of the culture group. Changing something in an existing group, without knowledge of what might result from that change, has been deemed unethical. The ethnography *Dancing Skeletons* (Detwyler, 1993) is an example of a medical intervention in an African village with good intentions but little understanding of the group. Inoculations were introduced for infants and children under 5. The ethnographer found that the increased population, due to the surviving infants and children, had caused a severe food crisis. The children were starving to death. No plans had been made to help the villagers increase their food supply to accommodate the population increase.

Ethnography (the term is used both for the field method as well as the subsequent publication), describing context, is best served in book form such as Germain's (1979) *The Cancer Ward*, Gazaway's (1974) *The Longest Mile*, Dougherty's (1978) story of rural Black women, or Kayser-Jones's (1981) comparison of nursing care in two nursing homes—one in Scotland and the other in San Francisco. Glittenberg, in her 1984 book (reissued by Waveland Press in 2004), described her years of research in Guatemala on the same population, beginning with her doctoral research.

Nursing literature using Traditional Ethnography in the past 20 years

Over 7000 articles and books, in English, have been labeled "Ethnography" in the past 20 years. Not all were written by nurses. Finding traditional ethnographies written by nurses from within this plethora of publications meant limiting the search. Reports using descriptors such as Focused Ethnography, Critical Ethnography, Meta-Ethnography, Mini-Ethnography, Institutional Ethnography or Ethnonursing were excluded. Any publication that was primarily an applied or an action anthropology approach was also excluded. These methods are discussed elsewhere. Studies that stated they only used one method of data collection, such as interviewing or focus groups, offered no evidence of participant observation or based the research on some form of researcher-created sample rather than a naturally occurring group, were excluded. Publications that included grounded theory or phenomenology were also excluded.

The concern in this chapter is with nursing research reports labeled "ethnography" which met the criteria for a Traditional Ethnography. Despite all the delimiters, there were innumerable articles on ethnography by nurses. The futility of mentioning them all is apparent.

Some articles discussed ethnography as a field method (Yang & Fox, 1999; Oliffe, 2005; Roberts, 2009; Thomson, 2011). These articles cover the same general material as covered in the Robertson and Boyle (1984) article. Other methods articles described the experience of the author in collecting data (Simmons, 2007), insider–outsider relationships during field work (Allen, 2004), emotions and feelings of the ethnographer during field work (Pellatt, 2003), the hospital ward as a valid field setting for ethnography (Long, Hunter, & van der Geest, 2008) or working with translators and interpreters (Baird, 2011).

Traditional Ethnography is a valuable field method for discovering what nurses actually do. Nursing has always claimed that "care" was their special province as opposed to "cure." Although nurses participate with physicians in the curative aspects of health care (some of whom spend most of their time in curative work), nursing insists that care is its special province. Care is elusive. If care is, in fact, what nurses do, then the discovery of what constitutes care will come about only through the observation of nurses' behavior in a variety of groups and settings.

Ethnography is the best way to describe patient populations as they are, whether in the community or in health care settings. Nursing interactions within these settings inform us of nurses' work. The holistic nature of ethnography brings people alive and tells their stories in a way not possible with other research methods. People are not a composite of cultural traits and do not always conform to expectations on how they will behave in certain circumstances. Clues to the inexplicable behavior of both nurses and patients come from ethnography.

Some ethnographies were set in hospital wards or clinics. Lauzon (2008) described how nurses assessed pain on two different nursing hospital units concluding that it was the ward setting itself that set the criteria for the particular pain assessment practice. Sheridan (2010) described routine nursing practice on a labor ward while Deitrick, Bokovoy, and Panik (2010) compared the differences in nurses' responses to call bells depending upon whether the patient was in a private room or a ward. Other settings included the operating room (Graff, Roberts, & Thornton, 1999), an adolescent ward (Hutton, 2008), a medical assessment unit (Griffiths, 2011), an intensive care unit (Bastos, 2001; Coombs & Ersser, 2004) and an HIV hotel (Carr, 1996). All these studies described nursing that occurred within particular settings.

Topics emerging from ethnographies included nursing rituals (Holland, 1993), nurses' decision-making processes (Hancock & Easen, 2006) or nurses working within a union in a rural psychiatric facility (Breda, 1997). Others included a description of a culture-bound syndrome (Juntunen, 2005), humor and laughter (Dean & Gregory, 2004), time as perceived by the patients on a nursing ward (Golander, 1995), and comfort concerns of older persons (Tutton & Seers, 2004). Bray (1999) spoke to the discomfort of nurses between what they wanted to do with their feeling that what they wanted to do was not right. Waters (2008) studied children living with renal illness on a hospital renal unit. Compliance with treatment was a major issue with this population.

Papers with international settings included a community mental health program in Northern India (Jain & Jadhav, 2009), rural maternity care in Swaziland (Thwala, Jones, & Holroyd, 2011), a nursing home in Iceland (Emilsdóttir & Gústafsdóttir, 2011), and a Taiwanese nursing home (Chuang & Abbey, 2009). A rather unique paper by Cashin, Newman, Eason, Thorpe, and O'Discoll (2010) described forensic nursing culture in a prison hospital ward in Australia.

Nurses reported continuing restrictions on nurses' professional role behavior. Coombs and Ersser (2004) found nurses' decision-making in intensive care was disregarded and undervalued. Nursing within the health care system of Sri Lanka continues to be curtailed by the system in which it operates (De Silva & Rolls, 2010). The discouragement of community health nurses working in two Northern Ireland communities was directly attributable to the health care policies within which they worked (Mason, Orr, Harrison, & Moore, 1999).

Ethnography remains the best way to discover the dimensions of nursing care in every setting where nurses practice. Whether nurses practice in prisons or hospitals, community health centers or private homes, there is distinctiveness about what nurses do for and with people that can be observed and documented. From these observations can be built nursing theory that explains and describes just what nursing care involves.

As with any science, nursing science is built bit by bit, based upon individual studies that add to our knowledge base of nursing and the people nurses encounter. Ethnography as a research approach can and should yield the kind of data useful for building a science of nursing care. The studies cited above, and others like them, help to tease out just what is similar and what is different about nursing care in different countries and different settings. What is that elusive thing we call *care*? Is it consistent across cultures? Is it culture bound? Is it restricted or enhanced by the environment in which it occurs? To what extent is it politically driven? Ethnography should add to the knowledge base of nursing, as it exists, in order to answer these questions.

Future directions of Traditional Ethnography in nursing

Judging from the publications in nursing journals over the past 20 years, Traditional Ethnography is fading from the American nursing research literature but will continue to be published in the clinical nursing literature and in the nursing research literature published in other countries. Perhaps it is the difference in these cultures.

American nurses tend to do research projects that are more theoretically driven, more time-limited, or lend themselves to a series of short articles on the same project. Funding agencies in the US tend to support problem-oriented, hypothesis-driven projects over qualitative projects. Junior faculty at American universities find the expectation to write grants and publish extensively, as the road to promotion and tenure, limits their choices. Ethnography beyond their doctoral research does not meet their professional needs.

Another explanation for the paucity of ethnography reported in American nursing research journals involves the requirements for the submission of research papers. American nursing research journals limit manuscript length. American nursing research journals also require a standard format for reporting research which includes a theoretical or conceptual framework, the purpose of the study or hypothesis being tested, detailed description of methods of data collection and analysis, issues of reliability and validity, ethical review procedures, results and conclusions. Because ethnography is a description of a group and its behavior, it is almost impossible to do justice to an ethnographic description in three or four manuscript pages.

Although American nurses are still receiving their doctoral degrees in anthropology, few seem to have embraced Traditional Ethnography for their research programs. Whether this is due to a lessening of interest by American anthropology for Traditional Ethnography; whether applied anthropology or action anthropology projects are more familiar and comfortable for nurse-anthropologists; or, whether American nurses do not find ethnography a way to answer their research questions, is difficult to say.

British nursing journals appear to allow for more flexibility in reporting the results of research. The *Journal of Advanced Nursing* has published a number of ethnographies based upon ward or clinic culture as well as papers set in other countries. British midwifery journals also report ethnographies. Perhaps it is the flexibility of reporting requirements, or nurses in other countries find ethnography a useful way to answer their research questions or are more concerned with the context in which nursing care is delivered. For whatever reason, Traditional Ethnography appears to be thriving outside of the United States.

References

Aamodt, A. M. (1972). The child's view of health and healing. *Communicating Nursing Research, WCHEN,* 5, 38–54.

Aamodt, A. M. (1982). Examining ethnography for nurse researchers. *Western Journal of Nursing Research,* 4(2), 209–221.

Aamodt, A. M., Taylor, J., Kayser-Jones, J. S., Kay, M., Evaneshko, V., Byerly, E. L., & Van Arsdale, P. (1979). Ethnography and nursing research. *Communicating Nursing Research, 12,* 77–85.

Agar, M. (1980). *The professional stranger: An informal introduction to ethnography.* San Diego: Academic Press.

Allbutt, H., & Masters, H. (2010). Ethnography and the ethics of undertaking research in different mental healthcare settings. *Journal of Psychiatric and Mental Health Nursing, 17*(3), 210–215.

Allen, D. (2004). Ethnomethodological insights into insider–outsider relationships in nursing ethnographies of healthcare settings. *Nursing Inquiry, 11*(1), 14–24.

Baird, M. B. (2011). Lessons learned from translators and interpreters from the Dinka tribe of Southern Sudan. *Journal of Transcultural Nursing, 22*(2), 116–121.

Bastos, M. A. (2001). Ethnography: Methodologic strategy used to conceptualize the cultural scenario in an intensive care center at a university hospital [Etnografia: estratégia metodológica utilizada para contextualizar o cenário cultural do CTI de um hospital universitário]. *Revista da Escola de Enfermagem da U S P, 35*(2), 163–171.

Bauwens, E. E. (Ed.) (1978). *The anthropology of health.* St. Louis, MO: The C. V. Mosby Co.

Bowen, E. S. (1961). *Return to laughter.* New York: Doubleday and Co., Inc.

Bray, J. (1999). An ethnographic study of psychiatric nursing. *Journal of Psychiatric and Mental Health Nursing, 6*(4), 297–305.

Breda, K. L. (1997). Professional nurses in unions: Working together pays off. *Journal of Professional Nursing, 13*(2), 99–109.

Brink, P. J. (1969). The Pyramid Lake Paiute of Nevada. Unpublished doctoral dissertation, Boston University, Boston.

Brink, P. J. (1976). *Transcultural nursing: A book of readings.* Englewood Cliffs, NJ: Prentice-Hall, Inc.

Brink, P. J. (1991).Issues of reliability and validity. In J. Morse (Ed.), *Qualitative nursing research: A contemporary dialogue* (pp. 163–186). Newbury Park, CA: Sage.

Byerly, E. L. (1969). Nurse researcher as participant-observer in a nursing setting. *Nursing Research, 18*(3), 230–236.

Byerly, E. L., & Brink, P. J. (1979). Model course V: Cultural variation in nursing practice: A course for upper division undergrad. students in nursing. In H. F. Todd, Jr. & J. L. Ruffini (Eds.), *Teaching medical anthropology: Model courses for graduate and undergraduate instruction* (pp. 55–66). Society for Medical Anthropology Special Publication, No. 1.

Cahill, I. D. (1967). Child rearing practices in the culture of poverty. *NLN Convention Papers. 1,* 1–4.

Carr, G. (1996). Ethnography of an HIV hotel. *Journal of the Association of Nurses in AIDS Care, 7*(2), 35–42.

Cashin, A., Newman, C., Eason, M., Thorpe, A., & O'Discoll, C. (2010). An ethnographic study of forensic nursing culture in an Australian prison hospital. *Journal of Psychiatric and Mental Health Nursing, 17*(1), 39–45.

Chuang, Y.-H., & Abbey, J. (2009). The culture of a Taiwanese nursing home. *Journal of Clinical Nursing, 18*(11), 1640–1648.

Committee of the Royal Anthropological Institute of Great Britain and Ireland. (1967). *Notes and Queries on Anthropology*. London: Routledge & Kegan Paul.

Coombs, M., & Ersser, S. J. (2004). Medical hegemony in decision-making: A barrier to interdisciplinary working in intensive care? *Journal of Advanced Nursing, 46*(3), 245–252.

Dean, R. A., & Gregory, D. M. (2004). Humor and laughter in palliative care: An ethnographic investigation. *Palliative & Supportive Care, 2*(2), 139–148.

Deitrick, L., Bokovoy, J., & Panik, A. (2010). The "dance" continues . . . evaluating differences in call bell use between patients in private rooms and patients in double rooms using ethnography. *Journal of Nursing Care Quality, 25*(4), 279–287.

De Silva, B. S. S., & Rolls, C. (2010). Health-care system and nursing in Sri Lanka: An ethnography study. *Nursing and Health Sciences, 12*(1), 33–38.

Detwyler, K. A. (1993). *Dancing skeletons: Life and death in West Africa*. Long Grove, IL: Waveland Press, Inc.

Dougherty, M. (1978). *Becoming a woman in rural Black culture*. New York: Holt, Rinehart & Winston.

Emilsdóttir, A. L., & Gústafsdóttir, M. (2011). End of life in an Icelandic nursing home: An ethnographic study. *International Journal of Palliative Nursing, 17*(8), 405–411.

Ford, V. (1973). Cultural criteria and determinants for acceptance of modern medicine among the Teton Dakota, Rosebud Indian Reservation, South Dakota. *Communicating Nursing Research, 6*, 41–62.

Gale, C. (1973). Walking in the aide's shoes. *American Journal of Nursing, 73*(4), 628–631.

Gazaway, R. (1974). *The longest mile: A vivid chronicle of life in an Appalachian Hollow*. New York: Penguin.

Germain, C. (1979). *The cancer unit: An ethnography*. Wakefield, MA: Nursing Resources Inc.

Germain, C. (1986). Ethnography: The method. In P. Munhall & C. Oiler (Eds.), *Nursing research: A qualitative perspective*. Norwalk, CT: Appleton-Century-Crofts.

Glittenberg, J. (2004). *To the mountain and back: The mysteries of Guatemalan Highland family life*. Long Grove, IL: Waveland Press, Inc.

Golander, H. (1995). Rituals of temporality: The social construction of time in a nursing ward. *Journal of Aging Studies, 9*(2), 119–135.

Gortner, S. R. (1991). Historical development of doctoral programs: Shaping our expectations. *Journal of Professional Nursing, 7*(1), 45–53.

Graff, C., Roberts, K., & Thornton, K. (1999). An ethnographic study of differentiated practice in an operating room. *Journal of Professional Nursing, 15*(6), 364–371.

Griffiths, P. (2008). Ethical conduct and the nurse ethnographer: Consideration of an ethic of care. *Journal of Research in Nursing, 13*(4), 350–361

Griffiths, P. (2011). A community of practice: The nurses' role on a medical assessment unit. *Journal of Clinical Nursing, 20*(1–2), 247–254.

Hancock, H. C., & Easen, P. R. (2006). The decision-making processes of nurses when extubating patients following cardiac surgery: An ethnographic study. *International Journal of Nursing Studies, 43*(6), 693–705.

Holland, C. K. (1993). An ethnographic study of nursing culture as an exploration for determining the existence of a system of ritual. *Journal of Advanced Nursing, 18*(9), 1461–1470.

Hutton, A. (2008). An adolescent ward; "In name only?" *Journal of Clinical Nursing, 17*(23), 3142–3149.

Jain, S., & Jadhav, S. (2009). Pills that swallow policy: Clinical ethnography of a community mental health program in Northern India. *Transcultural Psychiatry, 46*(1), 60–85.

Juntunen, A. (2005). Baridi: A culture-bound syndrome among the Bena peoples in Tanzania. *Journal of Transcultural Nursing, 16*(1), 15–22.

Kay, M. (1974). Using ethnographic semantics in nursing research. In L. Notter (Ed.), *Proceedings of the Ninth ANA Nursing Research Conference*.

Kay, M. A., & Evaneshko, V. (1982). The ethnoscience research technique. *Western Journal of Nursing Research, 21*, 485–490.

Kayser-Jones, J. S. (1981). *Old, alone and neglected: Care of the aged in Scotland and the United States*. Berkeley: University of California Press.

Lauzon, C. L. M. (2008). An ethnography of pain assessment and the role of social context on two postoperative units. *Journal of Advanced Nursing, 61*(5), 531–539.

Leininger, M. (1967). Nursing care of a patient from another culture. *Nursing Clinics of North America, 2*, 747–762.

Leininger, M. (1971). *Nursing and anthropology: Two worlds to blend.* Hoboken, NJ: John Wiley & Sons, Inc.

Long, D., Hunter, C., & van der Geest, S. (2008). When the field is a ward or a clinic: Hospital ethnography. *Anthropology & Medicine, 15*(2), 71–78.

MacGregor, F. C. (1967). Uncooperative patients: Some cultural implications. *American Journal of Nursing, 67*, 88–89.

Malinowski, B. (1922). *Argonauts of the Western Pacific: An account of native enterprise and adventure in the Archipelagoes of Melanesian New Guinea.* London: George Routledge and Sons.

Malinowski, B. (1967). *A diary in the strict sense of the term.* New York: Harcourt, Brace and World.

Mason, C., Orr, J., Harrisson, S., & Moore, R. (1999). Health professionals' perspectives on service delivery in two Northern Ireland communities. *Journal of Advanced Nursing, 30*(4), 827–834.

Oberg, K. (1954). *Culture shock.* Indianapolis: Bobbs-Merrill Co., Inc.

Oliffe, J. (2005). Why not ethnography? *Urologic Nursing, 25*(5), 395–399.

Omery, A., & Sarter, B; (1988). Ethnography. In *Paths to knowledge: Innovative research methods for nursing* (pp. 17–31). New York: National League for Nursing.

Osborne, O. H. (1968). The Egbado of Egbaland. Unpublished doctoral dissertation, University of Washington, Seattle, WA.

Pearsall, M. (1965). Participant observation as role and method in behavioral research. *Nursing Research, 14*, 37.

Pellatt, G. (2003). Ethnography and reflexivity: Emotions and feelings in fieldwork. *Nurse Researcher, 10*(3), 28.

Pelto, P. J. (1970). *Anthropological research: The structure of inquiry.* New York: Harper and Row.

Ragucci, A. T. (1972). The ethnographic approach and nursing research. *Nursing Research, 21*(6), 485–490.

Reid, M. B. (1969). Persistence and change in the health concepts and practices of the Sukuma of Tanzania, East Africa. Unpublished doctoral dissertation, Catholic University of America, Washington, DC.

Roberts, T. (2009). Understanding ethnography. *British Journal of Midwifery, 17*(5), 291–294.

Robertson, M. H. B., & Boyle, J. S. (1984). Ethnography: Contributions to nursing research. *Journal of Advanced Nursing, 9*, 43–49.

Roper, J. M., & Shapira, J. (1999). *Ethnography in nursing practice.* London: Sage.

Schatzman, L., & Strauss, A. L. (1973). *Field research: Strategies for a natural sociology.* Englewood Cliffs, NJ: Prentice-Hall.

Schwartz, M., & Schwartz, C. (1955). Problems in participant-observation. *American Journal of Sociology, 60*, 343–353.

Sheridan, V. (2010). Organisational culture and routine midwifery practice on labour ward: Implications for mother–baby contact. *Evidence Based Midwifery, 8*(3), 76–84.

Simmons, M. (2007). Insider ethnography: Tinker, tailor, researcher or spy? *Nurse Research, 14*, 4–7.

Spradley, J. (1979). *The ethnographic interview.* New York: Holt, Rinehart & Winston.

Spradley, J. (1980). *Participant observation.* New York: Holt, Rinehart & Winston.

Spradley, J., & McCurdy, D. W. (1972). *The culture of experience: Ethnography in complex society.* Chicago: Science Research Associates.

Thomson, D. (2011). Ethnography: A suitable approach for providing an inside perspective on the everyday lives of health professionals. *International Journal of Therapy and Rehabilitation, 18*, 1.

Thwala, S., Jones, L., & Holroyd, E. (2011). Swaziland rural maternal care: Ethnography of the interface of custom and biomedicine. *International Journal of Nursing Practice, 17*(1), 93–101.

Tutton, E., & Seers, K. (2004). Comfort on a ward for older people. *Journal of Advanced Nursing, 46*(4), 380–389.

Van Gennep, A., Vizedon, M., & Caffee, G. L. (1961). *Rites of passage.* Chicago: University of Chicago Press.

Waters, A. L. (2008). An ethnography of a children's renal unit: Experiences of children and young people with long-term renal illness. *Journal of Clinical Nursing, 17*, 3103–3114.

Wax, R. (1986). *Doing fieldwork: Warnings and advice.* Chicago: University of Chicago Press.

Whiting, B. B. (1963). *Six cultures: Studies of child rearing.* New York: John Wiley and Sons.

Whiting, J. W. M, Child, I. L., & Lambert, W. W. (1966). *Field guide for the study of socialization.* New York: John Wiley and Sons.

Yang, L., & Fox, K. (1999). Ethnography in health research and practice. *Ambulatory Child Health, 5*(4), 339.

16

Ethnonursing method of Dr. Madeleine Leininger

Marilyn A. Ray, Edith Morris, and Marilyn McFarland

Historical introduction

The ethnonursing method was developed by the renowned nursing scholar, Dr. Madeleine Leininger. Ethnonursing was the first open inquiry discovery method designed for nurse researchers to study and advance nursing phenomena from a human science philosophical perspective and through the qualitative analytical lens of culture and care (Leininger, 1978, 1985, 1990, 1991, 1995, 1997, 2002, 2006a, 2006b, 2006c; Leininger & McFarland, 2002, 2006). The method was presented in the *Culture Care Diversity and Universality: A Worldwide Theory of Nursing* (Culture Care Theory) (CCT) (Leininger & McFarland, 2006) to study the nursing dimensions of culture care that include care phenomena, research enablers, and the social structural factors (e.g., kinship and social; cultural values, beliefs, and lifeways; religious and philosophical; economic; educational; political/legal systems; technological; and environmental context, language, and ethnohistory), and three modes of care action and decision (Leininger & McFarland, 2002, p. 78). As a human care scientist and educator, the first nurse-anthropologist, and qualitative nursing ethnographer, Leininger created new insights into the nature of culture, care, and transcultural nursing by presenting ways to describe, interpret, discover, and understand the diverse meanings and patterns of health and illness, care and healing, survival, and ways of facing and understanding death or disability by diverse cultural groups. Leininger created this new ethnonursing method through her innovative spirit, and her vast knowledge of human beings and nursing, human care, cultural theories, ethnography, ethnoscience, and other field research methods that are used primarily in the discipline of anthropology. What is distinct about Leininger's ethnonursing method is the emphasis on the patterns of phenomena of interest to nursing, including care, health, culture, and environmental context. She initiated a systematic way to generate knowledge (patterns and themes) of culture care by studying the lifeways and cultural patterns of human beings and care phenomena within their environmental context including the nurse–patient or researcher–informant care relationship. The method provides a way to discover how specifically Leininger's transcultural theory of Culture Care Diversity and Universality (CCT) with its culture care modes could be applied and analyzed in research with the goal of providing culturally congruent care to people of similar and diverse cultures (Leininger, 1990, 1991, 2002, 2006a, 2006b, 2006c; Leininger & McFarland, 2002, 2006). Moreover, the ethnonursing method facilitated opportunities for the discovery of new transcultural nursing methods such as the meta-ethnonursing method of McFarland, Wehbe-Alamah, Wilson, and Vossos (2011).

The aim of this chapter is to present the philosophical and human science foundations of Leininger's ethnonursing method, the blending of nursing and anthropology, and the progression of the discipline of transcultural nursing and Leininger's theory with an evolutionary development of the state of the science of nursing. Leininger's transcultural nursing views, the CCT, and the ethnonursing method will be outlined and highlighted in terms of complexity science, complex caring dynamics, and translational science. Finally, a discussion will ensue regarding future directions highlighting research studies that incorporate Leininger's ethnonursing method, and the new meta-ethnonursing research method (McFarland et al., 2011), which facilitate overall advancement and translation of Leininger's and other transcultural nurses' conceptual ideas and theories for further understanding of evidence, and implementation of transcultural care decision-making in clinical practice for culturally congruent care (McFarland et al., 2011; Polit & Beck, 2011).

Philosophical and theoretical foundations of Leininger's ethnonursing method

Human science paradigm

A human science paradigm focuses on the study of human beings and human phenomena. This scientific view was advanced primarily in the twentieth century although one of the approaches, hermeneutics or interpretation, is an ancient form of exegesis. As a contrast to the natural sciences which focus on the objects of nature, things, or natural events (van Manen, 1997), human science focuses on human experience. The field of the human sciences includes symbolic interactionism, phenomenology, phenomenological sociology/anthropology, ethnography, ethnomethodology, critical theory, gender studies, semiotics, caring inquiry, grounded theory method, and others. These consist of approaches to research and theorizing which have their roots in European philosophy, sociological and anthropological perspectives, and caring science (Davidson, Ray, & Turkel, 2011; Polit & Beck, 2011; Ray, 1985, 1991, 1994, 2010a, 2010b, 2011, 2013; Strauss & Corbin, 2007; Ray & Turkel, 2012; van Manen, 1997). In nursing, human science is guided by views of human care and caring—nurses want and need to know what is most essential to their profession and to patients, families, and communities (Leininger, 1970; 1978; 1981, 1984, 1985, 1977; Ray, 1981a, 1981b, 1991, 2010a, 2010b, 2011; Davidson et al., 2011). Human science captures lived experiences through interviewing and observation (including digital formats), and by means of language and textual accounts to articulate a description of the subject matter of mind, thoughts, consciousness, values, beliefs, attitudes, feelings, emotions, actions, and purposes. Human science attempts to understand through interpretation the lived structures of the meanings of cultural experience and cultural institutions (van Manen, 1997). Human science thus involves description, interpretation, self-reflection, critical analysis or pattern/thematic analysis, and in some instances theory development.

Nursing and anthropology: dynamic disciplines that changed nursing practice

Over 50 years ago, Leininger (1970) stated that understanding the interrelationship between culture and care was the most crucial challenge of nursing. As a science and art, nursing is the primary discipline that focuses on care and caring, healing, health and illness, and well-being in the human–environment relationship (Leininger, 1970, 1978, 1981, 1984; Leininger & McFarland, 2006; Ray, 2010a, 2010b; Ray & Turkel, 2010; Davidson et al., 2011). Anthropology is the study of "culture [as] the blueprint for man's [human's] way of living, and only by understanding culture can we hope to gain the fullest understanding of man [human] as a social and cultural being" (Leininger, 1970, p. vii). By blending the disciplines of nursing and anthropology and research into a reciprocal relationship, Leininger changed the face of nursing education, administration, research, and practice. Leininger (1970) stated that there was a need to blend the two worlds of *culture* and *human care* to form new pathways in thought and research. Just as caring is the "most unifying, dominant, and intellectual and practice focus of nursing" (Leininger, 1981, p. 13), the theorist added that culture care is the broadest, most holistic means to know, explain, interpret, and predict nursing care phenomena to guide nursing care practices. Nursing's central commitment is authentic caring presence—being there to interpret, discover, and seek understanding of the values, cultural lifeways, and well-being of self and others within situations, events, or contexts (Leininger, 1978, 1981, 2002; Leininger & McFarland, 2002, 2006; Ray, 2010a, 2010b; Smith, Turkel, & Wolf, 2013). As such, nursing blends wholly with the discipline of anthropology as a scientific and humanistic field of study of human beings. Anthropology seeks to discover through archaeological or ethnographic means, ways of living from prehistory and history, or the past and present from a longitudinal view. It identifies and records social and cultural change and dynamic emergence within human-historical, bio-physical, psychological, linguistic, and social and cultural environments. Anthropologists' theoretical and ethnographic orientation is grounded in and based upon the assumption that culture is learned and the shared meanings that are co-created among members of a group which, if studied, can be described, interpreted, and understood (Leininger, 1970; Ray, 2010a; Andrews & Boyle, 2011). Human beings have advanced cultural norms and created social forms with many symbols and rituals. Within these social forms, human beings have identified and created social structures, for example, kinship, philosophical, religious, ethical, legal, political, economic, and technological systems including health care systems which allow groups of people to live together. Just as nursing and the concepts of care and caring have many definitions, so too has culture (Leininger, 1970, 1978; Ray, 1981a, 1981b, 1989, 2010a, 2010b). As stated, the most significant is shared systems of meaning that are transmitted from one group to the other (Leininger, 1970, 1978). A new way of looking at culture as the world is increasingly interconnected and global through networks of communication is with a new metaphor of dynamic complexity and emergence (Ray, 2010a): "Cultures survive because of genetic heritage, loyalty to traditions, reciprocal cooperation, and willingness of people to care and make social sacrifices for each other" (Ray, 2010a, p. 94). Cultures overlap and transform because of "the growing desire to *choose* to belong to a world community that is committed to the preservation of humanity and the rich cultures [and traditions] that have evolved through the centuries" (Ray, 2010a, p. 11). The anthropological insights gained from the study of human beings in the most distant places in the world, in the streets of our present-day cities, in organizational cultures (Ray, 1981a, 2010a; Ray & Turkel, 2012) and in contemporary rural areas provide a uniquely diverse yet comparative and transcultural view of human beings (Leininger, 1970, 2002, 2006a, 2006b, 2006c; Leininger & McFarland, 2006).

Blending nursing and anthropology became a passion of Leininger. After observing cultural difference in children and families in the 1950s as a clinical specialist in a pediatric clinic in Cincinnati followed by doctoral study in cultural anthropology and her own scholarly research of folk care practices, ethnohistory, and ecology among the Gadsup Akuna people of the Eastern Highlands of New Guinea in the early 1960s, Leininger (1970, 1978, 1991, 2006a, 2006b, 2006c) developed a heightened interest in blending nursing and anthropology. She created both a theory and a method to study culture care phenomena and predicted that care beliefs and practices impact the health, well-being, or illness decisions of all people. After receiving her PhD, she directed the nurse scientist program at the University of Colorado in the latter half of the 1960s where she introduced students to a new way of looking at nursing, health, and culture. She was familiar with the method used to gather anthropological/cultural data of human beings in diverse contexts. She began to contemplate and integrate concepts in nursing and society and determine how to advance a new method for nursing. Leininger was familiar with the anthropological methods of *ethnography* and *ethnoscience* as well as direct informant-observation in select small-scale societies or natural settings and how they are marked by the classification of emic and etic data. *Emic knowledge* is interpreted from the insider (key) informant point of view. *Etic knowledge* is from the outsider (general) informant point of view, and can also be observational or historical information from the researcher point of view. The synthesis of the emic and etic data provides holistic culturally relevant and comparative knowledge of a culture or cultures. Gathering data directly gave Leininger as a nurse anthropologist insight into many nursing care and cultural systems of meanings or transcultural knowledge (Andrews & Boyle, 2011). The blending of nursing and anthropology provided the pathway to discover and understand many different cultures and illuminate how cultural care, illness, health and healing knowledge emerge. Through awareness of anthropology and ethnographic research, and the evolution of her ideas of care and caring, Leininger (1978) created the substantive and comprehensive discipline called transcultural nursing and is recognized as its founding "mother." Captured at the same time was the creation of her theory of culture care diversity and universality (CCT) and her ethnonursing method.

Transcultural nursing is the dominant formal area of study using ethnonursing which explores and compares and contrasts cultural concepts, theories, social structural characteristics, and research findings and incorporates or translates them into nursing care practices (Leininger, 1978). Leininger's Theory of Culture Care Diversity and Universality (Aronoff, 2010; Leininger, 1991, 2002, 2006a, 2006b, 2006c; Leininger & McFarland, 2002, 2006) is one of the central theories that is used to guide or enhance transcultural nursing research, specifically by means of the ethnonursing method.

Evolution of the state of nursing science

In the process of creating transcultural nursing and the ethnonursing method, the idea of care and caring within and outside of transcultural nursing became increasingly more important in the evolution of the state of nursing science. Leininger (1977, 1981, 1984) identified *care* within transcultural nursing as a central construct. In the late 1960s and 1970s, the state of nursing science revolved around changes in the educational development of professional nursing, the nature of nursing's scientific paradigm, the development of theories of nursing, and the way that nursing phenomena would be studied. In graduate education, consideration was given to the development of actual Doctor of Philosophy programs *within* the discipline of nursing. Leininger had a great impact on this development. In the late 1960s, doctoral degrees were acquired by means of nurse scientist programs grounded in other disciplines, such as psychology, sociology, physiology, and anthropology using diverse quantitative and qualitative methods. As director of the nurse scientist program at the University of Colorado which led to a Doctor of Philosophy (PhD) degree, Leininger saw the need first-hand to develop a *nursing* PhD. Her transcultural nursing doctorate came to fruition in 1977 when she became Dean of the University of Utah College of Nursing. During that period of nursing history, Leininger declared that *caring was the essence of nursing* and highlighted the fact that archaeologists recognized that caring for self and others is one of the oldest forms of human expression. The concept of *care* was established in nursing from the beginning by Florence Nightingale and early nursing theorists; the idea of *caring* ensued thereafter (Davidson et al., 2011; Leininger, 1977, 1978, 1981, 1984, 1978; Smith, Turkel, & Wolf, 2013; Ray, 1981a, 1981b, 2010a, 2010b). The view of caring as a philosophy and science began to take hold and was advanced by Leininger herself (1977, 1981, 1984) and by many others: for example, Watson (1979, 1985, 2008); Gaut (1984); Ray (1981a, 1981b, 1984, 1989, 2010a, 2010b, 2011, 2013); Ray & Turkel (2012); Ray, Turkel, & Cohn (2011); Roach (2002); Swanson (2010). Within the decades of the 1960s and 1970s while founding and creating the discipline of transcultural nursing, Leininger also founded the Council on Nursing and Anthropology, the Transcultural Nursing Society, and the International Association for Human Caring.

The establishment of the International Association for Human Caring and the Transcultural Nursing Society with their annual conferences facilitated the growth and development of care and caring knowledge in its many forms and manifestations. *Caring in the human health experience* became the central maxim for the state of nursing science in 1991 (Newman et al., 1991). Critiques emerged and questions were raised as to whether or not the science of caring and transcultural care should be the legitimate foci for nursing science. The nursing theorist Martha Rogers initially opposed the concept of caring as the theoretical basis of nursing in favor of her conceptual system of unitary human beings which highlighted the complexity and dynamism of the human–environment relationship (Rogers, 1970; Davidson et al., 2011). Later, Rogers addressed and justified caring as the concept of love within her own philosophical position (Watson & Smith, 2002).

"Connectedness, conflict, choice, and transformation are hallmarks of change or continual emergence" (Ray, 2010a, p. 108). Progress in science and nursing science unfolds, not only with research, but also with conflict and opposition. Each generates questions and some answers. Science was changing rapidly during the 1980s and 1990s. The new science was revealing that "science begins [first] with our relationship to nature" (Peat, 2002, p. 208). Complexity sciences with holographic and chaos theories emerged over more than 50 years from the theories of relativity and quantum mechanics. The principle of uncertainty in science (the revelation of the observer being involved in the process of the research or what was observed) by Heisenberg (as cited in Peat, 2002) in the 1920s began to manifest itself more and more within the new sciences of complexity. The scientist Bohr (as cited by Peat, 2002, p. 16) argued that

> The properties we observe are in a certain sense the product of the act of measurement itself. Ask a question one way and Nature has been framed into giving a certain answer. Pose the question in another way and the answer will be different . . . [thus], the answer to a quantum measurement is a form of co-creation between the observer and the observed . . . Until the advent of quantum theory physicists had thought about the universe in terms of models, albeit mathematical ones.
>
> *(p. 22)*

Quantum theory revealed that we all are participants in the universe. Complexity science, more specifically, complexity sciences manifest tenets of interconnectedness, belongingness, consciousness, holism, and dynamism characterized by *relationship* (Peat, 2002; Wheatley, 2006; Ray, 2011). Now, science was beginning to acknowledge the subjective role of the researcher and communication in the conduct of research (Peat, 2002). Human science was flowing into the natural sciences. Scientists were both actors and spectators in discovering answers to questions just as in anthropological or qualitative research. Language thus became important to science. The philosopher Wittgenstein (as cited by Peat, 2002) argued that language itself has meaning and allows us to say things about the world which facilitate knowledge, choice, and ultimately harmony. Hence, the earth is a type of living creature rather than inert matter (O'Murchu, 1997) where moral choice is necessary for health and healing of the planet and people on it. Caring about the universe and the language of love are permeating science and science is responding (Arntz et al., 2005). The current views of science show us a new type of unification—science as a human science within a humanistic, linguistic and environmental framework. This view is not unlike Leininger's position of human science in nursing.

In the state of nursing science revisited, Newman, Smith, Dexheimer-Pharris, and Jones (2008) articulated the meaning of contemporary nursing science. The scholars acknowledged phenomena associated with the new sciences of complexity; the ideas are rooted in Rogerian science and also are similar to Leininger's historical views of transcultural nursing. The critical nature of the *unitary-transformative paradigm* and *relationship* as the central foci of nursing was articulated. This perspective of nursing as relational is characterized as: *Health*: the intent of the relationship; *Caring*: the nature of the relationship; *Consciousness*: the informational pattern of the relationship; *Mutual process*: the way the relationship unfolds; *Patterning*: the evolving configuration of the relationship; *Presence*: the resonance of the relationship; and *Meaning*: the importance of the relationship (Newman et al., 2008). The state of nursing science is consistent with concepts of complexity sciences in terms of notions of emergent, evolving phenomena which are knowledge-in-process as opposed to deterministic, stable, and rigorous information (Peat, 2002). In both science and the state of nursing science *relationship* is acknowledged. And through relationship, "[as] participants in the universe, we seek to belong" (Ray, 2010a, p. 43) by way of our relationships and the choices we make in terms of others. The notion of nursing as a human and cultural science, the moral ideal of respect, protection, and harmony brought to light by Jean Watson, and the idea of relational caring complexity, meaning, and choice-making (Leininger, 1977, 1981; Watson, 1985, 2008; Davidson & Ray, 1991; Leininger & McFarland, 2006; Newman, Smith, Dexheimer-Pharris, & Jones, 2008; Davidson et al., 2011; Ray, 2011) is continually unfolding. While transcultural care was not fully expressed in the state of the nursing science accounts, it is implied within the concept of health experience or relationship outlined by the scholars. In nursing education today, care and culture are considered important constructs. The focus also is on cultural diversity, cultural competency, vulnerable patients, local health care needs, and global millennial goals. Thus, in nursing education, *culture care* or *care* of the vulnerable are regarded as essential components of the discipline and are firmly established in most undergraduate and graduate schools of nursing. As nurses are learning more about cultural competency, they are learning more about how the scientific and humanistic discipline of transcultural nursing emerged and how Leininger's Culture Care Theory should be understood. Translational science, implementation science, and evidence-based practice (Leininger, 2002, 2006a, 2006b; Damschroder et al., 2009; Aronoff, 2010; Polit & Beck, 2011; Morris, 2012) advocated today already showed in Leininger's foresight as she blended nursing and anthropology into transcultural nursing. This discipline facilitates a primary role for nurses to respond to the call of fulfilling the mission of the Transcultural Nursing Society; that is, to provide culturally congruent, competent, and equitable care worldwide. As communicated, Leininger was aware of these ideas from the outset of her scholarship well over 50 years ago. She was a pioneer! Leininger highlighted human science, linguistics, and sociocultural phenomena to secure knowledge of what it means to be human, caring, and culturally aware. She understood patterns of relationship and caring; she identified the fact that nurses must be aware of themselves as cultural beings as they relate to patients and families as cultural beings to facilitate moral choices related to health, healing and well-being, and a peaceful death. Moreover, she understood the meaning of societies as both micro and macro cultures, in essence complex systems (Leininger, 1970; Ray, 1981a, 2010a, 2010b, 2011). She also knew the meaning of future nursing needs—

the call to be local and global, to be culturally relevant, congruent, and competent, and by recognizing the political processes of organizations and nations her work reflected the notion of protection for all people, and thus, protection of the human rights of all people.

Through transcultural nursing and the ethnonursing research method, scholars are grasping the meaning of a complex world governed by perceptions of globalization and transnationalism rather than purely assimilation or acculturation (Leininger & McFarland, 2006; Ray, 2010a). Leininger's historical ideas of culture care diversity and universality and ethnonursing method are validated at every turn (Davidson et al., 2011; Ray, 2010a, 2010b). Leininger's CCT and ethnonursing method lead the way in understanding more fully the view of evidence-based practice, that is, by translating research into practice—implementing culturally congruent care for patients, families, and professionals by means of knowledge and understanding of culture care expressions, beliefs, decisions, and actions in practice in complex health care organizations. Moreover, her ethnonursing method has led the way to the development of a meta-ethnonursing method (McFarland et al., 2011).

Ethnonursing and meta-ethnonursing research methods

As communicated, the goal of qualitative research and particularly, ethnographic research is to document and interpret as fully as possible the totality of a domain of inquiry (DOI) and its particular context from the emic (insider) and etic (outsider) cultural viewpoints of a people (Leininger, 1985, 1991, 2006a, 2006b). Ethnography and other qualitative methods are used to discover in-depth, full, and accurate truths about a phenomenon of interest (domain of inquiry). The ethnonursing method as a specific qualitative ethnographic method assists the researcher in eliciting in-depth *culture care* knowledge from informants (the term *participant* can be used with the theory or method) about a particular domain of nursing inquiry (Leininger 1991, 2002, 2006a; Leininger & McFarland, 2006).

Overview of the ethnonursing nursing research method

Ethnonursing as a comprehensive method allows for epistemic, ontologic, and historical discoveries about transcultural care phenomena (Leininger, 1991, 2002, 2006a, 2006b, 2006c; Leininger & McFarland, 2002, 2006). Leininger developed the ethnonursing research method as a means to study and analyze local or indigenous people's viewpoints and practices about nursing care phenomena and processes relative to designated cultures (Leininger, 1985, 1991, 2002a, 2002b, 2006a, 2006b, 2006c). The ethnonursing research method is a means of discovering, knowing, and confirming people's knowledge about care, ways they keep well, or how they view care when they become ill or disabled. As identified, the method was tailor-made to fit with the theory of Culture Care Diversity and Universality in order to obtain meaningful emic data about the phenomenon or particular domain of inquiry from key informants and to advance transcultural nursing knowledge through the discovery of embedded, covert, and largely unknown culture care knowledge (Leininger, 2002; Leininger & McFarland, 2002, 2006). In addition, attention is given to the etic perspective so as to provide a holistic view of the culture and people and to confirm the emic data from the outsider's points of view. The goal is to achieve a broad gestalt on people's worldview or cultural perspective on care, lifeways, and health (Leininger, 1991, 2002, 2006a, 2006b, 2006c; Leininger & McFarland, 2002, 2006; McFarland et al., 2012).

The process of the ethnonursing research method

The ethnonursing research method is a respectful process in that it honors its informants as knowers of care knowledge who have invited the researcher in as a guest to learn about the daily and nightly lifeways of the culture. It reminds the researcher of how to behave as a privileged and invited guest in another's culture. Once the domain of inquiry has been conceptualized within the Culture Care Theory, the ethnonursing method readies the researcher for entry into the culture whereby acceptance by the people can be gained; a critical first step in learning the "truth" about the domain as well as obtaining credible data. The researcher openly discusses the goal and aims of the study with the people and becomes more immersed (accepted) by the people as a trustworthy "friend."

Once the researcher has taken the time to become a "trusted friend" of the people, informant selection can begin based on the inclusion criteria established by the researcher and in congruence with the ethnonursing method and the domain of inquiry. Informed consent may be sought at this time, although with the ethnonursing method, this is an ongoing process. The ethnonursing researcher willingly and openly continues to discuss the purpose and aims of the study and nondefensively answers any questions that the people raise. At the same time the researcher makes it clear to the people that he or she is a learner about their care and cultural lifeways. As immersion continues to deepen, the indigenous customs, beliefs, and care practices become genuinely valued by the researcher. Authenticity is achieved through mutual respect between the researcher and the people. Respect is maintained throughout and beyond the study. At this level in the relationship between the researcher and the informants, a systematic process of data collection and confirmation begins. Data bearing on the domain of inquiry and the Culture Care Theory are collated and analyzed beginning with the first encounter. The researcher begins to notice that certain words are used frequently by the informants (key words). Over time and with more informants, these key words begin to form patterns that describe the domain of inquiry. The final step is the formation of major universal and diverse care themes that emerge from the patterns.

Appreciation and reverence are offered to the cultural community and to the informants for their sharing in the research study. As data are saturated or when no new data are emerging, the researcher makes plans for exiting the community as a researcher. As with any period of time in a community, one develops friendships. In essence, the relationship with the informants may continue even though the research has ended. Both the researcher and the informant need to be clear that the relationship, should it continue, is not within the realm of researcher to informant, but rather friend to friend. This phenomenon has occurred in several of the ethnonursing studies including with Leininger herself, who returned to visit the Gadsup Akuna of Papua, New Guinea, several times as a friend after her research had been concluded.

Enablers to support the ethnonursing method

Leininger (1991, 2006b) developed *enabler guides* over time to assist in explicating data about specific culture care practices, meanings, and lifeways related to health and well-being related to nursing phenomena. These guides, although transformed over time, were designed to assist the ethnonursing researcher in conducting the study in an organized, systematic, and effective manner. *Six enablers* associated with the method are presented: the Sunrise Enabler; the Stranger to Trusted Friend Enabler; the Observation-Participation-Reflection Enabler; the Domain of Inquiry Enabler; the Acculturation Enabler; and the Data Analysis Enabler. While these regularly used enablers were developed by Leininger, she encourages the researchers to develop enablers specific to their phenomena of interest that will assist them in obtaining useful and credible data. For example, if a researcher wants to study the importance of art or music from a particular culture, he or she may develop an enabler that will assist in explicating care phenomena that may be found in the artistic modes of that particular culture.

The Sunrise Enabler

Leininger (1985) first developed the Sunrise Model/Enabler to depict the various components of the theory of Culture Care Diversity and Universality based upon her knowledge of social structural factors and care dimensions in cultures (Leininger, 1985, 1991). Calling the Sunrise Enabler a model made it seem too much like it was something to be tested and measured from a hypothetical deductive paradigm, rather than a depiction of the theory that may be inductively explicated, thus, the change to Sunrise *Enabler*. The Sunrise Enabler's purpose is to assist the ethnonursing researcher in viewing care phenomena holistically and to discover care meanings and expressions which are embedded in the social structure factors of the culture being studied. These include the kinship and social factors, cultural values, beliefs and lifeways, educational factors, political and legal factors, and so forth (Leininger & McFarland, 2006). Through the lens of the interrelatedness of the social structure factors, the researcher can better understand and ultimately explain the responses of the informants about care, health, and well-being (Leininger, 1991, 2002; Leininger & McFarland, 2002, 2006). The informant dialogue against the backdrop of these contextual factors allows care expressions, patterns, and practices to emerge from the data, thereby revealing the worldview of the informant about health, illness, and death within the culture being studied. The researcher then identifies with the informants the generic or folk care practices within the culture as well as any professional care practices (Leininger, 1991; Leininger & McFarland, 2006). At this point the Sunrise Enabler guides the researcher (or practitioner if used in practice) in making transcultural decisions and actions about how culturally congruent care can be provided through the use of the three modes of care action and decision; the translational, evidence-based practice or research utilization aspect of the method (Polit & Beck, 2011; Morris, 2012). The three modes of care action and decision are preservation and/or maintenance; accommodation and/or negotiation; and repatterning and/or restructuring (Leininger, 1991, 2002; Leininger & McFarland, 2002, 2006).

Preservation and/or maintenance examines which current care practices within the culture (folk remedies) are beneficial to health and can be maintained in comparison to which generic care practices may be harmful to the health of an individual and need to be restructured and/or repatterned into healthier care practices collaboratively with the client (Leininger, 1991, 2002, 2006a, 2006b). Additionally, the researcher or practitioner examines what health care rituals are important to the people but are not optimal and may need to be negotiated and/or accommo-dated so as to promote health and well-being (Leininger 1991). By addressing the culture care modalities, Leininger was able to foresee the need for translational research/science or evidence-based practice well before their rise to prominence today. The culture care modalities provide the means for moving research findings about care directly into practice in order to promote health and well-being among individuals of various cultures worldwide.

Stranger to Trusted Friend Enabler

This enabler assists the ethnonursing researcher from the point of being a distrusted "outsider" to that of being a "trusted friend" to whom truths of the culture may safely be revealed. Prior to using this guide, the researcher should assess his or her own cultural beliefs, values, and behaviors. Continued use of this enabler throughout the research process is recommended so that the researcher may remain sensitive to her or his own behaviors in relation to that of the informant as s/he moves along the continuum of becoming a trusted friend (Leininger & McFarland, 2002, 2006). Indicators that the researcher is in the stranger phase include a sense of distrust on the part of the informants; "testing" by the informants in order to observe the stranger's behavior in relation to certain customs and rituals of the culture; and the avoidance of sharing secrets, stories, and local cultural information (Leininger & McFarland, 2002, 2006). Once the researcher has become a trusted friend of the informants, rich emic data will be shared as it is important to the informants that the culture be understood accurately (Leininger & McFarland, 2002, 2006).

Observation-Participation-Reflection Enabler (O-P-R)

The O-P-R Enabler delineates a plan for the researcher to begin the data collection process and is designed to be used simultaneously with the Stranger to Trusted Friend Enabler. Leininger (1991, 2006b) outlines four phases to the O-P-R Enabler to assist the ethnonursing researcher in moving from largely the observation phase within the culture (beginning of the immersion) to an active participation phase to a reflection of what has occurred while the researcher has been immersed in the culture. *Phase I* includes observing and listening without any active participation, followed by *Phase II* which continues the observing/listening process with some limited participation. In this phase, the ethnonursing researcher may begin asking some questions that are of a comfortable nature to the informants. In *Phase III*, the researcher moves the primary focus to active participation within cultural conversations and rituals, and at this time experiences a complete immersion into the culture. Though in-depth observations continue, observations are confirmed with the people. Reconfirming observations and findings with the key informants completes *Phase IV* or the Reflection portion of the enabler (Leininger, 1991; Leininger & McFarland, 2002, 2006). Though this enabler as well as the Stranger to Trusted Friend Enabler are divided into phases, the phases are fluid in that the researcher moves back and forth between the phases as needed to maintain the respect of the informants, maintain the trusted friendship, and ultimately to be allowed to share in the "secrets" of the culture.

Domain of Inquiry Enabler (DOI)

This enabler is developed by the ethnonursing researcher as a guide to studying the Domain of Inquiry of the proposed study. It is important that this enabler be developed in such a manner so as to examine and analyze in-depth cultural phenomena from the domain of inquiry. In-depth data about the domain become visible in light of the care practices of the culture as well as the beliefs and values that are embedded within the social structure factors of the culture. It is important to remember that this enabler serves as a guide for the researcher to answer questions and discover cultural care beliefs, values, and practices about the domain of inquiry (Leininger, 1991; Leininger & McFarland, 2002, 2006). It is *not* a survey tool to be used verbatim with the informants. Given that beliefs and values about care are embedded in the social structure factors explicated by the CCT and depicted in the Sunrise Enabler, the ethnonursing researcher may want to categorize the questions by kinship and family, religious and philosophical, technological, educational, and/or political and legal factors (McFarland et al., 2012).

Acculturation Health Care Assessment Enabler

This enabler is important to the ethnonursing researcher in terms of the ability to assess how acculturated the informants are into the culture under study. The researcher uses this enabler to assess whether informants are traditionally acculturated or non-traditionally acculturated in relation to the values, beliefs and lifeways of the culture. By using this enabler one can more precisely assess the informant's identity in relation to their culture or the culture under study, and it assists to further exemplify any cultural variability in values, beliefs, and practices (Leininger, 2006b; Leininger & McFarland, 2002).

Four phases of the Data Analysis Enabler

This enabler promotes systematic and rigorous analysis of the data in relation to the Domain of Inquiry. Data are analyzed from the beginning of the data collection phase of the study. During *Phase I*, the raw data are collected, described and documented with the use of a field journal, a digital or tape recorder, or a computer. During *Phase II*, descriptors are identified and categorized. Patterns and context analysis are generated simultaneously during *Phase III*. Finally, *Phase IV* is where major themes, research findings, theoretical formulations, and recommendations are identified and presented (Leininger, 2006b).

Criteria for evaluation of qualitative ethnonursing research

Leininger (1991, 1991, 2006b) developed six criteria for evaluating qualitative ethnonursing research. These criteria are credibility; confirmability; meaning-in-context; recurrent patterning; saturation; and transferability. *Credibility* refers to securing the truth of the findings which derives largely from the emic findings throughout the observation-participation-reflection (O-P-R) phases of the study. *Confirmability* refers to the repeated descriptions from key and general informants and reaffirms the researcher's O-P-R. *Meaning-in-Context* refers to the significance of the findings within the emic environment of the informants. *Recurrent patterning* refers to the repeated experiences and lifeways of informants designating patterns that are repeated over time. *Saturation* refers to taking in all that was known or understood about the phenomena under study and determining that there are no further new discoveries emerging from the data. *Transferability* refers to whether or not the findings from the study would have similar meanings with similar environments, contexts, or circumstances.

Future directions

Advancing scholarship: The meta-ethnonursing method

McFarland, Wehbe-Alamah, Wilson, and Vossos (2011) developed the *meta-ethnonursing research method* after analyzing and synthesizing 23 dissertations (see Table 16.1) conceptualized within the theory of Culture Care Diversity and Universality using the ethnonursing research method. These studies illuminate the variety of research generated historically by the use of the integration of Leininger's CCT and the ethnonursing method.

McFarland et al.'s meta-ethnonursing method is recognized as a groundbreaking study which explores generic and professional care discoveries within completed dissertations with the goal of being able "to synthesize generic and professional culture care meta-themes that promote health, well-being, and beneficial lifeways for people of similar and diverse cultures" (McFarland

Table 16.1 Dissertations analyzed for the meta-ethnonursing study using Leininger's theory

Author	Year	Title of study	University	Publication status
Berry, A.	1995	Culture care statements, meanings, and expressions of Mexican American women within Leininger's culture care theory	Wayne State University, Detroit, MI	(Unpublished doctoral dissertation)
*Ehrmin, J.	1998	Culture care meanings and statements, and experiences of care of African American women residing in an inner city transitional home for substance abuse	Wayne State University, Detroit, MI	(Unpublished doctoral dissertation)
Farrell, L. S.	2001	Culture care: Meanings and expressions of caring and non-caring of the Potawatami who have experienced family violence	Wayne State University, Detroit, MI	(Unpublished doctoral dissertation)
Fox-Hill, E. J.	1999	The experiences of persons with AIDS living-dying in a nursing home	University of Tennessee Health Science Center, Memphis	(Doctoral dissertation)
*Gates, M.	1988	Care and meanings, experiences and orientations of persons dying in hospitals and hospital settings	Wayne State University, Detroit, MI	(Unpublished doctoral dissertation)
*Gelazis, R.	1994	Lithuanian care: Meanings and experiences with humor using Leininger's culture care theory	Wayne State University, Detroit, MI	(Unpublished doctoral dissertation)
*George, T.	1998	Meanings and statements and experiences of care of chronically mentally ill in a day treatment center using Leininger's culture care theory	Wayne State University, Detroit, MI	(Unpublished doctoral dissertation)
Higgins, B.	1995	Puerto Rican cultural beliefs: Influence on infant feeding practices in Western New York	University of Colorado Health Sciences Center, Denver	(Doctoral dissertation) UMI 9604699, retrieved from ProQuest
Johnson, C.	2005	Understanding the culture care practices of rural immigrant Mexican women	Duquesne University, Pittsburgh, PA	(Doctoral dissertation) UMI 3175853, retrieved from ProQuest
Kelsey, B. M.	2005	Culture care values, beliefs, and practices of Mexican American migrant farmworkers related to health promoting behaviors.	Ball State University, Muncie, IN	(Doctoral dissertation) UMI 3166257, retrieved from ProQuest

Table 16.1 Continued

Author	Year	Title of study	University	Publication status
*Lamp, J.	1998	Generic and professional care meanings and practices of Finnish women in birth within Leininger's theory of culture care diversity and universality	Wayne State University, Detroit, MI	(Unpublished doctoral dissertation)
*Luna, L.	1989	Care and cultural context of Lebanese Muslims in an urban US community within Leininger's culture care theory	Wayne State University, Detroit, MI	(Unpublished doctoral dissertation)
*MacNeil, J.	1994	Cultural care: Meanings, patterns, and expressions for Baganda women as AIDS caregivers within Leininger's theory	Wayne State University, Detroit, MI	(Unpublished doctoral dissertation)
*McFarland, M. R.	1995	Cultural care of Anglo and African American elderly residents within the environmental context of a long-term care institution	Wayne State University, Detroit, MI	(Unpublished doctoral dissertation)
*Miller, J. E.	1996	Politics and care: A study of Czech Americans within Leininger's theory of culture care diversity and universality	Wayne State University, Detroit, MI	(Unpublished doctoral dissertation)
*Morgan, M.	1994	African American neonatal care in northern and southern contexts using Leininger's culture care theory	Wayne State University, Detroit, MI	(Unpublished doctoral dissertation)
*Morris, E.	2004	Culture care values, meanings, and experiences of African American adolescent gang members	Wayne State University, Detroit, MI	(Unpublished doctoral dissertation)
Prince, L.	2005	Culture care and resilience in minority women residing in a transitional home recovering from prostitution	Loyola University of Chicago, IL	(Doctoral dissertation) UMI 3174259, retrieved from ProQuest
*Rosenbaum, J.	1990	Cultural care, culture health, and grief phenomena related to older Greek Canadian widows with Leininger's theory of culture care	Wayne State University, Detroit, MI	(Unpublished doctoral dissertation)
Schumacher, G. C.	2006	Culture care meanings, beliefs, and practices of rural Dominicans in a rural village of the Dominican Republic: An ethnonursing study conceptualized within the culture care theory	Duquesne University, Pittsburgh, PA	(Unpublished doctoral dissertation)
Webhe-Alamah, H.	2005	Culture care of Syrian American immigrants living in Midwestern United States	Duquesne University, Pittsburgh, PA	(Unpublished doctoral dissertation)

Table 16.1 Continued

Author	Year	Title of study	University	Publication status
Wekselman, K.	1999	The culture of natural childbirth	University of Cincinnati, OH	(Doctoral dissertation) UMI 9936027, retrieved from ProQuest
*Wenger, A. F.	1988	The phenomenon of care of old order Amish: A high context culture	Wayne State University, Detroit, MI	(Unpublished doctoral dissertation)

Note: * Mentored by Leininger.

et al., 2011, p. 2). Additionally, the meta-ethnonursing method identified ways to facilitate and provide culturally congruent care to people of diverse cultures using Leininger's three care modes of nursing action and decision (1991, 2002; Leininger & McFarland, 2006).

Developing the meta-ethnonursing method

The development of the meta-ethnonursing method began as stated with a review of select ethnonursing research studies which included thoroughly reading and re-reading the studies (McFarland et al., 2011). The data progression continued toward a synthesis with the researchers who advanced this method, confirming one another's coding and analysis. Once each dissertation was coded, analyzed, and confirmability was established, the data were uploaded into the qualitative software data analysis package, NVivo 8. At this point, the researchers looked for recurrent patterning and data saturation among the combined themes from each of the dissertations. From these combined data, the themes and patterns were then synthesized to form meta-patterns and meta-themes leading to meta-care modalities with the goal to provide a higher level of care to individuals of similar and diverse cultures. This higher level of abstraction of themes is important to continue building the dynamic theory of Culture Care Diversity and Universality. Using the CCT as a guide, culture care action and decision *meta-modes* were discovered which were focused on providing culturally congruent nursing care among culture groups (McFarland et al., 2011). Discovering data from these meta-modes supported the translational science/research component of not only Leininger's Culture Care Theory, but also the meta-ethnonursing method. As described, translational research or implementation science is the foundation for research utilization or in modern parlance, *evidence-based practice* (Polit & Beck, 2011). The meta-ethnonursing method contributes directly to the promotion of health and well-being of individuals in similar and diverse cultures at the bedside, in the community, and the global culture-at-large. New findings or theories can emerge from the original and synthesized ethnonursing studies which can make substantive contributions to building culture care knowledge for the discipline of nursing (McFarland et al., 2011). This new meta-ethnonursing method promotes the overall expansion and conceptual development of culture care in general, as well as specifically, the further explication, substantiation and evolution of Leininger's theory of Culture Care Diversity and Universality and the ethnonursing research method (McFarland et al., 2011).

Conclusion

A presentation of Leininger's ethnonursing method illuminates the fact that this unique research method has the potential to build and expand transcultural nursing knowledge and understanding of diverse culture groups in all settings at local and global levels. As a unique method, it offers a research approach that highlights life as a cosmic web of interconnections where participation and cooperation and scholarship are essential. Through use of the culture care theory (CCT) and the ethnonursing method with its three care modes of action and decision, translational science/implementation science/evidence-based practice is co-created. "[T]the quality of culturally congruent, competent, and equitable care, as such, results in improved health and well being for people worldwide" (Transcultural Nursing Society, 2012). Ethnonursing research confirms understanding of the commonalities and diversities of cultures worldwide, and thereby gives rise to opportunities for humanized health care in the global community (Leininger, 1970, 2002, 2006a, 2006b, 2006c; Leininger & McFarland, 2006; Ray, 2010a; McFarland et al., 2011; Morris, 2012). The emergence of the new meta-ethnonursing method demonstrates the forward thinking of Leininger's mentees who participated in the use and evolution of the ethnonursing method by analyzing and synthesizing ethnonursing research that emerged over time (see the 23 dissertations presented in Table 16.1) (McFarland et al., 2011). Years ago, Leininger saw the truth of culturally congruent and competent care through nursing research and knowledge discovery. Although the state of the nursing science account may have left out Leininger's many significant contributions to understanding the nature of the human–environment relationship, her voice lives on through advancing the theory of Culture Care Diversity and Universality and the use of the ethnonursing research method in nursing and health care research (McFarland, Mixer, et al., 2012), illumination of translational science or evidence-based practice applications, the meta-ethnonursing method, and transtheoretical evolution (Ritzer, 1992; McFarland, Webhe-Almah, et al., 2011; Polit & Beck, 2011; Ray, & Turkel, 2012). Thus, the ethnonursing research method will continue to inspire and create knowledge and promote awareness and understanding of transcultural care in a diverse, dynamic, and complex world.

References

Andrews, M., & Boyle, J. (2011). *Transcultural concepts in nursing care* (6th ed.). Philadelphia, PA: Lippincott, Williams & Wilkins.

Arntz, W., Chase, B., & Vicente, M. (2005). *What the bleep do we know!?: Discovering the endless possibilities for altering your everyday reality.* Deerfield Beach, FL: Health Communications Inc.

Aronoff. S. (2010). *Translational research and clinical practice: Basic tools for medical decision making and self-learning.* Oxford: Oxford University Press

Damschroder, L., Aron, D., Keith, R., Kirsh, S., Alexander, J., & Lowery, J. (2009). *Fostering implementation of health services research findings into practice: A consolidated framework for advancing implementation science.* Retrieved from http://www.implementationscience.com/content/4/1/50.

Davidson, A., & Ray, M. (1991). Studying the human–environment phenomenon using the science of complexity. *Advances in Nursing Science, 4*(2), 73–87.

Davidson, A., Ray, M., & Turkel, M. (Eds.). (2011). *Nursing, caring and complexity science: For human–environment well-being.* New York: Springer Publishing Company.

Gaut, D. (1984). A theoretic description of caring as action. In M. Leininger (Ed.), *Care: The essence of nursing and health.* Thorofare, NJ: Slack, Inc.

Leininger, M. (1970). *Nursing and anthropology: Two worlds to blend.* New York: John Wiley & Sons.

Leininger, M. (1977). The phenomenon of caring: Caring: The essence and central focus of nursing. *American Nurses' Foundation, 2,*14.

Leininger, M. (1978). *Transcultural nursing: Concepts, theories, and practices.* New York: John Wiley & Sons.

Leininger, M. (Ed.). (1981). *Caring: An essential human need.* Thorofare, NJ: Charles B. Slack, Inc.

Leininger, M. (Ed.). (1984). *Care: The essence of nursing and health.* Thorofare, NJ: Charles B. Slack Inc.

Leininger, M. (Ed.). (1985). *Qualitative research methods in nursing*. New York: Grune & Stratton.

Leininger, M. (1990). Ethnomethods: The philosophic and epistemic bases to explicate transcultural nursing knowledge. *Journal of Transcultural Nursing, 1*(2), 40–51. doi: 10.1177/104365969000100206.

Leininger, M. (1991). Ethnonursing: A research method with enablers to study the theory of culture care. In M. M. Leininger (Ed.), *Culture care diversity and universality: A theory of nursing* (pp. 73–117). New York: National League for Nursing Press.

Leininger, M. (1995). *Transcultural nursing: Concepts, theories, research, and practice* (2nd ed.). New York: McGraw-Hill.

Leininger, M. (1997). Overview of the theory of culture care with the ethnonursing research method. *Journal of Transcultural Nursing, 8*(2), 32–52.

Leininger, M. (2002). The theory of culture care and the ethnonursing research method. In M. M. Leininger & M. R. McFarland (Eds.), *Transcultural nursing: Concepts, theories, research, and practice* (3rd ed., pp. 71–98). New York: McGraw-Hill.

Leininger, M. (2006a). Culture care diversity and universality theory and evolution of the ethnonursing method. In M. Leininger & M. R. McFarland (Eds.), *Culture care diversity and universality: A worldwide nursing theory* (2nd ed., pp. 1–42). Sudbury, MA: Jones and Bartlett Publishers.

Leininger, M. (2006b). Ethnonursing: A research method with enablers to study the theory of culture care [Revised reprint]. In M. Leininger & M. R. McFarland (Eds.), *Culture care diversity and universality: A worldwide theory of nursing* (2nd ed., pp. 43–82). Sudbury, MA: Jones and Bartlett Publishers.

Leininger, M. (2006c). Culture care of the Gadsup Akuna of the Eastern Highlands of New Guinea: First transcultural nursing study [Revised reprint]. In M. M. Leininger & M. R. McFarland (Eds.), *Culture care diversity and universality: A worldwide nursing theory* (2nd ed., pp. 115–157). Sudbury, MA: Jones and Bartlett Publishers.

Leininger, M., & McFarland, M. R. (Eds.). (2002). *Transcultural nursing: Concepts, theories, research and practice* (3rd ed.). New York: McGraw-Hill.

Leininger, M., & McFarland, M. R. (Eds.). (2006). *Culture care diversity and universality: A worldwide theory of nursing* (2nd ed.). Sudbury, MA: Jones & Bartlett Publishers, Inc.

McFarland, M. R., Mixer, S. J., Webhe-Alamah, H., & Burk, R. (2012). Ethnonursing: A qualitative research method for all disciplines. *Online International Journal of Qualitative Methods, 11*(3). University of Alberta, Canada.

McFarland, M., Wehbe-Alamah, H., Wilson, M., & Vossos, H. (2011). Synopsis of findings discovered within a descriptive meta-synthesis of doctoral dissertations guided by the culture care theory with use of the ethnonursing research method. *Online Journal of Cultural Competence in Nursing and Healthcare, 1*(3), 24–39.

Morris, E. (2012). Respect, protection, faith and love: Major care constructs identified within the subculture of selected urban African American adolescent gang members. *Journal of Transcultural Nursing*, April 3. doi: 10.1177/1043659612441014.

Newman, M., Sime, M., & Corcoran-Perry, S. (1991). The focus of the discipline of nursing. *Advances in Nursing Science, 14*(1), 1–6.

Newman, M., Smith, M., Dexheimer-Pharris, M., & Jones, D. (2008). The focus of the discipline of nursing. *Advances in Nursing Science, 31*(1), 16–27.

O'Murchu, D. (1997). *Quantum theology: Spiritual implications of the new physics*. New York: The Crossword Publishing Company.

Peat, F. (2002). *From certainty to uncertainty: The story of science and ideas in the twentieth century*. Washington, DC: Joseph Henry Press.

Polit, D., & Beck, C. (2011). *Nursing research: Generating and assessing evidence for nursing practice* (9th ed.). Philadelphia, PA: Lippincott, Williams & Wilkins.

QSR International. (2007). *N-VIVO*. Retrieved on May 28, 2012 from http://www.qsrinternational.com/products_nvivo.aspx.

Ray, M. (1981a). A study of caring within the institutional culture. Unpublished doctoral dissertation), University of Utah, Salt Lake City.

Ray, M. (1981b). The philosophy of care and caring. In M. Leininger (Ed.), *Caring: An essential human need*. Thorofare, NJ: Charles B. Slack, Inc.

Ray, M. (1984). The development of a nursing classification system of caring. In M. Leininger (Ed.), *Care: The essence of nursing and health* (pp. 93–112). Thorofare, NJ: Charles B. Slack Inc.

Ray, M. (1985). A philosophical method to study nursing phenomena. In M. Leininger (Ed.), *Qualitative research methods in nursing*. New York: Grune & Stratton, Inc.

Ray, M. (1989). A theory of bureaucratic caring for nursing practice in the organizational culture. *Nursing Administration Quarterly, 13*(2), 31–42.

Ray, M. (1991). Caring inquiry: The esthetic process in the way of compassion. In D. Gaut & M. Leininger (Eds.), *Caring: The compassionate healer* (pp. 181–189). New York: National League for Nursing Press.

Ray, M. (1994). The richness of phenomenology: Philosophic, theoretic, and methodologic concerns. In J. Morse (Ed.), *Critical issues in qualitative research*. Thousand Oaks, CA: Sage Publications.

Ray, M. (2010a). *Transcultural caring dynamics in nursing and health care*. Philadelphia: F. A. Davis Company.

Ray, M. (2010b). *A study of caring within an institutional culture: The discovery of the Theory of Bureaucratic Caring*. Saarbrücken, Germany: Lambert Academic Publishing.

Ray, M. (2011). Complex caring dynamics: A unifying model of nursing inquiry. In A. Davidson, M. Ray, & M. Turkel (Eds.), *Nursing, caring, and complexity science: For human-environment well-being*. New York: Springer.

Ray, M. (2013). Caring inquiry: The esthetic process in the way of compassion. In M. Smith, Z. Wolf, & M. Turkel (Eds.), *Caring in nursing classics: An essential resource* (pp. 339–345). New York: Springer.

Ray, M., & Turkel, M. (2010). The theory of bureaucratic caring. In M. Smith & M. Parker (Eds.), *Nursing theory and nursing practice* (3rd ed.). Philadelphia, PA: F.A. Davis Company.

Ray, M., & Turkel, M. (2012). A transtheoretical evolution of caring science within complex systems. *International Journal for Human Caring, 16*(2), 28–49.

Ray, M., Turkel, M., & Cohn, J. (2011). Relational caring complexity: The study of caring and complexity in healthcare hospital organizations. In A. Davidson, M. Ray, & M. Turkel, (Eds.), *Nursing, caring, and complexity science: For human–environment well-being* (pp. 95–117). New York: Springer Publishing Company.

Ritzer, G. (1992). *Metatheorizing*. Newbury Park, CA: Sage Publications.

Roach, M. (2002). *Caring, the human mode of being* (2nd rev. ed.). Ottawa, ON: The Canadian Hospital Association.

Rogers, M. (1970). *An introduction to the theoretical basis of nursing*. Philadelphia, PA: F.A. Davis Company.

Smith, M. C., Turkel, M. C., & Wolf, Z. R. (2013). *Caring in nursing classics: An essential resource*. New York: Springer.

Strauss, A., & Corbin, J. (2007). *Basics of qualitative research: Techniques and procedures for developing grounded theory* (3rd ed.). Thousand Oaks, CA: Sage.

Swanson, K. (2010). Kristen Swanson's theory of caring. In M. Parker & M. Smith (Eds.), *Nursing theories and nursing practice* (3rd ed., pp. 428–438). Philadelphia, PA: F. A. Davis Company.

Transcultural Nursing Society (2012). Mission Statement. Retrieved from www.tcns.org.

van Manen, M. (1997). *Researching lived experience. Human science for an action sensitive pedagogy* (2nd ed.). London, ON: The Althouse Press.

Watson, J. (1979). *The philosophy and science of caring*. Boston: Little, Brown and Company.

Watson, J. (1985). *Nursing: Human science, human care*. Norwalk, CT: Appleton-Century-Crofts.

Watson, J. (2008). *The philosophy and science of caring* (2nd rev. ed.). Boulder, CO: University of Colorado Press.

Watson, J., & Smith, M. (2002). Caring science and the science of unitary human beings: A transtheoretical discourse for nursing knowledge development. *Journal of Advanced Nursing, 37*(5), 452–461.

Wheatley, M. (2006). *Leadership and the new science*. San Francisco: Berrett-Koehler Publishers, Inc.

17

Critical ethnography

Karen Lucas Breda

Overview of critical ethnography

Critical ethnography is a methodology that came about in the 1960s and 1970s as an outgrowth of *traditional* or *conventional* ethnography.[1] It was the result of the desire by ethnographers to create a form of ethnography that was reflective as well as analytical in nature and that focused on "the relationships among knowledge, society and political action" (Thomas, 1993, p. vii).

Critical ethnography can be considered a product of traditional ethnography. However, unlike traditional ethnography, it is intrinsically critical in nature. It assumes the position that unequal power relationships exist among the social and cultural groups under study and it aims, in part, to uncover those inequities. Critical ethnographers often strive for democracy and social justice-oriented changes as the outcomes of their research projects.

While *traditional* ethnography is usually considered having a value-free approach to knowledge, critical ethnography views knowledge as contested and driven by the interests of the dominant society. Critical ethnography intentionally uses the premises of critical theory (critical social theory or another critical theoretical framework) to inform its development and execution.

Thomas has described critical ethnography as "conventional ethnography with a political purpose" (1993, p. 4). To grasp the meaning of this statement it is necessary to intimately understand both the philosophical underpinnings of ethnography as an important qualitative approach to research and critical theory as the conceptual basis of critical ethnography. Both of these topics will be dealt with later in this chapter.

Because of its relevancy to real-life issues of power and disenfranchisement and for its ability to engender change in the status quo, critical ethnography is a good fit for the applied sciences. For these reasons, critical ethnography has been adopted by nursing and related disciplines (especially education) for about two decades. Nursing has used critical ethnography to address clinical issues specific to practice (Street, 1992; Martin, 2006; Harrowing, Mill, Spiers, Kulig, & Kipp, 2010), in settings such as long-term residential care agencies (Bland, 2007; Baumbusch, 2010) and with vulnerable populations such as the rural elderly (Averill, 2002, 2005, 2006), the terminally ill (Allen, Chapman, Francis, & O'Connor, 2008); women experiencing menopause (Elliott, Berman, & Kim, 2002) and women subjected to violence (Mikandawire-Valhmu, Rodriquez, Ammar, & Nemoto, 2009). Because of its ability to inform important debates on issues of urgency in health care and quality of life, the method of critical ethnography can be particularly useful to the evolution of nursing research and theory.

Why should you read this chapter?

The purpose of this chapter is threefold. First, the chapter will describe the historical evolution, value and relevance of critical ethnography within the family of critical qualitative research methodologies and the broader theories from which they emanate. Second, the chapter will analyze the body of nursing literature using critical ethnography, including any controversial applications of the method and, third, it will discuss the future directions of critical ethnography in nursing and how nursing can benefit the most from using the method.

What is critical ethnography?

Even though today a number of disciplines in the social and applied sciences use many forms of ethnography as a research method, it behooves us to look specifically to cultural anthropology for its original meaning and usage. Additionally, we would do well to keep in mind the idea that qualitative research methods are not static. Rather, they are in flux and dynamic in as much as they continually respond to societal changes and to theoretical developments within the disciplines that create them. In essence, growth and evolution in science produce shifts and movement in both theoretical and methodological approaches.

The method that researchers have come to call "critical ethnography" evolved from ethnography, a research method that existed earlier and was well established in the social sciences (particularly in anthropology and sociology) before critical ethnography was created. To distinguish it from more specialized types of ethnography developed at a later point in time, some analysts refer to the original form of ethnography as traditional, classic, contemporary or conventional ethnography.

Anthropology, specifically cultural anthropology, is ethnography's original home. Hence, the conceptualizations of ethnography and the role of the ethnographer emerged from the internal logic of the discipline of anthropology. Ethnography was not only embedded within an anthropological paradigm, but also it emerged from a way of seeing the world that was unmistakably anthropological. In effect, it privileged culture and an *emic*, a local or insider's worldview. Having sufficient time to conduct ethnographic research is one of the most important elements of ethnography for anthropologists. Observing and participating in the everyday life of the groups being researched without imposing one's values, beliefs and concepts of the world are another unique and critical component of ethnography. Together these elements facilitate the ethnographer's goal of understanding ways of life, traditions and the link between culture and behavior.

Critical ethnography and traditional ethnography share the fundamental rules of fieldwork, data collection and recording. The methods differ in that critical ethnography actively attempts to solve problems and to change society. To do this, critical ethnographers assume a political and an activist position. At the same time, critical ethnographers are acutely aware of their own biases, role and values in respect to the group under study.

To be more specific, critical ethnographers search for and reveal hidden power relations and contradictions in society. These contradictions are ones that exploit and oppress groups which lack power and influence. The topics of interest to critical ethnographers are usually the "fundamental questions of social existence often ignored by other approaches" (Thomas, 1993, p. 3). In researching these issues, which are often overtly political in nature, critical ethnographers seek to change them to make relations more fair and equitable. Necessary in the method is the element of reflexivity that requires researchers to self-reflect on their own position in society, particularly their positions of privilege.

Critical ethnography emerged during a period when much social upheaval and experimentation was taking place. It is safe to say that critical ethnography is still in the process of development and that it will continue to evolve over the next decades. Here is a bit of its origin.

Becoming critical

The 1970s and 1980s represented a period of time when cultural anthropology began a major shift or even, in Thomas Kuhn's terminology, a *scientific revolution* in the discipline's paradigm or way of seeing the world (Kuhn, 1970). This period of "blurred genres" is typified by anthropologist Clifford Gertz's suggestion that "all anthropological writings were interpretations of interpretations" (Denzin & Lincoln, 1994, p. 9). Anthropologists, at least critical anthropologists, began to question traditional ethnography as a method and to critique the role of ethnographers as researchers. This period of questioning was part of a larger movement in academe that extended beyond anthropology; it was part of a theoretical shift in a number of disciplines toward critical perspectives.

Among other things, the movement called for self-critique and increased reflexivity by researchers. Reflexivity, in part, is when qualitative researchers pay special attention to the influence they have as researcher on the research process and take this information into account in the data analysis. Interestingly and importantly, traditional ethnography as a method came into question primarily by anthropologists themselves, members of the discipline that created it. This critique of ethnography was part of a broader process of methodological and theoretical critiques occurring within the science of anthropology.

To better understand this movement it is important to know that the theoretical basis for the questioning and the ultimate paradigm shift emanated from the influence of critical theory. "Critical theory" is an umbrella term used to describe a way of thinking that focuses on a critique of power structures in society and culture. It grew out of an anti-positivist view of science and has many factions, sub-schools of thought and prominent theorists associated with it (notably scholars from the Frankfurt School who incorporated elements of Marx, Gramsci, Kant, etc. into their work). While traditional or orthodox science attempts to understand and explain society, critical science attempts to *critique* society and ultimately to *change* it.

Various forms of critical theory permeated the intellectual thought of the late twentieth century and in the course influenced research methods and methodological theory first across the social sciences and humanities and later in the applied sciences.[2] The emerging field of critical anthropology began to treat traditional ethnography as *constructions* and viewed it as being influenced by the prejudices, preconceptions and convictions of the ethnographic researcher. Critical anthropologists saw the privileged social and class position of the ethnographer as interfering with the "objectivity" of the researcher. Even lowly graduate students often had a higher status than the groups they studied and even if they did not, they had the power to exclusively interpret the ethnographic data as they saw fit. Ultimately, critical anthropologists began to think of the traditional ethnographic method as an example of positivist science and sought to change it.

While Clifford and Marcus (1986) were not the first to question traditional ethnography, they were among the first to write about it. In their landmark book, *Writing Culture: The Poetics and Politics of Ethnography*, they present a collection of essays that critique the ethnographic narrative. The volume challenged the assumption that ethnographic writings represent unquestionable truths and that ethnography was by default a kind of "cultural reality." The book was controversial, to say the least. But, within the controversy it bared a set of shared concerns and set off a firestorm of debate and exploration in anthropology into the ways in which ethnographic texts are created, viewed and interpreted. The ideas put forth in the volume by Clifford and Marcus began what some call the "writing culture movement."

During that general period a number of anthropologists were experimenting with the traditional ethnographic form to allow various degrees of voice, input and power to the research participant (e.g. Asad, 1986; Crapanzano, 1986; Rabinow, 1986; Rosaldo, 1986, Tyler, 1986). While different theories influenced the specific direction of the experimentation (e.g. critical feminist theories spurred research on gender issues while critical race theory spurred research on racial issues), the notion of objectivity took centerstage among all forms as ethnographers themselves changed their perspectives.

Because the changes and innovations were taking place in many parts of the world, the notion of ethnographers as "insiders" or "outsiders" changed as well. Previously, ethnography was conducted by a person who was foreign to and outside the culture. This guaranteed, it was thought, a degree of objectivity. But as scholars from the Global South emerged on the international arena, the idea of the "indigenous ethnographer" emerged. This is a person, an ethnographer from the target culture who studies his or her own culture. With the new view, the idea of cultural insiders vs. cultural outsiders was turned on its head. For the first time, the potential benefit of insiders studying their own culture could be imagined.

The argument was made that indigenous ethnographers might better understand dynamic changes in culture because of their lived experience in the culture and their knowledge of the history and change in the culture over time. Cultural insiders may, in fact, write more reflexively and with greater understanding of the dynamics of their own cultures than non-indigenous ethnographers. With this new view, the benefit of insiders studying their own culture could be seen. Clifford (1986) claimed that the presence of indigenous ethnographers could possibly increase the degree of vision and understanding of a population and maintained that "[a]nthropology no longer speaks with automatic authority for others defined as unable to speak for themselves ('primitive,' 'pre-literate,' 'without history')" (p. 10). The whole idea of cultures being dynamic and in constant flux with the environment as well as the opening to a global reality lent itself to the tenor of this period. Clifford solidified the *culture in flux* perspective when he wrote somewhat humorously that "cultures do not hold still for their portraits" (p. 10).

The *writing culture* movement (and parallel developments) spurred anthropologists to adopt a more reflexive attitude with regard to their ethnographic writings. Anthropology used this time of rich debate to evolve new methods and methodological theories that align well with the new perception of how best to study and to interpret human phenomena. All of the critical qualitative research methods (including critical ethnography which had already developed but had not undergone widespread testing or diffusion) became increasingly relevant and important during this period. The new methodologies allowed researchers to adopt research methods that were in sync with the theoretical lenses that they were using to conceptualize problems.

A number of theories aided the crafting of the methodologies. In addition to critical theory or critical social theory, other critical perspectives used include "hermeneutics," "structuralism," "history of Mentalities," "neo-Marxism," "genealogy," "post-structuralism", "post-modernism," "pragmatism" (Clifford, 1986, p. 10). Additional related schools of thought are feminism, post-feminism, eco-feminism, post-colonialism, critical race theory, and more. Some of the assumptions and tenets of the theories overlap and scholars may adopt aspects of more than one conceptual lens. Even though similarities exist, critical scholars (even within the same school of thought) often disagree on certain aspects of a theory. Theoretical development in general is not an orderly or consensus-driven process. Debate and contestation abound even among scholars from similar persuasions. More often than not, healthy arguments foster further examination of suppositions and they ultimately add to the depth and advancement of both theory and methods.[3]

Critical ethnography is not without controversy (Atkinson & Hammersley, 1994). As disciplines (particularly anthropology and sociology) adopted more critical methods, they experimented with different research aspects and approaches and they sought out appropriate terms to refer to the new systems of conducting research they were creating. Theoretical and methodological development is asynchronous and uneven with different aspects of new approaches being studied and developed at different rates. Furthermore, because applied science seeks innovation and discovery, it is not a precise practice. Nuances abound in critical ethnography and in other qualitative methods. Nursing can benefit from learning about and becoming comfortable with the ambiguity inherent in the field. One way to do this is to read widely on the topic both inside and outside of nursing to better understand how other disciplines view and engage in qualitative methodology.

The evolution of critical ethnography

Despite its existence for over two decades, critical ethnography is in the relatively early stages of development. Well known and used in certain limited circles, it is not yet widely adopted or generally well understood. Nonetheless, critical ethnography has great potential for further development and use as a methodology and even as a methodological theory in nursing.

The general consensus is that critical ethnography was shaped and continues to be informed by several traditions including the neo-Marxist, post-structuralist, and postmodernist perspectives (Kincheloe & McLaren, 1994). Others would add feminist, critical race theorists and post-colonialists to the list (Madison, 2012). What all of these critical perspectives have in common and follow are a set of given suppositions concisely gathered here. While not every critical researcher would agree, most of them would concur with the following ideas that

all thought is fundamentally mediated by power relations that are social and historically constituted; that facts can never be isolated from the domain of values or removed from some form of ideological inscription; that the relationship between concept and object and between signifier and signified is never stable or fixed and is often mediated by the social relations of capitalist production and consumption; that language is central to the formation of subjectivity (conscious and unconscious awareness); that certain groups in any society are privileged over others and, although the reasons for this privileging may vary widely, the oppression that characterizes contemporary societies is most forcefully reproduced when subordinates accept their social status as natural, necessary, or inevitable, that oppression has many faces and that focusing on only one at the expense of others (e.g. class oppression versus racism) often elides the interconnections among them; and, finally that mainstream research practices are generally, although often unwittingly, implicated in the reproduction of systems of class, race, and gender oppression.

(Kincheloe & McLaren, 1994, in Denzin & Lincoln, 1994b, pp. 139–140)

Most critical perspectives recognize that the above injustices and inequities permeate society and the broad genre of critical research puts in place some strategy to highlight societal injustices and attempts to give power to those who lack it. In the development of critical research methods in ethnography, no labels or names were given at first to new forms of ethnography. Later categories emerged with terms such as "critical ethnography," "post-modern ethnography," "post-structuralist ethnography" and "Marxist ethnography."

Critical ethnography emerged alongside other critical methodologies in a response to the disenchantment of anthropologists with traditional ethnography. Traditionally, anthropologists studied other cultures in remote locations and more often than not those populations were oppressed and exploited by colonial or post-colonial rulers. A British anthropologist studying an indigenous tribe, a clan or population group in Africa is an example of a powerful researcher from the dominant colonial British culture studying a less powerful group. Even the example of Native Americans in North America (so often studied by anthropologists) fit the description of a colonized, exploited group. In part, to extricate itself from being perceived in the role of oppressor and, in part, in response to a theoretical shift toward critical social science, anthropology developed more self-scrutinizing research methods. Critical ethnography is one of several "critically oriented" methodological strategies produced during this period.

Current debates and controversies regarding critical ethnography

While anthropology is ethnography's original disciplinary home, ethnography is used often by other disciplines, especially sociology and more recently the applied sciences.[4] This is also true for critical ethnography. One aspect of critical ethnography that makes it difficult to understand is the fact that it has been adopted by several different disciplines which then have interpreted and developed critical ethnography in slightly different ways. Disciplines create what Kuhn (1970) called a "disciplinary matrix" or paradigm to view their reality and the world. These internal traditions and epistemologies of individual disciplines can lend themselves to different interpretations of theory and methods. While this can ultimately be good for the development of methodologies and theories, different interpretations are confusing and misleading for the newcomer.

Additionally, the use of the term "critical ethnography" has been contested over the years with some scholars preferring to use broader terms. For example, in the text *Critical Ethnography in Educational Research: A Theoretical and Practical Guide*, Phil Carspecken (1996) uses the term "critical qualitative research" instead of "critical ethnography," even though "critical ethnography" is in the title of the book. The author explains his use of the term "critical qualitative research" instead of "critical ethnography" in a footnote in his book. About his decision not to use the term "critical ethnography," Carspecken writes: "[t]he term 'qualitative' is actually more appropriate to my mind than 'ethnography.' Hence, I will use 'qualitative' much more often than 'ethnography' in this book, despite the title" (p. 22). While for all intents and purposes, the method Carspecken outlines in his book would be considered critical ethnography by most, he does not use the term "critical ethnography" in the book, only in the title.

As mentioned earlier, basic ethnography and the science that supports it, including "what it *is* and what it *is not*," have a long history of contestation and controversy (see also the excellent discussion by Brink on this topic; see Chapter 15, this volume). Lastly, it is important to remember that critical ethnography is a product of traditional ethnography and that it shares many common elements, such as data collection and analysis strategies, with ethnography. In reality, critical ethnography is so entwined in the logic of ethnography that it simply would not exist if ethnography did not exist (Thomas, 1993).

Today, the method of critical ethnography is often used by the applied sciences. The discussion now moves to how critical ethnography as a research method was adopted by nursing and nurse researchers including controversies and idiosyncrasies of the method to the discipline of nursing and the trajectory the method will most probably take over the next decade.

Critical ethnography in nursing research

A body of literature on critical ethnography emerged in the social sciences in the 1990s together with several methodological books and book chapters focusing on critical ethnography and the broader topic of critical qualitative research (Thomas, 1993; Denzin & Lincoln, 1994; Kincheloe & McLaren, 1994; Carspecken, 1996; Madison, 2005). This allowed researchers to follow an effective methodological format for critical ethnography while paying attention to issues of validity and reliability. Interest in critical ethnography grew outside of the social sciences as it became clear that the method had great promise for the applied sciences and the professions. Nurse researchers, along with those in the other health professions, education and social work began to adopt critical ethnography as a legitimate and effective methodological approach.

Australian nurse scholar Annette Fay Street's 1992 landmark text *Inside Nursing: A Critical Ethnographic Study of Clinical Nursing Practice* brought critical ethnography to the fore and to the attention of the nursing and applied health science community. Street aptly used critical social theory, critical pedagogy and feminist theory to inform her study of nursing in a large metropolitan hospital in Melbourne, Australia. Street's book-length monograph examined the relationship between nursing knowledge and practice by paying particular attention to "oral culture" and to "practical knowledge" in nursing. Street used critical ethnography to situate nursing in its cultural and historical contexts and considered nursing "as a site in which the intersection of power, politics, knowledge, and practice gives rise to a contested terrain of conflict and struggle" (Street, 1992, p. 2). A goal of the study was to help nurses and other health care workers "to develop more enlightened and liberating health care practices" (Street, 1992, pp. 5–6).

Street's work followed the tenets of critical ethnography in that it directly uncovered the unequal power relations present in the health care system and strove for democratically oriented changes and greater autonomy for nurses. As a method of transformation Street's critical ethnography deconstructed many of the taken-for-granted gender and social class rooted assumptions in the context of the setting. Street described her methods at length in the text and demonstrated how she followed good ethnographic practice in her use of participant observation, field notes and data analysis. Madison (2012) reminds us that the critical ethnographer has an "ethical responsibility to address processes of unfairness or injustice within a particular *lived* domain" (p. 5) and subsequently to attempt to rectify or ameliorate those conditions in some way. Street accomplished these objectives admirably.

During the same period in the early 1990s in Northern Ireland, nurse sociologist Sam Porter agued for the introduction of reflexivity into nursing research and challenged the assumption that objective and unbiased knowledge is possible in nursing research (Porter, 1993). His critique of the philosophy of "naïve realism" opened a formidable debate within the discipline of nursing *and* between sociology and nursing. Porter encouraged nurse researchers to turn their attention to the wider social issues of import in health and illness through the use of methods such as "critical realist ethnography" (Porter & Ryan, 1996, p. 413).

In a critical realist ethnographic study on the theory–practice gap, Porter and Ryan (1996) showed that the theory–practice gap (so often attributed to nurses' lack of interest in or antipathy toward theory) was actually attributable to a lack of resources available to nurses. In their study site they found that time constraints, lack of professional nursing staff and pressure to "get the job done" permeated everyday nursing practice. Study participants actually did understand theory and held positive ideas about how theory could influence their practice. However, participants reported an inability to adequately implement theory due to a lack of sufficient time and resources. Ultimately, findings showed that the theory–practice gap was related primarily to structural issues within the organizational setting where the study was conducted and to broad political economic issues prevalent in the hospital system.

Porter and Ryan's (1996) work demonstrate how power and resources influence the everyday execution of nurses' work and how "the formation of economic structures impinges upon the possibility of nursing action" (p. 419). Power relations are integral to the production process in health care settings. Educator and critical qualitative theorist Phil Carspecken, in his book *Critical Ethnography in Educational Research: A Theoretical and Practical Guide* urges researchers to pay special attention to power relations in all forms of qualitative research. Drawing from Giddens' concept of power Carspecken considers all acts as "acts of power" and urges qualitative researchers to "examine power relations closely to determine who has what kind of power and why" (1996, p. 129).

Emphasis on understanding power relations is a particularly important aspect of all critical ethnographic studies. Porter and Ryan's critical ethnography raised the level of discourse by focusing not only on the experiences of individuals (which can be gleaned through traditional ethnography), but also by exploring those relationships in the context of human *agency* (the ability of individuals to make free choices) and social *structure* (recurring social patterns in society which influence the choices possible).

These early works by researchers set the stage for more critical qualitative and critical ethnographic studies in nursing. Critical theory and method are connected and contribute jointly to knowledge, so critical theory and methods are developed concurrently. A tradition in both critical theory and methods in nursing made their deepest inroads in Australia, New Zealand, Canada, Latin America, and Great Britain.[5] In the United States a solid tradition of critical theory and critical ethnographic research in nursing is still not present. While isolated studies using critical ethnography were located (e.g. Averill, 2002, 2005, 2006) and a formidable multi-disciplinary work by Mikandawire-Valhmu, Rodriquez and Amman (2009), the use of critical ethnography connected to advanced critical theory is rare in the U.S. nursing literature.

Following Annette Street's work, other nurse researchers in Australia carried out studies using critical ethnography. Allen, Chapman, Francis, and O'Conner (2008) wrote a joint paper which examined the field strategies used in critical ethnography. The team reviewed their own study entitled "End-of-Life Care and Palliative Care for Aged-Persons within a Residential Multi-Purpose Service: A Critical Ethnographic Study," spelling out the procedures they used in their study, including every step of the research process.

A thorough understanding of how to carry out a critical ethnographic study is central because the method is relatively new to nursing. But it is also important to know that much variability exists in the way critical ethnography is implemented. Because the primary intention of critical ethnography is to uncover "the political, social and material disempowerment of individuals and disadvantaged groups in order to elicit change" (Allen et al., 2008, p. 228), study participants are offered an active role in the research process. To some degree, the voice of the participants determines the implementation style for the critical ethnographer. Additionally, the specific theoretical framework adopted in the study guides the methodological procedures.

Using critical ethnography, Marian Bland (2007) explored the nature of comfort, discomfort, individualized care and disempowerment in New Zealand nursing homes. Patients' loss of independence, the inability to determine their own care as well as the "one-size-fits-all" mentality of nursing home staff were a constant source of discomfort for nursing home patients. In this study, critical ethnography proved to be an excellent method to flesh out the rich descriptive quality of the human interactions, the pathos of the patient experience, the myriad contradictions present in nursing home life and the complex demands made on both staff and the institution. Bland sums up the expectations made on staff and the institution as being "extraordinarily complex and almost unattainable demands, especially as much of that care was provided by caregivers, often with only rudimentary preparation for so exacting and important a role" (p. 941). This effective critical ethnography is the kind of report that should be read by regulatory boards and high level administrators to let them know of the struggle for care in this type of institution.

A strong tradition of critical ethnographic studies exists in Canadian nursing. Papers by Baumbusch (2010), Harrowing, Mill, Spiers, Kulig, and Kipp (2010) and Elliott, Berman, and Kim (2002) are examples of this practice. In a study of long-term residential care (LTRC), Baumbusch addresses the issue of trustworthiness via five well-defined criteria: credibility, reflexivity, reciprocity, voice and praxis. Fleshing out the criteria on trustworthiness with critical ethnography gives Baumbusch a powerful complement to her post-colonial feminist framework and Foucauldian epistemology.

Harrowing and colleagues (2010) use critical ethnography informed by a critical constructivist perspective to explore the concept of *cultural safety* and the conduct of nursing research internationally. Considering the team was interested in understanding the dynamics of power, politics and justice when researchers from high-income countries study low- and middle-income countries, critical ethnography was a particularly good methodological choice. Studies such as this one bring to light ethical, as well as safety issues for participants from the Global South when they take part in research projects.

This review of works is intended to offer a lens into a selection of the more interesting critical ethnography studies conducted by nurse researchers. The review is not exhaustive and any omissions are unintentional. The following section looks a bit at the debates occurring in nursing in regard to critical ethnography.

Controversial applications of critical ethnography in nursing

One of the drawbacks of critical ethnography is the historical lack of materials explaining how to implement the method. This fact makes its application particularly problematic and difficult for researchers in the applied sciences such as nursing who look to critical qualitative methodologies for direction and guidelines by which to carry out such research. Several nursing papers (Manias & Street, 2001; Smyth & Holmes, 2005; Vandenberg & Hall, 2011) have analyzed critical ethnography to consider its strengths and areas of deficiency. The papers critique the method and look specifically for gaps, potential biases and other limitations.

Manias and Street (2001) bring to light the many useful aspects of critical ethnography while citing three methodological concerns: "researcher/participant subjectivity; the movement from empowerment to reflexivity and the construction of one form of ethnographic 'truth'" (p. 235). Although the authors recognize that in critical ethnography the "participants are considered central to the process of doing collaborative research" (p. 235) and that the method can "provide a forum for consciousness-raising" to change oppressive conditions, they also note that together researchers and participants seek and find some kind of "absolute truth" (p. 235). Absolute truths are problematic for critical researchers in general, and in particular for critical ethnographers who find absolute truth antithetical to their basic assumptions. The fear is that by seeking one absolute truth researchers could unwittingly propagate authoritarian positions with participants (p. 241). Manias and Street advocate the use of a post-structural analysis to aid in the analysis of critical ethnographic data to reverse or completely avoid issues of subjectivity, reflexivity and absolute truths.

Smyth and Holmes (2005) offer an excellent synopsis of Carspecken's approach to critical ethnography. They find important strengths that make critical ethnography a good fit for nursing and recognize the appeal of Carspecken's work to nurses. Smyth and Holmes chose Carspecken because his is the most common reference text on critical ethnography used by nurse researchers. The only weakness they identified is that he can be "unnecessarily verbose and occasionally obscure" (p. 73).

Vandenberg and Hall (2011) critique Carspecken's interpretation of critical ethnography and alert researchers to what they view as methodological weaknesses and potential deficiencies in his approach. Primarily, they fault Carspecken for failing to adequately address "how researchers can minimize researcher biases and dominance when studying power relations" (p. 25). This could be remedied, they posit, by the researcher "giving participants equal power in decision making and taking action toward social justice" (p. 25). Vandenberg and Hall maintain that "reflexivity, relationality and reciprocity" are vehicles researchers can use to avoid reinforcing dominant power relations in critical ethnography (p. 26).

The controversy and criticisms found in the nursing literature related to critical ethnography are legitimate and discussions such as these serve to bring attention to areas of need in the method. Presenting strategies to modify and fine-tune elements can enhance and improve the method. It may be the case that certain aspects of critical ethnography can be specifically adapted for nursing. Ongoing critique of all qualitative methods is welcomed and needed for methodological growth and progress.

Each year more literature on critical ethnography is made available. It is by reading widely about critical ethnography in both the nursing and non-nursing literature and by engaging in in-depth study of both method and theory that nurse researchers will gain the expertise to implement the method in rigorous scientific studies. No single manual or guide is sufficient to understand the intricacies of a methodological tradition, particularly a qualitative methodology. To gain familiarity with critical ethnography, researchers can begin by studying the reference texts (Thomas, 1993; Carspecken, 1996; Madison, 2012) and by reading some classic critical ethnographies (Willis, 1981; Street, 1992). From there, they can put forth more sophisticated and comprehensive analyses.

Future directions of critical ethnography in nursing

Critical ethnographic studies are increasing in popularity in the nursing literature, particularly in Canada and Australia, with the fastest increase present after the year 2000. More and more, nurse scholars who are skilled and knowledgeable in both critical theory and methods are able to serve as mentors and guides to graduate students in the field. As the method becomes better understood, new generations of scholars using critical ethnography will emerge in nursing.

Nursing is progressively more committed to addressing health and social issues that are unequal and exploitative of population groups. The desire to right those wrongs and for fundamental social change harkens back to Florence Nightingale and her efforts for social justice.

Using a critical research process allows researchers not only to describe social processes, but also to take action that can ultimately change social conditions for disenfranchised groups. While critical ethnography is only one of several critical qualitative methodologies with an emancipatory role, researchers who adopt a critical theory as a conceptual lens and who seek methods with an openly critical dimension can benefit from learning to use critical ethnography and from gaining competency in the method. Because research methods are always in a state of dynamic change, the disciplines that adopt them can help shape their continued development. Nursing can benefit from using the method of critical ethnography, by gaining expertise in its implementation, and by adding to its growth and evolution. This process will inform the discipline of nursing both methodologically and theoretically, open the doors for a more rigorous nursing science, and allow nursing to contribute to a broad, transdisciplinary intellectual dialogue.

Notes

1   Conventional ethnography, stemming from the field of cultural anthropology, is also called traditional, classic, or contemporary ethnography.
2   Critical theory has marginally influenced nursing science. Use of theory generally follows the theoretical

and intellectual trends of the local environment. Today, nursing writings and research using critical theory are found more often in areas where critical theory is better understood and accepted both in academe and in the general population (e.g. Latin America, Australia, New Zealand, Canada and Great Britain).

3   For a recent example, the slightly different interpretations of a critically applied medical anthropology by Merrill Singer and Hans Baer (Baer, Singer, & Susser, 2003; Singer & Baer, 1995), on the one hand, and Nancy Scheper-Hughes (1993, 2001), on the other, add to the general evolution of the field of critical theory and to the particular theory of Critical Medical Anthropology (CMA) put forth by Singer and Baer.

4   Ethnography (and subsequently critical ethnography) originated in the social sciences, particularly in anthropology and sociology. Much later it spread to the applied sciences such as education, social work, nursing, library science, and computer science.

5   I was not able to adequately review the nursing literature in Spanish or Portuguese and unfortunately studies in those languages are not represented in this chapter. See Chapter 36 in this volume (on Latin America and Brazil) for more detail, and refer also to the text by Breda (2009).

References

Allen, S., Chapman, Y., Francis, K., & O'Connor, M. (2008). Examining the methods used for a critical ethnographic enquiry. *Contemporary Nurse, 29*, 227–237.

Asad, T. (1986). The concept of cultural translation in British social anthropology. In J. Clifford & G. E. Marcus (Eds.), *Writing culture: The poetics and politics of ethnography* (pp. 141–164). Berkeley, CA: University of California Press.

Atkinson, P., & Hammersley, M. (1994). Ethnography and participant observation. In N. Denzin & Y. Lincoln (Eds.), *Handbook of qualitative research* (pp. 248–261). Thousand Oaks, CA: Sage.

Averill, J. (2002). Voices from the Gila: Health care issues for rural elders in south-western New Mexico. *Journal of Advanced Nursing, 40*(6), 654–662.

Averill, J. (2005). Multicultural aging. Studies of rural elderly individuals: Merging critical ethnography with community-based action research. *Journal of Gerontology Nursing, 31*(12), 11–18.

Averill, J. (2006). Getting started: Initiating critical ethnography and community-based action research in a program of rural health studies. *International Journal of Qualitative Methods. 5*, 2, Retrieved January 31, 2012 from http://www.ualberta.ca/ijqm/backissues/pdf/5_2/averill.

Baer, H., Singer, M., & Susser, I. (2003). *Medical anthropology and the world system* (2nd ed.). Westport, CT: Praeger.

Baumbusch. J. (2010). Conducting critical ethnography in long-term residential care. *Journal of Advanced Nursing, 67*(1), 184–192.

Bland, M. (2007). Betwixt and between: A critical ethnography of comfort in New Zealand residential aged care. *Journal of Clinical Nursing, 16*, 937–944.

Breda, K. L. (Ed.). (2009). *Nursing and globalization in the Americas: A critical perspective*. Amityville, NY: Baywood.

Carspecken, P. F. (1996). *Critical ethnography in educational research: A theoretical and practical guide*. New York: Routledge.

Clifford, J. (1986). Introduction: Partial truths. In J. Clifford & G. E. Marcus (Eds.), *Writing culture: The poetics and politics of ethnography* (pp. 1–26). Berkeley, CA: University of California Press.

Clifford, J., & Marcus, G. (Eds.) (1986). *Writing culture: The poetics and politics of ethnography*. Berkeley: University of California Press.

Crapanzano, V. (1986). Hermes' dilemma: The masking of subversion in ethnographic description. In J. Clifford & G. E. Marcus (Eds.), *Writing culture: The poetics and politics of ethnography* (pp. 51–76). Berkeley: University of California Press.

Denzin, N. K., & Lincoln, Y. S. (Eds.) (1994a). *Handbook of qualitative research*. Thousand Oaks, CA: Sage.

Denzin, N. K., & Lincoln, Y. S. (1994b). Introduction: Entering the field of qualitative research. In N. Denzin & Y. Lincoln (Eds.), *Handbook of qualitative research* (pp. 1–17). Thousand Oaks, CA: Sage.

Elliott, J., Berman, H., & Kim, S. (2002). A critical ethnography of Korean Canadian women's menopause experience. *Health Care for Women International, 23*, 377–388.

Harrowing, J. N., Mill. J., Spiers, J., Kulig, J., & Kipp, W. (2010). Critical ethnography, cultural safety, and international nursing research. *International Journal of Qualitative Methods, 9*(3), 240–251.

Kincheloe, J. L., & McLaren, P. L. (1994). Rethinking critical theory and qualitative research. In N. Denzin & Y. Lincoln (Eds.), *Handbook of qualitative research* (pp. 138–157). Thousand Oaks, CA: Sage.

Kuhn, T. S. (1970). *The structure of scientific revolutions* (2nd ed.) Chicago: University of Chicago Press.

Madison, S. (2005). *Critical ethnography: Methods, ethics, and performance.* Thousand Oaks, CA: Sage.

Madison, S. (2012). *Critical ethnography: Methods, ethics, and performance* (2nd ed.). Los Angeles: Sage.

Manias, E., & Street, A. (2001). Rethinking ethnography: Reconstructing nursing relationships. *Journal of Advanced Nursing, 33*(2), 234–242.

Martin, D. E. (2006). Aboriginal nursing students' experiences in two Canadian schools of nursing: A critical ethnography. University of British Columbia (Canada). *ProQuest Dissertations and Theses,* 352 p. Retrieved from http://search.proquest.com/docview/304904915?accountid=11308.

Mikandawire-Valhmu, L., Rodriquez, R., Ammar, N., & Nemoto, K. (2009). Surviving life as a woman: A critical ethnography of violence in the lives of female domestic workers in Malawi. *Health Care for Women International, 30,* 783–801.

Porter, S. (1993). Nursing research conventions: Objectivity or obfuscation. *Journal of Advanced Nursing, 18,* 137–143.

Porter, S., & Ryan, S. (1996). Breaking the boundaries between nursing and sociology: A critical realist ethnography of the theory-practice gap. *Journal of Advanced Nursing, 24,* 413–420.

Rabinow, P. (1986). Representations are social facts: Modernity and post-modernity in anthropology. In J. Clifford & G. E. Marcus (Eds.), *Writing culture: The poetics and politics of ethnography* (pp. 234–261). Berkeley: University of California Press.

Rosaldo, R. (1986). From the door of his tent: The fieldworker and the inquisitor. In J. Clifford & G. E. Marcus (Eds.), *Writing culture: The poetics and politics of ethnography* (pp. 66–97). Berkeley: University of California Press.

Scheper-Hughes, N. (1993). *Death without weeping: The violence of everyday life in Brazil.* Berkeley: University of California.

Scheper-Hughes, N. (2001). *Saints, scholars and schizophrenics.* Berkeley, CA: University of California Press.

Singer, M., & Baer, H. (1995). *Critical medical anthropology.* Amityville, NY: Baywood.

Smyth, W., & Holmes, C. (2005). Using Carspecken's critical ethnography in nursing research. *Contemporary Nurse, 19,* 65–74.

Street, A. F. (1992). *Inside nursing: A critical ethnography of clinical nursing practice.* Albany, NY: State University of New York Press.

Thomas, J. (1993). *Doing critical ethnography,* Qualitative Research Methods Series 26. Newbury Park, CA: Sage

Tyler, S. A. (1986). Post-modern ethnography: From document of the occult to occult document. In J. Clifford & G. E. Marcus (Eds.), *Writing culture: The poetics and politics of ethnography* (pp. 122–140). Berkeley: University of California Press.

Vandenberg, H., & Hall. W. (2011). Critical ethnography: Extending attention to bias and reinforcement of dominant power relations. *Nurse Researcher, 18*(3), 25–30.

Willis, P. (1981). *Learning to labor: How working class kids get working class jobs.* New York: Columbia University Press.

18

Institutional ethnography

Janet M. Rankin

Introduction

Institutional ethnography (IE) is a method that supports nurse researchers to examine issues that arise in the institutional and organizational arrangements of nursing work and patient care. IE is a relatively new sociological method of inquiry that has been under development since the mid-1970s. Characterized as a "sociology that talks back" (Campbell & Manicom, 1995), it is designed to support researchers to better understand features of contemporary social organization that create problems for people (Smith, 1987, 1990a, 1990b, 1999, 2005, 2006). The aim of IE is to explore how people's activities and problems are coordinated. It describes and examines links between people's local experiences and those things going on at a distance from direct practice, in order to discover how everyday practices and difficulties are put together. IE research "extends people's ordinary knowledge as practitioners of their everyday lives into realms of power and relations that go well beyond their everyday lives" (Howard, Risman, & Sprague, 2005, p. xi).

This chapter is an introductory overview. It includes a brief discussion of the philosophical and theoretical underpinnings of IE and the methodological fit of IE for nursing. Selected IE contributions to nursing are described, including examples from my own research, which are used to demonstrate the pragmatics of formulating an IE project.

Philosophical and theoretical underpinnings of institutional ethnography

Institutional ethnography is a method of inquiry that selectively draws from scholars of sociology and philosophy. A variant of constructionism (McCoy, 2008) it examines how social realities are organized and how knowledge about what is going on is constructed. It is a method that makes claims of truth about the social world, asserting that social activities arise within "concerted sequences of action among people . . . always in time and always in action . . . that potentiates a world in common" (Smith, 1999, p. 127). In other words, there are activities going on in the world that have a materiality that we can observe, describe and agree on (e.g. "the infant rolled over").

Feminist roots

The method was developed by Canadian sociologist Dorothy Smith (1987) who formulated the method during second-wave feminism. Smith's experiences as mother and scholar drew her attention to how society is organized by gendered processes that "perform a routine, generalized, and effective repression" (p. 26) of the knowledge practices that arise in "the endless detailing of particulars" (p. 6) that characterize the domestic sphere. She noted that the daily, always contingent, always dynamic and uncategorical aspects of her everyday work—the knowledge she used in the home—went on invisibly and unremarked. As an academic, Smith noted that she was participating "in a sociology put together by men" (1974, p. 7) wherein there was a distinct rupture between her knowledge of her everyday domestic work and the "authorized" discourse in women's studies she was teaching.

Marx's materiality

Smith's reading of Marx informed her development of IE. Specifically she relied on Marx and Engel's (1968) writings about materiality and work. Marx contrasted the "material world" of labor with "ideological" knowledge about society and its machinations. Using Marx, Smith refers to "ideological practices" to denote knowledge practices that circulate as abstractions. They are practices of knowing, that are distanced from, and often contradictory to what is "really" going on within the *material* features of people's experiences. Ideological practices rely on techniques of researching and writing that "replace the actual with the conceptual" (Smith, 2005, p. 54). They operate at a meta-level (across disciplinary, professional, national and international spheres of activity) to coordinate and organize local settings. Often they organize "feedback loops" that become circular and impenetrable. They inscribe interests of the people who occupy particular positions (social locations) within experiences of gender, race and class (Smith, 1990a). Frequently understood as neutral, objective, or "common sense," ideological practices leave behind what people do, building up authorized logics, that circulate as "conceptual practices of power" (Smith, 1990b).

Ruling relations

In IE, references to power are not abstract. Rather, as with everything in an IE project, power must be understood as something happening, having empirical features that can be chronicled and tracked. In order for researchers to use this core ontology of IE, "power" is referred to as "ruling" or, more specifically, as "ruling relations." This nuanced IE language emphasizes that power is a practice embedded in everyday living. It is produced and reproduced by ordinary people, often in mundane and unthinking ways. People's work (work defined as *all* the purposeful things that people do that take time) is infused with ruling relations that are observable and traceable. People cannot step outside ruling relations. We are all implicated, often simultaneously both as the ruler and the ruled. In IE, actions that generate people's social world are called "social relations." When social relations carry powerful and authoritative coordination into people's lives and activities they are 'relations of ruling.'

Exactly how relations of ruling arise in people's lives depends on people's *social location* within the broad institutional activities where they live and work. In IE research this is referred to as a person's "standpoint." Each person's standpoint determines how their purposeful activity is organized; *there* in *that* location within social relations. For example, a licensed practical nurse occupies a different location within relations of ruling than does a registered nurse. A hospitalized patient occupies yet a different social location, and a housekeeper's location is different again. Each of these social locations is specifically situated within various institutional activities (labor union agreements, professional regulation, insurance benefits, and so forth). Thus, when people undertake work in a hospital, the ruling relations they are engaged in and are subject to are different depending upon the social location (patient, nurse, pharmacist). The problems that arise for them will be similarly dependent upon their standpoint within particular aspects of the managing and ordering of a hospital; these are the sorts of complexes of social and ruling relations that an IE researcher sets out to understand.

Texts and textual analysis

Key to Smith's method is her critical appraisal of how information (knowledge) is circulated through texts. What people can know about what is going on at the standpoint location depends upon whether one knows from being in the setting or whether one knows more abstractly, that is, from interpreting data and reports. IE pays attention to texts (organizational forms, reports, research papers, statistical analysis, and so forth). In such texts, the contingencies of what goes on in everyday work are selected, categorized and tidied up; losing sight of what people are actually doing. Textual practices produce authorized forms knowledge. For example, nurses theorize their observations, employing concepts from health discourses to turn what they notice and what they do into categories offered by texts. Moreover, people replicate and circulate these texts—coordinating activities across different occasions and locations. As nurses, we use admission forms, transfer forms, patient indexing programs, electronic medication records, and so forth. This work with texts organizes, standardizes *and represents* the things that nurses do.

Within the dominance of textually mediated knowledge important details that do not fit the categories are left out. Nonetheless, texts are taken to represent facts. Textual knowledge becomes institutionally and professionally approved. In IE these textual constructions of knowledge are framed as "ideological." They are practices of knowing and acting that may leave people with problems that remain unseen within social policies and administrative and professional practices. They are ideological insofar as they introduce and rely on conceptions that insert institutional interests while at the same time covering over and subordinating other things going on.

Congruent with the central assumption of IE—that the social world only exists in the practices of people—in IE, textual analysis focuses on people. Texts are written by people. Texts are read by and worked on by people. People are accountable to textual representations of work required or work done. People have "text-reader conversations" as they read and respond to the ideas carried in texts. These conversations can be discovered, described and analyzed; examining how directions are organized and activities generated.

Of note is the way a text is "fixed" even if people respond differently to a text, the text itself is constant. People *activate* texts when they replicate and distribute the set features of texts across time and geography. The wide circulation of textual forms of knowledge contributes to the methodological importance and emphasis on texts and textual practices. Texts feature centrally in ruling relations. Smith (2005) writes:

> *It is the replicability of texts* that substructs the ruling relations; replicability is a condition of their existence. The capacity to coordinate people's doings translocally depends on the ability of the text, as a material thing, to turn up in an identical form wherever the reader, hearer, or watcher may be in her or his bodily being . . . Texts suture modes of social action organized extralocally to the local actualities of our necessarily embodied lives. Text-reader conversations are embedded in and organize local settings of work.
>
> *(p. 166, original italics)*

Texts are visible material links that connect people's work across time and location.

Institutional ethnography: a valuable addition to qualitative research in nursing

Methodological fit for nursing

Nursing, a historically gendered occupation, is characteristically accomplished within "endless details and particulars." Nurses create and hold together worksites that are filled with the contingency, individuality and distinctiveness of people's health and illness. The patients, families, communities and populations to whom nurses provide care, experience their needs for nursing services within dynamic, complex features of daily living that interface with numerous institutional practices. Institutional ethnography provides a way to display how nurses and the recipients of nursing care negotiate their work within poorly understood, frequently contradictory practices and to trace how these tensions are organized by broad institutional goals.

Situating institutional ethnography in the qualitative paradigm in nursing

IE is characterized as an "alternate" (Smith, 2005, p. 2) approach to doing social research. As such, the habits of thinking that IE researchers need to establish are not always congruent with the "common essential elements" (Streubert & Carpenter, 2011, p. 18) that dominate the qualitative paradigm in nursing.

One example of how IE diverges from qualitative analysis rests in a particular understanding of "multiple realities" that circulates widely within the descriptive and interpretive qualitative approaches. In a text on qualitative research, Streubert and Carpenter (2011) write:

> The idea that multiple realities exist and create meaning for the individuals studied is the fundamental belief of qualitative researchers ... Qualitative researchers believe that there are always multiple realities (perspectives) to consider when trying to fully understand a situation.
>
> *(p. 20)*

IE researchers have a subtly different view related to the philosophical claim of "multiple realities." While recognizing that people's experiences are multiple and varied, for IE, the essential element rests in the assumption that "human realities" arise in concrete happenings that "originate[s] in people's *bodily being and action*" (Smith, 2005, p. 224, emphasis added). IE is not focused on interpreting people's experiences, rather, it is focused on building an analysis about how experience is organized. This is an important modification when contrasted to the conventional way the phrase "multiple realities" is invoked by nurses—as a way to consider people's feelings, or to learn about the *multiple meanings* people make of experience.

It is important to see how IE researchers make use of experience differently than other qualitative researchers. IE research insists on an empirical analysis resolutely linking experience to the material evidence of its coordination. Because it rejects, as analysis, a researcher's interpretation, IE rejects thematic analyses that slot ethnographic data into conceptual categories.

The evolution of IE in nursing

One of the key contributors to the IE project in nursing is Marie Campbell who studied with Smith when Smith was developing institutional ethnography in the 1970s and 1980s. Campbell, a former nurse, conducted institutional ethnographic research on the early use of patient classification systems. She went on to do several more institutional ethnographies of nursing and health care (1984, 1988a, 1988b, 1992, 1994, 1995, 1998, 2000a, 2000b).[1] This work provided the foundation for a historical tracking of the "managerial turn" in nursing. My own research conducted under Campbell's supervision during the mid-1990s and early 2000s explicated the pervasive intrusion of "accounting logic" into the practices of nurses, and the serious consequences this has for nurses and patients (Rankin & Campbell, 2006).

According to Smith (2005), different IE studies conducted in diverse places and looking at different topics have the capacity to "begin to add up" (p. 212). She elaborates:

> We are exploring a complex of interrelations that cannot readily be bound within one corporate entity, agency or even one institutional complex. Once we begin to see how to locate and analyze texts ethnographically as integral to institutional organization it becomes possible to trace connections that might otherwise be inaccessible.
>
> *(p. 213)*

IE research being conducted by nurses expands what can be known about nursing work. Cumulatively the studies being amassed reveal serious flaws in how nursing is organized, known about and taught. There are generalizing social and ruling relations that pull nurses into contradictory work across a variety of settings. In large part these are standardizing processes that overlook what nurses actually do at work. There are a growing number of IE studies conducted from the standpoint of nurses. Melon (2012) conducted an IE inquiry looking at emergency room triage. Hamilton and Campbell (2011) and Hamilton et al. (2010) used IE to explicate nurses' work to better understand high mortality rates during "off peak" hours in hospitals,[2] while Clune (2010, 2011) took up IE to examine nurses' return to work following disability leave. MacKinnon (2011) investigated the social and ruling relations that organize nurses in rural practice. McGibbon, Peter and Gallop (2010), McGibbon and Peter (2008) and McGibbon (2004) published a series of studies that combined IE with other research approaches to focus on nurses in pediatric intensive care. Quance (2007) studied nurses' work during childbirth. Benjamin (2011) took the standpoint of unregulated nursing aides to investigate the social organization of elderly residents' diminished physical ability following a move into residential care. IE research explicitly taking the standpoint of patients includes Lane (2007, 2011) who investigated care systems for older adults who experience mental illness; MacKinnon (2006) who studied pregnant women's work to prevent preterm labor; and Angus (2001) who studied women's experiences after aortocoronary bypass surgery. The standpoint of nursing students and that of nurse educators has been studied by Rankin, Malinsky, Tate and Elena (2010) and Paterson, Osborne and Gregory (2004). Limoges (2010) used the theoretical framework of IE to explore the ruling relations of nursing education as they arise in high fidelity simulation. Cumulatively the growing body of IE research maps a complex set of interrelations being generated across nurses' professional regulation, health care administration and education. It is compelling evidence; a rich resource upon which to make different sorts of "evidence-based" decisions.

Exploring ruling relations in nursing: how to proceed with an IE project

Positioning the study in relation to the literature

In IE, the analytical process starts when the researcher is reading about the topic. The literature is an important clue that can provide preliminary insight into how an issue is being socially organized. At the outset of the project the researcher looks for papers that confirm that there is a problem; other researchers homing in on the same topic. This supports the researcher's credibility and may validate the significance of the proposed study. However, rather than reading for the gaps in the literature as an entry to a research topic, institutional ethnographers treat the literature as a terrain of knowledge that is part of how the world is both already organized and known. It is often the case that an IE researcher is conceptualizing an issue very differently than other researchers and it may be that, even when something has been studied recurrently, there is scant literature that maintains the IE stance in the materiality of the "everyday world." Thus, the institutional ethnographer's entry to a topic is not *from* the literature. However, what is discovered ethnographically is brought back to the literature in order to determine the discursive home in which practices may be nested and organized.

While IE explicitly avoids theorizing a topic, it can be helpful to understand how the topic is being theorized by others. The critical effort required by IE researchers is to avoid being captured by the theories of others and to maintain the ontological stance in something happening. The researcher is aware that theorized language and terms can obscure people's activities.

For example, when Andrea Ingstrup began to frame her MN research project (currently underway) into healthy infant development in Canadian Aboriginal First Nations communities, she was immersed in theories of "parental child attachment" which was an "official" organizer of the parenting programs she had been implementing. Ingstrup's work and training drew her into a theorized view of parents (most often mothers) and their infants. Despite her confidence in attachment theory as a way to address the issues, her early exposure to IE provided a lens through which to acknowledge that some of the attachment literature made her uneasy. She began to critically interrogate the theoretical knowledge she had relied upon to develop parenting programs to teach parents how to effectively respond to their baby's cues. She began to notice how, socially organized within attachment theory, the problem of inadequate infant care could only be framed in relation to parents' skills, or lack of thereof. Parents were the problem to be worked with.

Ingstrup began to see how she had been "captured" (Smith, 2005, p. 155) by the theoretical framework of attachment. Using IE, her reading approach changed. As she read about attachment, she contrasted what actually happened in her work as a frame, noting where her own knowledge and experience were displaced. She began to understand how the challenges of her work in First Nations communities were not (and could not) be described within the research being done on attachment. Even though some researchers had endeavored to include the multiple factors that influence mothers' and infants' attachment (depression, maternal age, gestational age, addictions, family structures, cultural and ethnic background, income, and so forth), there was no research explicating what she knew about the problems and complexities of her work with First Nations' families such as unstable funding, difficulties recruiting families into the parenting classes, issues regarding transportation and food security, and some disarray among service providers and programs. These realities were not addressed in the literature she was reading.

IE gave her the tools to interrogate the literature, as an expert knower of her own work processes. She began to identify where government reports and research "worked up" her own experiences and, in so doing, overlooked a great deal of what she (and the parents and infants with whom she worked) grappled with or knew about. Thus, when she designed a study to explore the ruling relations organizing First Nations mothers and their infants, she entitled the study "The social organization of the mothering work of a First Nations woman." The expression of a problem, that does not import a theory of that problem, is a critically important step.[3]

Thus, the reading skills required to conduct and institutional ethnography are more complex than just reading broadly and synthesizing what is being said. They require readers to interrogate their own comprehension. The IE reader/researcher consistently pays attention to how she or he is responding to the literature to consider how that reading is socially organized.

Starting with people and things happening: deciding on a standpoint and a question

Choosing a standpoint within a matrix of social relations is an important step in an IE study; to explicate *from there* how things are socially organized. The standpoint is the anchor for data collection and analysis. Smith, Mykhalovskiy and Weatherbee (2006) took the standpoint of people with HIV/AIDS to explore their location within HIV/AIDS services. They asked:

> How is this relation socially organized? In particular we want to examine the legislation, regulations, policy directives and standard paperwork practices that organize the interface between people with HIV/AIDS and social agencies from the institutional side. What characteristic problems emerge? How are such problems generated by the interplay between the HIV/AIDS configuration of life problems and the institutional structure within which social service agency employees work? How do the conditions of the everyday work of living with HIV/AIDS, the organization of that work, and its relation to social service agencies vary with the different social locations (e.g., class, gender, injection drug use, ethnicity, race, etc.) of these people? And lastly, what effect does the stage of someone's illness have on this organizational matrix?
>
> *(p. 168)*

The research questions in an IE project are used to frame the topic of study within a broad interest in "how does it happen?" The questions direct research attention to the problems of the people who occupy the standpoint and may also gesture towards institutional practices.

Formulating the problematic(s)

In IE, the formulation of research "problematic(s)" is a useful orienting device. Problematics are encountered in the field and are vested in data. They are formulated through preliminary analysis and rely on descriptions of things actually happening. While the research questions may refer broadly and nonspecifically to the issues and problems encountered by the people occupying the standpoint, the research problematics point more specifically and empirically to things going wrong. The problematics draw attention to the actual contradictory practices that exist between the everyday demands and goings on in the standpoint informants' work and the institutionalized processes that coordinate and/or represent those activities. Problematics arise in institutionally sanctioned practices that organize life in a way that does not make sense for what is needed *there*. For nurses, problematics may be located inside practices that are understood to produce good nursing care but, when closely examined, go against what nurses know about how to support people's health and well-being. Problematics describe practices that do not seem to make sense or that build conflicting accounts of things going on.

The problematic(s) may become evident in the intersections between fundamentally different kinds of knowledge practices; dissimilar ways of understanding something going on in the world. They are junctures where the researcher can describe people situated "on one side of a line of fault separating them from the objective bureaucratic domain of a politico-administrative regime" (G. Smith, 1995, p. 20) where the researcher discovers the "ruptures" in ideological accounts. These may be occasions when the language use contradicts how "people know a situation to be otherwise on the basis of their everyday experiences" (G. Smith, 1995, p. 20).

There will likely be a variety of problematics emerging from small pieces of data. It is useful to note all those problematic occasions when knowledge among differently situated people clashes. These may point to a broad ruling frame of practices that "hold" the features of the variety of contradictions being described. When a broad frame is identified, there may be a process of choosing which clues to follow into the broad institutional practices.

When Karen Melon (2012), an experienced emergency nurse, took the standpoint of nurses doing triage in urban emergency departments, she wanted to study new systems of fast-tracking non-urgent patients. She believed fast-tracking undermined the standards and practices established in the Canadian Triage and Acuity Scale (CTAS) which, she understood, were fundamental to ensuring that the sickest patients are treated first.

What Melon discovered was a series of problematics. She discovered that despite nurses' faith in the CTAS standards, that were congruent with other authorized views about how CTAS works, that CTAS is only a small component of what nurses know and what they do to "get the sickest patients in." She identified numerous other informal knowledge practices and systems that nurses use to triage, monitor and juggle patients. Moreover, she noted that the CTAS score nurses assigned to patients never changed, while patients did. This contradicted how CTAS scores were monitored and how they were being used to make decisions to reorganize emergency care. Specifically she discovered an authorized knowledge about patients who scored "three" on CTAS; that they are non-urgent patients who wait too long to receive care in emergency. This was a view shared by a majority of nurses. Melon's descriptions of what triage nurses *really* know about "threes" (CTAS 3s) contradicted this view. CTAS 3s are unpredictable; they can change quickly, for the better or the worse. Melon analytically linked this problematic with another one—the authorized view that "waiting" is empty of activity. This was a view that was at odds with Melon's field notes describing triage nurses' skilled monitoring of all the contingencies of the waiting room *especially as it unfolded for CTAS 3s.* Using these problematics she could begin to examine how authorized managerial knowledge being invoked to eliminate delays was disrupting how nurses keep waiting patients safe. These problematics guided her analysis and her capacity to display how nurses' work on behalf of patients who are "waiting" is being reorganized within processes that "perform a routine, generalized, and effective suppression" (Smith, 1987, p. 26) of the knowledge and work of triage nurses. Melon's analysis and argument are built on her identification of taken-for-granted, but nonetheless puzzling, components of triage work. It relies on recognition that these were problematics that held traces of institutional practices.

In my view, the problematics are analytically indispensable. Discovered in the data they provide an empirical ground to guide researchers to ruling relations that can be described and verified. In formulating problematics, the researcher must remain open to surprising twists and turns—paying attention to what the data are showing. Often this means letting go of what one might expect to find, in order to be able to see what is really going on.

For example, Kathleen Benjamin (2011) took the standpoint of nursing aides to investigate what happens when long-term-care residents lose physical capacity. Surprisingly, when she reviewed her field notes her attention was drawn to mealtimes. She noted how the aides hurried and, most often, transported people to the dining room. Her field notes included descriptions of the aides' subsequent work helping people to eat. She turned her attention to describing the social organization of mealtimes where she discovered an ideological construction of a "pleasant dining experience." This construction seriously disrupted the aides' capacity to support patients to walk to the dining room. Moreover, the construction of the pleasant dining experience became quite bizarre when contrasted to the description of how mealtimes actually unfolded. This finding linked into a second line of analysis related to how caregivers' work (and the texts that guided it) constructed residents' activity as "extra" to activities of daily living—formulated as "exercise" to be parceled off, at designated times, to experts. Uncovering the social organization of mealtimes was a surprising finding; not what Benjamin had expected to focus her research on. Nonetheless, her findings provide insight into how to collaborate with the aides to organize their work differently in order to accommodate residents' walking and dining. Formulating the problematics provide direction to move beyond what the standpoint informants can explain from their stance inside the work setting.

Observations and interviews

It is not imperative that fieldwork include both observations *and* interviews. Diamond (1995) found employment as a care aide and relied predominantly on field observations to study the forces shaping aged care in the USA. Hamilton (Hamilton et al., 2010; Hamilton & Campbell, 2011) relied exclusively on interviews to develop insight into what happens during "off-peak" hours in hospitals. In both projects the researchers looked for the social and ruling relations; both projects directed attention to texts.

In IE fieldwork, the researcher is always looking *for* something—observations and interviews consistently focus on work processes and work knowledge. As well, even at the outset, observations and interviews are designed to notice traces of institutional processes, apparent in the setting, but not fully visible there. It is not by chance that nurses show up at work. There are myriad institutional arrangements organizing nurses' arrival for a shift of duty. Noting what happens at change of shift and talking to nurses about their schedules opens an entire field of activity related to clerical work, administrative work, unions, contracts, and so forth. Of course the broad research topic organizes what the researcher notices but, as with Benjamin's (2011) study on physical activity, it could not have been predicted at the outset that her focus would be drawn to dining room protocols. Because she was not looking for "physical activity" as a category, she was able to pay attention to *all the people and all the things going on* within an understanding that all the activities of any social setting are linked together. Things that, at first seem unrelated to the topic may, in fact, be key organizers.

Using IE's generous conception of work, fieldwork using interviews and/or observations develops rich descriptions of all the purposeful activity that people are engaged in; learning from them how they know how to proceed. The researcher is attentive to the occasions of work that do not contribute to what is needed in the setting; the activities that take time and energy but seem unrelated to the work at hand. These are the junctures of work that the researcher will ask more about. For those of us who are "insiders" to our topics, this can be challenging. We tend to gloss over things we take for granted (for nurses, this may be double signing narcotics, completing admission forms, and so forth). As well, the theoretical habits of our education need to be noticed and interrogated. Nurses' conceptualizations of patients are organized by theoretical language that carries preconceived ideas about things such as "activities of daily living" or "pain management" that blind us to things being done. Smith (1987) advises that we need to render the settings we enter "fundamentally mysterious" (p. 92). Concerning everyday experiences, she writes:

> If we cease to take them for granted, if we strip away everything we imagine we know of how they come about (and ordinarily that is very little), if we examine them as they happen within the everyday world, they become fundamentally mysterious.
>
> *(p. 92)*

Nurse researchers must be cognizant not to gloss over practices that seem so normal and natural as to be unremarkable.

It is important to pay attention to the tensions and frustrations of the standpoint informants. For example, in my own research into nursing work in hospitals, I observed a nurse completing an admission form. This was rather a mundane feature of the work that I had observed several times. I had collected sample admission forms for my files. In this instance the nurse was in a hurry. She was also annoyed. There was a requirement for the form to be completed within 24 hours of admission, the patient had been in the emergency department for three days and the form had not been completed. She was asking the patient about where he lived and who would be coming to collect him. She was noting his answers in tick boxes and hastily filling in names and telephone numbers. I asked her about this afterwards. She was annoyed because the emergency nurses consistently missed the "discharge planning" section of the form. For her, this was important. She explained how it was part of holistic care. However, the rushed form filling exercise I had observed seemed at odds with "holistic practice." The patient seemed well able to organize his own plans to get home. Also, it seemed unrealistic to expect the emergency nurses to gather this information. This is a rich piece of IE data. It contains a work process, a textual practice, a regulatory requirement and several contradictions. Observations like this are useful to formulate problematics. As well, they point to other potential informants whose work is linked into the form. It has traces of other texts (the rules about admission forms), which may lead to texts related to accreditation or quality and safety. The data also has traces of nurses' ideological, theorized knowledge (holistic care and timely discharges).

It should be noted that IE interviews can vary from formal, prearranged audio-recorded interviews to ongoing questioning that runs alongside observations. DeVault and McCoy (2002) write: "'interviewing' in institutional ethnography is better described as 'talking to people'" (p. 22). Rather than following a pre-established list of questions, the interview focuses on what the informant knows about their work and how it unfolds. This is the informant's "expert knowledge" that the researcher needs to learn about. There may be a few standard questions to start, but it is up to the researcher to listen and to formulate questions as the interview proceeds. Interviews are structured analytically. As an informant describes his or her work, the researcher identifies the traces and threads of the tensions.

It is important to ask the informant to provide examples of things that happened, especially in the absence of observations. One of the challenges for conducting IE interviews is the propensity for informants to discuss their work broadly, omitting important details that are key to the researcher's capacity to describe and trace the empirical threads. Below is an example from an interview conducted by Nicole Snow who, taking the standpoint of nurses working in mental health, is studying legally imposed treatment for people who experience severe persistent mental illness (Community Treatment Orders). The interview was with a nurse caseworker who was explaining a challenge in her work:

> Unfortunately, what happens a lot of times, you identify these people in the community, and at the end of the day they're reluctant to get treatment, sometimes, unfortunately, you do have to get police involvement to actually apprehend them, to bring them into a psychiatric facility involuntarily. Of course, that makes for bad relations, because if you end up following this client, when they are discharged from hospital, it's very difficult to maintain a close therapeutic relationship with them because they know that you're the one that called the cops on them sort—of thing, right—that in itself is very challenging.

There is a lot of the caseworker's knowledge embedded in this description, and a lot of other implied knowledge to dig down into as well. The informant broadly describes "these people" and situates the challenge as one of maintaining a "therapeutic relationship", but this is not the whole story. Buried in the term "therapeutic relationship" (an example of professional, ideological language) are a whole set of work processes. The analytic interviewer listens carefully and asks follow-up questions to learn about those features of the work that are being covered over. One way to do this would be to ask the informant for an example; an actual situation when the police were called. The interviewer would listen carefully and ask about the details of calling the police. How does this work? Are there forms to be filled out, reports to be generated? What are the laws and processes that link the caseworker with police work? How does the person with mental illness know that it was the caseworker who called the police? Is the caseworker present when the police arrive? What are the social relations of "involuntary"? Does the caseworker have work to do while the patient is hospitalized? How does this unfold? What is the work of a "therapeutic relationship"? Are there other rubs going unnoticed? Asking for a description of a case supports the researcher to gather empirical data and to detail these aspects of the caseworker's practice.

Analysis

Throughout this chapter I have emphasized the *materiality* of IE and IE's core ontology that requires researchers to keep people and people's practices at the centre of the research. This stance is especially critical when doing analysis and, in my experience, it is during analysis that researchers can be pulled off track and fall back to using an ideological frame as a lens through which to examine the data.

Despite the fact that nursing is a practice profession and that people's doings (and people's bodies) are at the center of that practice, our language often loses sight of "people's doings." When nurses discuss caring, moral distress, burnout, or even assessment, we bundle our descriptions of nurses' unfolding activities into broad representations that can never recover the detail of what was going on; the sequences of action; the things nurses actually do. Smith (2005) describes how language conventions that cross disciplinary boundaries establish words and language practices (the discursive practices of each discipline) that lack any specific content, remaining empty, waiting for us to fill them in with pre-formulated understandings. She calls these "shell words" (p. 112). These capture analysts. It is as though we have an empty basket (a shell) that we unwittingly carry into our analytic processes. A shell word may be "attachment," "bullying," "transition" or "uncertainty." Basket in hand, we go gathering those data excerpts that fit our conceptual pre-understanding. Using these processes we lose our capacity to describe something that happened, how it unfolded (social settings where there are other people speaking and moving about), and the material traces of the coordinating relations.

Early in my own research I wobbled during my analysis when the shell term "respect" captured me. The nurses I was working with understood that, fundamentally, the problems they were encountering in their workplaces were happening because managers did not respect them. Their accounts of things going awry in their work became instances of "lack of respect." I became captured by the nurses' persuasive explanation. Framed within this "shell" there was no going back. Analytically, I lost touch with actual nurses and managers, concerting activities within the material conditions of a workplace. "Lack of respect" had no materiality, it could not be used to formulate a problematic wherein I could track different practices of knowledge. It has no empirical links into the social organization of nurses' work.

With the risk of being captured in mind, it is useful to find venues to talk about the data and to articulate the emerging analytic threads (Benjamin & Rankin, under review) and to engage in analytic conversations with people who share IE's core ontology. In the absence of this, the novice researcher needs to identify when they are being pulled into theorized accounts of the data (this may happen with an academic advisor who is unfamiliar with IE) and, instead, learn to think about the data in the unique way that IE research demands. When the researcher is drawn to theoretical explanations it is useful to treat theorized responses to data as *more data*. The work of the IE analyst is to consistently redirect attention to the ethnographic data. It is up to the researcher to establish the accounts of people's doings, to describe what takes their time, what they worry about, what the hassles are.

In doing analysis, the researcher will begin to be able to identify broadly organized practices. These lead to a rough mapping of the variously located work practices and texts and to writing "analytic chunks." These activities begin to establish what can be made of the data and what is missing. Analytic writing and mapping include talk and activities. It makes use of texts, describing where they are generated and where they move. It may include other social relations where work is being hooked together (e.g. the directions a clerk gives an immigrant on the telephone). As the broad terrain of things happening begins to emerge, people's work behind the scenes will become visible, as will junctures of contested knowledge.

Analysis builds a "case" for readers to follow that reliably echoes (but also expands) what people know. It must be a warrantable account. Readers must be able to follow the links, to understand for themselves the social organization that joins people's practices across time and place.

Louise Dyjur (Folkmann & Rankin, 2010) is studying nurses' medication work. The authorized view is that nurses administer medications in a stepwise, organized fashion. Even as she entered the field, Dyjur had a hunch that "medication administration" is a theoretical perspective; too narrow to accommodate all the medication work that nurses do. Her descriptions support her hunches. Observations of medication work reveal it is contingent and emergent.

As analysis proceeds, Dyjur is writing analytic chunks. She is describing nurses' choreography around medication carts. She is writing analytically about the largely taken-for-granted processes related to medication administration records; the authorized view, as it contrasts with what she is observing. She is writing about the work of pharmacists, pharmacy managers and nursing managers. She notes how these people discuss nurses' work, what they need from nurses and their understandings about what nurses lack. She is writing analytically about what she is reading in the quality and safety discourse that is bringing attention to the number of time nurses are interrupted during their medication work. She is puzzling over the category of an "interruption" that is lifted out of the ongoing, contiguous "interruption" that characterizes a nurse's workday. She notes how the quality and safety literature upholds assumptions about medication work, that it can be made systematic and orderly. The analytic chunks are not yet a cohesive explication of how medication work is organized, but the process of writing and mapping are bringing both the problematics and the analytic threads into view.

IE analysis is challenging and absorbing. There is no step-wise recipe for how to proceed. There are various ways to manage the data and a variety of software programs that can support the researcher to organize field notes, interviews and texts that help to systematically review data and make excerpts easier to retrieve. In sum, the most important things to keep in mind when doing analysis are: (1) stay materially grounded in people and their doings (avoiding theoretical categories or phenomenological interpretation); and (2) once you have good descriptions of the practices that are puzzling and/or contradictory, move the analytical gaze to the broad institutional practices that organize and coordinate what is going on.

Conclusion

Nurses are drawn to IE because of its pragmatism and its capacity to provide a ground upon which to validate and articulate their knowledge about what is going on in their everyday practice. It also offers down-to-earth ways to support the patients and populations who are the recipients of nursing care. IE builds knowledge to illuminate how current health care arrangements (and the ways those arrangements are authorized and known about) create consistent problems for front-line caregivers and the people who need care. IE offers refreshingly new understanding to entrenched problems. A robust body of IE nursing research has much to contribute to the discipline.

Notes

1 Campbell and Gregor (2002) published a highly accessible guide to conducting institutional ethnography entitled *Mapping social relations: A primer for doing institutional ethnography*.
2 Looking at weekends, evenings and nights.
3 A paradox in IE is that, although IE directs researchers to reject theories and theory building as the analytic project, IE is not atheoretical. The social organization of knowledge is the important theoretical framework that underpins IE.

References

Angus, J. (2001). The material and social predicaments of home: Women's experiences after aortocoronary bypass surgery. *Canadian Journal of Nursing Research, 33*(2), 27–42.

Benjamin, K. (2011). The social organization of personal support work in long-term care and the promotion of physical activity for residents: An institutional ethnography. Unpublished doctoral thesis, University of Ottawa, Ottawa.

Benjamin, K., & Rankin, J. (2012). Reflections of a novice institutional ethnographer. (Under review.)

Campbell, M. L. (1984). Information systems and management of hospital nursing: A Study in the social organization of knowledge. Unpublished PhD thesis, University of Toronto, Toronto.

Campbell, M. L. (1988a). Management as ruling: A class phenomenon in nursing. *Studies in Political Economy, 27*, 29–51.

Campbell, M. L. (1988b). Accounting for care: A framework for analyzing change in Canadian nursing. *Political Issues in Nursing: Past, Present and Future, 3*, 45–69.

Campbell, M. L. (1992). Nurses' professionalism in Canada: A labour process analysis. *International Journal of Health Services, 22*(4), 751–765.

Campbell, M. L. (1994). The structure of stress in nurses' work. In B. Singh Bolaria & Harley D. Dickinson (Eds.), *Health illness and health care in Canada* (2nd ed., pp. 592–608). Toronto: Harcourt Brace and Co.

Campbell, M. L. (1995). Teaching accountability: What counts in nursing education? In M. Campbell & A. Manicom (Eds.), *Knowledge, experience, and ruling relations: Studies in the social organization of knowledge* (pp. 211–233). Toronto: Toronto University Press.

Campbell, M. L. (1998). Institutional ethnography and experience as data. *Qualitative Sociology, 21*(1), 55–73.

Campbell, M. L. (2000a). Knowledge, gendered subjectivity, and the restructuring of health care: The case of the disappearing nurse. In S. M. Neysmith (Ed.), *Restructuring caring Labour: Discourse, state practice and everyday life* (pp. 187–208). Don Mills, ON: Oxford University Press.

Campbell, M. L. (2000b). Research on health care experiences of people with disabilities: Exploring the social organization of service delivery. *Research in Social Science and Disability, 1*, 131–154.

Campbell, M., Copeland, P., & Tate, B. (1998). Taking the standpoint of people with disabilities in research: Experiences with participation. *Canadian Journal of Rehabilitation, 12*(2), 95–102.

Campbell, M., & Gregor, F. (2002). *Mapping social relations: A primer on doing institutional ethnography*. Aurora, ON: Garamond Press.

Campbell, M. L., & Manicom, A. (Eds.). (1995). *Knowledge, experience, and ruling relations: Studies in the social organization of knowledge*. Toronto: University of Toronto Press Inc.

Clune, L. (2010). The social (dis)organization of "Return to work" from the standpoint of the injured nurse: An institutional ethnography. *Sigma Theta Tau International*, Indianapolis, IN. Retrieved from http://hdl.handle.net/10755/15210.

Clune, L. (2011). *When the injured nurse returns to work: An institutional ethnography*. Published doctoral dissertation, Lawrence S. Bloomberg Faculty of Nursing, University of Toronto, Toronto, Canada. Retrieved from https://tspace.library.utoronto.ca/bitstream/1807/29519/1/Clune_Laurel_A_201106_PHD_thesis.pdf.

DeVault, M., & McCoy, L. (2002). Institutional ethnography: Using interviews to investigate ruling relations (pp. 751–776). In J. F. Gubrium & J. Holstein (Eds.), *Handbook of interview research: Context and method*. Thousand Oaks, CA: Sage.

Diamond, T. (1995). *Making gray gold: Narratives of nursing home care*. Chicago: University of Chicago Press.

Folkmann, L., & Rankin, J. (2010). Medication work: What do nurses know? *Journal of Clinical Nursing, 19*(21–22), 3218–3226.

Hamilton, P., & Campbell M. (2011). Knowledge for re-forming nursing's future: Standpoint makes a difference. *Advances in Nursing Science, 34*(4): 280–296. doi: 10.1097/ANS.0b013e3182356b6a.

Hamilton, P., Mathur, S., Gemeinhardt, G., Eschiti, V., & Campbell, M. (2010). Expanding what we know about off-peak mortality in hospitals. *Journal of Nursing Administration, 40*(3), 124–128.

Howard, J. A., Risman, B., & Sprague, J. (2005). Foreword. In D. E. Smith, *Institutional ethnography: A sociology for people* (pp. ix–xii). Walnut Creek, CA: AltaMira Press.

Lane, A. (2007). The social organization of placement in geriatric mental health. Unpublished doctoral dissertation, University of Calgary, AB, Canada.

Lane, A. (2011). Placement of older adults from hospital mental health units into nursing homes: Exploration of the process, system issues and implications. *Journal of Gerontological Nursing, 37*(2), 49–55.

Limoges, J. (2010). An exploration of ruling relations and how they organize and regulate nursing education in the high-fidelity patient simulation laboratory. *Nursing Inquiry, 17*(1), 58–64.

MacKinnon, K. (2006). Living with the threat of preterm labor: Women's work of keeping the baby in. *Journal of Obstetric, Gynecologic, and Neonatal Nursing, 36*(6), 700–708.

MacKinnon, K. (2011). Rural nurses' safeguarding work: Re-embodying patient safety. *Advances in Nursing Science, 34*(2), 119–129.

Marx, K., & Engels, F. (1932/1968). *A critique of the German ideology* (Trans. T. Delaney & B. Schwartz). Moscow: Progress Publishers. Available at: Marx/Engels Internet Archive (marxists.org) 2000. http://www.marxists.org/archive/marx/works/download/Marx_The_German_Ideology.pdf.

McCoy, L. (2008). Institutional ethnography and constructionism. In Y. Lincoln & N. Lincoln (Eds.), *Handbook of constructionist research* (pp. 701–715). New York: Guilford Press.

McGibbon, E. A. (2004). Reformulating the nature of stress in nurses' work in pediatric intensive care: An institutional ethnography. Unpublished doctoral dissertation, University of Toronto, ON, Canada.

McGibbon, E., & Peter, E. (2008). An ethnography of everyday caring for the living, the dying, and the dead: Towards a biomedical technography. *Qualitative Inquiry, 14*(7), 1134–1156.

McGibbon, E., Peter, E., & Gallop, R. (2010). An institutional ethnography of nurses' stress. *Qualitative Health Research, 20*(10), 1353–1378.

Melon, K. (2012). Inside triage: The social organization of emergency nursing work. Unpublished master's thesis, University of Calgary, AB, Canada.

Paterson, B. L., Osborne, M., & Gregory, D. (2004). How different can you be and still survive? Homogeneity and difference in clinical nursing education. *International Journal of Nursing Education Scholarship, 1*(1), 1–13.

Quance, M. (2007). The social organization of nurses' labour pain work. Unpublished doctoral dissertation, University of Calgary, AB, Canada.

Rankin, J., & Campbell, M. (2006). *Managing to nurse: Inside Canada's health care reform.* Toronto: University of Toronto Press.

Rankin, J. M., Malinsky, L., Tate, B., & Elena, L. (2010). Contesting our taken-for-granted understanding of student evaluation: Insights from a team of institutional ethnographers. *Journal of Nursing Education, 49*(6), 333–339.

Smith, D. E. (1974). Women's perspective as a radical critique of sociology. *Sociological Inquiry, 44*(1), 7–13.

Smith, D. E. (1987). *The everyday world as problematic: A feminist sociology.* Boston, MA: Northeastern University Press.

Smith, D. E. (1990a). *Texts, facts, and femininity: Exploring the relations of ruling.* London: Routledge.

Smith, D. E. (1990b). *The conceptual practices of power: A feminist sociology of knowledge.* Boston, MA: Northeastern University Press.

Smith, D. E. (1999). *Writing the social: Critique, theory, and investigations.* Toronto: University of Toronto Press.

Smith, D. E. (2005). *Institutional ethnography: A sociology for people.* Walnut Creek, CA: AltaMira Press.

Smith, D. E. (2006). *Institutional ethnography as practice.* Lanham, MD: Rowman & Littlefield.

Smith, G. (1995). Accessing treatments: Managing the AIDS epidemic in Ontario. In M. Campbell & A. Manicom (Eds.), *Knowledge, experience, and ruling relations: Studies in the social organization of knowledge* (pp. 18–35). Toronto: University of Toronto Press.

Smith, G., Mykhalovskiy, E., & Weatherbee, D. (2006). A research proposal. In D. Smith (Ed.), *Institutional ethnography as practice* (pp. 165–179). Lanham, MD: Rowman & Littlefield.

Streubert Speziale, H., & Rinaldi Carpenter, D. (Eds.). (2011). *Qualitative research in nursing: Advancing the humanistic imperative* (5th ed.). Philadelphia, PA: Lippincott, Williams & Wilkins.

19

Historical research in nursing

A current outlook

Sandra B. Lewenson

Nursing educator Bertha Harmer ended her 1926 edition of *Methods and Principles of Teaching the Principles and Practice of Nursing* by instructing the reader that the written language was indispensable to the progress of society and likewise to the "progress of the nursing profession" (p. 135). By writing down thoughts, ideas, plans, aims, or results gained from work experience, Harmer explained, nurses could study the meaning of what was done, what was felt at the time it was done, and consider what could be changed in the future. Harmer (1926) wrote that:

> [W]ritten facts can be tested and verified; they may be classified and analyzed; comparisons may be made and new relationships and principles revealed. Records serve as a future reference and guide and by systematic review and checking up, they enable us to evaluate the soundness of our methods and the progress made in both content or knowledge and in methods of work.
>
> *(pp. 135–136)*

Harmer looked at how the written word could support nursing progress. She saw documentation and record keeping as a means to move forward. Similarly, historians look at the documentation (or the lack thereof) to illuminate the past. The same documentation that Harmer sought to propel nursing forward offers historians a glimpse of what nursing did in the past and how it has progressed. In historical research, the researcher seeks documentation to explain what happened, couched within the framework of a particular period in time. They examine the context in which something happened, the contingencies that influenced the event under study, and analyze the data for meaning. Historians look at evidence that earlier nurses left behind in their letters, books, nurses' notes, diaries, journals, records, documented oral histories, and stories that tell us what may have happened. Like Harmer, historians look to what nurses did to help explain events and make adjustments for the future. Historians selectively "impose meanings" (Gaddis, 2002, p. 24) on evidence that is left behind by former generations. This chapter explores the meaning and significance of historical research, the progress that has been made in this type of research, and the influence that the various organizations, centers, and archives have had on advancing the study of nursing history.

Why study nursing history?

History provides nursing a collective memory that can shape our professional identity (Lynaugh, 1996; Padilha & Nelson, 2011; Toman & Thifault, 2012). D'Antonio (2004) writes that nurse historians are "in the process of proclaiming history as an overarching intellectual paradigm for a practice discipline that draws its strengths from its contextual specificity and ideological flexibility" (p. 1). She wonders if history will serve as a "new paradigm for nursing knowledge" (p. 1).

Knowing the history of nursing supports understanding of nursing practice, education, and research. This knowledge socializes nurses into the profession; provides a context in which to examine the health care system; offers insight into past nursing innovations and practice; and renders critique that informs the work nurses do today. In order to know the history of nursing, however, the profession must consider how this knowledge is transmitted. Historical research offers a way to study and transmit historical knowledge. The layered patterns of the past, compared, contrasted, and critiqued within the boundaries of time and space offer a nuanced understanding. Each historian views the data from their own unique perspective, situates the data within a framework, analyzes the data, and writes a narrative.

The written records described earlier by Harmer (1926) can serve as rich primary sources for historians when placed within a contextual framework and historiographical critique. Toman and Thifault (2012) explain that historians must learn "how to 'read' primary sources critically, how to examine the evidence, and how to question various interpretations of that evidence" (p. 187). Historians read the documentation that nurses have left behind found in archives and attics; in schools and clinical settings; in organizational minutes, in patient records, in professional journals, and in the stories and oral histories collected. But reading the past records critically and recognizing the significance to nursing does not come easy, as history and historical methodology have often been omitted in most nursing curricula (Lewenson, 2004; Toman & Thifault, 2012). Yet, if nursing history is to become the overarching paradigm as D'Antonio (2004) suggests, then nurses must learn to value history as well as the historical method that will provide evidence for practice, research, and education.

Relevance of historical research

In practice

Fairman and D'Antonio (2008) contend that nursing is "as central to the history of clinical practice as it is already to our health care system" (p. 7). Evidence for clinical practice can exist within the history of a particular nursing intervention, within the relationships that existed at a particular point in time, and within the clinical wisdom of the practitioners (D'Antonio & Lewenson, 2011). Gaddis (2002) describes the historian's ability to travel through time viewing the "past from the perspective of the present" (p. 25) as simultaneity. Using the vantage point of the present, historians can study the way nurses cared for patients with bedsores, as we see, for example, in Helen Zuelzer's (2011) work "'An Obstinate and Sometimes Gangrenous Sore': Prevention and Nursing Care of Bedsores, 1900 to the 1940s." Zuelzer begins her historical narrative with a story about the former actor Christopher Reeve and his struggle with bedsores, an outcome of a riding accident that left him paralyzed and disabled. Although privileged and well cared for, Zuelzer writes, "despite his access to excellent care, Christopher Reeve died from an infected ulcer" (p. 44). She researched how nurses cared for patients with bedsores by reviewing the nursing literature on this topic between the 1900s and the 1940s, allowing the evidence to show the interventions nurses used to keep bedsores in check. The significance of understanding care of bedsores in the past, and comparing them with care today, offer us additional evidence as nurses explore interventions today.

In education

Just as history provides evidence for practice, history explicates the education of nurses at all levels. History provides a "sense of identity" and supports the ability of nurses to think critically (Madsen, 2008, p. 525; Toman & Thifault, 2012). By observing the landscape of nursing education from a distance that time affords, historians can "understand and, more significantly, *compare* events" (Gaddis, 2002, p. 24). Comparing events surrounding the education of nurses offers the profession a narrative describing, for example, nursing's efforts to standardize practice through education. It also shows the development of nursing scholarship and the knowledge generated from such scholarship grounded in practice. Within the history of nursing education lie the contextual relationships between and among the various stakeholders in this endeavor including educators, physicians, hospitals, students, patients, and private and governmental funders. Studying the history of nursing education using the perspectives of class, race, and gender also offers greater understanding and meaning.

Historians try to understand and explain the disparate meaning history can bring to the present and the future. It must be noted here that the significance of the history of nursing education, or all history, does not enable us to predict the future. Instead, as Gaddis (2002) believes, history "is to *prepare* you for the future by expanding experiences, so that you increase your skills, your stamina—and, if all goes well, your well, your wisdom" (p. 11). Thus, studying the development of nursing scholarship in the United States following World War II as historian Julie Fairman (2008) did in her study "Context and Contingency in the History of Post World War II Nursing Scholarship in the United States," for example, provides us with experiences that scholars today can use to support their efforts to advance nursing science, practice, and education. Fairman (2008) underscores the idea that "contextual and contingent factors shape nursing scholarship" (p. 10); the evolving ideas about theories, frameworks, and practice changed according to the period of time and those engaged in the development of these ideas. Factors such as the number of baccalaureate prepared nurses, the doctoral programs producing nursing scholars, the funding sources available, the social and cultural milieu contribute to the understanding of scholarship development in nursing. The ability to understand how nursing scholarship developed in the past infuses wisdom into today's discussions about scholarship and education.

Power, politics, and leadership

Historical research in nursing education and scholarship, such as Fairman's (2008) work, can prepare us for the future (Gaddis, 2002). History can inform us about what happened in the past and provide us with the wisdom to make decisions today that influence the profession and the care nurses will provide in the future. The significance of historical research extends beyond practice and education that include relevancy to ideas related to power, policy, and leadership. Historical research explores what happened at a particular point in time, within a space bordered by boundaries that intersect with political, cultural, and social factors. Without studying the historical antecedents, the profession misses the nuances that led us to some of our issues today. And, perhaps more importantly, lack of historical understanding creates a void in the knowledge and wisdom that the profession needs in order to advance. A good example of this is demonstrated in the work of D'Antonio et al. (2010) that challenges the predominant paradigm that sees nursing as being "relatively powerless" (p. 207). These authors acknowledge the "invisibility and gender biases" that nursing has endured over time, yet they see the strength and power that nurses have wielded as nurses established this profession over time (p. 207). The authors use contextual case studies as exemplars to provide alternative ways of understanding the power nurses wielded in practice, education, and within the profession. One example examined the history of private duty nursing where nurse-run registries organized and negotiated the work of private duty nurses. Nurses, faced with competition by others to control these registries, often operated nurse-run registries successfully. The ability of these nurse-run registries to shape the work of private duty nurses demonstrated a typically unacknowledged power nurses held (D'Antonio et al., 2010). The authors argue that historical inquiry into the work of these nurses offers insight that can be overlooked when using a twenty-first century perspective about authority, professionalism, and health care delivery. These "contextualized case studies" permit the historian to examine the events within a timeframe where social, political, and economic factors intersect and shape meaning for historians.

Use of frameworks

Analysis of the past requires historians to use frameworks in which to organize, reflect, and interpret the data. Frameworks provide the particular lens in which the historian views the data and "brings methodological discipline and coherency to the processes of reading, researching, representation, and writing" (D'Antonio, 2008, p. 18). Frameworks guide historians in their research. The guide selected depends on the questions raised, the primary and secondary sources found, the researchers' knowledge, their individual understanding, and biases (Lewenson, 2008). Lewenson (2008) wrote that "organizing the evidence preserved by posterity is necessary in order to place the data, whatever data there is, in some form of contextual framework" (p. 38). The frameworks commonly used in historiographical studies include social, cultural, policy, and biographical (Buck, 2008). Frameworks, as Buck (2008) explains, "help to recapture and make sense of out of the past" (p. 45). The framework directs the kinds of questions raised, the data used, the process used in the analysis of the data, and the way in which the contextual analysis in relation to time and space occurs (Buck, 2008). The narrative emerges from the researchers' interpretation of the data within the chosen framework. The selection of a framework, therefore, is crucial to the outcome of the study, and dependent on several variables including the researchers' own bias and beliefs.

Policy framework

A policy background by other researchers' work such as Cindy Connolly's (2011a) "Determining Children's 'Best Interests' in the Midst of an Epidemic: A Cautionary Tale from History" or Joy Buck's (2004) "Home Hospice Versus Home Health: Cooperation, Competition, and Co-optation," influences the way they question and analyze the data in their respective studies. Buck, for example, looked at the history of the policies that developed that would provide end-of-life care to patients and families. She did this by questioning the local and national policies that affected the American hospice movement. Connolly returned to an earlier epidemic and the policies society developed to control that epidemic. She explored these policies in light of social and political control of certain populations and related her findings with the way policies are being established today in relationship to another epidemic today.

The use of a policy framework in historical research emerged to a greater extent in the 1970s, where history was used to inform policy-makers (Buck, 2008), although, Buck notes, the use of this framework by historians studying nursing and nurses' role within the health care environment has been limited. Yet, those that have placed their historical study within a political framework can better respond to inquiry about how policies influence practice and health care; how nurses who are often marginalized, for example, participate in policy decisions that relate to public health and safety, licensure laws, or a myriad of other responses where nurses can add to the discussion and decisions made in both the public and professional arena. Connolly (2011b) asks historians to place "[their] work clearly in the time stream of history while also translating it into narratives to [sic] that speak to issues that matter, not just to nurses, but to the broader American society as well as policymakers" (p. 12).

Social framework

A social framework, often closely tied to a policy framework, challenges the earlier twentieth century consensus[1] paradigm to be more inclusive of those people and structures that were typically studied. No longer would those who held elite positions be the focus of historical research, instead focus would shift to those from diverse backgrounds and who were rarely deemed important enough to study, such as women, children, and minorities (Connolly, 2004). This shift emerged in the 1960s and 1970s and continues to be among the frameworks that nurse historians can use to frame their studies. Connolly (2004) describes in greater depth, however, the polarization that social history brought to historical research contending that these "culture wars" among historians and the fall-out from these disparate approaches were evidenced in the later part of the twentieth century.

Nurse historians participated in this shift towards a social/political framework as early as the 1950s. For example, mid-century *American Journal of Nursing* editor and historian, Mary Roberts (1954) provided an examination of the history of nursing structures, organizations, and great leaders in the United States through a social/political lens in her text, *American Nursing: History and Interpretation*. Nursing leader Lucile Petry Leone (1954) wrote a description of the book in the Foreword, noting that Roberts' book offered "more information, deeper analysis, and a broader view of the society which nursing served and challenges which nursing met" (p. vii).

Roberts' book predated the women's movement of the 1960s and 1970s, but she moved history of nursing away from the more traditional formats that typically showcased the professionalization of nursing and the leaders who led this change and provided a detailed account of twentieth century nursing (Lynaugh, 2009).

The women's movement of the 1960s, along with other cultural shifts nationally and internationally, contributed to the change in how historians approached historical research. Social and political histories rose in popularity throughout the last four decades of the twentieth century. Interest in studying society from a "grassroots," "bottom-up" perspective allowed history to include more than the great "white" leaders (Buck, 2008). Studying the origins of nursing in the United States, for example, lent itself to studying about the work nurses did at the bedside, instead of the typically studied "leaders" of the profession.

This change in focus evolved during the latter part of the twentieth century and continues today. A series of historians wrote about the changes in historical research, moving from one of chronicling the professionalization of nurses to the more nuanced studies of the past. D'Antonio (1999) wrote about this change in a paper entitled "Revisiting and Rethinking the Rewriting of Nursing History," reflecting on the histories that were being produced as a result of this move towards framing history from a social and political perspective. Ellen Condliffe Lagemann (1983), for example, had published a set of essays on the history of nursing, presented at a two-day conference in 1981 at the Rockefeller Archive Center in Pocantico, New York, which showcased a broader perspective about the work done by nurses. Lagemann wrote that the history of nursing was "very much in ferment" (p. 1) suggesting an increasing interest in women's history as well as the history of professions prompting this new focus. Histories, conducted by researchers from a variety of disciplines also broadened the view about nursing and nurses and how this group of workers fit within health care. This new direction, Lagemann asserted, while still unknown, would lead to new "research questions, designs, and strategies" (p. 4).

Celia Davies, who first wrote *Rewriting Nursing History* in 1980, returned to this theme in a paper she presented for the Monica Baly Memorial Lecture[2] and published as "Rewriting Nursing History – Again?" in the 2007 edition of *Nursing History Review*. Davies reminds the reader of the changes in how historians approached the history of nursing, and were now using a broader lens in which to frame its history. She explored her own foray into nursing history as a sociologist and the progress that had been made in historical research in nursing, identifying several significant essays that addressed this progress including: Janet Wilson James's (1984) essay, "Writing and Rewriting Nursing History," D'Antonio's (1999) essay, "Revisioning and Rethinking the Rewriting of Nursing History," Sioban Nelson's (2002) "The Fork in the Road: Nursing History Versus the History of Nursing," and Barbara Mortimer's (2005) "The History of Nursing: Yesterday, Today and Tomorrow." Davies (2007) lays out a "new agenda" (p. 19) for the history of nursing. First, she calls for an internationalism of nursing history that will include finding new ways in which to "generate real comparative understanding across national boundaries" (p. 20); second, she suggests histories that focus attention on how health care policy, nursing, and the state intersect; third, doing historical research that furthers the understanding of how professional identity of nurses (and other health care professions) developed in relation to gender, ethnicity, class, and race; and finally, examining nursing practice, knowledge, and caring as a means of understanding and moving us beyond earlier, ideas about caring and society's value (or lack thereof) of the care provided. Davies wrote that each generation engages in "rewriting history, and the rewritings that we produce will be affected by our identities, our subject positions, and the discourses of the day" (p. 25). This piece of wisdom holds true for historians as they embrace biographical and oral histories to understand the diversity of ideas held by nurses from all different parts of the world, as they embrace identities of who and where nursing fits into the policies that influence the health of the society in which they live. Historians need to be comfortable writing to larger audiences than just other nurse historians as Davies (2007) suggests a larger public, including nurses, the general public, and other historians, awaits.

Cultural framework

Buck (2008) describes the use of a cultural framework as a "blend of history and anthropology to explore cultural interpretations of the past and cultural traditions in the present" (p. 46). Like social history, cultural history replaced some of the earlier histories' use of the great "leaders" with more focused questions and analysis on the relationship of nurses living in a particular culture. Newer revisionist historical narratives trend toward examining the lives of the more "unknown" rather than the known and famous; it examines events and rituals that are typically shared by the "nonelite" as well as explores the meaning of concepts like power, ideology, and perception (Buck, 2008, p. 46).

Biographical

Along with the social, political, and cultural frameworks, one can also study history using a biographical framework. Biographical frameworks offer historians a way of telling the story that fills in the larger history with stories about individuals. Biography can " 'connect the dots,' linking individuals to the events of the period in which they lived" (Lewenson, 2006, p. 1). Following the trends in social, political, and cultural frameworks, biographies of lesser-known figures in nursing can tell stories that capture the essence of everyday life. For example, Wanda Hiestand (2006) studied the life of nurse educator Frances Reiter who was active in nursing education in the 1950s and 1960s, and started one of the early Master's level entry programs in nursing at the New York Medical College. Hiestand (2006) writes about what Reiters refers to as the "whiskey file," where whiskey was kept in one of the drawers of her file cabinet, thus showing a human side to this relatively unknown but visionary nurse educator. Hiestand explains that we "would learn infinitely more if we study the lives of our nursing leaders as human beings instead of icons that we worship" (personal interview on June 29, 2004, Lewenson, 2006, p. 3).

Grypma (2008) considers the biography an important and necessary method to use to study someone's life and calls for biographers to expand the range of the people studied. Studying nurses working in different settings, different geographical locations, from different ethnicities and backgrounds allows for greater diversity of questions and topics that might be explored. Hiestand's study of Frances Reiter opened up discussions about graduate education, entry into practice, collaboration with other health professions, and reform in nursing education.

In order to be successful, the biographer must be able to access sufficient primary documents as well as understand the social, cultural, and political context in which these documents were produced (Grypma, 2008). The researcher needs to have sufficient understanding of background data to ask knowledgeable questions of the data. With sufficient knowledge of nursing education in the 1960s, for example, one can study Reiter's innovative curriculum within the context of what was happening in nursing and the broader society.

The biographer must also provide a "truthful portrait" (Grypma, 2008, p. 75) of the person's life. Immersion into the life of the individual requires the historian to engage fully in the life of the individual under study through the reading of the primary and secondary sources. Unveiling data, engaging the imagination, and creating a narrative that others would want to read challenges the biographer further. Developing bonds with the person being studied, while necessary, may lead the historian to question inclusion of data that may or may not be flattering to the subject and also consider the ethical ramifications.

Oral histories

As one nurse historian explained, oral histories provide the "icing on the cake" (pers. comm., Annemarie McAllister, January 20, 2012). This icing fills in and adds richness to the historical story, providing insights that other primary and secondary source material cannot give. Grypma (2008) acknowledges a debate exists among historians about the value of someone's recollections to historical research. While oral histories can "corroborate" and "clarify" disparate data, it can also be mired in personal bias and "selective memory" (p. 70). The use of oral histories to flesh out the data requires the historian to understand, as in other historical research approaches, the context in which the recollection fits (Nelson, 2002; Grypma, 2008).

Nelson (2002) distinguishes historical research from qualitative research, specifically the use of oral recollections. Unlike qualitative research that uses oral recollections of nurses to "analyze a particular phenomenon . . . historical data are rendered meaningful only through the analysis of historical context" (p. 181). Although oral histories offer a limited perspective of the person being interviewed, nowhere else can one hear the words of how an event was perceived the way one can in an oral history. For example, in historian Louise Fitzpatrick's videotaped interview of educator Mildred Montag, you hear (and see) how Montag viewed her creation of the associate degree in nursing movement and what she thought about nursing education (Interview with Dr Mildred Montag, 1983), Montag's words, captured on tape almost 30 years after initiating the associate degree program curriculum, could be assessed and analyzed within a mid-century American milieu (McAllister, 2012). Her words, influenced by the environment in which she formed her original ideas and later reflected upon in the interview, offer historians invaluable data in which to consider the broader story of nursing education. Historians then must be familiar with the pitfalls of oral history, biography, or any of the frameworks described above, so that they can be more adept at analyzing the data appropriately.

Bias, subjectivity, objectivity

As mentioned earlier, historians' background weighs heavily on the research process. Historians need to be reflective of who they are and know their biases. Knowing one's bias can help in several ways such as how it influences the selection of a framework for the study or even the subject under study. It also lets the reader know the lens that shaped the historian's perspective and the subjectivity that will permeate the work. Boschma, Grypma, and Melchior (2008) consider the issue of objectivity and subjectivity, concluding that all historians, whether writing biography, a social history, or oral history, must address similar challenges in balancing both. These authors explain, "if the former [objectivity] represents rigor toward the subject, the latter [subjectivity] represents relationship with it" (p. 118). Who we are—our own contextual background—influences the kinds of study we do, the questions we ask, the analysis we do, and the narrative we write. This author's research in studying the phasing out of the Bellevue and Mills School of Nursing and the expansion of Hunter College Department of Nursing in New York City in 1967 illustrates this point (Lewenson, 2013). This author selected this topic because of her background as a nurse educator and historian for over 20 years as well as her being part of Hunter's first class admitted into the Bellevue facility. Being raised in the Bronx, from a family that valued a college education where a diploma in nursing would never have been sanctioned, during the 1960s social unrest (Vietnam protests and the women's rights movement) contributed to the subjectivity this researcher brought to the study. The bias and subjectivity one brings to the study challenge the objectivity of the findings. Or perhaps, one can argue, objectivity can never be fully attained because the nature of any study (historical or not) retains the human element and thus, the bias. This is huge and cannot be overlooked. Conscience or unconsciously, one's background—gender, race, ethnicity, education, religion, work, and nationality—plays a role in historical research.

Progress made in historical research

Organizations, conferences, and centers

Much of the progress we have seen in historical research in nursing has been integrated in previous sections of this chapter. Yet reflection in this progress continues to be a topic of interest to historians. The American Association for the History of Nursing (AAHN), the premier nursing history organization in the United States, typically includes articles and editorials that reflect the changes in historical method in the yearly published *Nursing History Review* (*NHR*). Articles range from methodology on biography to oral histories and lectures on where historical research is heading. Continued examination of method and the state of historical research in nursing resonate among nurse historians in their search to be recognized as historians among their peers in nursing and the academy. The very establishment of the AAHN, whose history begins in 1978 as a historical methodology group (the association was briefly named the International History of Nursing Society), speaks to this interest in all aspects of nursing history (AAHN website, 2012).

Interest among historians lends itself to scholarly and collegial activities around the history of nursing and use of the historical method. Scholars come together to discuss the method, present their research, make connections between and among historians from other disciplines interested in the history of nursing, support the research (both financially and intellectually) of budding and seasoned historians alike, promote the collection and safekeeping of historical materials, reach out to broader audiences, and advocate inclusion of history in nursing curricula. The AAHN offers funding and award opportunities that the historical researcher need as little federal funding opportunities for this type of research exists for nursing. The AAHN website offers researchers a list of funding opportunities for pre-doctoral and post-doctoral studies. This organization, as well as others around the world like the Canadian Association for the History of Nursing, the Australian Nursing History & Midwifery Project, the British Columbia History of Nursing Group, the Canadian Association for the History of Nursing (CAHN), and the Danish Society of Nursing History, fills an important role in the promotion and dissemination of the history of nursing globally.

Increasing interest in international collaboration in nursing history became even more apparent when in 2010 historians from around the globe came together to study in the United Kingdom at the Royal Holloway College in Egham at the conference entitled "International Perspectives in the History of Nursing." Considered one of the largest international conferences in nursing history, the conference attracted over 300 participants (Lusk, 2011). The AAHN and the newly formed European Nursing History Group (ENHG), consisting of: the UK Centre for the History of Nursing and Midwifery; the Irish Centre for Nursing and Midwifery History; Kingston University, St. George's, University of London; and the Royal College of Nursing History and Heritage Committee organized this landmark event. This in itself demonstrated the power of global collaboration.

There continues to be a growing interest in the history of nursing as evidenced by the number of organizations, meetings, publications, and centers that address historical research in nursing. As each locality, nationally and internationally, addresses changes to health care, the history of nurses becomes increasingly visible and important to include in the mix. Useful to understanding history are the many nursing history and archival centers that have been established that include historical inquiry as part of its mission. Examples of three centers in the United States include the Bellevue Alumnae Center for Nursing (originally called the Foundation of New York State Nurses) (http://www.foundationnysnurses.org/aboutus/foundationataglance.php), the University of Pennsylvania Barbara Bates Center for the Study of Nursing History (http://www.nursing.upenn.edu/history/Pages/default.aspx), and the University of Virginia Eleanor Crowder Bjoring Center for Nursing Historical Inquiry (http://www.nursing.virginia.edu/research/cnhi/). Each one offers archival collections, forums, and opportunities for study. The reader is encouraged to check out the websites for more detailed description of these and other centers around the world.[3]

Global initiatives

In the last few decades of the twentieth century and into the twenty-first century, nursing and international interest in nursing history and the historical method continue to expand. Organizations like the International Council of Nursing as well as Sigma Theta Tau International both include history among the many papers delivered at recent conferences. In the summer of 2012, the Danish Society of Nursing History and the Danish Museum of Nursing History convened an international conference on the history of nursing. The planned keynote speakers included historians from the United States, England, and Germany and papers were presented on themes including: Medieval and Renaissance Nursing, Nursing in Modern Times, Religious and Secular Nursing, Gender, Culture and Ethnicity, Professionalization and Education, Disaster and War, Clinical Nursing, and Nursing Ethics. The conference shows the increasing global interest and recognition of nursing history.

Yet the difficulties in doing international historical research require the historian to be even more aware of many of the same issues that affect historical research in general, and global history, in particular. Historians engaging in international historical research require sensitivity to the variations of culture, politics, and language that will affect the ability to do the research and the outcomes of that research. Ethical issues that all historians face become even more pertinent in global nursing history, as researchers may be confronted with data containing unflattering descriptions of the events. Including the names of participants of an oral history, a part of the historical process, contrasts with the anonymity afforded to oral interviewees in other forms of qualitative research. Balancing how much critique and how much celebration to include, as Grypma and Wu (2012) writes, brings into play the researchers' own background and skill. Grypma and Wu (2012) discuss methodological issues in doing international historical research by using their own work examining the China mission experience. Historian Eleanor Herrmann (2008) explains the challenges in doing international historical research, especially in developing countries, that the researcher needs to consider. For example, having an advocate or host for you in the country where you are doing the research will go a long way in identifying source materials, building trust among participants (e.g. oral histories), and obtaining official documents. Speaking the language that the documents are written in and understanding the nuances that affect meaning or working with someone who can interpret the data are necessary to understand and interpret data. Using bilingual and binational teams, as suggested by Grypma and Wu (2012), will expand the ability to more accurately interpret the data, taking into account more than one perspective. Being reflective of one's own gendered, religious, national, and cultural self becomes even more relevant when participating in global historical initiatives.

Final thoughts

If, in fact, "history teaches us who we are" (Lewenson & Herrmann, 2008, p. 2), and if we are to value what nursing history has to offer, then we need to teach future generations about its history as well as its value to the profession. Yet in order to value historical evidence and engage in historical thinking, a focused effort is required (Toman & Thifault, 2012). Integrating nursing history into the curriculum has been an ongoing concern for many in nursing, because without it we will not be raising new nurses with respect for the historical data that can inform their work, nor will we be developing new historians that can continue the progress made in historical research (Lewenson, 2004). Keeling writes that knowledge of history and the historical method offers students "cognitive flexibility that will be required for the formation and navigation of tomorrow's health care environment" (Keeling, n.d.). The knowledge of the historical method and value for the outcomes of this kind of research is necessary to make nursing a more visible citizen of the history of health care, nationally and internationally.

Historical research requires thought, reflection, and a place among research methods used by nurses. It has changed over time from the celebratory recording of chronological events, or memories of leaders and experiences, to a critique of the past, requiring reflection and critical thinking. Historical research in nursing has also changed, demanding the researcher to continually search for understanding and meaning about events or people in the past. Harmer's (1926) request

265

in the past for nurses to write succinct notes, in order to create records for review in the future, requires the historian to be ready to contextualize and analyze this record. Nurse historians, historians from other disciplines studying nursing and health care, local, national, and globally situated, contribute to this ongoing discussion about the use of the historical method; and as it has changed throughout the twentieth century, it will continue to progress into the twenty-first century.

Notes

1 Consensus history, as described by Connolly (2004), frames the history as a united story, without exploring the differences among the various individuals or groups studied.
2 Davies presented the Monica Baly Lecture at the "Nursing History: Profession and Practice" conference at the University of Manchester on November 18, 2005. The conference was organized by the United Kingdom Centre for the History of Nursing and Midwifery, the University of Manchester, and by the History of Nursing Society of the Royal College of Nursing. A revision of this lecture was published in *Nursing History Review*, 2007, *17*, 12–27.
3 The AAHN website contains information about each of these centers and their websites as well as a host of other centers around the world with similar goals.

References

American Association for the History of Nursing (AAHN) website. Retrieved on February 8, 2012 from http://www.aahn.org/about.html.
Boschma, G., Grypma, S. J., & Melchior, F. (2008). Reflections on researcher subjectivity and identity in nursing history. In S.B. Lewenson & E. K. Herrmann (Eds.), *Capturing nursing history: A guide to historical methods in research* (pp. 99–121). New York: Springer:
Buck, J. (2004). Home hospice versus home health: Cooperation, competition, and co-optation. *Nursing History Review*, *12*, 25–46.
Buck, J. (2008). Using frameworks in historical research. In S. B. Lewenson & E. K. Herrmann (Eds.), *Capturing nursing history: A guide to historical methods in research* (pp. 45–62). New York: Springer.
Connolly, C. (2004). Beyond social history: New approaches to understanding the state of and the state in nursing history. *Nursing History Review*, *12*, 5–24.
Connolly, C. (2011a). Determining children's "Best Interests" in the midst of an epidemic: A cautionary tale from history. In P. D'Antonio & S. B. Lewenson (Eds), *Nursing interventions through time: History as evidence*. New York: Springer.
Connolly, C. (2011b). Historians and health care reform: Avoiding the "ash heap." *Nursing History Review*, *19*, 11–14.
D'Antonio, P. (1999). Revisiting and rethinking the rewriting of nursing history. *Bulletin of the History of Medicine*, *73*, 268–290.
D'Antonio, P. (2004). Editor's note. *Nursing History Review*, *12*, 1.
D'Antonio, P. (2008). Conceptual and methodological issues in historical research. In S. B. Lewenson, & E. K. Herrmann (Eds.), *Capturing nursing history: A guide to historical methods in research* (pp. 11–23). New York: Springer.
D'Antonio, P., Connolly, C., Wall, B. M., Whelan, J., & Fairman, J. (2010). Histories of nursing: The power and possibilities. *Nursing Outlook*, *58*(4), 207–213.
D'Antonio, P., & Lewenson, S. B. (2011). *Nursing interventions through time: History as evidence*. New York: Springer.
Davies, C. (2007). Rewriting nursing history—Again? *Nursing History Review*, *15*, 12–28.
Fairman, J. (2008). Context and contingency in the history of post World War II nursing scholarship in the United States. *Journal of Nursing Scholarship*, *40*(1), 4–11.
Fairman, J., & D'Antonio, P. (2008). Reimagining nursing's place in the history of clinical practice. *Journal of the History of Medicine and Allied Sciences*, *63*(4), 435–446. Retrieved from http://www.ncbi.nlm.nih.gov/pmc/articles/pmc2730498 (1–7), doi: 10.1093/jhmas/jrn01810.1093/jhmas/jrn018.
Gaddis, J. L. (2002). *The landscape of history: How historians map the past*. New York: Oxford University Press.
Grypma, S. (2008). Critical issues in the use of biographic methods in nursing history. In S. B. Lewenson

& E. K. Herrmann (Eds.), *Capturing nursing history: Guide to historical methods in research.* New York: Springer.

Grypma, S., & Wu, N. (2012). China confidential: Methodological and ethical challenges in global nursing historiography. *Nursing History Review, 20,* 162–183.

Harmer, B. (1926). *Methods and principles of teaching the principles and practice of nursing.* New York: Macmillan Company.

Herrmann, E. K. (2008). Historical research in developing countries. In S. B. Lewenson & E. K. Herrmann (Eds.), *Capturing nursing history: A guide to historical methods in research* (pp. 123–128). New York: Springer.

Hiestand, W. (2006). Frances U. Reiter and the Graduate School of Nursing at the New York Medical College, 1960–1973. *Nursing History Review, 14,* 213–220.

Institute of Medicine. (2011). *The future of nursing: Leading change, advancing health.* Washington, DC: The National Academies Press.

Interview with Dr. Mildred Montag. (1983). Tape 1 and 2. Interview by Louise Fitzpatrick. [Videotape recording.] Archives of the Department of Nursing Education, Gottesman Library, Teachers College, Columbia University, New York. Available at: http://pocketknowledge.tc.columbia.edu/home.php/viewfile/103389.

Keeling, A. W. (n.d.) AAHN Position paper: Nursing history in the curriculum: Preparing nurses for the 21st Century. Retrieved on March 3, 2012 from: http://aahn.org/position.html.

Lagemann, C. E. (Ed.). (1983). *Nursing history: New perspectives, new possibilities.* New York: Teachers College Press,

Leone, L. P. (1954). Foreword. In M. M. Roberts (Ed.), *American nursing: History and interpretation* (pp. v–vii). New York: Macmillan Company.

Lewenson, S. B. (2004). Integrating nursing history in the curriculum, *Journal of Professional Nursing, 20*(6), 374–380.

Lewenson, S. B. (2006). Connecting the dots: Biography shapes nursing history. *Nursing History Review, 14,* 1–4.

Lewenson, S. B. (2008). Doing historical research. In S. B. Lewenson & E. K. Herrmann (Eds.), *Capturing nursing history: A guide to historical methods in research* (pp. 25–43). New York: Springer.

Lewenson, S. B. (2013). "Nurses training may be shifted": The story of Bellevue and Hunter College, 1942–1969. *Nursing History Review, 21,* 14–32.

Lewenson, S. B., & Herrmann, E. K. (2008). Why do historical research? In S. B. Lewenson & E. K. Herrmann (Eds.), *Capturing nursing history: A guide to historical methods in research* (pp. 1–10). New York: Springer.

Lusk, B. (2011). President's message (2011). *American Association for the History of Nursing Bulletin, 102,* 1–2. Retrieved on February 11, 2012 from http://www.aahn.org/files/AAHN_BULLETIN_winter11.pdf.

Lynaugh, J. E. (1996). Editorial. *Nursing History Review, 4,* 1.

Lynaugh, J. E. (2009). "In and out of favor": Scholarship and nursing history. Unpublished presentation given at the Randolph International Nursing History Conference, University of Virginia.

Madsen, W. (2008). Teaching history to nurses: Will this make me a better nurse? *Nurse Education Today, 28,* 524–529.

McAllister, A. (2012). R. Louise McManus and Mildred Montag create the associate degree model for the education of nursing: The right leaders, the right time, the right place: 1947–1959. Unpublished doctoral dissertation, Columbia University Teachers College, New York.

Mortimer, B. (2005). The history of nursing: Yesterday, today and tomorrow. In B. Mortimer & S. McGann (Eds.), *New directions in the history of nursing: International perspectives* (pp. 1–21). London: Routledge.

Nelson, S. (2002). The fork in the road: Nursing history versus the history of nursing. *Nursing History Review, 10,* 175–188.

Padilha, M. I., & Nelson, S. (2011). Networks of identity: The potential of biographical studies for teaching nursing identity, *Nursing History Review 19,* 183–193. doi: 10.1891/1062-8061.19.183.

Roberts, M. (1954). *American nursing: History and interpretation.* New York: Macmillan.

Toman, C., & Thifault, M.-C. (2012). Historical thinking and the shaping of nursing identity. *Nursing History Review, 20,* 184–204.

Wilson, J. J. (1984). Writing and rewriting nursing history. *Bulletin of the History of Medicine, 58,* 568–584.

Zuelzer, H. (2011). "An obstinate and sometimes gangrenous sore": Prevention and nursing care of bedsores, 1900 to the 1940s. In P. D'Antonio, & S. B. Lewenson (Eds.), *Nursing interventions through time: History as evidence.* New York: Springer.

20

Narrative inquiry

Patricia Hill Bailey, Phyllis Montgomery, and Sharolyn Mossey

In this chapter, narrative inquiry in nursing is situated within the broader context of natural inquiry during the last quarter century. Although stories are a phenomenon of interest across multiple research methodologies, this chapter was predominantly influenced by an ethnographic lens. The discussion focuses on individual stories, in particular, limited genre, a common form of social discourse identified within research data bases. We begin with the description of narrative inquiry from the perspective of major authors in this area. The common classifications and features of stories are then detailed, followed by models of narrative analysis. The ongoing controversy regarding the legitimacy of narrative as a research method is presented. We conclude the chapter with a discussion of the state of narrative inquiry within nursing research and an example of narrative inquiry.

Narrative inquiry

The foundational notions of narrative are attributed to the oldest traditions of storytelling dated to ancient literary work in humankind's quest to communicate the self. Narrative inquiry, a contemporary nursing research approach, originates from social scientists' reaction to the Enlightenment phase of knowledge development (Bochner, 2001; Bruner, 1991, 2004; Frank, 2010; Koch, 1998; Sandelowski, 1991). Narrative began to gain legitimacy as a strategy of inquiry following the recognition that all that is to be known about human health experience is not within the grasp of traditional science (Polkinghorne, 2007; Wiltshire, 1995). Narration, regardless of disciplinary orientation, is the process of constructing, reconstructing and communicating human experience, both the exceptional and the ordinary (Bruner, 1991, 2004; Clandinin & Connelly, 2000; Coffey & Atkinson, 1996; Connelly & Clandinin, 1986; Gee, 1991; Gubrium & Holstein, 2009; Labov, 1972; Langellier, 1989; Mattingly & Garro, 1994, 2011; Mishler, 1979, 1986, 1990, 2004, 2005; Ricoeur, 1981; Riessman, 1987, 1988, 1989, 1990, 1991a, 1991b, 1993, 1994, 2003, 2008; Riessman & Mattingly, 2005; Sacks, 1970; White, 1981; Wiltshire, 1995). Through narration, individuals select events that require relating an inner world of desire and motive to an outer world of observable actions and states of affairs (Mattingly & Garro, 1994).

Fundamental to narrative inquiry is the belief that individuals *most effectively* make sense of their world through narration. Gee (1985) asserts that "all human beings are masters of making sense of experience and the world through narrative" (p. 27). Thereby, narrative inquiry seeks to uncover the meaning embedded in communicated stories—the unit of analysis.

What constitutes story

Researchers must declare a definition of story so that the unit of analysis within individual studies is identifiable. Although the conceptualization of story is debated within the narrative inquiry literature (Langellier, 1989; Mishler, 1986; Riessman, 1993, 2008; Scholes, 1980; Scholes & Kellogg, 1966; Stivers, 1993; Wiltshire, 1995), a singular understanding remains elusive. Two broad categories of story, expanded and limited genre, however, can be identified across reports of narrative inquiry. Both categorizations are representative of diverse human experiences portrayed through identifiable plot and structure within a particular context but are differentiated by temporal and experiential specificity. These general categorizations assist both researchers and consumers to begin to articulate a cogent understanding of what is story in narrative inquiry.

Story structure, plot and context

All personal stories within narrative inquiry are structured around an explicit or implicit plot situated in a particular context. These three elements are central to any health care story, as dialogue unfolds sequentially in "clock time, of one thing after another . . . transformed by a plot" (Mattingly, 1994, p. 813). Structure defines the boundaries of a story. Plot specifies the components of a story and the context of its creation. According to Smith (1981), "No narrative version can be independent of a particular teller and occasion of telling" (p. 215). Bruner (1990) summarizes the interdependence and importance of these three features: "These constituents do not, as it were, have a life or meaning of their own. Their meaning is given by their place in the overall configuration of the sequence as a whole" (p. 43).

The combined presence of these elements differentiates stories from other forms of discourse such as reports or lists. In addition, narrative researchers contend that for discourse to be defined as story, it must have a "point" from the perspective of both the teller and the audience (Del Vecchio Good et al., 1994; Hunt, 1994; Riessman, 1993, 2008).

To adequately understand the intended point of stories, the "narrative environment" of their creation must be understood (Gubrium & Holstein, 2008). Individual stories are created within a social and cultural context defined by dominant narratives. As such, the researcher must be prepared to hear inherently political stories that counter dominant narratives (Kirkpatrick, 2008; Sandelowski, 1991). Attending to alternate narratives may generate new knowledge that challenges our entrenched understandings of human experiences.

Story as expanded genre and limited genre

Extensive in breadth and depth, expanded genre stories are constructed from multiple modalities inclusive of written, verbal and visual data often over the life course of an individual (Kleinman, 1988, 1992; Personal Narrative Group, 1989a, 1989b; Monks & Frankenberg, 1990, 1995; Polkinghorne, 1988; Riessman 2008; Sacks, 1970). From this orientation, the unit of analysis is all available data. This unit of analysis is necessarily broad in order to understand complex human and system interactions and context over time. Narrative researchers, guided by an explicit or implicit theoretical frame, interpret themes that thread through these extensive segments of data.

Circumscribed in breadth and depth, limited genre stories describe specific events embedded within longer segments of data (Mishler, 1986; Riessman, 1993, 2008). Comprehensive stories within this genre have an identifiable beginning, middle and end. An individual story is the unit of analysis. Limited genre stories are differentiated as first-person event-specific (Riessman, 1993), generic (Bennett, 1986; Riessman, 1991b), and kernel stories (Connelly & Clandinin, 1990; Kalčik, 1975; Kermode, 1981). All available research data will include a number of these story types. First-person event-specific stories are accounts that describe a single occurrence of a specific event experienced by the teller. Generic stories, also first-person accounts, present usual or recurring events. Riessman (1991b) adds that a generic story is identifiable in the data by linguistic elements that denote repetition and routinization. Third, kernel stories are partial accounts suggestive of comprehensive first-person experiences yet to be told; what Viney and Bousfield (1991) describe as "stories-begun-but-not-told." As a collective, individual limited genre stories are further identifiable within all available data by their inclusion of an evaluative component (Polanyi, 1979, 1985, 1989; Riessman, 1991a, 1991b; Schiffin, 1994).

Narrative in nursing

From a disciplinary perspective, the practice of storytelling as a means of relating is not new in nursing. Nursing narratives are frequently used to recount poignant health human experiences. Stories offer a familiar conduit for both the formal and informal communication of complex nursing phenomenon. For example, the colloquial titles of the following publications mask the complexity embedded within narrations: "A Way with Words" describes a personal story of attending the dying (McGarvey & Diekelmann, 1992); and "A Broken Promise," an intimate account about learning from a mistake (Fowler, 1992). Multiple comparable extended and limited story genres have been published in the nursing literature. Traditionally, such stories function to convey the hegemony of nursing conventions or illustrate practice dilemmas. Underlying these communicative efforts is the assumption that storied accounts effectively convey complex information in a way that is understood by the listener, frequently the neophyte nurse.

From a developmental perspective, the prolific use of storytelling in nursing education aligns with an appreciation of the merits of active learning (Benner, Sutphen, Leonard, & Day, 2010; Brown, Kirkpatrick, Mangum, & Avery, 2008; Diekelmann, 2001; Diekelmann & Scheckel, 2004; Ironside, 2006). Stories are a strategy to engage learners through the vicarious experience of events. Patient, family and health care provider stories pervade learning resources and contexts. It is essential to recognize that this ubiquitous use of storytelling clearly falls outside of the conventions of narrative inquiry. Narrative research, a "profoundly complex, technical, method-ological and even philosophical operation" (Thorne, 2009, p. 1184), departs from colloquial traditions of storytelling.

From a knowledge creation perspective, stories are used to examine a wide range of nursing phenomena. This includes, but is not limited to the following studies: the ambiguities experienced by infertile couples (Sandelowski, Holditch-Davis, & Harris, 1990); women and chronic illness (Koch, Turner, Smith, & Hutnik, 2010; Kralik & Koch, 2003; Montgomery, Mossey, Bailey, & Forchuk 2011); perceptions of schizophrenic patients and their carers (Hellzen, Norberg, & Sandman 1995); children's health (Knafl, Ayres, Gallo, Zoeller, & Breitmayer, 1995); Chronic Obstructive Pulmonary Disease as a chronic illness (Bailey, 2001, 2004); nurses' experiences and work life (Benner, 1991; Benner, Tanner, & Chesla, 1992; Bowers & Moore, 1997; Fenton & Brykczynski, 1993; Tanner, Benner, Chesla, & Gordon, 1993; Vezeau, 1993); HIV and lesbian health care issues (Hall, 1994; Stevens, 1993, 1994, 1996; Stewart, 1994); the meaning of long-term care (Crisp, 1995; Heikkinen, 1993; Heliker, 1997); cancer nursing (Mathieson & Stam, 1995); issues related to women's health (Facione & Dodd, 1995; Meleis, Arruda, Lane, & Bernal, 1994); and ethical issues in nursing care (Benner, 1991; Udén, Norberg, Lindseth, & Marhaugh, 1992).

The preceding works are cited to illustrate the broad use of "stories" for the construction of nursing knowledge. There is, however, limited reference to the manner in which an identified narrative model guided the process. It is our contention that all narrative works must be subject to the conventions of methodological adequacy (Koch, 1998; Thorne, 2009). The relative merit of this science is often called into question based on outstanding quality concerns. Wiltshire (1995) cautions that regardless of the nurse-researcher's definition of story,

> It should not be assumed that a narrative [story] form gives direct and unproblematic access either to the patient's condition, or the nurse's practice knowledge. One cannot think of a narrative [story] simply as a transparent window opening onto new epistemological realms of material and understanding. Windows have frames, and window panes that refract and reflect.
>
> *(p. 77)*

Alternately, stories have been presented without interpretation, begging the question "Is the story enough?" (Thorne, 2009). Can stories speak for themselves? For this reason, researchers and consumers alike must not only know what constitutes story, but also the indicators of quality in narrative inquiry.

Quality in narrative analysis

In the last two decades there has been a growth in the identification and/or construction of stories as evidence within qualitative research. This use of stories is based on the belief by some that stories are a unique entity for making sense of health and illness experiences (Frank, 2000, 2001, 2010). Stories allow for the study of human responses to health challenges often "bearing witness to the suffering of sick people" (Bochner, 2010, p. 662). Within the realm of natural inquiry, health care narratologists endeavour to address complex methodological and quality issues (Bailey, 1996; Mishler, 1986, 1990, 2005; Polkinghorne, 2007; Riessman, 1993, 2008).

As this body of science develops, it remains subject to the fundamental criticism of narrative inquiry originating within the social sciences (Atkinson, 1997, 2010; Atkinson & Delamont, 2006; Thorne, 2009). The ongoing acrimonious public debate addresses the legitimacy of personal stories as qualitative data and the robustness of narrative analytic processes (Atkinson, 1997, 2005, 2009, 2010; Atkinson & Delamont, 2006; Atkinson & Silverman, 1997; Bochner, 2001, 2010; Frank, 2010; Mishler, 2005; Sakalys, 2000, 2003; Thomas, 2010). Some critics censure narratives presented as qualitative data as romanticized, privileged illness stories, illegitimate counter-narratives to the dominant health care metanarratives, the providers' truth (Atkinson, 1997, 2010; Atkinson & Silverman, 1997; Stein, 1990).

Quality within the positivist paradigm is, in part, understood as validity and reliability. Within the interpretive paradigm, quality is conceptualized as credibility (Thorne, 2008). Within this frame, analytic transparency has been presented as a primary indicator of credibility (Bailey, 1996; Polkinghorne, 2007). This reformulation involves the demonstration of credibility throughout the research process, understanding quality not as a static objective reality, but rather as an auditable process of confirmation. A credibility orientation addresses "the uneasy realization that the concept of validity (objective truth) and reliability (the stability of findings over time) . . . [are] somehow inappropriate [for natural inquiry]" (Bailey, 1996, p. 188).

Demonstrating quality within narrative inquiry is an arduous responsibility. In part, this is attributable to narrative inquiry's void of absolute, singular interpretations. Rendering the analytic process overtly visible is intended to allow external judgment regarding the authenticity of the researcher's interpretive work, thereby enhancing trustworthiness and credibility (Bailey, 1996; Polkinghorne, 2007; Riessman, 1993). This necessitates reporting of a defined unit of analysis, a systematic analytic strategy, representative data and the interpreted product. Without this information, the reader's ability to critically appraise the quality of the work or draw alternate conclusions is forfeited. This may fuel the premise that the researcher is privileged as the sole interpreter of story. "Indeed, there is not just one correct interpretation of the structure, meanings or context of narratives" (Bailey, 1996, p. 191).

Models of narrative analysis

Using systematic analysis, narrative researchers contend that stories in qualitative interviews can generate meaningful and promising findings (Mishler, 1986). The two primary strategies used in the analysis of stories are thematic and structural. Thematic analysis is most common in narrative inquiry. Riessman (2008) identifies that this method attends to "'what' is said, rather than 'how,' 'to whom,' 'for what purposes'" (pp. 53–54). Alternatively, structural analysis, attends to not only the what, but also the who, how and why of telling within an identified story. In both methods, researchers use strategies to account for the context of events (Altheide & Johnson, 1994).

The following is an explication of one form of structural analysis as applied to limited genre stories. As identified, this type of story is a form of meaning-making talk embedded in interview data. Qualitative study participants have a natural impulse

> to tell a story that recounts the actions and events of interest in some kind of temporal sequence. Such a story, however, does more than simply outline a series of incidents: it places those incidents in a particular narrative [story] context, thereby giving them a particular meaning.
>
> *(Tappan & Brown, 1989, p. 185)*

Further stories within interview data reference a specific event (referential) as well as evaluate the significance of the event for the teller (evaluation) precipitating the researchers' interpretation (Labov & Waletzky, 1972). In order to analyze a story's meaning embedded within its structure to yield its function, each of these three elements will be described. As presented here, structural analysis makes visible the interplay between content and form to adequately ascertain meaning.

Story structure

An initial step in structural analysis of limited genre stories is the identification of story structure. Guided by Labov and Waletzky's (1972) functional analysis model, a story's structure is comprised of seven elements: story stimulus, abstract, orientation, complicating action, evaluation, resolution and coda (Table 20.1). These elements frame a story by defining its components and, by extension, its parameters. Parsing a story into it constituent parts exposes the teller's representation of a specific event. How the story is told is intricate to developing an understanding of the event as experienced by the storyteller. The process of outlining the story structure is critical to defining the boundaries of the unit of analysis. Not only does this facilitate the interpretation of the story's meaning, but it enhances credibility.

Table 20.1 Limited genre story elements

Story elements	Description of story phrases
Story stimulus	Initiates the telling of the story
Abstract	Provides a plot summary Defines the beginning boundary of the story
Orientation	Performs the referential function by identifying the events around which the story is based Usually placed at the beginning of the account
Complicating action	Defining element of a story Provides temporal retelling or portrayal of past events Involves the actual or implied use of the conjunction "then" between two story phrases Generally occurs after the orientation clauses and precedes the resolution segments of the story
Evaluation	Explicates the "point" or "significance" of the story Expresses the teller's interpretation of the recounted events
Resolution	Outlines the outcome of the narrative clauses Generally follows the evaluation statement(s)
Coda	Marks the end of the story Brings the storyteller and the listener back to the present Assists in defining the boundary of the story

Sources: Labov (1972), Labov and Waletzky (1972).

Story meaning

Story meaning explicates the significance of the account for the teller; the intended essence of the story. Why a story is told and what the storyteller is emphasizing are often found within the evaluation structure of the story (Labov & Waletzky, 1972). Storytellers relate the meaning of their recounted event not only through text but also discursive and rhetorical strategies. These techniques, inclusive of metaphors, direct quotations, matter-of-fact declarations, ideas, word or phrase repetition, variations in tone and volume, and references to a "like" other strengthen the identification of the story meaning, the purpose of the telling (Bennett, 1986). Some of these strategies are represented through transcription conventions. Story meaning is not isolated to a single story but rather emerges from a pattern of coherence in meaning (Agar & Hobbs, 1982, 1983) identifiable within a group of stories across the interview data base. This component further differentiates thematic and structural analysis by exposing the purpose of the telling.

Story function

The story function denotes the implications of the story that is told. By virtue of their different vantage points, the implications of the story may differ. For storytellers, the story functions to convey "the truth of *their* experience" (Bailey & Tilley, 2002, p. 581). Story function for

273

researchers involves the translation of shared meanings into a theoretical rendering. Function yields experientially grounded pragmatic nursing knowledge to inform practice.

Within this approach it is essential that story structure, meaning and function are integrated into an iterative analysis process. One such process involving five steps is outlined in Figure 20.1. Analysis begins with the identification of story types (first-person event-specific, generic, and

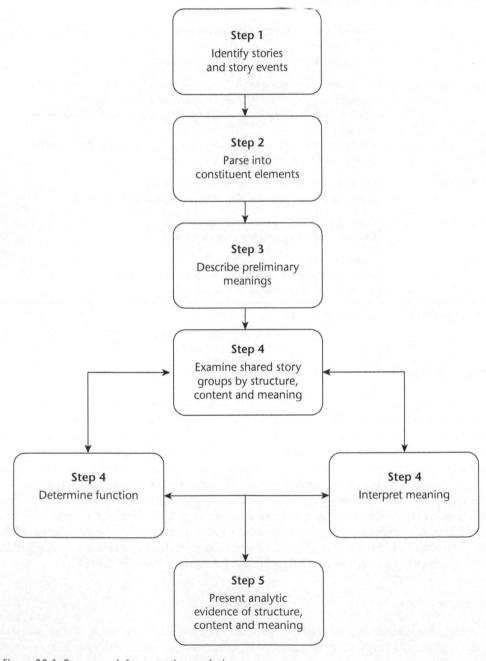

Figure 20.1 Framework for narrative analysis

kernel stories) from "untidied" interview transcripts inclusive of rhetorical and discursive devices. Common story events are identified within interviews and across the data set. Then each story is deconstructed to identify its constituent elements (Table 20.1). Next, interpretations of the essence of individual stories are identified to uncover initial story meanings. An example of a question at this step of analysis is: "Why is this story being told?" The fourth step is twofold. First, stories that share a common meaning, structure and for some a common event, are identified and grouped. Second, the stories' meaning and function are interpreted to develop an emic understanding of the phenomenon. Critical questions for consideration are: "Why is this grouping of stories told?" and "What are the implications of coming to know insiders' perspectives?" Finally, the integrity of this process is reflected in the presentation of the analytical evidence inclusive of story segments and a complete story. An appreciation of the narrative context informs interpretation throughout this process.

In the following case example a segment of narrative text is presented to illustrate the application of the above structural analytic framework (Figure 20.1). Through this process is the identification of a distinct story: parsing of the narrative into its constituent elements, interpreting the participant's intent of telling the story to reveal meaning, and constructing story function for both storyteller and listener from an emic perspective. The selected story was told by Mary during her participation in a study exploring mothering in the context of mental illness.

Case example

Like other participants in the study, Mary experienced enduring depression characterized by episodic exacerbation of symptoms. Amidst the accounts across the data base which detailed everyday experiences of mothering were depictions of escalating mental health challenges. As a group, these stories, that shared a common event, structure, function, and meaning were labelled "Just before the crisis." Mary's account is presented in Table 20.2.

Mary was diagnosed with depression as an adolescent. At the time of the interview, she was a young married mother of two healthy and energetic children under the age of 5. She lived with her children and her spouse of seven years at a distance from their extended families in subsidized housing within a rural community. As parents, Mary and her husband were committed to providing a stable and loving upbringing for their children. They both worked full-time in entry-level service industry jobs. With a meager combined income, they struggled to earn sufficient money to cover their daily expenses, purchase Mary's prescribed medications, save enough money for a downpayment on a home, purchase a family vehicle, and cover their rising credit debt.

As presented in Table 20.2, Mary's account is constituted by the inclusion of seven structural elements including: story stimulus, abstract, orientation, complicating action, evaluation, resolution and coda. Such a comprehensive presentation is not essential to the telling of a story; however, it assists the researcher in confirming the data's legitimacy as a complete story, and thus a credible unit of analysis within narrative inquiry. This particular unit of analysis is classified as a first-person event-specific limited genre story as it details a particular event experienced by Mary, the teller of the story, at one particular moment in time. Although commuting to work on public transportation was part of Mary's usual weekday routine, her experience on the bus ride recounted in this story was anything but typical. In essence, in a public venue, she privately experiences an escalation of her internal distress beyond what she can continue to independently manage.

Deconstruction of Mary's narrative allowed for the identification of four structural components (Table 20.2). The first component includes a recognition that illness "has gone too far" resulting

Table 20.2 "Just before the crisis story"

Story element	Story data	Structural components
Story stimulus	Interviewer: /your illness is showing itself	
Abstract/ Evaluation	Mary: /it has gone too far when I just don't know what to do anymore /like I'm [pause]/ I know it's too much /I know that I don't have much time left before I feel like I'm gonna completely be one of those people who are yellin' at people on the street	Impending sense of loss of control
Orientation	/it takes everything to be able to sit down and relax	Struggle to maintain composure
Complicating Action/Evaluation	/on the city bus /there's someone tappin' their fingers on the window /... it takes everything for me not to say "STOP IT" /you know /like /and I feel that soon that it's gonna happen /where I'm jus' gonna be /"like you are bugging me" /and you know	Heightened perceptual sensitivity
Evaluation	/and [I'm] just LOSING it	
Resolution	so then I just thought /"OK" /"something needs to be done now"	Urgency for action
Coda	/ "like RIGHT NOW"	

in an impending sense of loss of control. Further, she indicates her awareness that she doesn't "have much time left" to be well. She talks about how "it takes everything" she has to be able to maintain her composure in the midst of escalating symptoms of illness. Within this context, she has a heightened perceptual sensitivity. This is particularly bothersome as she identifies how seemingly inconsequential events, such as "someone tappin' their fingers on the window" in the bus, triggers disproportionately negative responses which contravene social conventions, such as yelling at strangers. Finally, she demonstrates insight into her vulnerability during the time period immediately before a crisis, identifying the urgent need for help to preserve her well-being. The structural composition of Mary's story aligns with all other stories about experiences "just before the crisis" across the dataset.

An initial interpretation of the essence of Mary's story further supports alignment with the "just before the crisis" story grouping. The meaning of her story is revealed in the evaluation element "and [I'm] just LOSING it," communicating that she has awareness of her diminishing control immediately prior to a crisis. She relates the essence of the recounted event not only through this text excerpt, but also discursive and rhetorical strategies such as direct quotations, repeated phrases, and variations in vocal volume. For Mary, and the other participants, these stories function to signal when they must seek help to preserve their wellness. A failure to attend to one's own sense of increasing loss of control, struggle to maintain composure, heightened perceptual sensitivity, and urgency for action may enable the unfolding of a crisis. For researchers, these stories function to develop an emic understanding of the phenomenon. Based on the interpreted function of these stories, practitioners are advised to attend to subtle cues suggestive of the need for immediate intervention. Health care professionals who engage women to allow for early disclosure of escalating illness symptoms concurrent with depleting adaptive resources may be best situated to intervene in a timely manner to preserve wellness and divert crisis. These stories thus have practical utility for both the storyteller and the listener.

Conclusion

Narrative inquiry has become prolific within nursing research over the last 20 years. This growth, however, is not matched by concurrent efforts to communicate the underlying methodological rigor. In this chapter we have argued for the differentiation of storytelling in everyday life and stories as units of analysis within narrative inquiry. Indeed, both have utility. To transform story beyond its colloquial use, however, the bond between stories and knowledge creation requires the explicit declaration and transparent demonstration of credible methodological processes.

References

Agar, M., & Hobbs, J. R. (1982). Interpreting discourse: Coherence and the analysis of ethnographic interviews. *Discourse Process*, *5*, 1–32.

Agar, M., & Hobbs, J. R. (1983). Natural plans: Using AI planning in the analysis of ethnographic interviews. *Ethos*, *11*, 33–48.

Altheide, D. L., & Johnson, J. M. (1994). Criteria for assessing interpretive validity in qualitative research. In N. L. Denzin, & Y. S. Lincoln (Eds.), *Handbook of qualitative research* (pp. 485–499). London: Sage.

Atkinson, P. (1997). Narrative turn or blind alley? *Qualitative Health Research*, *7*(3), 325–344.

Atkinson, P. (2005). Qualitative research: Unity and diversity. *Forum: Qualitative Social Research*, *6*(3), Art. 26.

Atkinson, P. (2009). Illness narrative revisited: The failure of narrative reductionism. *Sociological Research Online*. Retrieved from: http://www.socresonline.org.uk/14/5/16.html.

Atkinson, P. (2010). The contested terrain of narrative analysis: An appreciative response. *Sociology of Health & Illness*, *32*, 661–667.

Atkinson, P., & Delamont, S. (2006). Resulting narrative from qualitative research. *Narrative Inquiry*, *16*(1), 164–172.

Atkinson, P., & Silverman, D. (1997). Kundera's *Immortality*: The interview society and the intervention of the self. *Qualitative Inquiry*, *3*, 304–325.

Bailey, P. H. (1996). Assuring quality in narrative analysis. *Western Journal of Nursing Research*, *18*(2), 186–194.

Bailey, P. H. (2001). Death stories: Acute exacerbations of chronic obstructive pulmonary disease. *Qualitative Health Research*, *11*(3), 322–337.

Bailey, P. H. (2004). The dyspnea-anxiety-dyspnea cycle: COPD patients' stories of breathlessness: "It's scary/when you can't breathe." *Qualitative Health Research*, *14*(6), 760–778.

Bailey, P. H., & Tilley, S. (2002). Storytelling and the interpretation of meaning in qualitative research. *Journal of Advanced Nursing*, *38*(6), 574–583.

Benner, P. (1991). The role of experience, narrative, and community in skilled ethical comportment. *Advances in Nursing Science*, *14*(2), 1–21.

Benner, P., Sutphen, M., Leonard, V., & Day, L. (2010). *Educating nurses: A call for radical transformation*. San Francisco, CA: Jossey-Bass.

Benner, P., Tanner, C., & Chesla, C. (1992). From beginner to expert: Gaining a differentiated clinical world in critical care nursing. *Advances in Nursing Science*, *14*(3), 13–28.

Bennett, G. (1986). Narrative as expository discourse. *Journal of American Folklore*, *99*, 415–434.

Bochner, A. P. (2001). Narrative's virtues. *Qualitative Inquiry*, *7*(2), 131–157.

Bochner, A. P. (2010). Resisting the mystification of narrative inquiry: Unmasking the real conflict between story analysts and storytellers. *Sociology of Health & Illness*, *32*(4), 662–665.

Bowers, R., & Moore, K.N. (1997). Bakhtin, nursing narratives, and dialogical consciousness. *Advances in Nursing Science*, *19*(3), 70–77.

Brown, S. T., Kirkpatrick, M., Mangum, K. & Avery, J. (2008). A review of narrative pedagogy strategies to transform traditional nursing education. *Journal of Nursing Education*, *47*(6), 283–286.

Bruner, J. S. (1990). *Acts of meaning*, Cambridge, MA: Harvard University Press.

Bruner, J. S. (1991.) The narrative construction of reality. *Critical Inquiry*, *18*, 1–21.

Bruner, J. S. (2004). Life as narrative. *Social Research*, *71*(3): 691–710.

Clandinin, D. J., & Connelly, F. M. (1994). Personal experience methods. In N. L. Denzin & Y.S. Lincoln (Eds.), *Handbook of qualitative research* (pp. 413–427). London: Sage.

Clandinin, D. J. & Connelly, F. M. (2000). *Narrative inquiry: Experience and story in qualitative research.* San Francisco, CA: Jossey-Bass.

Coffey, A., & Atkinson, P. (1996). *Making sense of qualitative data: Complementary research strategies.* London: Sage.

Connelly, F. M. & Clandinin, D. J. (1986). On narrative method, personal philosophy, and narrative unities in the story of teaching. *Journal of Research in Science Teaching, 23*(4), 293–310.

Connelly, F. M. & Clandinin, D. J. (1990). Stories of experience and narrative inquiry. *Educational Researcher, 19*(5), 2–14.

Crisp, J. (1995). Making sense of the stories that people with Alzheimer's tell: A journey with my mother. *Nursing Inquiry, 2,* 133–140.

Del Vecchio Good, M., Munakata, T., Kobayashi, O., Mattingly, C., & Good, B. J. (1994). Oncology and narrative time. *Social Science & Medicine, 38*(6), 855–862.

Diekelmann, N. (2001). Narrative pedagogy: Heideggerian hermeneutical analysis of lived experiences of students, teachers, and clinicians. *Advances in Nursing, 23*(3), 53–71.

Diekelmann, N., & Scheckel. M. (2004). Teacher talk: new pedagogies for nursing. Leaving the safe harbor of competency-based and outcomes education: re-thinking practice education. *Journal of Nursing Education, 43*(9), 385–388.

Facione, N. C., & Dodd, M. J. (1995). Women's narratives of help seeking for breast cancer. *Cancer Practice, 3*(4), 219–225.

Fenton, M. V., & Brykczynski, K. A. (1993). Qualitative distinctions and similarities in the practice of clinical nurse specialists and nurse practitioners. *Journal of Professional Nursing, 9*(6), 313–326.

Fowler, S. (1992). A broken promise. *Nursing Times, 88*(45), 45.

Frank, A. W. (2000). The standpoint of the storyteller. *Qualitative Health Research, 10,* 354–365.

Frank, A. W. (2001). Can we research suffering? *Qualitative Health Research, 11,* 353–362.

Frank, A. W. (2010). In defence of narrative exceptionalism. *Sociology of Health and Illness, 32*(4), 665–667.

Gee, J. P. (1985). The narrativization of experience in the oral style. *Journal of Education, 167*(1), 9–35.

Gee, J. P. (1991). A linguistic approach to narrative. *Journal of Narrative and Life History, 1*(1), 15–39.

Gubrium, J. F., & Holstein, J. A. (2008). Narrative ethnography. In S. Hesse-Biber & P. Leavy (Eds.), *Handbook of emergent methods* (pp. 241–264). New York: The Guilford Press.

Gubrium, J. F., & Holstein, J. A. (2009). *Analyzing narrative reality.* Thousand Oaks, CA: Sage.

Hall, J. M. (1994). The experiences of lesbians in Alcoholics Anonymous. *Western Journal of Nursing Research, 16*(5), 556–576.

Heikkinen, R. L. (1993). Patterns of experienced aging with a Finnish cohort. *International Journal of Aging and Human Development, 36,* 269–277.

Heliker, D. M. (1997). A narrative approach to quality care in long-term care facilities. *Journal of Holistic Nursing, 15*(1), 68–81.

Hellzen, O., Norberg, G. A., & Sandman, P. O. (1995). Schizophrenic patients' image of their carers and the carers' image of their patients: An interview study. *Journal of Psychiatric and Mental Health Nursing, 2,* 279–285.

Hunt, L. M. (1994). Practicing oncology in provincial Mexico: A narrative analysis. *Social Science & Medicine, 38*(6), 843–853.

Ironside, P. M. (2006). Using narrative pedagogy: Learning and practicing interpretive thinking. *Journal of Advanced Nursing, 55*(4), 478–486.

Kalčik, S. (1975). ". . . like Ann's gynaecologist or the time I was almost raped": Personal narrative in women's rape groups. In C. R. Farrer (Ed.), *Women and folklore* (pp. 3–11). Austin: University of Texas.

Kermode, F. (1981). Secrets and narrative sequence. In W. J. T. Mitchell (Ed.), *On narrative* (pp. 79–97). Chicago: University of Chicago Press.

Kirkpatrick, H. (2008). A narrative framework for understanding experiences of people with severe mental illnesses. *Archives of Psychiatric Nursing, 22*(2), 61–68.

Kleinman, A. (1988). *The illness narrative: Suffering, healing and the human condition.* New York: Basic Books.

Kleinman, A. (1992). Local world of suffering: An interpersonal focus for ethnographies of illness experience. *Qualitative Health Research, 2*(2), 127–134.

Knafl, K. A., Ayres, L., Gallo, A. M., Zoeller, L. H., & Breitmayer, B. J. (1995). Learning from stories: Parents' accounts of the pathway to diagnosis. *Pediatric Nursing, 21*(5), 411–415.

Koch, T. (1998). Story telling: Is it really research? *Journal of Advanced Nursing, 28*(6), 1182–1196.

Koch, T., Turner, R., Smith, P., & Hutnik, N. (2010). Storytelling reveals the active, positive lives of centenarians. *Nursing Older People, 22*(8), 31–36.

Kralik, D., & Koch, D. (2003). "It's just the way I am": Life with schizophrenia. *Australian Journal of Holistic Nursing, 102*, 11–18.

Labov, W. (1972). *Language in the inner city: Studies in the Black English vernacular*. Philadelphia: University of Pennsylvania Press.

Labov, W., & Waletzky, J. (1972). Narrative analysis: Oral versions of personal experience. In J. Helms (Ed.), *Essays on the verbal and visual arts* (pp. 12–44). Seattle: University of Washington Press.

Langellier, K. M. (1989). Personal narratives: Perspectives on theory and research. *Text and Performance Quarterly, 9*(4), 243–276.

Mattingly, C. (1994). The concept of therapeutic "emplotment" . . . clinician and patient in the creation and negotiation of a plot structure within clinical time. *Social Science & Medicine, 38*(6), 811–822.

Mattingly, C., & Garro, L. C. (1994). Introduction: Narratives of illness and healing. *Social Science and Medicine, 38*(6), 771–774.

Mattingly, C., & Garro, L. C. (Eds.). (2011). *Narrative and the cultural construction of illness and healing*. Los Angeles: University of California Press.

Mathieson, C. M., & Stam, H. J. (1995). Renegotiating identity: Cancer narratives. *Sociology of Health & Illness, 17*(3), 283–306.

McGarvey, H., & Diekelmann, N. (1992). A way with words. *Nursing Times, 88*(45), 43.

Meleis, A. I., Arruda, E. N., Lane, S., & Bernal, P. (1994). Veiled, voluminous, and devalued: Narrative stories about low-income women from Brazil, Egypt, and Colombia. *Advances in Nursing Science, 17*(2), 1–15.

Mishler, E. G. (1979). Meaning in context: Is there any other kind? *Harvard Educational Review, 49*(1), 1–19.

Mishler, E. G. (1986). *Research interviewing context and narrative*. Cambridge, MA: Harvard University Press.

Mishler, E. G. (1990). Validation in inquiry-guided research: The role of exemplars in narrative studies. *Harvard Educational Review, 60*(4), 415–442.

Mishler, E. G. (2004). Historians of the self: Restorying lives, revisiting. *Research in Human Development, 1*(1&2), 1001–1021.

Mishler, E. G. (2005). Patient stories, narratives of resistance and the ethics of humane care: À la recherche du temps perdu. *Health, 9*(4), 431–451.

Monks, J., & Frankenberg, R. (1990). The presentation of self, body and time in the life stories and illness narratives of people with multiple sclerosis. Paper presented at the BSA Medical Sociology Conference, Edinburgh, Scotland.

Monks, J., & Frankenberg, R. (1995). "Being ill and being me": Self, body, and time in MS narratives. In B. Ingstad & S. Reynolds-White (Eds.), *Disability and culture*. Los Angeles: University of California Press.

Montgomery, P., Mossey, P., Bailey, P. H., & Forchuk, C. (2011). Mothers with serious mental illness: Their experience of "hitting bottom." *International Scholarly Research Network*, ID: 708318.

Personal Narratives Group (1989a). "Conditions not of her own making," In Personal Narratives Group (Ed.), *Interpreting women's lives: Feminist theory and personal narratives* (pp. 19–23). Bloomington: Indiana University Press.

Personal Narratives Group (1989b). Origins. In Personal Narratives Group (Ed.), *Interpreting women's lives: Feminist theory and personal narratives* (pp. 3–15). Bloomington: Indiana University Press.

Personal Narratives Group (1989c). Truths. In Personal Narratives Group (Ed.), *Interpreting women's lives: Feminist theory and personal narratives* (pp. 261–264). Bloomington: Indiana University Press.

Polkinghorne, D. E. (1988). *Narrative knowing and the human science*. Albany: State University of New York Press.

Polanyi, L. (1979.) So what's the point? *Semiotica, 25*(3–4), 207–241.

Polanyi, L. (1985). Conversational storytelling. In T. A. Van Dijk (Ed.), *Handbook of discourse analysis* (pp. 183–201). London: Academic Press.

Polanyi, L. (1989). *Telling the American story: A structural and cultural analysis of conversational storytelling*. London: MIT Press.

Polkinghorne, D. E. (1988). *Narrative knowing and the human science*. Albany: State University of New York Press.

Polkinghorne, D. E. (2007). Validity issues in narrative research. *Qualitative Inquiry, 13*(4), 471–486.

Ricoeur, P. (1981). Narrative time. In W. J. T. Mitchell (Ed.), *On narrative* (pp. 165–186). Chicago: University of Chicago Press.

Riessman, C. K. (1987). When gender is not enough: Women interviewing women. *Gender and Society, 1*(2), 172–207.

Riessman, C. K. (1988). Worlds of difference: Contrasting experience in marriage and narrative style. In A. D. Todd, & S. Fisher (Eds.), *Gender and discourse: The power of talk* (pp. 151–173). Norwood, NJ: Ablex Publishing Corporation.

Riessman, C. K. (1989) Life events, meaning and narrative: The case of infidelity and divorce. *Social Science and Medicine, 29*(6), 743–751.

Riessman, C. K. (1990). Strategic uses of narrative in the presentation of self and illness: A research note. *Social Science & Medicine, 30*, 1195–1200.

Riessman, C. K. (1991a). Personal troubles as social issues: A narrative of infertility in context. In I. Shaw & N. Gould (Eds.), *Qualitative research in social work* (pp. 73–82). Thousand Oaks, CA: Sage.

Riessman, C. K. (1991b). Beyond reductionism: Narrative genres in divorce accounts. *Journal of Narrative and Life History, 1*(1), 41–68.

Riessman, C. K. (1993). *Narrative analysis*. Newbury Park, CA: Sage.

Riessman, C. K. (1994). Narrative approaches to trauma. In C. K. Riessman (Ed.), *Qualitative studies in social work research* (pp. 67–71). London: Sage.

Riessman, C. K. (2003). Performing identities in illness narrative: Masculinity and multiple sclerosis. *Qualitative Research, 3*(1), 5–33.

Riessman, C. K. (2008). *Narrative methods for the human science*. Newbury Park, CA: Sage.

Riessman, C. K., & Mattingly, C. (2005). Introduction: Toward a context-based ethics for social research in health. *Health, 9*(4), 427–429.

Sacks, O. (1970). *The man who mistook his wife for a hat and other clinical tales*. New York: Touchstone.

Sakalys, J. A. (2000). The political role of illness narratives. *Journal of Illness Narratives, 31*(6), 1469–1475.

Sakalys, J. A. (2003). Restoring the patient's voice: The therapeutics of illness narratives. *Journal of Holistic Nursing, 21*(3), 228–241.

Sandelowski, M. (1991). Telling stories: Narrative approaches in qualitative research. *Image: Journal of Nursing Scholarship, 23*(3), 161–166.

Sandelowski, M., Holditch-Davis, D., & Harris, B. G. (1990). Living the life: Explanations of infertility. *Sociology of Health & Illness, 12*(2), 195–215.

Schiffin, D. (1994). *Approaches to discourse*. Oxford: Blackwell.

Scholes, R. (1980). Language, narrative, and anti-narrative. In W. J. Y. Mitchell (Ed.), *On narrative* (pp. 200–208). Chicago: University of Chicago Press.

Scholes, R., & Kellogg, R. (1966). *The nature of narrative*. London: Oxford University Press.

Smith, B. H. (1981). Afterthoughts on narrative. In W. J. T. Mitchell (Ed.), *On narrative* (pp. 207–231). Chicago: University of Chicago Press.

Stein, H. F. (1990). The story behind the clinical story: An inquiry into biomedical narrative. *Family Systems Medicine, 8*(2), 213–227.

Stevens, P. E. (1993). Marginalized women's access to health care: A feminist narrative analysis. *Advances in Nursing Science, 16*(2), 39–56.

Stevens, P. E. (1994). Lesbians' health-related experiences of care and noncare. *Western Journal of Nursing Research, 16*(6), 639–659.

Stevens, P. E. (1996). Struggles with symptoms: Women's narratives of managing HIV illness. *Journal of Holistic Nursing, 14*(2), 142–161.

Stevens, P. E., Hall, J. M., & Meleis, A. I. (1992). Examining vulnerability of women clerical workers from five ethnic/racial groups. *Western Journal of Nursing Research, 14*(6), 754–774.

Stewart, B. M. (1994). End-of-life family decision-making from disclosure of HIV through bereavement. *Scholarly Inquiry for Nursing Practice: An International Journal, 8*(4), 321–359.

Stivers, C. (1993). Reflections on the role of personal narrative in social science. *Signs: Journal of Women in Culture and Society, 18*(2), 408–427.

Tappan, M. B., & Brown, L. M. (1989). Stories told and lessons learned: Toward a narrative approach to moral development and moral education. *Harvard Educational Review, 59*(2), 182–205.

Tanner, C. A., Benner, P., Chesla, C., & Gordon, D. R. (1993). The phenomenology of knowing the patient. *Image: Journal of Nursing Scholarship, 25*(4), 273–280.

Thomas, C. (2010). Negotiating the contested terrain of narrative methods in illness contexts. *Sociology of Health & Illness, 32*(4), 647–660.

Thorne, S. (2008) *Interpretive description*. Walnut Creek, CA: Left Coast.

Thorne, S. (2009). Is the story enough? *Qualitative Health Research, 19*(9), 1183–1185.

Udén, G., Norberg, A., Lindseth, A., & Marhaugh, V. (1992). Ethical reasoning in nurses' and physicians' stories about care episodes. *Journal of Advanced Nursing, 17*, 1028–1043.

Vezeau, T. M. (1993). Storytelling: A practitioner's tool. *Maternal & Child Nursing, 18*, 193–196.

Viney, L. L., & Bousfield, L. (1991). Narrative analysis: A method of psychological research for AIDS-affected people. *Social Science and Medicine, 32*(7), 757–765.

White, H. (1981). The value of narrativity in the presentation of reality. In W. J. T. Mitchell (Ed.), *On narrative* (pp. 1–24). Chicago: University of Chicago Press.

Wiltshire, J. (1995). Telling a story, writing a narrative: Terminology in healthcare. *Nursing Inquiry, 2*, 75–82.

21

Discourse analysis

Michael Traynor

Introduction

A rumor went around the institution where I work, some while ago, that a tutor had told one of our Master's students who was working on a dissertation that she couldn't (read *shouldn't*) use discourse analysis when approaching the texts of mothers talking about their experience of childbirth. I don't know whether this actually happened but the implication was that there was a valuable realm of authentic experience that lay beyond the reach of discourse analysis. Some researchers hold assumptions that the overriding purpose of qualitative research is to investigate and bring to light the subjective experience of research participants. In reading articles which claim to be using a form of discourse analysis in nursing research journals, I have often sensed the influence of a kind of methodological gravity which is pulling down the trajectory of many articles. What starts off with strong methodological claims and reviews of discourse analytic theory ends up by reporting a series of themes derived from the meaning-making of participants and labeled "discourses." In addition to this specific problem a common-sense approach to human signification tends to focus on content rather than form, on meaning rather than structure. It is because of these problems that much of this chapter will focus on the *differences between* discourse analysis and most other qualitative research methods. Some readers, already familiar with discourse analysis, may find this emphasis unnecessary but I believe that in the context of this particular volume this is a good place to start. If you are not familiar with discourse analysis, I would recommend investigating it precisely because it presents a refreshing and sometimes radical alternative to other qualitative ways of doing research. As a former student of English literature, I find examining a text to see how it achieves its effect comes relatively naturally; however, I remember my astonishment when an experienced conversation analyst first demonstrated to me the structures and processes at work in "naturally occurring" conversation.

This chapter has three main parts: the first sets out the range of practices that go under the name of discourse analysis and discusses some of their different assumptions particularly about human subjectivity. It offers a simple typology of approaches. "Conversation analysis" is included in this discussion. Having set out this basic map, I will rehearse some of the debates, dilemmas and tensions within the field. The second section reviews the uptake of the various forms of discourse analysis by researchers in nursing and presents one particular example that I consider successful. The final section discusses the relationship between language and subjectivity by pushing into literature produced by writers including Julia Kristeva, Slavoj Žižek and Jacques Lacan, broadly, post-structuralist and psychoanalytic work. What I am not offering in this chapter is a recipe of "how to do" discourse analysis. Once the variety of different approaches to discourse analysis has been grasped, it will be clear why I am not doing this. In addition, it is far more important to have a sophisticated feel of the spirit and kind of thinking behind discourse analysis —in all its forms—than to know about and attempt to follow some procedures, or steps or stages, set out by any particular writer.

What are discourse analysis?

Please excuse my tortured grammar but there is plurality at work. Van Dijk in the introduction to *Discourse Studies* (van Dijk, 2006) writes: "Discourse Analysis is not a method of research, but a (cross) discipline" (p. 6). Van Dijk cannot even say it is anything as specific as a discipline. Taylor writes discourse analysis is best understood as a field of research rather than a single practice (Taylor, 2001). Most other writers who set out to introduce or describe discourse analysis inevitably start by talking about its broad scope and multidisciplinary origins. The fact that discourse studies have developed *in parallel* in different disciplines is both remarkably exciting and potentially bewildering. But before we grapple with the bewilderment, we need the starting point of a definition that is broad enough to include most if not all varieties of discourse analysis:

> Discourse analyses are investigations of *how* something is said or written (or performed in any other communicative way) not so much of *what it is* that is said or written. Its business is unearthing the mechanics of the text, *not* representing the life-world of those individuals who (appear to be) producing such a text.

Now we can return to the bewilderment. Discourse analysis has developed within different disciplines and though the practices of analysts within these different disciplines sometimes appear similar, they can be based on different theoretical assumptions and set out to contribute to different fields of knowledge, refer to different ranges of theorists, and answer particular questions specific to those disciplines. This can lead to confusion for the researcher who is unfamiliar with the field. In terms of involved disciplines, van Dijk draws attention to the "remarkably parallel developments in the humanities and social sciences between 1964 and 1974" (van Dijk, 2006, p. 1). According to his summary, anthropologists began to study communicative events, sociologists turned toward detailed analysis of interaction and conversation, linguists began to examine the situated text and talk of real language users, cognitive psychologists rediscovered the importance of knowledge and mental representations and their link with language production, social psychologists began to look at how discourse and interaction shaped reality and the mind while the field of communication studies, those who examined the mass media and political communication, had gradually taken on methods from discourse analytical and conversation analytical work.

Before summarizing two attempts at the categorization of different approaches to discourse analysis, it is worth pointing out to the uninitiated that it is the very process of devising systems of categorization that discourse analysis, or certain approaches within it, question. The founder of structural linguistics, Ferdinand de Saussure, writing in the late nineteenth century and early decades of the twentieth century, argued that language precedes the world, rather than the other way around; the language available to us determines how we are able to "carve up" the world, rather than simply describing what is already there. His evidence was the different language resources available to speakers of different languages. He claimed that both the linguistic sounds— the signifiers— and the mental concepts they referred to—signifieds—and their relationship to each other were in themselves arbitrary. They bear no relationship of equivalence to the world. What was important to language speakers, and the only thing that gives language its meaning, is the difference between the various signifiers. "Dog," for example, only comes to stand for our mental image of these animals because it is not "dig" or "dag." Language, therefore, was a formal system and words have their primary relationship to each other rather than to the non-linguistic world. Notes from the series of lectures on this topic, which de Saussure gave only three times towards the end of his life in 1913, were collated by his students and published as the *Course in General Linguistics* (de Saussure, 1974). His "structuralist" approach was taken up and adapted to different fields of inquiry such as anthropology, philosophy, literary studies and psychoanalysis and the lasting influence of de Saussure's ideas is perhaps stronger in these disciplines than in linguistics itself. His proposition had the radical effect of allowing subsequent thinkers to decenter the human subject and its intentions, because, as Roland Barthes was later to say, language makes people its slaves because it is only possible to speak about or conceive of what already exists in language. As he writes: "We do not see the power which is in speech because we forget that all speech is a classification, and that all classifications are oppressive" (Barthes, 1996, p. 365). It is the covert way that language makes particular constructions of the world appear natural that can be considered oppressive. But at this point there is no need to see particular groups or individuals behind the "oppressive" effect of language. This oppression is intrinsic to the structure of language. Though it may be exploited deliberately by certain groups, we inevitably participate in this oppression (and are ourselves "oppressed") simply by being speaking beings.

This is all by way of a warning that the following categorizations of the "varieties" of discourse analysis are not the only ones possible though they are intended to form a helpful introduction to the field.

In 2000, organizational researchers Mats Alvesson and Dan Karreman produced a discussion of some of the dilemmas facing discourse analytic researchers and readers of such research (Alvesson & Karreman, 2000) in organizational studies specifically, and social sciences more generally. I will save discussion of the problems that they raise for later. For now I want to draw on their representation of various approaches to discourse analysis as on two axes because that is how I intend to present it in this chapter. On one axis we can think of the "level" of discourse being attended to from the "micro" use in specific micro-contexts of an individual utterance or conversation, for example, to "mega" discourse—more or less standardized ways of conceptualizing certain phenomena at societal level. On the other axis is the extent to which discourse is understood as determining conceptualization, subjectivity and meaning, from being totally determining, at one end, to having very little or only very temporary effects at the other. As I mentioned above, many authors have offered categorizations of discourse analytic approaches and I want to leave this broad one floating in the background while I briefly describe another and then, with an impressive flourish, bring the two together. Stephanie Taylor proposes four models—what she calls "possible approaches"—of discourse analysis which I think can be understood as levels of focus (Taylor, 2001). Though the titles are my own, her four approaches are:

1 *"Identifying code": Language regularities and linguistics.* In this approach, analysts focus on the properties and structures of language, tending to work with formal experiments rather than "naturally occurring data." For example, Gillian Brown from the Research Centre for English and Applied Linguistics, at the University of Cambridge, UK asked one set of subjects to explain features and routes on a map to a second set of subjects, and tape recorded and analyzed the techniques of explanation (Brown, 1998).
2 *"Use and interaction": Conversation Analysis.* These studies feature investigations of language use in naturally occurring interactions with an attempt to bring to light the conventions that

any speaker is constrained by in ordinary conversation. Harvey Sacks, a sociologist who lectured at the University of California in the 1960s and 1970s, founded the practice of Conversation Analysis (CA). Sacks' intention was to build up a model of social life from an empirical understanding of actual linguistic events (Silverman, 1998) and in order to do this he identified a number of regular features of conversation which speakers attend to informally such as openings and closings, turn-taking and repairs (Sacks et al., 1974). He developed his work by means of an analysis of the tape recordings of a suicide counseling telephone service in Los Angeles. Although there are differences between his approach and ethnomethodology developed by Garfinkel (1967), Sacks, like Garfinkel, was concerned to investigate how people accomplish "being ordinary" in social life. He studied the local production of social order in great detail, building a "cumulative science of conversation" (Silverman, 1998, p. 41). Such an approach brings an increasing social context to the previous focus on language structure. The potential strength and interest of this kind of work are its close attention to actual text rather than to abstract "discourses" and its ability to bring to light features of interaction that are so taken-for-granted that they have become invisible.

3 *"Interpretive repertoires": Studies of particular activities.* The 1960s and 1970s also saw the development of studies of occupational groups and settings. This range of work focuses on how individuals develop, enact and maintain their membership of occupational—or other—groups in their talk and documentation and their "interpretive repertoires." Such studies may focus on the interaction between professionals and their clients (Atkinson & Heath, 1981; Drew & Heritage, 1992; Garfinkel, 1986; Marshall, 1994) or between different groups of professionals (Hughes, 1996; Traynor, 1996). Their characteristic focus is on talk-in-interaction "through which the daily working activities of many professionals and organizational representatives are conducted" (Drew & Heritage, 1992, p. 3). Language use is analyzed in particular social and cultural contexts rather than the context of particular interactions. Because of this locating of analysis within social and cultural contexts, this type of approach overlaps with the fourth.

4 *"Societal discursive practices": critical discourse analysis (CDA) and post-structuralism.* Taylor's fourth approach describes analyses which assume the "all-enveloping" character of discourse. This type of work investigates language use in the broadest of the four contexts. These analyses identify patterns of language and related practices and demonstrate how they constitute aspects of society and people within it. Such analysis submits "taken-for-granted" aspects of the social and natural world to historical and sociological analysis. In terms of the positioning of the analyst working within this approach, it is philosophically the most complex with obvious possibilities for fudging and self-contradiction. For example, Taylor talks about the language user as heavily constrained in their choice of language and action and "struggling" with their own social and cultural positioning but this is to see the individual as exercising some agency outside of or beyond discourse. For me, the full conclusion of the "all enveloping" view of discourse (i.e. that all that can be felt, thought or talked about has to already be available within language) leaves no place at all for a "freedom" to speak and act outside of discourse.

A slight diversion: some specific approaches

Before returning to our classification of different approaches within discourse analysis, I want to linger on some specific forms within Taylor's fourth approach as they are popular among researchers in nursing and offer particular theoretical interests.

The first is Critical Discourse Analysis or CDA. In the United Kingdom it has been associated with the work of Norman Fairclough and particularly his *Language and Power* (Fairclough, 2001a), first published in 1989. The focus of CDA has typically been on political topics such as the persuasive techniques apparent in the speeches of political leaders (for example, Fairclough, 2001c). Fairclough summarizes: "CDA is analysis of the dialectical relationships between discourse (including language but also other forms of semiosis, e.g. body language or visual images) and other elements of social practices" (Fairclough, 2001b, p. 231).

Fairclough's influential approach features the linking of close textual and sociological analysis (Fairclough, 2003) and focuses on issues of power, resistance and identity. For Fairclough and other practitioners of CDA, the hidden "oppression" of language must be linked to political domination, via ideology. French Marxist discourse analysts have argued that language has come to be structured in a way that closely corresponds to social and economic structures, hence the study of language can give authoritative insights into its ideological effects. The most notable name in this field is that of Michel Pêcheau who set out to empirically investigate ideological practices that were theorized by Louis Althusser (Pêcheau, 1995). Because of the link between the concept of ideology and sign-making, the importance of language and other forms of signification has been understood by Marxists since the early decades of the twentieth century and the reader who is interested is recommended to explore the archive pages of the website, www.marxists.org, where a number of important and surprisingly contemporary texts are translated into English, including Joseph Stalin's views about language. Marxism is highly critical of idealist philosophies, insisting that it is material conditions that determine the character of consciousness and of course the rest of social practice. Because of this, the critical discourse analyst will always attempt to link discourse with social and material practices and to understand discourse as such practice.

> Signs also are particular, material things; and, as we have seen, any item of nature, technology, or consumption can become a sign, acquiring in the process a meaning that goes beyond its given particularity. A sign does not simply exist as a part of reality—it reflects and refracts another reality . . . The domain of ideology coincides with the domain of signs. They equate with one another. Wherever a sign is present, ideology is present, too. *Everything ideological possesses semiotic value.*
>
> *(Vološhinov, 1929)*

A second popular label applied to published discourse analysis is "Foucauldian" discourse analysis. Michel Foucault was interested in the social and discursive practices that have contributed toward the formation of the human subject since the eighteenth century in Europe. His broad investigations are of institutions and practices of modern European government. For him, different institutions, for example, those concerned with penal and medical arrangements, became associated with systems of thought and kinds of statement-making that set out the boundaries for knowledge development at particular points in history. Foucault linked these to their practices for controlling and ordering populations through various forms of classification of individuals (Foucault, 1973, 1977). He proposed that at particular points during the eighteenth and nineteenth centuries, various discursive rules determined what could be said and by whom, i.e. linking knowledge with power. Foucault's use of the term discourse and the way he links this to the modern human subject involve a denial that there is an essential, unchanging core to human nature. The modern subject, he famously suggested, is like a figure sketched in sand, recently drawn and likely to be highly temporary. He argues that various liberal humanist political systems valorize the uniqueness of the individual as part of the process of ordering and controlling populations. Central to his project has been investigations of the points in history when it became possible to talk about "the individual" in this way (Foucault, 1973). Such critical anti-essentialist historical studies of the development of discourse have become known as genealogies, after the term was taken up in this way by Nietzsche.

Many contemporary pieces of research that comment on power relations describe themselves as Foucauldian. Although his *Archaeology of Knowledge* (Foucault, 1972) is seen as his "methods" text, it does not, unsurprisingly, set out a formal procedure so "Foucauldians" tend to identify with Foucault's particular interests rather than adopt recognizable and reproducible techniques.

The general approach of discourse analysis as sceptical of settled meanings has resonance with post-structuralist examinations of meaning, text and identity, sometimes linked with so-called "deconstruction." Deconstruction, originally associated with the philosophical and literary writing of Jacques Derrida (1930–2004) has been highly influential, though controversial, across literary theory, legal studies, psychoanalysis and other disciplines (Culler, 1997). For example, much contemporary literary criticism includes discussion of the possibility that: (1) language constitutes the world that it purports merely to describe; (2) the meaning of a text cannot be fixed, even by reference to the intention of its author and, (3) a text can be deconstructed by identifying the hierarchical oppositions upon which it relies (e.g. reason/emotion, serious/non-serious, central/peripheral) and that it is possible to reverse this hierarchy to produce a reading "against the grain" of a text's face-value or "official" reading (Norris, 1991; Derrida, 1976; Barry, 2002). In similar vein, discourse analysis has the potential to destabilize particular ideologies by showing, through close analysis of ideological claims, that alternatives are equally possible. For example, work on managerialism in the UK health service showed managers and nurses constructing hierarchical pairs to denigrate each other's activities (and identities) and enhance the importance of their own (Traynor, 1999).

As I sum up this section of the chapter, it is important to remember that attempts to categorize approaches to DA will be confounded by specific examples which combine elements from a number of "different" approaches. Sometimes the proponents of one particular approach exaggerate the differences between them in order to argue their corner.

I now bring these two systems, that of Alvesson and Karreman and Stephanie Taylor together in Figure 21.1. The approaches to discourse analysis remain represented on two axes, following Alvesson and Karreman. Axis A–D represents theoretical assumptions regarding the relationship between the individual and language. Position A. indicates a view of the human individual as having autonomous control over language which they employ to represent their thoughts. Position D. reflects the post-structuralist position of proposing that even human individuality is always a result of available ways of thinking and talking about the human subject, i.e. is an effect of discourse. Axis C–B sets out various foci of discourse analytic studies, from a focus on the competencies involved in conversation at B. to an understanding of language as a mechanism and reflection of ideology at C. In an attempt to represent the fact that analysts who are concerned with the constraints on possibilities of identity of discourse may well also emphasize political and other social structures within their analysis (Chouliaraki &Fairclough, 1999), the two axes are not orthogonal. In a similar way analyses that focus on the characteristics of successful communication tend not to question understandings of the autonomous self and its mastery over language (Brown, 1998).

To add to the detail of the conceptualization, four boxes numbered 1–4, based on Taylor's (2001) four broad approaches, are superimposed upon the first schema in appropriate positions.

Debates, dilemmas and tensions in the field

Two of the main debates within the field or, rather, certain segments of the field, foreshadowed in the schematization detailed above, concern the relationship of "discourse" to the non-discursive realm and the relationship between the "agency" of discourse and human agency. In a response to a subsequent paper by Alvesson and Karreman (2011), Rick Iedema summarizes

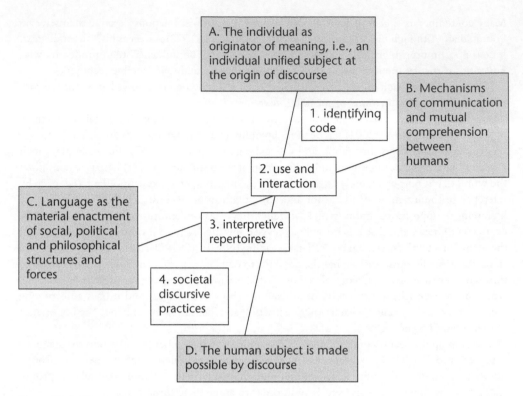

Figure 21.1 Dimensions of discourse analysis

Source: Based on Alvesson and Karreman (2000) and Taylor (2001). Reproduced by kind permission of the *Journal of Advanced Nursing.*

the main aspects of the first problem (Iedema, 2011). First, he says, "the field does not come as text" (p. 1). Interview transcripts cannot bring into the frame the materialities of "pre-discursive" emotions, energies, resistance to discourse and historical contexts of their production. This argument is also made by Bargiela-Chiappini in her own response to the same paper (Bargiela-Chiappini, 2011). In fact, she argues, there is an uneasy border between text, as focus of study, and "context" which lies beyond the text and runs the danger of being excluded from study or at least marginalized. So, there is anxiety among some analysts that discourse analysis can sometimes claim too much for the role of "discourse" in providing the key to understanding social and political situations at the expense of material factors. Iedema's text is full of the search for a "pre-discursive," a-signifying world, of affect perhaps that discourse cannot encompass. Turning to the second, related, problem, Iedema takes issue with the seductive phrase "discourse constitutes the real" (2011, p. 6). With the basis for this agency ascribed to discourse inadequately defined, he argues that this is too often taken as a starting assumption for researchers when it should be a problem to be investigated. Both of these problems question the limits of social constructionism and call on discourse analysts to be far more thorough when making such claims. However, in practice, it is not uncommon for analysts, including Iedema, to withdraw from such unequivocal positions and instead offer understandings of the relationship between the agency of humans and the "agency" of discourse where the individual is left, in some form or other, to "choose" or "use" or "have skill in" discourses. For example, in her investigation of teamwork and professional divisions in operating theaters, Finn, in her Introduction claims:

> Social actors are creative and strategic in their use of language as a resource, trying to invoke particular versions of the world that suit their interests in particular contexts, in ways that appear plausible, legitimate and factual.
>
> *(Finn, 2008, p. 109)*

Much discourse analysis, critical discourse analysis and ethnomethodology, even though it talks of "performing" identity rather than accepting essentialist views of the self, still implies a unquestioned self at the heart of decisions, even if habitual or highly constrained, about such performances. At the end of this chapter I will talk about work that has developed from a philosophical tradition that is radically critical of this view of the human individual. It is important to understand that different theoretical and operational orientations give rise to different "problems." "Organizational" discourse analysts are applying discourse analysis to enable them to find out "what's really happening" in the organization, while social psychologists will have different concerns (see the final section discussing Pavon Cuellar's arguments with "mainstream" social psychology). I will now present a brief review of discourse analytic studies on topics of relevance to nursing. Many of these display the inconsistencies and weaknesses discussed above.

Discourse analysis in use in nursing research

A search of PubMed in August 2011 using search terms "nurs★" and "discourse" and "analysis" for articles published in English between the years 1991 and 2010 produced 256 hits after false positives were eliminated after reading the abstracts of articles. There is a clear upward trend in articles identified over this time period with 54 being published from 1991 to 2000 compared with 202 between 2001 and 2010. Among these are two reviews of discourse analytic papers published in nursing journals. These are one article by me (Traynor, 2006) and one by Niels Buus (Buus, 2005).

Buus identified papers by searching CINAHL using the thesaurus terms ("'discourse analysis' and 'nurs★'") limited to journal articles in English published between 1996 and 2003 and, after removing inappropriate papers, reviewed 74 articles. Buus found that in 34 of these studies, the object of analysis was previously published text, interview transcripts were used to construct text for analysis in 32 studies and in 14 studies interaction or conversation was analyzed. He argued that as the interview data were not studied in terms of social interactions, the choice of data used in these studies reflected a preference for studying the social through textual analyses rather than through real-time social interaction and practice. He described most articles as "front heavy," i.e. presentations of the theoretical approaches to discourse were lengthy and of high theoretical density. In most of the articles containing a definition of discourse, he found the emphasis was on the functions of discourse rather than on formal characteristics of discourse. Discourse was most often conceptualized as patterns of representation and as linked to social practice. The unit of analysis, in other words, of how the actual object of analysis was delineated, was often inadequately described or appeared to be constructed in some common-sense way. Claimed links between the words of informants and "underlying" discourses were often speculative. Buus found in the analyses confusion between topic "themes" and linguistic categories such as "discourses." He noted many references to Michel Foucault's work, either in the form of his theories of power/knowledge and discourse or his concepts were used to contextualize findings; for example, discourses of surveillance or notions of subjectification. He commented that this particular theorist's influence was so powerful that the categories from an inductive analysis were constructed as exact matches to his concepts, therefore functioning as a reification of Foucault's concepts.

My review focused on one prominent generalist nursing journal, the *Journal of Advanced Nursing* so includes only a proportion of published studies in all journals. Using the search term "discourse analysis," 41 papers were identified from the Blackwell Synergy electronic database between 1996 and the time of the review, October 2004. Some 17 papers were excluded which were book reviews, replies, editorials or research papers and which did not state that they used discourse analysis. Apart from five published in 2003 and four in 2000, the number appearing in any one year was between one and three. Fifteen were from authors with a UK or Ireland address, seven from Australasia and one from the United States of America. All of the authors appeared to use discourse analysis in order to reveal influences on the character of nursing or its practices or education. The approaches ranged from a focus on individual nurse–patient interaction to "nursing discourse" or "contemporary discourse" at the most general level. Most authors declared an orientation to critical discourse analysis or a slightly differently worded description of a critical project. All but one of the papers described some aspect of the theoretical foundations of discourse analysis, although this varied greatly in length and emphasis, some providing little detail. Six authors stated that they used Foucauldian discourse analysis, or referred to his ideas about discourse while five stated that they used discourse analysis alongside another method, or methods. Central to discourse analysis is the demonstration of the operation of discourse within the talk or text under analysis; however, apart from two notable exceptions (Adams, 2000; Hardin, 2003), it was rare that authors provided the reader with a close analysis of their material. I will return to Adams' paper in a moment. This lack of visible discourse analysis and reliance on identification of themes characterized approximately half of the papers. Such thematic analysis is a characteristic of any broadly qualitative research method. As Alvesson and Karreman point out, an interest in discourse can signal a "started but not completed linguistic turn" where other phenomena such as ideas or meanings are included within the term (Alvesson & Karreman, 2000, p. 1129).

So, Niels Buus and I, in partially overlapping reviews, both found considerable interest in discourse analysis among the authors of nursing research often linked, on the part of the authors, to a desire to investigate the operation of various sources of power on nurses and their work. However, such research did not always reveal close analysis of sources or clarity about links between "discourses" and social practices. Since these reviews, as I have pointed out, nearly 150 papers have been published claiming to apply discourse analysis to a nursing topic and an updated review is called for.

I mentioned a paper by Trevor Adams and I want to briefly summarize why I think it is a good example of a discourse analytic paper. First, the author focuses the paper on one specific text—the transcription of a complaint made by the carer of a patient with severe dementia in a conversation with a psychiatric nurse responsible for her care—rather than some unspecified "discourse" which operates in a distant and shadowy way. We have the lengthy transcript to allow us to interrogate the author's analysis and judge how convincing it is. The analysis focuses in part on "identities" taken up by the carer—what some have referred to as "subject positions"— and how these frame and to an extent justify the criticisms subtly made. These claims spring from a close examination of the text. The author contextualizes the findings within the context of policy of the time which encouraged "shared decision-making" between people with dementia, their carers and professionals involved, showing an example of how "shared decision-making" can be achieved. Finally, the analysis is prefaced by a review of ethnomethodological views of identity construction in talk. Such consistency between the theoretical orientation announced in the review and methods sections and the practice of the analysis is surprisingly rare in the collection of papers reviewed.

Future directions: discourse, language and subjectivity

I want to end this chapter by showing how the concerns and theoretical position related to certain approaches to discourse analysis provide a gateway to a field of inquiry that, like discourse analysis, foregrounds the structuring effects of language on the human psyche and human activity. The links between discourse analysis and some varieties of psychoanalytic theory are complex, but close. From a post-structuralist point of view, we have already heard Barthes saying we are "slaves" to language because it determines, generally without our realizing it, what we can say and conceive of. Such claims can be seen as part of a tradition of European philosophy that includes the work of German philosophers Friedrich Hegel (1770–1831) and Nietzsche (1844–1900) that questions the reality of the individual as autonomous and fully conscious to itself. The notion of the unconscious, first systematically investigated by Sigmund Freud (1856–1939), radically undermines this version of the human psyche with the claim that the individual has a dimension to their own being that is inaccessible to themselves and beyond their control. However, it was Jacques Lacan (1901–1981) who famously brought structuralist linguistics to bear on Freud's psychoanalytic theory and founded a new approach to understanding the human psyche. In line with much post-structuralist thinking, Lacan's human subject was not the unified Cartesian self who surveys the world around him but a fragmented subject haunted by a sense of loss. He proposed an understanding of the unconscious as "the discourse of the Other," that is, society's system of signification, and particularly language, that inescapably has a structuring effect upon us as subjects and over which we have no ultimate control (Lacan, 1980). According to Sean Homer, Lacan's "big Other" is "the symbolic order, that foreign language that we are born into and must learn to speak if we are to articulate our own desire." The unconscious can be understood as the "discourse of the Other" in as far as "we are condemned to speak our desire through the language and desires of others" (Homer, 2005, p. 70). As the developing infant acquires language, it cannot but be positioned by the fundamental system of separating classifications intrinsic to language: me/other, man/woman, etc. The term subjectivity has been used by Lacan and those working alongside and after him, such as Julia Kristeva, to explain people's relationship to language—language produces speaking beings who are its subjects (McAfee, 2004). Kristeva has particularly explored the implications of broadly Lacanian thought to topics widely discussed by feminists, for example, explorations of sexual difference, motherhood (Kristeva, 1996) and the question of whether there can be masculine and feminine language. However, she has been much criticized by some feminists. For example, Nancy Fraser has accused her of developing her own essentialist stereotype of femininity (Fraser, 1992).

Lacan's work has been discussed and, in combination with Hegelian and Marxist concerns, applied to a number of contemporary political and cultural problems and events by Slovenian philosopher and psychoanalyst Slavoj Žižek. Žižek makes it clear that his analyses are very different to discourse analysis, informed as they are by a psychoanalytic critique of "subject positions," for example (Žižek, 2005). His readings of film, as an example of cultural object, feature a level of critique, wit and understanding of the context and style of production that makes some "discourse analysis" of such artifacts dull and irrelevant by comparison as they slavishly follow a codified and uninspired system of analysis and entirely fail to conceive of the sophistication in individuals' interactions with such artifacts.

Finally, Pavon Cuellar, in a book edited by Ian Parker, whose own early initiatives in discourse analysis and critiques of traditional social psychology are much cited by discourse analysts, interrogates the relationship between discourse analysis in social psychology and Lacanian psychoanalysis (Pavon Cuellar et al., 2010). His detailed examination and re-examination of a political speech by a Mexican revolutionary fighter provide his running example. For him, the symbolic world—the realm of language and signifying practice—has a radical primacy over the realm of the imaginary. Language, he argues, is open to analysis in a way that the realm of the imagination is not. When his revolutionary uses the word "pillar" in his political statement, "his" "pillar" and the "pillar" in the reader's imagination may be broadly similar but are not the same, however, the *word* "pillar" will always be identical to itself, the identity of any word to itself along with its difference to other words (as you will remember) being the key feature of language according to structuralist linguistics. Pavon Cuellar's title *From the Conscious Interior to an Unconscious Exterior* describes the contrast between conventional psychology and Lacanian psychoanalysis.

Conclusion

In this chapter we have taken, hopefully together, quite a journey. My starting point was that discourse analysis can present a problem to researchers who are steeped in an unwitting—or witting—allegiance to humanist assumptions. I have tried to make clear that across the breadth of discourse analytic practices, some are inconsistent with such assumptions. Nearly every writer on discourse analysis comments that the field is complex and goes on to present a system for understanding the differences within it. I have added my own here which is based on two of the most useful classifications that I am aware of, though I have reminded the reader that any way of carving up the world, or anything in it, is done more for convenience than as an innocent reflection of how things are. I have not taken the time to mention that the field is fractional, not so much in terms of explicit disagreement and conflict between the champions of different approaches, but through silence and omission. Something of the longstanding split between Anglo-Saxon and Continental philosophy is at work here,[1] with some writers who operate more or less in one tradition conspicuously failing to cite the work of theorists from the other even though they clearly have relevance. This omission is possibly the most confusing thing for the researcher who is naïve to the field. I have outlined some of the debates engaged in by some who practise discourse analysis partly simply to rehearse them but partly to emphasize that any (interesting) practice is far from settled and perfectly codified and that difference of opinion characterizes any non-moribund research area. I have very briefly discussed the uptake of various forms of discourse analysis by those presenting research to do with nursing. Drawing on a paper by Buus and my own review, I noted that critical and Foucauldian approaches have been the most popular but that the approaches were often applied inconsistently with definitions of "discourses" and how they might operate often only vaguely specified. But these reviews need updating. I pointed to one particular paper from the earlier review where the author adopted a type of discourse analysis successfully. I ended by pointing to a field of theoretical literature with connections to discourse analysis that I believe offers an exciting though challenging basis for further research focusing on language and subjectivity.

Note

1   If by any chance you are not familiar with this divide, see Simon Critchley's highly readable *Continental Philosophy* (2001).

References

Adams, T. (2000). The discursive construction of identity by community psychiatric nurses and family members caring for people with dementia. *Journal of Advanced Nursing, 32*, 791–798.

Alvesson, M., & Karreman, D. (2000). Varieties of discourse: on the study of organisations through discourse analysis. *Human Relations*, *53*, 1125–1149.

Alvesson, M., & Karreman, D. (2011). Decolonializing discourse: Critical reflections on organizational discourse analysis. *Human Relations*, *64*, 1121–1146.

Atkinson, P., & Heath, C. (Eds.). (1981). *Medical work: Realities and routines*. Farnborough: Gower.

Bargiela-Chiappini, F. (2011). Discourse(s), social construction and language practices: In conversation with Alvesson and Kärreman. *Human Relations*, *64*, 1177–1191.

Barry, P. (2002). *Beginning theory. An introduction to literary and cultural theory*. Manchester: Manchester University Press.

Barthes, R. (1996). Inaugural lecture at the Collège de France. In R. Kearney & M. Rainwater (Eds.), *The continental philosophy reader*. London: Routledge.

Brown, G. (1998) *Speakers, listeners and communication: Explorations in discourse analysis*. Cambridge: Cambridge University Press.

Buus, N. (2005). Nursing scholars appropriating new methods: The use of discourse analysis in scholarly nursing journals, 1996–2003. *Nursing Inquiry*, *12*, 27–33.

Chouliaraki, L., & Fairclough, N. (1999). *Discourse analysis in late modernity: Rethinking critical discourse analysis*. Edinburgh: Edinburgh University Press.

Critchley, S. (2001). *Continental philosophy. A very short introduction*. Oxford: Oxford University Press.

Culler, J. (1997). *Literary theory: A very short introduction*. Oxford: Oxford University Press.

Derrida, J. (1976). *Of grammatology*. Baltimore, MD: Johns Hopkins University Press.

De Saussure, F. (1974). *Course in general linguistics*. London: Fontana.

Drew, P., & Heritage, J. (Eds.). (1992). *Talk at work: Interaction in institutional settings*. Cambridge: Cambridge University Press.

Fairclough, N. (2001a). *Language and power*. Harlow: Pearson Education.

Fairclough, N. (2001b). The dialectics of discourse. *Textus*, *14*, 231–242.

Fairclough, N. (2001c). The discourse of New Labour: Critical discourse analysis. In M. Wetherell, S. Taylor, & S. Yates. (Eds.), *Discourse as data: A guide for analysis*. London; Sage/Open University Press.

Fairclough, N. (2003). *Analyzing discourse: Textual analysis for social research*. London: Routledge.

Finn, R. (2008). The language of teamwork: Reproducing professional divisions in the operating theatre. *Human Relations*, *61*, 103–130.

Foucault, M. (1972). *The archaeology of knowledge*. London: Routledge.

Foucault, M. (1973). *The birth of the clinic*. London: Tavistock.

Foucault, M. (1977). *Discipline and punish*. Harmondsworth: Penguin.

Fraser, N. (1992). The uses and abuses of French discourse theorists for feminist politics. In N. Fraser & S. Lee Bartky (Eds.), *Revaluing French feminism: Critical essays on difference, agency and culture*. Bloomington: Indiana University Press.

Garfinkel, H. (1967). *Studies in ethnomethodology*. Englewood Cliffs, NJ: Prentice Hall.

Garfinkel, H. (Ed.). (1986). *Ethnomethodological studies of work*. London: Routledge & Kegan Paul.

Hardin, P. K. (2003). Constructing experience in individual interviews, autobiographies and on-line accounts: A poststructuralist approach. *Journal of Advanced Nursing*, *41*, 536–544.

Homer, S. (2005). *Jacques Lacan*. London: Routledge.

Hughes, D. (1996). NHS managers as rhetoricians: A case of culture management? *Sociology of Health & Illness*, *18*, 291–314.

Iedema, R. (2011). Discourse studies in the 21st century: A response to Mats Alvesson and Dan Kärreman's "Decolonializing discourse." *Human Relations*, *64*, 1163–1176.

Kristeva, J. (1996). Women's time. In R. Kearney & M. Rainwater (Eds.), *The continental philosophy reader*. London: Routledge.

Lacan, J. (1980). *Ecrits/Jacques Lacan: A selection translated from the French by Alan Sheridan*. London: Tavistock.

Marshall, H. (1994). Discourse analysis in an occupational context. In C. Cassell & G. Symon (Eds.), *Qualitative methods in organisational research*. London: Sage.

McAfee, N. (2004). *Julia Kristeva*. London: Routledge.

Norris, C. (1991). *Deconstruction: Theory and practice*. London: Routledge.

Pavon Cuellar, D., Carlo, D., & Parker, I. (2010). *From the conscious interior to an exterior unconscious: Lacan, discourse analysis, and social psychology*. London: Karnac Books.

Pêcheau, M. (1995). *Automatic discourse analysis*. Amsterdam: Rodopi.

Sacks, H., Schegloff, E., & Jefferson, G. (1974). The simplest systematics for the organisation of turn-taking in conversation. *Language*, *50*, 697–735.

Michael Traynor

Silverman, D. (1998). *Harvey Sacks: Social science and conversation analysis*. Cambridge: Cambridge University Press.

Taylor, S. (2001). Locating and conducting discourse analytic research. In M. Wetherell, S. Taylor, & S. Yates (Eds.), *Discourse as data: A guide for analysis*. London: Sage/Open University Press.

Traynor, M. (1996). A literary approach to managerial discourse after the NHS reforms. *Sociology of Health and Illness, 18*, 315–340.

Traynor, M. (1999). *Managerialism and nursing: Beyond profession and oppression*. London: Routledge.

Traynor, M. (2006). Discourse analysis: Theoretical and historical overview and review of papers in the *Journal of Advanced Nursing*, 1996–2004. *Journal of Advanced Nursing, 54*, 62–72.

Van Dijk, T. A. (Ed.). (2006). *Discourse studies: A multidisciplinary introduction*. London: Sage.

Vološhinov, V. N. (1929). Marxism and the philosophy of language. In *Marxism and the Philosophy of Language*. New York: Seminar Press, in liaison with the Harvard University Press and the Academic Press Inc., 1973.

Žižek, S. (2005). Beyond discourse analysis. In *Interrogating the real* (pp. 271–284). London: Continuum.

22

Interpretive description

Sally Thorne

Introduction

Interpretive description is a qualitative research approach that draws upon the philosophical structure of applied disciplinary knowledge for its interior logic and design decisions. It was first articulated in 1997 in response to the expressed wish of many qualitative nurse researchers to break free of the constraints imposed by conventional qualitative methodological orthodoxies and restrictions in order to more effectively build the kind of knowledge their discipline required. This chapter describes the origins and development of an applied methodological approach explicitly designed to capitalize on the angle of vision that nursing brings to the rigorous qualitative study of the kinds of complex human health concerns that are inherent to its disciplinary mandate.

Rationale for a disciplinary approach to qualitative inquiry

In order to position an understanding of why a credible and rigorous new approach was needed, it is instructive to remind ourselves of the world of health science in which qualitative nursing research emerged. Around 1980, when nurses first began to explore the possibilities of a non-quantitative paradigm of formal research, they were striving for credibility within a highly biomedically oriented health science environment. In those early days, when generic description was understood as a prelude to method and not method itself in health science research, borrowing a formal (i.e., named) methodological tradition from their social science colleagues was a strategic way for nurses to justify the scholarliness of their qualitative inquiry projects. However, eventually, that affinity for social science credibility came back to bite them. Because they typically had to modify some aspects of the methods and techniques that had been designed to suit the demands of other disciplines in order to really get at the kinds of questions that concern nurses, their scholarly products were vulnerable to being judged by the disciplines claiming ownership over the methods as lacking (Thorne, 2001). Thus, qualitative nursing research was caught in a considerable predicament between methodological traditions imperfectly suited to the unique features of nursing's "ways of knowing."

Unlike the social sciences, which essentially exist to theorize, nursing theorizes in order to act. It is in the nature of nursing knowledge to expect that any idea worth having might potentially be taken up in a practice context, influencing human experiences in ways that enact the moral agency of the professional practice (Pesut & Johnson, 2013; Rodney et al., 2011; Sellman, 2011). Nursing knowledge inherently and unambiguously reflects a dialectic between the general and the particular (Reed, 2006; Rolfe, 2011). Knowledge in the general exists not to control, or to claim truths, but to inform the complex and individualized considerations that application to practice always entails. The thought structure of nursing seeks not to codify human universals, but rather to know how to apply generalities within an infinite variety of unique cases (Thorne & Sawatzky, 2007). And it is the professional responsibility of the nurse researcher to recognize and account for that practice world in which the ideas generated on the basis of research may have impact (Thorne, 2008). Thus, it seems natural that certain elements of the way thoughtful nurses wanted to build knowledge would depart from the methodological rule structures that were invented toward an entirely different purpose.

Method as logic model in an applied context

Whether they formalize it in a nursing framework or work more generally from a conceptual scheme such as the nursing process, the work of all nursing follows a kind of logic model. In a dynamic and cyclical manner, it engages, assesses, interprets, plans, acts and evaluates. It can be characterized as inherently complex and messy, dealing with an infinite range of possible variables that may enter into relevance from time to time. No matter how extensive our general knowledge of a phenomenon, we cannot enter into a case of it with absolute confidence in which variables are likely to come into play, and we cannot assume that, because we have seen something like it before, we know what to do with it. So nursing always works with the question of generalities, because we do require textbook knowledge, but with the understanding that general claims must be framed as amenable to the variance of the practice context.

In the more population-based or theoretical worlds, it suffices and serves the purpose to focus upon commonalities, sometimes even obscuring and ignoring differences. It may seem a subtle difference, but it is one that is highly important to this discussion, that nurses whose sights are too firmly fixed on the search for commonalities may lose their way with regard to their disciplinary logic. Similarly, nurses who become too confident in any one way of understanding a phenomenon run the risk of becoming overly narrow in their thinking. In the more postmodern/poststructural tradition of scholarship, deconstruction helps reveal the implications of particular ways of considering phenomena (Kagan, Smith, Cowling, & Chinn, 2009). However, unfettered critical reflection for its own sake defeats the fundamental purpose of a practice discipline, making it difficult to land upon any justification for action (Munhall, 2012). While these quite distinct inquiry techniques can make an important contribution to disciplinary knowledge, I would argue that the good nurse researcher who understands his or her disciplinary tradition will always have the intellectual proclivities of a nursing target audience in mind, such that in the shape and form of the research we can discern awareness of and respect for that ultimate practice mandate (Cheek, 2000). In other words, the nursing disciplinary mind never truly accepts standardization; it always seeks to ensure that there is room for necessary variation. It never rests with indulgence in the esoteric; it always envisions directionality. And because it never stops at the simple telling, but is always drawn toward the "so what," the term "interpretive description" was coined as a legitimizing maneuver to justify a range of solid and rigorous approaches to qualitative methodological application that draw heavily on the distinctive attributes and logical form of nursing knowledge (Thorne, Reimer-Kirkham, & MacDonald-Emes, 1997).

Overview of use within nursing research

Having entered the methodological lexicon at a time when many applied researchers were straining to find language to defend the design variations they required to tackle many of their disciplinary questions in an intelligent manner, interpretive description has been enthusiastically take up by researchers in such fields as public health (Kenny & Duckett, 2004; O'Connor, 2007), human kinetics (Clark, Spence, & Holt, 2011), clinical medicine (Davison & Simpson, 2006), gerontology (O'Connor, 2007) and integrative medicine (Mulkins & Verhoef, 2004) to name a few. Within nursing, it has been used to draw attention to particular features of human health experiences such as bereavement (Koop & Strang, 2003) or uncertainty (Oliffe, Davison, Pickles, & Mróz, 2009) as they are explained by those affected. It has been applied to the work of sensitizing practitioners to the complexities inherent in patient experience associated with specific clinical contexts and conditions, such as understanding symptoms before, during and after treatment for lymphoma (Johansson, Wilson, Brunton, Tishelman, & Molassiotis, 2010), managing chemotherapy-induced peripheral neuropathy (Bakitas, 2007), or coping with therapeutic isolation associated with thyroid cancer treatment (Stajduhar et al., 2006). It has also been used as a means to stimulate reflection upon the complex nature of enacting nursing practice in diverse contexts, such as the complexities of communicating with culturally and linguistically diverse clients (Cioffi, 2003), or enacting the moral obligations inherent in intensive care nursing (Cronqvist, Theorell, Burns, & Lützén, 2004). In general, it has been of particular relevance in discerning and making sense of patterns and variations across the beliefs, attitudes and opinions that persons with various conditions may bring to a particular care situation the ways they make sense of and manage the indignities and complexities of illness, and to expand a professional imagination about ways of being, thinking, feeling and acting when one is confronted with various health challenges. In this manner, by bringing illustrative exemplars to light within the context of human variation, it helps to guide nurses in their capacity to contextualize disease within the experiential, spiritual, sociocultural and geopolitical worlds of human living.

An important attribute of interpretive description is that it implies no attachment to being singularly responsible for method. Just as nursing shamelessly borrows and skillfully adapts any available theory that seems to show promise for solving the problems of practice, interpretive description explicitly celebrates the wealth of research technique that may be extracted and extrapolated from the extant methodical traditions. If it makes sense for a nurse scholar in the context of a particular inquiry project to draw inspiration from Spradley's ethnographic interviewing guidance (Spradley, 1979), Strauss and Corbin's basic approach to grounded theory coding technique (Strauss & Corbin, 1990) and Colaizzi's global steps for phenomenological data analysis (Colaizzi, 1978), and these elements of technique can be credibly explained within a coherent logic model that serves the discipline, then interpretive description can serve as referee, running interference against the challenges of methodological purists. Claiming interpretive description as the methodological underpinning of a study does not sentence the researcher to prescriptive method, but rather frees the applied research mind to do—and to defend—good scholarship.

Design options and approaches

As will be evident from these preliminary comments, interpretive description implies no fixed design elements. However, in that there is quite a solidly coherent intellectual structure to a discipline such as nursing (as is the case for other disciplines in which it is also being taken up as a useful method), there often are familiar features between the various kinds of studies claiming interpretive description as method. These are depicted here to provide suggestions, not limits, on the possible ways that good nursing minds can approach important nursing questions.

Articulating a research question

The form and structure of a qualitative research questions betray a lot about the assumptive base that the researcher is taking into the study. When a question is expressed as "What is the lived experience of . . .?" we are drawing from a phenomenological position having to do with "essential" elements of being human (van Manen, 1990). Similarly a question expressed as "What is the process of . . .?" signals the perspective derived from the symbolic interactionist heritage of grounded theory methodology that the socially constructed self, not the self accessible to conscious thought, explains why patients act as they do (Pascale, 2011). Since the mind driven by a nursing logic takes care never to understand all patients as experiencing something in a particular manner, and values patients' perspectives on their situation, the very launching point for the research sets up a tension within the study that makes it difficult to meet both masters. For this reason, interpretive description studies are typically set up in a syntax that reflects what the discipline might wonder. Questions beginning with: "What are the common ways in which patients experience . . .?," "How do patients describe their experience with . . .?" "What kinds of experiences with . . .?" are more generically reflective of the kind of knowledge domains that will draw meaning from interpretation among and between patient accounts and allow for both pattern recognition and variance detection throughout the research process.

Theoretical and positional scaffolding

The notion that all research must be positioned within a specific theoretical tradition is one that derives from the conventions that have emerged in the formalization of scientific method within the Western tradition. Because of a deeply held mistrust of subjectivity, theory operates within that tradition as the link that aligns ideas. Without explicit theoretical positioning, expressed as a hypothesis to be falsified, scientific knowledge cannot progress. In this way, quantitative science has evolved with a fixation upon a procedural accuracy that demands precision and clarity as to which theory is being tested. In order to justify their work as science, rather than some more fuzzy form of thinking, the fields of study we now consider social sciences developed their methodological traditions with a heavy reliance upon theory. If their scholarship was firmly rooted within a theoretical position, then it qualified as a science. Indeed, as the disciplines evolved within the academic context, theorizing became their driving motivation.

Early qualitative research in nursing adhered to this tradition as best it could. Certainly there are various sociological or psychological theories that helped scaffold some of our studies, but we were rarely engaging with those theories in anything like the manner that our social science colleagues did (Sandelowski, 1993). For the most part, taking a theoretical position served as a hollow launching pad from which we would leap into our more disciplinary way of organizing ideas for the remainder of the study. Occasionally, various social theories would be again brought out of the closet and tried on as we discussed the meanings one might make of what we had found in the field. Thus, the requirement for aligning with a theoretical position has not served nursing in the generation of rigorous applied research, and our attempts to weave theory into many of our studies have been somewhat awkward and unproductive.

The history of thought in nursing also includes a significant chapter in which "nursing theory" meant the adoption of a particular framework for putting the puzzle pieces of patient assessment together in a comprehensive "nursing" manner. As conceptual models of the complex thinking structure of the discipline, these "theories" were impossible foundations upon which to base the majority of our disciplinary research questions. Thus, we have paradoxically shied away from nursing theories while uncritically sprinkling a collection of non-nursing theories into our justification for research. What interpretive description attempts to do is reclaim not the individual "theories" of nursing but the foundational intellectual character of nursing thought. Drawing on the insights about our unique angle of vision that have been informed by an increasingly sophisticated body of philosophical thinking about the discipline, I believe we have sufficiently matured to be able to quite easily grasp and articulate those core reasoning elements that characterize what nursing represents epistemologically. And thus, the disciplinary thought structure, and one's capacity to make explicit which elements of it are being brought to the fore in any particular inquiry, are what makes the scaffolding of an interpretive study solid and credible. It becomes the foundational position from which the logic that explains all other design decisions will derive.

Data sources and samples

Nurses often ask research questions about patients, and require extensive knowledge about how they think, feel and respond to various conditions because those insights are important to their capacity to practice well. Thus, many interpretive description studies are oriented to discovering patterns and themes discernible by observing or interacting with patients. However, interpretive description imposes no limits as to alternative data sources that might be applicable to address a nursing question. For example, beyond that which individual patients might understand about their own experience in a particular context, experienced nurses might be ideally positioned to provide insights and interpretations across time and experience with multiple patients in similar circumstances. Patterns in clinical wisdom can become a powerful tool for clarifying the nature of certain health contexts and in generating strategic directions toward knowledge building. Depending on the kind of question that is being posed, interpretive description would be amenable to retroactive reflective interviewing, to cross-sectional reporting, or to longitudinal follow-up over time. Recognizing that the act of rendering experience into narrative for the purpose of communicating it to a researcher may prompt further sense-making and interpretation, the method lends itself to both single-exposure and multiple-exposure approaches, again depending upon the kind of question being posed and the level of depth and detail that will be relevant to the question at hand.

Although the direct human encounter associated with interviews, participant observations, and focus groups may hold special experiential appeal for nurse researchers, it is important not to neglect alternative data sources that may have tremendous value for primary or collateral material. Textual material such as patient records, published testimonials, lay autobiography, public press and policy documents may yield important and meaningful insights on aspects of professional practice or human health experience. In addition, existing data bases obtained for the purposes of research or quality improvement may contain valuable ingredients for a secondary analysis. The key is to understand the nature of the data source in relation to the nature of the question that has been posed—specifically to deeply consider both the attributes and the limitations in what exists, including a critical reflection on what it reveals as well as what it might conceal.

The question of sample size is also one that must be considered in alignment with the nature of the phenomenon under study. In nursing, we understand the value of the well-selected anecdote or exemplar (Benner, 1983), and in some instances the single case study approach may be a particularly powerful means by which to convey important experiential meanings. More often, we recognize that clinical phenomena are inherently variously experienced, and therefore would tend to solicit multiple and diverse perspectives in order to feel comfortable that theoretical constructions proposed on the basis of our inquiries were not unduly influenced by the unique features of individual cases. The sample size will also depend upon interpretation of the state of the science related to a clinical circumstance, and the expected level of theoretical development that the study might achieve. If we are wanting to document relatively superficial similarities and differences across cases in order to begin the work of understanding a novel clinical circumstance, then a smaller sample and briefer exposure may be appropriate. Alternatively, if the field is maturing, and what is called for is a more nuanced, comprehensive depiction of multiple facets of a clinical circumstance, then a more robust and extensive interpretive description would seem warranted. Thus, the obligation of the researcher on behalf of the discipline is to understand what is known, and on what basis, in setting the design for a study. Where something has already been well documented, a small qualitative study may not be defensible, and to embark on one may reflect more a matter of personal indulgence than an act of professional scholarship. So again, the key is a solid appreciation for the relationship between the sample size and the kinds of interpretations that can appropriately be made on the basis of it.

Technique options

The interview is something of a mainstay in nursing qualitative research, likely because nurses feel quite competent and comfortable in the interview context (at least they do until they begin to understand that the researcher role requires that they approach the study participant as an informed learner, rather than an expert practitioner). Nurses have been challenged with an over-reliance on the open-ended interview as their mainstay data source (Silverman, 1998), and this is a fair critique, given our recognition that narrative and truth are decidedly different knowledge propositions (Sandelowski, 1996).

Beyond individual interviewing in a more open-ended and iterative manner, various forms of structured engagement can also yield valuable material. Examples might include case studies from which a set of conditions or questions arises, hypothetical situations from which decisional approaches might be ascertained, or theoretical propositions used to provoke informed patient responses. The key to using a structured method well is always to understand its nature and limitations, much as nurses ought to understand the scope and confines of the clinical assessments they perform in the practice context—always an informed beginning point, but never the final answer.

Dyadic and triadic interviewing, and group data collection approaches, can also be highly productive for generating certain forms of data that might not be revealed in the individual interview context. In each instance, just as in the clinical context, it behoves the nurse to understand that human dynamics are at play, and to account for the manner in which they influence what is exposed. Since much of the ordinary reality of illness experience is played out in a social context, engaging with people, conversations and processes can be highly informative of content. And since so much of what we think, believe and perceive about what we encounter in relation to our health is shaped and molded by public discourses, much can be learned from observing cross-talk and consensus/dispute formations. These represent but a smattering of the possible options open to the nurse using interpretive description, since the only truly meaningful boundaries will be creativity, integrity and professionalism. As we progress in our comfort zone with adapting and manipulating qualitative technique to our disciplinary purposes, I am confident we can support a broad range of rigorously applied, thoughtfully depicted, and credibly defended qualitative techniques.

The role of the researcher in interpretive description will always be shaped by the disciplinary knowledge creation agenda. This positions the nurse as simultaneously both informed and open to the possibility that prior information is inadequate. Thus, a role that presumes a blank slate (*tabula rasa*) or brackets all preconceptions is not really appropriate, since the question ought to have derived from a practice understanding of why it is being asked. At the other end of the spectrum, a more presumptive conceptual structure, such as a content analysis framework into which new information will be placed, would also be inappropriate to the kind of problem that begs an inductive inquiry. Thus, the nurse's role will combine clarification of that which is known in the sense of having generated the questions and a genuine desire for new possibilities in structuring knowledge that may alter how prior knowledge has been interpreted. This intellectual stance departs from the clinical assessment interview role more familiar to nurses in that it explicitly engages study participants with the expectation that current knowledge will be strengthened and informed through the additional perspective that experiences such as theirs can contribute. The nurse researcher is never pretending not to be a nurse, but is positioning that nursing expertise in suspension for the purpose of inquiry.

Analytic alternatives

In general, interpretive description implies an analytic process in which the collection or generation of data takes place concurrently and iteratively with reflecting upon it, asking questions about it, and considering options for what sense one might make of it (Thorne, Reimer-Kirkham, & O'Flynn-Magee, 2004). Its general direction will be iterative analysis allowing the mind of the researcher (rather than the qualitative data software system) to ponder, challenge, chew on, wrestle with and massage pieces of data until they can be formed into parts that seem individually and collectively to tell us something we did not know previously about the phenomenon, or we did not appreciate in that particular manner. As multiple options for how parts might be conceptualized emerge, it becomes possible to consider them in relation to one another, seeking to determine what each configuration might reveal or narrate differently from each other. This process continues until a sense of clarity as to a preferred organizational structure can be justified on the basis of where it is taking the findings. And once this aspect is clarified, then a second phase of examining relationships between these parts begins to yield insights about the logic and flow of the display of findings that will lead toward the most appropriate or satisfying conclusion, given the question that was posed. Considering where the study began and where it will go when it is completed, the form and structure of the outcome are aligned with an understanding of the intended audience. Thus, interpretive description would rarely conclude with a metaphoric claim intended to capture the essence of a complex phenomenon, or a finite set of conditions meant to represent all cases, but rather take the form of a grounded interpretive structure through which a clinician might make sense of what is both seen and not seen in the clinical world, in all of its commonalities and variations.

To facilitate working with data until they become findings, various tools and techniques can be useful. While coding can certainly support the process, it should never dominate, and the primary directional influence will be the ongoing capacity of the professional to interrogate the data with increasing levels of understanding and questioning, such that premature coding can impede the process. The flow of the analytic process in interpretive description moves from the self-evident to that which was not previously apparent, from variation to similarity and back again, wondering why the data are as they are, but never forgetting the disciplinary lens that will allow us to recognize that what we have seen is never all that we need to know. For example, the nurse using interpretive description would have the potential to theorize exceptions on the basis of practice knowledge without having seen them in the research context, thereby safeguarding against premature closure or over-generalization (McPherson & Thorne, 2006). Although it is easier to be definitive about what not to do in the analytic process than it is to clearly explain what one does do (Thorne & Darbyshire, 2005), the over-riding aim of the work will be to generate an outcome that actually does move thinking forward in the manner that was envisioned when the research question was proposed. So if the question was thoughtfully located within a practice problem or health puzzle, it will provide ample direction to inspire the form within which the findings will be most effective. Thus, the product may not look quite like an ethnography, or a phenomenological product, but it will look like nursing knowledge.

Issues in the conduct of interpretive description

Disciplinary logic and emergent design

As has been apparent from the description of methodological elements, interpretive description takes the best of what qualitative technique has to offer and considers its application and implications within the logic of disciplinary epistemology. As we know from several generations now of nursing theorists and philosophers, there is no singular and comprehensive way to define and delineate what nursing does when it does it well. At the same time, when we study the history of nursing thought, we recognize an inherent core of values, processes, and capacities that become recognizable as nursing excellence even across theoretical languaging and clinical fields. In other words, nursing has a nature that exists and is recognizable, even if it is remarkably difficult to "nail it down" definitionally. The excitement about interpretive description is that it is asking for this same kind of intellectual coherence within the context of a wide range of conditions, expressions and circumstances, challenging us to imagine the theoretical disciplinary audience and to address our findings to its essential nature and structure. Thus, while various studies claiming to use interpretive description for methodological guidance may look quite different in terms of data sources, extraction approaches and analytic techniques, they will resemble one another in being intellectually auditable to an informed disciplinary audience. Just as one nurse conveys only pieces of an exemplar narrative to another, but effectively makes the point, the good interpretive description will draw the (critically) informed reader into an understanding of how a nurse has reasonably come to the conclusions that have been formed and the interpretations that have been offered. And it is this adherence to the logic structure of "how the discipline thinks" that makes it possible to be expansive about design options without sliding into the "anything goes" of sloppy scholarship.

The art of logical conclusions

Nursing demands of its members a commitment to responsible, responsive and justifiable intellectual processes. While we most certainly value the intuitive and the emotive, we recognize that they never replace the commitment to the logical and defensible in our clinical judgments. So too in qualitative inquiry, since we explicitly capitalize on inductive reasoning, iterative analysis and interpretive curiosity, but expect that what professionals conclude on the basis of scholarly processes will be characterized by the rigor and trustworthiness that are a hallmark of scholarly excellence. Ideas outside of that context may play a role in advancing our thinking, but they become points of departure rather than research conclusions.

In nursing, because we respect the inherent complexity and messiness of the business we are in, findings are rarely definitive, and in most cases they prompt additional (and hopefully even better informed) questions. But we do appreciate the kinds of findings that offer enhanced understandings, more possibilities, and the capacity to capture more complexity than what we had before. Thus, the form of our conclusions takes us back to the state of the science, that which is known and not known by the profession, and engages us with a new opportunity for applying it. For this reason, the quality criteria appropriately used to judge the product of interpretive description are more inherently aligned with the purpose and nature of applied knowledge than would be the case of the field of qualitative inquiry in general. They include such qualities as epistemological integrity, representational credibility, analytic logic, interpretive authority, and moral defensibility, as well as disciplinary relevance, pragmatic obligation, and contextual awareness (Thorne, 2008). Each of these is articulated as a lens with which to guide both researcher and audience in developing an aptitude for critical and disciplined reflection on where ideas come from, how they are made, and where they are going.

An exemplar

One of my favorite exemplars of the kind of research that interpretive description aspires to is a delightful study by Marie Bakitas (2007) on chemotherapy-induced peripheral neuropathy published in *Nursing Research* in 2007. Recognizing that conventional quality of life measurement studies significantly under-represent what would be important for understanding and supporting what patients were going through, Bakitas sought a better way to explain what it was really like for patients to try to make sense of and cope with the intense tingling, burning, numbness and painful sensations of the feet and hands that arise as a predictable side effect of some chemotherapeutic agents. Her design involved strategic sampling from the diverse contexts and experiential effects that might be encountered in practice, and she gathered data in an iterative dialectic process that included steps to engage both patients and professionals in assuring the relevance and credibility of her evolving interpretations. The results of the study were conveyed within a neatly constructed and highly evocative metaphoric depiction of these symptoms as "background noise" capable of producing functional, emotional, and social cacophony for these patients, but also amenable to strategic attempts to face the music, adjust the volume, or tune it out. The metaphor works as an interpretive frame because it would be immediately recognized by a nursing audience as an effective organizing heuristic for the layering of complexity of patient experience and of the processes by which patients can learn how to cope. Each element of the findings is rigorously derived, elegantly explained, logically argued, and intelligently ordered so that the study becomes a comprehensive yet accessible depiction that, having read it, changes your grasp of why and how this phenomenon matters in practice.

State of the science

From an interpretive description perspective, findings become part of the ongoing search for knowledge to inform the applied discipline across its various activities. From a nursing professional perspective, new knowledge is never definitive, but part of this relentless march forward into better and more effective ways to enact the unique contribution of the discipline. Since nursing exists within the context of a world captivated by the idea of evidence-based practice, and indeed that is what justifies most of the research we do, it is important to try and locate the products of our inquiry within that larger context.

The politics of competing traditions

Interpretive description does not imply a positioning against any of the marvelous intellectual and methodological traditions from which nursing has drawn inspiration, but it does challenge the notion that, in their conventional forms, they necessarily serve the needs of knowledge advancement within the discipline (Thorne, 2011). Epistemologically, nursing sits squarely in the middle ground between post-positivism and constructivism, recognizing the relevance of both as "standpoints" from which to consider the complexity that is nursing, but rejecting both extremes as insufficient. Therefore, various critical social theorizing perspectives may well prove useful to nursing to take apart that which has not been thoughtfully examined, and postmodern theorizing can help take us beyond the fixed positions that some theoreticians have attempted to stake out, but the manner in which either is used will be somewhat different from the applications expected in the non-applied or more purely theoretical disciplines. Interpretive description exists as an option to nurses to align various approaches within an interior logic that speaks to the knowledge needs of the discipline. By framing a study as interpretive description, or by using interpretive descriptive logic to explain modifications on conventional method, the method becomes a tool to inform and justify processes of relevant inquiry without planting them solidly in an unsatisfying tradition.

Application to the evidentiary context

Qualitative researchers have long been embroiled in debates about how to position the products of their research "as evidence" (Miller & Fredericks, 2003; Upshur, 2001). Similarly, nursing literature has been fraught with confusing and contradictory claims about how qualitative and quantitative products ought to feature within evidence claims (Thorne & Sawatzky, 2007). Interpretive description implies no particular stature in the evidence hierarchy, but instead becomes an instrument through which evidence bits derived from the full spectrum of method can be considered, examined, tested, and challenged within the context of practice reality. Instead of competing for equivalence as a knowledge form, it becomes the approach within which the other puzzle pieces can be displayed, linked, interpreted and potentially aligned. As such, it can form the "glue" that binds the universe of available scientific evidence and clinical wisdom and knowledge from alternative sources such as patient perspective into a cohesive and more fulsome understanding. If we have positioned our research explicitly and purposively with the gaps and inadequacies of biomedical science in mind, for example, then the products of our studies can increasingly approach solutions to the questions that were driving the science in the first place and that those who wish to apply the science need to have answered. Interpretive description works far better as the challenger, illuminator, variance interpreter, gap-filler, and humanizer that corrects the course of what quantitative science is capable of yielding than a competing form of "truth." Having this ultimate aim in mind helps firmly position our inquiries within the world of where science is going, and where this kind of inductive inquiry can best contribute.

Nursing's role in the evolving field

To me, it comes as no surprise that nursing has played such a leading role in the development of qualitative research methodologies within the health field over the last generation or two, or that it is advancing the broader field of methodological application. It is in the nature of nursing to embrace complexity, to recognize the evolving contexts within which health and illness experience take place, and to accept a profoundly social and indeed moral mandate for why knowledge matters. What we do is informed by conventional science, but it is not conventional science, and the science we create has been creatively and marvelously influenced by our awareness of the unique perspective on the world that the discipline demands. I fully believe that which we learn and discover in the attempt to wrestle with knowledge generation can be shared with and taken up by our colleagues in other applied disciplines, but that it will be important for us to accept a mantle of responsibility for the advancement and refinement of method over time. Having come through a long period characterized by the kinds of theoretical disputations that made us tear our hair out, we are emerging into a new place in which our understanding of the philosophy of science, the implications and limitations of its methods, and the inherent complexity of the business we are in has placed us legitimately in a new intellectual leadership role. These are exciting times, and through these discussions about method we are making significant headway.

Future directions for nursing inquiry

Integrating social justice, moral agency, complexity, integrative holism, contextual embedded-ness, with what we understand of human frailty, vulnerability, resilience and strength, we are transitioning into a new era of being able to rigorously grapple with the ideas that will shape the practice of our discipline. This will be an era characterized by critically informed thinking, an appreciation for the very real social and material determinants of health, honoring the individuality of experience, and balancing the realities of costs and constraints with the ideals of health for all, regardless of circumstance. What I see in the future is a new generation of nursing research capable of weaving into its fabric the full scope of the mandate that nursing stands for. I see an era in which it is the mandate of the discipline that drives our inquiry, in which method becomes possibility instead of limitation and we capitalize on the full set of our empirical and reasoning tools. Interpretive description seems well positioned to be part of the process that takes us there.

References

Bakitas, M. (2007). Background noise: The experience of chemotherapy-induced peripheral neuropathy. *Nursing Research*, *56*, 323–331.

Benner, P. (1983). Uncovering the knowledge embedded in clinical practice. *Image: The Journal of Nursing Scholarship*, *15*(2), 36–41.

Cheek, J. (2000). *Postmodern and poststructural approaches to nursing research*. Thousand Oaks, CA: Sage.

Cioffi, R. N. J. (2003). Communicating with culturally and linguistically diverse patients in an acute care setting: Nurses' experiences. *International Journal of Nursing Studies*, *40*, 299–306.

Clark, M. I., Spence, J. C., & Holt, N. L. (2011). In the shoes of young adolescent girls: Understanding physical activity experiences through interpretive description. *Qualitative Research in Sport, Exercise and Health*, *3*(2), 193–210.

Colaizzi, P. F. (1978). Psychological research as the phenomenologist sees it. In R. S. Valle & S. King (Eds.), *Existential-phenomenological alternatives for psychology* (pp. 48–71). New York: Oxford University Press.

Cronqvist, A., Theorell, T., Burns, T., & Lützén, K. (2004). Caring about-caring for: Moral obligations and work responsibilities in intensive care nursing. *Nursing Ethics*, *11*(1), 63–76.

Davison, S. N., & Simpson, C. (2006). Hope and advance care planning in patients with end stage renal disease: Qualitative interview study. *BMJ Online*. Retrieved from doi: 10.1136/bmj.38965.626250.55.

Johansson, E., Wilson, B., Brunton, L., Tishelman, C., & Molassiotis, A. (2010). Symptoms before, during and 14 months after the beginning of treatment as perceived by patients with lymphoma. *Oncology Nursing Forum*, *37*(2), E105–113.

Kagan, P. N., Smith, M. C., Cowling, W. R., & Chinn, P. L. (2009). A nursing manifesto: An emancipatory call for knowledge development, conscience, and praxis. *Nursing Philosophy*, *11*(1), 67–84.

Kenny, A., & Duckett, S. (2004). A question of place: Medical power in rural Australia. *Social Science & Medicine*, *58*, 1059–1072.

Koop, P. M., & Strang, V. R. (2003). The bereavement experience following home-based family caregiving for persons with advanced cancer. *Clinical Nursing Research*, *12*(2), 127–144.

McPherson, G., & Thorne, S. (2006). Exploiting exceptions to enhance interpretive qualitative health research: Insights from a study of cancer communication. *International Journal of Qualitative Methods*, *5*(2). Retrieved on March 1, 2012 from http://www.ualberta.ca/~ijqm/backissues/5_2/pdf/mcpherson.pdf.

Miller, S., & Fredericks, M. (2003). The nature of "evidence" in qualitative research methods. *International Journal of Qualitative Methods*, *2*(1 Article 4), Retrieved on March 5, 2012 from http://www.ualberta.ca/~iiqm/backissues/2_1/html/miller.html.

Mulkins, A., & Verhoef, M. J. (2004). Supporting the transformative process: Experiences of cancer patients receiving integrative care. *Integrative Cancer Therapies*, *3*(3), 230–237.

Munhall, P. L. (2012). Epistemology in nursing. In P. L. Munhall (Ed.), *Nursing research: A qualitative perspective* (5th ed., pp. 69–94). Sudbury, MA: Jones & Bartlett.

O'Connor, D. L. (2007). Self-identifying as a caregiver: Exploring the positional process. *Journal of Aging Studies*, *21*, 165–174.

Oliffe, J. L., Davison, B. J., Pickles, T., & Mróz, L. (2009). The self-management of uncertainty among men undertaking active surveillance for low-risk prostate cancer. *Qualitative Health Research*, *19*(4), 432–443.

Pascale, C.-M. (2011). *Cartographies of knowledge: Exploring qualitative epistemologies*. Thousand Oaks, CA: Sage.

Pesut, B., & Johnson, J. (2013). Philosophical contributions to nursing ethics. In J. L. Storch, P. Rodney, & R. Starzomzki (Eds.), *Toward a moral horizon: Nursing ethics for leadership and practice* (2nd ed., pp. 41–58). Toronto: Pearson.

Reed, P. G. (2006). The practice turn in nursing epistemology. *Nursing Science Quarterly*, *19*(1), 36–38.

Rodney, P., Kadyschuk, S., Liaschenko, J., Brown, H., Musto, L., & Synder, N. (2011). Moral agency: Relational connections and support. In J. L. Storch, P. Rodney, & R. Starzomzki (Eds.), *Toward a moral horizon: Nursing ethics for leadership and practice* (pp. 160–187). Toronto: Pearson.

Rolfe, G. (2011). Practitioner-centred research: Nursing praxis and the science of the unique. In P. G. Reed & N. B. Crawford Shearer (Eds.), *Nursing knowledge and theory innovation: Advancing the science of practice* (pp. 59–74). New York: Springer.

Sandelowski, M. (1993). Theory unmasked: The uses and guises of theory in qualitative research. *Research in Nursing & Health*, *16*, 213–218.

Sandelowski, M. (1996). Truth/storytelling in nursing inquiry. In J. F. Kikuchi, H. Simmons, & D. Romyn (Eds.), *Truth in nursing inquiry* (pp. 111–124). Thousand Oaks, CA: Sage.

Sellman, D. (2011). *What makes a good nurse*. Thousand Oaks, CA: Sage.

Silverman, D. (1998). The quality of qualitative health research: The open-ended interview and its alternatives. *Social Sciences in Health*, *4*(2), 104–118.

Spradley, J. P. (1979). *The ethnographic interview*. New York: Holt, Rinehart & Winston.

Stajduhar, K. I., Neithercut, J., Chu, E., Pham, P., Rohde, J., Sicotte, A., & Young, K. (2000). Thyroid cancer: Patients' experiences of receiving iodine-131 therapy. *Oncology Nursing Forum*, *27*(8), 1213–1218.

Strauss, A., & Corbin, J. (1990). *Basics of qualitative research: Grounded theory procedures and techniques*. Thousand Oaks, CA: Sage.

Thorne, S. (2001). The implications of disciplinary agenda on quality criteria for qualitative research. In J. M. Morse, J. Swanson, & A. Kuzel (Eds.), *The nature of qualitative evidence* (pp. 141–159). Thousand Oaks, CA: Sage.

Thorne, S. (2008). *Interpretive description*. Walnut Creek, CA: Left Coast Press.

Thorne, S. (2011). Toward methodological emancipation in applied health research. *Qualitative Health Research*, *21*(4), 433–453.

Thorne, S., & Darbyshire, P. (2005). Landmines in the field: A modest proposal for improving the craft of qualitative health research. *Qualitative Health Research*, *15*, 1105–1113.

Thorne, S., Reimer-Kirkham, S., & MacDonald-Emes, J. (1997). Interpretive description: A non-categorical qualitative alternative for developing nursing knowledge. *Research in Nursing & Health*, *20*(2), 169–177.

Thorne, S., Reimer-Kirkham, S., & O'Flynn-Magee, K. (2004). The analytic challenge in interpretive description. *International Journal of Qualitative Methods*, *3*(2). Retrieved on March 12, 2012 from http://www.ualberta.ca/~iiqm/backissues/3_1/html/thorneetal.html.

Thorne, S., & Sawatzky, R. (2007). Particularizing the general: Challenges in teaching the structure of evidence-based nursing practice. In J. Drummond & P. Standish (Eds.), *The philosophy of nursing education* (pp. 161–175). New York: Palgrave Macmillan.

Upshur, R. E. G. (2001). The status of qualitative research as evidence. In J. M. Morse, J. M. Swanson, & A. J. Kuzel (Eds.), *The nature of qualitative evidence* (pp. 5–26). Thousand Oaks, CA: Sage.

van Manen, M. (1990). *Researching lived experience: Human science for an action sensitive pedagogy*. Albany: State University of New York.

23
Focus groups
Denise Côté-Arsenault

Brief history of focus groups

Focus groups were first mentioned in the literature prior to World War II, and later disseminated by Robert K. Merton in 1956 as an alternative to individual interviews. During World War II focus groups were used to determine the impact of propaganda films on civilians in the US. Merton was a researcher using this new technique (that he called the "focused interview") to explore sensitive topics and affective responses to the topics within the military (Merton, Fiske, & Kendall, 1990). Merton found that participants opened up within a safe, group environment with others who experienced the same film, radio broadcast, or whatever. The basis of the usefulness of such interviews was the social interaction around a topic to elicit understanding of the group's responses to similar experiences.

Interviews of the time consisted primarily of close-ended questions. The most obvious disadvantage was that the interviewer was in charge of what was said, leaving the interviewee as a respondent but not an informant. Social scientists began to question the usefulness of the traditional interview; focus groups, or group interviews, were a new strategy for obtaining more pertinent and valuable information.

This early work often consisted of quantitative data of responses, with the explanations for the responses elicited through what we now call focus groups. Despite Merton's work and publications on the topic, focus groups and qualitative research in general were not embraced or accepted within academia at the time. However, marketing researchers used them extensively to sell products in the post-war era. Focus groups continue to be used today for marketing and development.

Within the academy, it was the social scientists (anthropologists, sociologists, etc.) who used qualitative methods in the 1970s. Beyond Merton, focus group methodology handbooks and articles have been prominently written by Richard A. Krueger (1998), David L. Morgan, Mary Anne Carey, and Jenny Kitzinger, among others. Stewart and Shamdasani wrote a Sage monograph in 1990 in the Applied Social Research Methods Series; Morgan's (1997) monograph in the Sage qualitative research methods series was already a second edition.

Early nurse scientists used research methods learned in doctoral programs, which were in fields other than nursing, or in nursing education. Research methods from anthropology, sociology and other fields were applied to nursing problems. It follows then that qualitative methods were among the research traditions applied to nursing questions. The initial adoption of focus groups by nurse researchers was seemingly inconspicuous, with noted increased popularity in the 1990s that mirrored the increasing acceptance and use of qualitative research in general. Indeed, focus groups are now commonly used in qualitative research studies in nursing.

The method

Focus groups, used for the purpose of collecting qualitative data within a research study, are *planned groups brought together for discussing a specific topic among 5–10 people who have a key characteristic in common.* Within a comfortable environment, focus groups capitalize on group interaction, and the fact that individuals are influenced by each other. Focus groups are also known as a "group interview." Thus, it follows that the unit of analysis is the group; it is therefore imperative to conduct more than a single focus group with each type of participant. For example, if the population of interest is adolescents 13–19 years of age, it is best to stratify group composition by age groups, such as 13–16 and 17–19 to make sure that the participants around the table are on a similar developmental level. Two or more sessions should be held with the younger and the same with the older age group to insure that the findings (i.e. categories or themes) were not a product of group think or unusual group dynamics.

The basic format of a focus group is as follows: groups should be held in a quiet, comfortable room with a central table, or a circle of chairs, that the moderator and participants sit around. Participants are greeted as they arrive by the moderator and a second research team member, the informed consent process needs to be verified (done on site or previously), and then participants are directed to their seats. The focus group discussion generally needs to be recorded for later transcription, so one or two recorders need to be placed in the center or on either side of the table, and explained to the participants. Use of name cards, drinks and other refreshments are optional but recommended. (See details in other sources, including Côté-Arsenault & Morrison-Beedy, 1999.) The moderator guides the discussion using a prepared interview guide, adding prompts to elicit more details as needed. The moderator decides when the discussion should be ended, based on coverage of all desired topics or the end of the allotted time. After participants leave, the moderator and the second research team member should hold a debriefing session, that is also audio-recorded, to review what was heard, how the group went, and plan on any changes for the subsequent group. The recordings should then be slated for transcription.

Kitzinger (1995) makes it clear that conversation in focus groups should be between and among the participants, not simply responses to the moderator's questions. She asserts that focus groups are most useful in going beyond what people think to how and why they think the way they do. So, to gain the most from the method, interaction must be facilitated and achieved. Often individuals are not clear about their thinking, until they talk with others with differing perspectives. This is the essence of the most important advantage of focus groups: that within the group experience participants express their views with greater clarity because of the social processes that occur in conversation around a topic.

A word of caution needs to be inserted here. Focus groups are often touted as a quick, easy, straightforward, and valid means to do research. In truth, focus groups are a method of data collection, not a complete research method, and there is a great need for careful planning and execution in order to obtain trustworthy data. The choice of research design and other procedures for sampling, analysis and interpretation of findings should be congruent with the use of focus groups. *The main focus here is the use of focus groups as the sole method of data collection; examples of mixed methods uses are provided as alternative uses.*

An example of the inappropriate use of focus groups would be to call the design grounded theory and all that it entails. For example, stating that what was done was theoretical sampling, conducting two focus groups (one group of newly diagnosed individuals and a second 2–5 years out from diagnosis), followed by constant comparative analysis with open, selective and theoretical coding, and that the findings included the identification of the basic social process and a newly defined theory. This would not be possible. Grounded theory requires more on-going, and likely more diverse data collection than would be possible within focus groups. That said, if used in conjunction with other means of data collection so that theoretical sampling could be done and individual stories heard, focus group data could contribute a great deal to such a study. See Table 23.1 for a listing of other advantages and disadvantages of focus groups.

Foundational frameworks or assumptions

Focus groups are based on the understanding that humans are social beings, and that we are influenced by those around us (the underlying principle of the social sciences such as social psychology). The assumption is that people talk with one another, sometimes about topics of interest, and that they will listen to what others have to say, compare it to their own comments,

Table 23.1 Advantages and disadvantages of focus groups

Advantages	Disadvantages
• Very flexible method that can be used on multiple topics	• Scheduling less flexible to accommodate individual's timetable
• Observe interaction among several people in a short period of time	• Requires keen observation skills to capture responses of many at once
• More in-depth knowledge gained than individual interview	• Cannot learn individual stories
• Facilitates synergy among participants as they react to and build upon the responses of others	• Responses from members of the group are not independent of one another
• Data collection period may be much shorter	• More difficult to transcribe with numerous voices and potential overlap
• Participants do not need to be literate	• Member checking more challenging
• Results are easy to understand	• Moderator could bias the responses (unknowingly)
• Provides direct information about similarities and differences between individuals quickly	• Limited generalizability
• Less costly than other means of data collection	• Transcription is more time-consuming due to multiple speakers on the recording
• Provides large amounts of rich data in their own words	• Analysis may be more time-consuming due to within and between analyses
• Yields a great deal of self-report data on topics that could not be gleaned from other methods	• Results could be biased by one loud or opinionated participant
• May be more acceptable than individual interviews by vulnerable groups	• Open nature could make summarizing and interpreting the data more difficult

and add to or adjust their response. What other people in the conversation say triggers a comparative analysis and a subsequent response. As such, this implies that results from a group interview will differ from a series of individual interviews—even if these were with the identical participants.

There is no single theory or conceptual framework that guides all focus groups, but many theories and frameworks are compatible with this basic assumption that humans are social beings.

Sample characteristic considerations

Considerable thought needs to be given when making decisions about group composition for focus groups because the success is dependent on group interaction.

Homogeneity or heterogeneity in the study in general and within discrete groups requires careful planning. Inclusion and exclusion criteria must be applied as in most research, then group formation is done. Knowledge of the population is required to determine upon which characteristics homogeneity should be based. Unlike individual interviews, participants in focus groups affect the others in the group. The participants in a group must be comfortable talking as peers with the other group members; consider gender, age, race, education, socioeconomic status, experience, diagnosis, etc. In a study of women's experiences of pregnancy after perinatal loss, gestational age of loss was not considered critical to separating groups but rather was important to provide heterogeneity; the key variable of homogeneity was their history of loss. The women relished the opportunity to share their experiences with each other and the researchers. Had the focus been on events at the time of loss, gestational age (miscarriage versus stillbirth versus neonatal death) would have been critically important as a variable by which to form separate groups.

When forming groups, it is critical to avoid power differences within a group. For example, combining RNs and nurses' aides in a group discussing areas of dissatisfaction with skin care of nursing home residents would likely not have either group feeling safe to open up about their true concerns. It is far better to have separate focus groups of RNs only and others of only nurses' aides.

The choice of sampling method, convenience, purposive, or probability, should be dependent on the study purpose, research questions, and transferability concerns (samples may or may not be representative of the target population).

An interesting question that deserves pondering is whether or not participants in the group can know each other. Focus groups are usually temporary then disbanded, but knowledge of others in the group can occur within many areas of interest to nurse researchers. If two people within a group know each other well, seating arrangements could be made to blend them in with those who are strangers in order to facilitate group cohesion and avoid side-by-side sharing between friends. To go one step further, should pre-existing groups be used as a focus group? This latter question is dependent on the research topic and purpose, and the type of group being considered. In order to achieve the most open discussion, the likely answer is generally "No" because within existing groups there are already established rules, roles, and relationships that would likely dictate group behaviors. Thus, the individuals around the table might not share their opinions as openly with people they would see again, either at work or church, or elsewhere. There are likely exceptions to this, however, when the topic is not sensitive or laden with controversy. For example, this author moderated focus groups of hospital staff who attended monthly meetings that focus on emotions (i.e. Schwartz Center Rounds®). Nurses (staff and managers), speech and physical therapists, social workers, administrators, members of the patient transport team, all talked about their experiences attending these sessions. It seemed to work quite well, but it is hard to know what was not said. Physicians could never commit to a group, so they were interviewed individually. One could only speculate about how the discussion with physicians included might have been different.

Another alternative group is a family; could a single family form a focus group? An example of this in the literature is the work of Kean (2010) who conducted group interviews with families coping with one of their members being brain-injured and in intensive care. Given the stressful situation, it is likely that the family being together was best for them but it is also likely that family dynamics influenced who said what, and the way it was said. Direct and open communication is often not the norm in families, and thus would not be possible within a focus group. If examining family dynamics is part of the study, focus groups could be ideal. On the other hand, if the research goal is to understand individual coping, focus groups would not be the method of choice. Interpretation of results always needs to take these issues into consideration.

There are several examples of studies with cultural groups who are suspicious of research and researchers (Pavlish & Ho, 2009; Rodehorst-Weber, Wilhelm, Stepans, Tobacco, & de la Paz, 2009; Scharff, Mathews, Jackson, & Hoff, 2010). In these instances, the researchers reported that focus groups provided a safe environment with others from their ethnic group. Access was thus possible only with focus groups, and therefore the discussion was likely the best possible way to gain entrée into the population.

Group and sample size

Many resources on focus groups suggest group sizes of 8–12 participants. While that may work ideally in marketing-oriented focus groups, researchers seeking more detailed responses will typically find it is far better to have 5–8 participants per group. This ensures adequate time to hear from everyone around the circle, and minimizes the risk of more quiet or timid participants feeling intimidated by the size of the group. There is always a risk of no-shows but reminder phone calls, emails, or facilitating attendance by supplying transportation or child care will likely reduce this problem. Having too many attendees, which can happen if the topic is of great interest, will cause numerous logistical and validity dilemmas. Too few participants could negate the idea of group interaction but with a topic of intensity even a group of three plus the moderator could create good interaction and yield rich data.

The issue of how many groups should be planned is dependent on the topic, the diversity within the population of interest, and the availability of participants. Ultimately, however, when the moderator hears the same thing over and over again, saturation has been reached and data collection is over. This requires a minimum of two groups, but it could be a great many more than that with heterogeneous groups.

Research team

Each focus group should be run by two research team members: the moderator and a second person such as one of the researchers or a research assistant. These two individuals need to have a solid understanding of the research study's focus and purpose. They are the first to begin data analysis, which occurs simultaneously with data collection, through a debriefing after each group session, and they should participate throughout the analysis process.

Moderator

The moderator (aka the facilitator) is the key to success or the source of failure in a focus group. Ideally, this person should not be the researcher, but should be someone with excellent listening and people skills, sensitive to body language and nuance, as well as moderately knowledgeable about the topic under discussion (so as not to ask inappropriate questions or respond ignorantly to comments). The moderator must focus on the group dynamics, what each individual is saying and how others are reacting to what is being said. Reactions to conversation, both positive, negative, or indifferent, should be followed up with clarifying questions to insure that the reasons for the reactions is understood by all in the group. An insider joke or the moderator's misinterpretation of an issue requires further inquiry, particularly early on in the session because further conversation builds on what has been said previously. The moderator must keep the purpose and questions of interest in the fore, and steer conversation back to those intentions if they go afield. That said, a good moderator must allow and encourage the sharing of various viewpoints, respectful conflicts, and differences of opinion to be voiced and captured while maintaining civility and focus.

The choice of moderator based on age, gender, race, or culture is not clear-cut. At the most basic level, participants must feel comfortable with the moderator. The researcher must be very knowledgeable about the population of interest as to which characteristics are essential (e.g. adolescent girls talking about sex require a young female moderator) and which have little or no impact (e.g. group of men and women responding to a satisfaction with care survey).

From the perspective of the participants, the moderator is the leader. It therefore follows that the moderator should begin a session by thanking everyone for participating, explaining the role of the second research team member in the room, stating the ground rules for the session (see Table 23.2), explaining how things will proceed, encourage discussion to be between each other not directed to the moderator, and why he or she might need to redirect conversation along the way. The moderator brings the session to an end, again thanking everyone for their time and contributions.

Table 23.2 Suggested ground rules

Main point	Follow-up explanation
1 Please speak one at a time.	What you have to say is important to us and we want to hear you and capture it on our recording.
2 Although I am asking the questions, please share your thoughts and opinions with each other, around this circle.	Our goal here is to learn about ___ from all of you; you are the experts. Having a discussion back-and-forth among you will provide us with our best information.
3 Be respectful towards each other.	It is likely that your experience or opinion is different from others here, and we want to hear those differences. Respectfully share your own point of view without criticizing that of others.
4 What you *say* in this room should *stay* in this room.	Although we cannot guarantee anonymity because you can all see who is here, we would like everyone to feel comfortable sharing their true feelings and opinions.
5 When addressing each other, please use the name on each person's name card.	Each of you has provided us with a name you would like used in this session. Please know that no names will be included in our transcript.

Second team member

The second person of the research team in the focus group wears several hats: greeter, field note taker, manager of the digital recorder, analyzer, problem-identifier. This person could be the principal investigator or a designated assistant and is one of the essential ingredients of focus groups (Table 23.3). It is possible that the moderator could get caught up in the conversation and lose focus on the purpose of the discussion. This was the case with a known study about people living with osteoporosis. When the transcripts were read, it became quite clear that the moderator had not picked up on the fact that the participants were talking about their pain as a problematic symptom but the source of the pain was from arthritis. Without the specification of osteoporosis, the data were essentially worthless. The second team member who is tasked with seeking answers for the research questions should have picked up on this discrepancy and helped to steer the moderator back on track.

Field note taking is another role for this team member. If it is important to be able to match each comment with the participant who said it, then the field notes need to include a record of who spoke, and in what order. If this is done carefully in the beginning by creating a seating chart on paper and numbering the speakers in turn, then voices can be matched to the digital recording. It is also helpful if the people who were in attendance either do the transcription or at least verify its accuracy within a short period of time of the focus group. The goal here is not to have individual stories, but to be able to interpret comments from individuals based on what they said previously.

Clear audio recordings are critical to data collection and accurate transcripts so it is important to hold focus groups in relatively quiet surroundings with no outside interruptions. Therefore, all cell phones should be turned off and overhead announcements should not be made in the room. It is best to have two digital recorders, placed at opposite ends of the table or circle with extra batteries, and check the pick-up prior to each focus group. As part of ground rules presented in the beginning of the session, ask that individuals speak one at a time.

Various approaches

Research design

Focus groups are most commonly used in exploratory or descriptive studies where they are the single method of data collection. The findings may provide new knowledge in a field of study in and of themselves, or may be a formative step in preparation for future studies. Formative uses of focus groups include the generation of items for instrument development, or as a means of

Table 23.3 Essential ingredients of focus groups

- Several individuals as participants
- Have key characteristics (relevant to the research) in common
- Safe, comfortable, quiet environment
- Seating arrangement that allows participants to see others
- Skilled moderator
- Alert and informed second research team member taking field notes
- Interview guide that begins with a warm-up question that involves every participant, then moves to more complex questions
- Ask questions that quickly pull participants in because they can relate to them
- Debriefing immediately after session to capture key findings and general gestalt

---

gaining feedback about components of an intervention that is being developed. In these latter uses, focus groups provide a structured and rigorous means of rapidly hearing from members of the target population. The level of inquiry can vary according to the purpose of the study, even though focus groups are used for all. Some research questions can be answered by participants in a straightforward way, and others require a longer period of time, with more prompts, more participants, and with more intensive analysis. Sensitive topics, such as sexual risk-taking, require a slower approach so that trust is gained with the moderator and within the group. On the other hand, seeking feedback on items for a patient satisfaction survey may be more content-driven and less personal.

However, there are recent examples of various uses of focus groups in combination with other data collection methods: mixed methods including studying the content and effects of the group discussion as an intervention; as one component of participatory action research; or as part of an ethnography. In all of these instances, other data, qualitative or quantitative, were collected in several ways. The group interaction is capitalized on to gain insiders' knowledge or to make individuals comfortable because they are with others who are like themselves.

Lambert and Loiselle (2008) provide a critical reflection on the differences of data and findings gained from individual interviews and focus groups through their own method triangulation in a grounded theory study. Use of both data collection methods (individual and focus group interviews) was originally done for pragmatic reasons—they could not get everyone scheduled for focus groups so they resorted to individual interviews. They later utilized these two methods to evaluate data convergence, divergence, and complementarity. Keeping in mind that neither approach is better, they found that focus groups provided more contextual data and led to their initial model of the phenomenon of interest. In contrast, individual interviews showed the exact decision-making processes of the participants. Data analysis was iterative between data from individual interviews and group interviews. Together, these authors suggest that the triangulation of two qualitative data collection methodologies enhanced their resulting description of their phenomenon's structure, as well as its essential characteristics. The in-depth examination of this triangulation illuminates some key issues to consider and as such is a promising approach.

Data analysis

When using focus groups alone to collect data, only group data can be reported. Individual stories, percentage of opinions, etc. are not possible due to the inherent group interaction in focus groups. Therefore, the unit of analysis is the group. Each group will have its own characteristics due to the unique nature of the participants and the discussion that ensued among those participants. As such, analysis should first be done of each group's data as a whole; a *within group analysis*. After all groups have been analyzed separately, a *between group analysis* should be done to compare and contrast what was learned from each group. This approach allows the researchers to discern commonalities across all groups, and unique findings within groups (Morrison-Beedy, Côté-Arsenault, & Feinstein, 2001). The unique findings could obviously be due to a single participant's overpowering influence, for example, or be due to group composition differences such as gender, age, or job descriptions. As a clarifying example, a study of sexual abstinence in adolescent girls required recruitment of female participants aged 13–19. Two focus groups were conducted with 13- to 15-year-olds and two others with 16- to 19-year-olds. After the within group analyses were done, where categories and themes were identified, analysis moved to between groups. It was found that the 13- to 15-year-olds had similar data, as did the older girls, but when younger and older girl groups were compared, there were many differences found in their view of themselves, their parents, and the how and why of their sexual abstinence. These differences were consistent with developmental theory of adolescence, thus the data from the two age groups were not combined. Rather, they were reported with the same categories across all groups but with different themes for the younger and older girls due to their developmental levels. Combining all of the data would have lost the rich findings of developmental differences and reduced the usefulness in future development of interventions for different-aged adolescents.

Focus group data are textual and include recordings/transcripts from the focus group conversations, field notes, debriefing sessions, artifacts surrounding the topic. After data collection the next critical step is transcription. *Transcripts must be complete!* They need to accurately convey what was said, with the exact words, and the way in which it was said. Transcripts should include accurate emotions, body language, interpersonal exchanges such as touch, nods or eye contact, tone of voice, sarcasm or humor. Field notes, memory, and debriefing sessions should be used to add details and interpretive notes. Some statements' intended meaning would not be known from the words alone. A single word such as "Really" could be a question (?) accompanied by a skewed facial expression, or an explanation of surprise (!) or pleasant agreement of understanding. The transcript should make the meaning clear with notes in brackets within the transcript. The transcript should be verified by research team members through listening to the recording with the typed transcript and field notes in front of them.

How these data are analyzed must be determined by the purpose of the study; therefore the purpose statement must be kept front and center (perhaps up on the wall in large letters!). Textual data can be analyzed using variations of content analysis, thematic analysis, or question analysis (of responses to specific questions). Repetition of words or phrases can be counted; prevalence or absence of certain color codes can be noted. Analysis can be cursory or in-depth; some research questions are quickly and easily answered and others require many iterations of readings and ponderings. There are many choices described elsewhere but, as Krueger and Casey state, analysis should always be "systematic, sequential, verifiable, and continuous" (2000, p. 128).

As with all qualitative data analysis, it should occur simultaneously with data collection. Impressions, surprises, connections, and even verification of expectations should all be noted and dated in memos. Analysis can be done using cut-up transcripts, colored markers, envelopes or piles; computer programs may be useful with very large quantities of data. If hard copies of transcripts are cut up, color code each transcript by group and number each line. This then allows the researcher to identify where each quote came from, and context can be regained to truly understand its meaning.

What should not be done is treat these data as if they were transcripts of individual interviews, where the conversation can be tracked from interviewer and interviewee. Nor should changes in group composition be seen as trivial; on-going groups should be intact or assume that missing individuals will change the dynamics of the groups.

Trustworthiness

Issues of trustworthiness apply to focus group data just as with any other qualitative research project. Credibility, dependability, confirmability and transferability are all important to the rigor of the entire research study (Lincoln & Guba, 1985). Gaining member checks of research findings may require some creativity, because it is probably difficult to reconvene a group to review the tentative findings. Once again, the study purpose should guide one's choices of how to confirm that the findings reflect what participants intended. The added challenge is the group perspective, so it is helpful to ask "Is this what you heard in the group?" rather than "Did I capture what you were trying to say?"

Current controversies

A current controversy surrounding the use of focus groups is whether or not findings need to include a description of the nature of the interaction within the research report, or whether the interaction is assumed to be inherent in the results. Morgan (2010) responds directly to this question: "saying that the interaction in focus groups produces the data is not the same as saying that the interaction itself is the data." He argues that the goal of the project should dictate the focus of the analysis, and that a focus on what is said would yield different results than an analysis of how things are said. Morgan goes further and makes a very reasonable suggestion: the use of "lead ins" and "follow outs" to sandwich a quote, to provide context and interaction description. This approach acknowledges the interaction and shifts in interaction patterns while limiting the text to fit the publication's length limits.

When reviewing submitted journal manuscripts or searching the literature, studies were found where focus groups are misused as a complete research method or where focus groups alone are not appropriate for data collection. In addition, interpretation of findings from focus group data are sometimes stated as findings about individuals, such as case findings from group members, rather than the collective findings from the group. There appears to be a lack of knowledge of the limitations of focus group use.

Webb and Kevern (2001) agree that published nursing studies represent misuse of focus groups. They note that some authors of published studies state that grounded theory, phenomenology, or ethnography was done when using only focus group data transcripts—focus groups are incompatible with several components of these mainstream research methods. It is not possible to do theoretical sampling, participant observation, or capture individual's lived experiences when only collecting data with focus groups.

Current state of nursing science in the use of focus groups

Webb and Kevern (2001) reviewed Cumulative Index of Nursing and Allied Health Literature (CINAHL) citations for focus group use in publications 1990 to 1999 and found that, out of 124 articles that mentioned focus groups, there were only 33 data-based studies that used focus groups. In order to do a more current comparison, this author went to CINAHL and searched for publications from 2000 to 2010 that were research, with at least one nurse author, and where the abstract included the term "focus group." Of the 104 results, the vast majority of studies used focus groups appropriately as a data collection method; 8–10 of the 104 stated that they did grounded theory or ethnography in the abstract. These qualitative methods are not appropriate for focus group data collection alone and were deemed inappropriate.

An important caveat must be made: not all research studies done by nurses using focus groups were found in CINAHL. There are others that are known to this author that were not indexed by CINAHL, however, as a means of comparison with Webb and Kevern's review that limit was placed. It certainly appears that focus groups are being used in nursing research much more now than in the 1990s and the use is most commonly as a data collection method. Here is a list of the uses of focus groups found in the literature from 2000 to the present:

1 Descriptive studies
2 Focus groups as an intervention
3 For the development of an instrument; either for item generation or item evaluation
4 To see the change of opinions, over time
5 Participatory action research, as part of a mixed methods study

6 Grounded theory
7 Ethnography
8 Phenomenology/hermeneutics.

Exemplars

Two examples of well-done studies using focus groups are highlighted here. Murrock, Higgins, and Killion (2009) report on a mixed methods intervention pilot combining dance and peer support to improve physical measures of diabetes (Type II) status for African American women. This two-group, pretest–posttest study used the bio-physical measures of blood pressure, A1C,weight and body fat for individual outcomes. Peer support inherent in dance class was explored in focus groups to answer the question, "What is the role of peer support in this intervention?" Group responses were appropriately analyzed for themes for the collective women. The authors found that the integration of quantitative and qualitative findings yielded greater understanding of the effects of the 12-week dance intervention, including the role of peer support.

Amar, Bess, and Stockbridge (2010) conducted a study with college women about inter-personal violence, victimization, and seeking help. Focus groups were the only data collection method; the design was described as "qualitative," which is non-specific, but the rest of the audit trail is quite clear, including a paragraph on trustworthiness. Data analysis was stated as "group as the unit of analysis" with four themes that emerged from the data. This is an exemplar write-up of an appropriate use of focus groups with the study purpose driving the methods and analysis.

Conclusion

Focus groups are a useful and accessible means of collecting qualitative data that is often of interest to nurse researchers. Care should be taken to use focus groups within a research design that is congruent with their use. While focus groups may yield rich data quickly, they are only worthwhile if their planning and conduct are meticulous, and the analysis of group data rigorous. Appropriate use of focus groups should be included in doctoral education. Use of focus groups will enrich the knowledge generated in our nursing research studies.

References

Amar, A. F., Bess, R., & Stockbridge, J. (2010). Lessons from families and communities about interpersonal violence, victimization, and seeking help. *Journal of Forensic Nursing, 6*(3), 110-120. doi: 10.1111/j.1939-3938.2010.01076.x.

Côté-Arsenault, D., & Morrison-Beedy, D. (1999). Practical advice for planning and conducting focus groups. *Nursing Research, 48*(5), 280–283.

Kean, S. (2010). Children and young people's strategies to access information during a family member's critical illness. *Journal of Clinical Nursing, 19*(1–2), 266–274.

Kitzinger, J. (1995). Introducing focus groups. *BMJ, 311*(July 29), 299–302.

Krueger, R. A. (1998). *Analyzing and reporting focus group results.* Thousand Oaks, CA: Sage.

Krueger, R. A., & Casey, M. A. (2000). *Focus groups: A practical guide for applied research* (3rd ed.). Thousand Oaks, CA: Sage.

Lambert, S. D., & Loiselle, C. G. (2008). Combining individual interviews and focus groups to enhance data richness. *Journal of Advanced Nursing, 62*(2), 228–237. doi: 10.1111/j.1365-2648.2007.04559.x.

Lincoln, Y. S., & Guba, E. G. (1985). *Naturalistic inquiry.* Newbury Park, CA: Sage.

Merton, R. K., Fiske, M., & Kendall, P. L. (1990). *The focused interview: A manual of problems and procedures* (2nd ed.). New York: The Free Press.

Morgan, D. L. (1997). *Focus groups as qualitative research* (2nd ed.). Thousand Oaks, CA: Sage.

Morgan, D. L. (2010). Reconsidering the role of interaction in analyzing and reporting focus groups. *Qualitative Health Research, 20*(5), 718–722.

Morrison-Beedy, D., Côté-Arsenault, D., & Feinstein, N. F. (2001). Maximizing results with focus groups: Moderator and analysis issues. *Applied Nursing Research, 14*(1), 48–53.

Murrock, C. J., Higgins, P. A., & Killion, C. (2009). Dance and peer support to improve diabetes outcomes in African American women. *Diabetes Educator, 35*(6), 995–1003. doi: 10.1177/0145721709343322.

Pavlish, C., & Ho, A. (2009). Displaced persons' perceptions of human rights in southern Sudan. *International Nursing Review, 56*(4), 416–425. doi: 10.1111/j.1466-7657.2009.00739.x.

Rodehorst-Weber, T. K., Wilhelm, S. L., Stepans, M. B. F., Tobacco, R., & de la Paz, F. (2009). Screening Native American children for asthma: Findings from focus group discussions. *Issues in Comprehensive Pediatric Nursing, 32*(4), 200–209. doi: 10.3109/01460860903281382.

Scharff, D. P., Mathews, K. J., Jackson, P., Hoffsuemmer, J., Martin, E., & Edwards, D. (2010). More than Tuskegee: Understanding mistrust about research participation. *Journal of Health Care for the Poor & Underserved, 21*(3), 879–897. doi: 10.1353/hpu.0.0323.

Stewart, D. W., & Shamdasani, P. N. (1990). *Focus groups: Theory and practice,* Applied Social Research Methods Series, Vol. 20. Newbury Park, CA: Sage.

Webb, C., & Kevern, J. (2001). Focus groups as a research method: A critique of some aspects of their use in nursing research. *Journal of Advanced Nursing, 33*(6), 798–805.

24

Participatory Action Research

A new science for nursing?

Lynne E. Young

As a doctoral student in the 1990s I was introduced to Participatory Action Research (PAR) and Participatory Research (PR) at the UBC Institute of Health Promotion Research (UBCIHPR) during sessions capably facilitated by Dr. L.W. Green, an internationally esteemed health promotion researcher and scholar. At the time, the IHPR was preparing a White Paper for the Royal Society to guide the evaluation of the quality of participatory approaches to research that would be used to guide researchers and peer-reviewers to navigate this new and, to many people, mysterious, terrain of science of health promotion. As a group of researchers, post-doctoral fellows, and graduate students, during these sessions we engaged in lively conversations about "What is PAR/PR?" "How is this research?" Concurrently, as a doctoral student in nursing, I was grappling with definitions of health-promoting nursing practice[1] in the midst of what seemed to me were a plethora of unclear and conflicting definitions. As the IHPR conversations progressed, there was resonance between what I was coming to understand were key principles of health-promoting nursing practice and participatory approaches to research such as PAR and PR. Discovering this synchronicity between practice and research was thrilling for me. As a nurse, I began to see how I might not only generate knowledge for health-promoting nursing practice, but how the research process itself could be health promoting! This aha moment launched me on a journey of understanding, applying, and critiquing the relevance of PAR for my nursing research practice.

Defining PAR: a moving target

PAR is a strand of Action Research (AR)[2] that holds to a view of knowledge generation that assumes that participation in research by those most affected by it democratizes research and therefore has transformative potential. Here, researchers work collaboratively with those most affected by the problem through an iterative cycle of fieldwork or practice, reflection, planning, education, research, and action (Fals Borda, 2001; Green et al., 1995; Greenwood & Levin, 2007; Kemmis & McTaggart, 2003; Maguire, 1987; Pavlish & Pharris, 2012; Reason & Bradbury, 2001; Stringer & Genat, 2004). PAR specifically focuses on the concerns and issues of oppressed people, for example, the landless, women, subjects of racism and genocide, the disabled, the homeless and many others (Greenwood & Levin, 2007), whereas Action Research has a broader reach, for example, organizational change. PAR is an approach to research where participatory principles guide researchers and participants to collaborate to co-generate knowledge that addresses a practical problem. These principles over-arch a research process that employs qualitative or a mixed methods designs.

Action Research originated with Kurt Lewin's 1930s inquiries designed to demonstrate how greater productivity in factories and improvements in law and order in communities could be achieved through democratic participation rather than autocratic coercion. Lewin espoused that Action Research was designed to enable minority groups to overcome problems arising from their histories of exploitation and colonialism (Adelman, 1993). Freire's (1970) emancipatory pedagogy added to understandings of how knowledge generation could elicit the voices of the silenced and marginalized to catalyze social and political transformation for their betterment. Freire's approach, like others with a political intent, generally excludes the holders of power from the inquiry (Greenwood & Levin, 2007). Maguire (1987) enriched thinking about participatory approaches offering a design she refers to as Feminist Participatory Research. When Maguire was a student engaged in PR, she noticed that "women occupy a peripheral, even hidden place in most participatory research literature" (p. 4). In response, she articulated a feminist approach to PR in her classic book entitled *Doing Participatory Research: A Feminist Approach*. Researchers apply not only feminist lenses to their PAR designs but apply other critical lenses such as a post-colonial lens. Critical lenses such as feminist and post-colonial lenses sensitize researchers to attend intentionally to the diversity of voices and perspectives in participatory designs (Pavlish & Pharris, 2012).

PAR is located within an emerging paradigm of science, the aim of which is to understand a system as a focus of inquiry as characterized by interconnectedness where dynamic relational processes are in constant flux (Wheatley, 1994). From this holistic perspective on human nature and reality, it is assumed that the world is complex, subjectivity is valued, information is a creative force, truth depends on context, and the world is a comprised of circular, dynamic relationships (Watkins & Mohr, 2001). Consistent with this view of science, PAR is designed to be transformative and empowering; knowledge is co-created; inquiry is educative when meaning is negotiated; and change can be mobilized to generate or evaluate new practices or policies (Fals Borda, 2001; Green et al., 1995; Kemmis & McTaggart, 2003; Maguire, 1987; Stringer & Genat, 2004; Watkins & Mohr, 2001). Khanlou (2010) refers to participatory approaches to research as "passionate research with a blurring of theoretical, methodological, pragmatic, and researcher–participant boundaries" (p. 281).

Located within a paradigm that radically differs from the underlying assumptions about human nature, truth, and reality characteristic of classical liberal theory that have shaped Western science since the seventeenth century, participatory approaches to inquiry challenge PAR researchers (Watkins & Mohr, 2001; Williams, 1989). Classical liberal theory is based on three key assumptions: abstract individualism, rationalism, and egoism (Williams, 1989). Abstract individualism considers human beings as solitary, self-sufficient, and self-determining beings that exist independent of social relationships. Rationalism assumes that there is a separation between mental faculties and the physical and emotional. Related to this is the assumption that a complete set of facts can be isolated from emotions and values, and that this set of facts will reveal the truth. Egoism assumes that individuals are the sole agents of their situations, with social life assumed to be a choice. The new science is a move away from dichotomous thinking, objectivity, predictability, and the search for one truth (Watkins & Mohr, 2001). PAR researchers apply a new approach to science, one that is in sharp, if not dramatic, contrast to dominant scientific discourses that are deeply embedded in Western thought.

With its roots in the social and political sciences and organizational change literature, PAR is well suited to questions of interest to nursing. The emancipatory and educational aims of PAR resonate with the principles of health-promoting nursing practice defined as a process that enables people to increase control over and to improve their health (Choudhry et al., 2002; Green et al., 1995). With its focus on addressing practical problems, PAR has the capacity to address questions related to the practice of nursing (Doane & Varcoe, 2005). Thus, PAR is embraced by nurse researchers who engage communities in research, work with marginalized groups, address health inequities, health system effectiveness, and clinical practice. Philosophically, PAR resonates with holistic views of nursing; for example, Roger's (1970) science of unitary human beings where Rogers posits that the mission of nursing is fulfilled through the union of theory and practice (Barrett, 2010). Thus, the ontology and epistemology of the unitary paradigm of nursing and PAR align. As well, Roger's view on nursing and PAR align ethically. For Rogers, the art of nursing is in the creative use of nursing for the betterment of human beings, and this occurs through practice (Barrett, 2010; Butcher, 2006/2008). The moral aim of participatory approaches, characterized as "inquiry in the pursuit of worthwhile purposes, for the flourishing of persons" (Reason, 2006, p. 187) resonates with the ethical position assumed by Rogers in her position on nursing. Within and beyond nursing, PAR is increasingly embraced by researchers who hold to a holistic view of the world (Bradbury, 2004).

In spite of the exciting promises of PAR, it may be viewed by conventional researchers as unsystematic, primarily storytelling, and atheoretical (Dick, 2006; Greenwood & Levin, 2007; Gustavsen, 2003). Even conventional scientists who see the potential of participatory research find it esoteric when compared with traditional scientific methods (Gustavsen, 2003). Thus, its acceptance in the halls of academia may be compromised. And, participation as a process is not without critics (Kesby, 2005). Cooke and Kothari (2001) point to the dark side of participation, noting that participation may impose rather than overcome power relations and that participation itself engenders practical and theoretical tensions. To add to these critiques, currently there is a proliferation of labels for approaches to research that resemble PAR. Nurses label their participatory research in new ways such as participatory health research and community-based collaborative action research, often without delineating to readers how their approach is similar to, or different from, traditional participatory designs, thereby contributing to the linguistic challenges of understanding this approach to research.

In the following section, I provide examples of research that align with the key principles of PAR to illustrate how these designs have been used by nurses in their research practice. Note that not all studies presented here are labeled Participatory Action Research, but all align the principles of participation that guide participatory approaches to research: the inquiry addresses a practical or practice problem; some of those under study participate actively with the researchers throughout the research process along a continuum from some involvement to extensive involvement (see Table 24.1); participants and researchers co-generate knowledge using a collaborative process; and the social purpose of the research is to transform and/or empower (Green et al., 1995; Greenwood & Levin, 2007).

Feminist Participatory Action Research (FPAR): advancing the social mandate of nursing

An interprofessional team of researchers that included a nurse, Salmon, Browne, and Pederson (2010), designed a feminist Participatory Action Research design (FPAR) to improve health care practice for women who use drugs in a marginalized community in Vancouver, BC, the Downtown East Side (DTES). The researchers and DTES women collaborated throughout the research process to reveal the women's experiences with primary health care services with the intent to change practice. FPAR, the authors note, aligns with the social mandate of nursing

Table 24.1 Guidelines for rating participatory research

1. Participants and the nature of their involvement:
   a) Is the community of interest clearly described or defined?
   b) Do members of the defined community participating in the research have concern or experience with the issue?
   c) Are interested members of the defined community provided opportunities to participate in the research process?
   d) Is attention given to barriers to participation, with consideration of those who have been underrepresented in the past?
   e) Has attention been given to establishing within the community an understanding of the researchers' commitment to the issue?
   f) Are community participants enabled to contribute their physical and/or intellectual resources to the research process?
2. Origin of the research question:
   a) Did the impetus for the research come from the defined community?
3. Purpose of the research:
   a) Can the research facilitate learning among community participants about individual and collective resources for self-determination?
   b) Can the research facilitate collaboration between community participants and resources external to the community?
   c) Is the purpose of the research to empower the community to address the determinants of health?
   d) Does the scope of the research encompass some combination of political, social and economic determinants of health?
4. Process and context – methodological implications:
   a) Does the research process apply the knowledge of community participants in the phases of planning, implementation and evaluation?
   b) For community participants, does the process allow for learning about research methods?

Source: Modified from Green et al. (1995).

envisioned as a concern for people who are marginalized with a commitment to "redress power inequities, hierarchies, and health and social inequities" (Salmon, Browne, & Pederson, 2010; VANDU Women's Care Team, 2009). Salmon, Browne, and Pederson note that PAR has been used successfully in a variety of health services and policy-oriented research.

In this example of FPAR, the DTES women were included in every phase of the research, from the identification of research questions to writing the final report. The initiative was entitled the VANDU (Vancouver Drug Users) Women CARE (VANDU Women's Care Team, 2009). Using FPAR enabled a research process where the women's voices were elicited and given space for expression, the power hierarchies of traditional research were disrupted, the women developed research and analytical skills, and the women were paid for their work. There was an intent in this study to use FPAR not only for its emancipatory potential but also as a strategy for changing practice.

This FPAR study is reported in a research report (VANDU, 2009). With the three academic researchers, 32 DTES women designed the research and 11 women were trained as peer interviewers. Fifty DTES women's experiences were documented during individual interviews. These 50 women were 20–70 years old with 62% of participants Aboriginal. All of these women had used drugs in the Downtown East Side (DTES) and all had accessed primary health care services in the preceding 12 months. Qualitative and quantitative data were gathered to provide a thorough description of the women's experiences. In the report, there is little information about how the qualitative method was used in this research, or how data from the two paradigms illuminated or augmented each other. Initial findings of the study were presented at Dialogue Day where the research team, including DTES women participants, health care providers, and policy-makers involved in the DTES were convened. Findings of the study are compelling, touching, and informative. The research report is organized into two main sections: "Women's experiences and use of primary care" and "Going the extra mile together to improve primary care for women who use drugs in the downtown eastside." The report documents in detail the health problems and health care needs of the women, and how they used primary health care services. The authors theorized that for DTES women "being known" was a key to effective health care relationships. The study led the team to a radical conclusion: that primary health care must be redefined.

Salmon, Browne, and Pederson (2010) reflect on the challenging, and often disturbing, realities of working in partnerships with marginalized women, challenges noted elsewhere by a nurse researcher (Varcoe, 2006). For example, the authors report that while FPAR was effective in generating knowledge about the lived experiences of DTES women, the participation of the women was hampered by the extreme demands of their lives, lives frequently consumed by basic survival and/or supporting friends and family through crises such as incarceration, illness, and death. In this reflection on using FPAR, these researchers note that they were less effective in fostering change than they had envisioned they might be. Nonetheless, at the individual level, there was evidence that was empowering in that women's confidence increased and they came to realize that their experiences with primary health care were a result of system-level issues and failures rather than their own shortcomings. This courageous example of FPAR aligns with the key principles of PAR in its focus on: collaboration, participation, eliciting lived experiences, giving voice, and empowering marginalized women. Furthermore, FPAR as employed in this study aligns with nursing's social justice mission.

Critical Participatory Research: partnering with Aboriginal people to improve care

Undertaking research with Aboriginal people is complex and controversial as it is located in a history of exploitation and abuse. In this section, I feature a study designed using a critical postcolonial stance with the principles of Participatory Research to address the issue of Aboriginal women and their family's access to prenatal care "'Making a Difference': A New Care Paradigm for Pregnant and Parenting Aboriginal People" (Smith, Edwards, Martens, & Varcoe, 2007).[3] That Aboriginal women's participation in prenatal care is less than optimum and they experience less desirable outcomes of care when compared to the general population are the practical problem addressed by this research. Research with Aboriginal communities designed to measure health benefits from the researchers' and health care stakeholders' perspectives reveals numerous benefits from involving the Aboriginal community throughout the inquiry process, for example, early access and participation in care. Yet, there is a paucity of research that identifies the health benefits of prenatal care from the perception of Aboriginal people. Thus, the researchers collaborated with Aboriginal people and health care providers to reveal the health benefits of care from the perspective of Aboriginal women and their families.

In this inquiry, the researchers applied the principles of Participatory Research using a post-colonial lens to ensure that colonization processes were visible. This design, the researchers claim, enabled the inclusion of different value systems, sensitivity to difference, appreciation of all forms of knowledge, and the capacity to generate knowledge relevant to stakeholders that is useful for solving practical problems (Smith et al., 2007). Case study design that followed the tradition method proposed by Yin (2003) guided data collection and the analysis of qualitative data. The cases included both one urban and one rural Aboriginal health care delivery organization that were reputed to offer effective approaches to prenatal care. In reviewing this study, it is instructive to note that Canadian researchers undergo an extensive ethics approval process when working with Aboriginal people because of the history of exploitation and abuse of Aboriginal people in Canada. Ethical approval for this study was required from the university ethics review board, the Board of Directors of the Health Organization, the ethical review committee of the participating Tribal Council, and the Chiefs and Councils of the participating communities.

Network sampling was the sampling strategy employed in this study so that data would represent a variety of perspectives from community members, providers, and leaders. Participants often had multiple roles, for example, a leader could be a provider and community member. One-to-one exploratory interviews and small group discussions were used to collect data with interviews lasting from 45 to 120 minutes. Fifty-seven men and women participated in the study, 61% of participants were Aboriginal identified and 50% were women. One member of the research team analyzed the data using interpretive description. Participants were convened to provide input into the preliminary analysis.

In the peer-reviewed article in which this study is reported, the interpretation was presented according to three themes: (1) acknowledging progress over the long term; (2) using a strengths-based approach; and, (3) recognizing relevant outcomes. "Acknowledging progress over the long term" speaks to the importance of health professionals recognizing and respecting Aboriginal clients' recovery from the impact of the residential school system. "Using a strengths-based approach" facilitated a collaborative model of care that enabled clients to speak up, speak out and find their voice. The theme, "recognizing relevant outcomes" was presented as a list of items that were located in a conceptual framework. The conceptual framework presents the findings along an "upstream/downstream" health care continuum. Findings were supported with an array of compelling quotes, thus giving voice to participants, and the results of the study were presented in the participants' communities, creating another arena for participants' voices to be heard.

Participatory principles were used effectively in this compelling study, one that appears to be somewhat more researcher-driven than participant-driven when compared to the Salmon, Browne, and Pederson (2010) study. Nonetheless, the interpretation reflected input from participants, participants' voices were amply represented, and presenting the results of the study in participating communities was a strategy for opening a space for conversations about caring for prenatal Aboriginal women and their families. Like the Salmon, Browne, and Pederson (2010) study, this study aligns well with the social justice perspective on nursing while addressing a practice problem.

Participatory Action Research: ethics in action

In a study by Doane, Storch, and Pauly (2009), the research team implemented a design that they label Participatory Action Research to theorize an epistemology of ethics in everyday nursing work. This study differs from the previous two studies reviewed as it focuses on nursing work rather than on the health care needs of marginalized people, thus demonstrating how PAR can be used to generate knowledge for nursing practice. The study reports on the epistemological and methodological insights gained. The goal of this research was "to purposefully enlist the knowledge, ideas, and expertise of the nurses [nurse participants] to develop further knowledge and simultaneously affect the intrapersonal, interpersonal, and contextual elements that shaped their ethical practice" (p. 234). The inquiry was informed by deconstructive hermeneutics that rests on the assumption that knowledge is interpretive and experiential. The researchers immersed themselves in the everyday of nursing work on a medical oncology unit, buddying with nurses to gather data that were then analyzed to reveal the particulars of situations and contexts.

In this PAR, the research team pursued this inquiry over a prolonged period of time, 2.5 years. The academic researchers and staff nurses on a medical oncology unit collaborated during buddy shifts and once a month during meetings. The academic researchers gathered data, summarized their analysis, and presented the analysis to staff nurses for feedback. The authors claim that this process empowered the nurses to find words to describe their experience of ethical practice while contributing to the construction of an authentic interpretation of their ethical practice:

> The inquiry process enabled them to critically consider particular situations within the context of their nursing values and obligations, more intentionally listen to their inner rumblings that told them "this isn't right", and continually "find" and develop their own resourcefulness and capacity to recreate themselves and their practice to respond to the difficulties and challenges that arose.
>
> *(p. 237)*

Overall, the most significant finding was that ethical practice constantly changes in response to personal, interpersonal, and contextual influences.

As an elegant example of the use of PAR in nursing research, this study exemplifies a respectful engagement between staff nurses and academic nurses throughout a prolonged engagement of inquiry into ethical nursing practice. The PAR was collaborative in that nurses were involved through all phases of the research, with the academic researchers taking the lead initially and gradually turning the lead over to the staff nurses. Staff nurses participated in developing the design of the research, for example, suggesting buddying as a data collection strategy. And the staff nurses and academic researchers engaged in dialogue about the academic researchers' interpretations of the data to sharpen and enrich the analysis. Staff nurses were given voice during regular meetings of staff nurses and the academic researchers. Learning about ethical nursing practice was a key feature of this research for the staff nurses and academic researchers. Similar to other studies using a PAR design, the political influence of the study was limited. However, in this study, what appeared to be powerful and lasting was the development of networks through which ethical knowledge flowed. Gustavsen (2001) posits that AR as inquiry is a relationship among three discourses: (1) a discourse on theory; (2) a discourse on practice; and (3) a mediating discourse on how to link them. Gustavsen (2001, 2003) notes that fostering networks of social relationships among stakeholders opens spaces wherein "mediating" discourses have transformative potential. This inquiry reflects Gustavsen's claims related to the power of creating networks to mediate between theory and practice.

To summarize, all three studies presented in this chapter drew on participatory principles in their inquiries. In each study, the inquiry addressed a practice problem relevant to nursing, participants were involved in some way in the inquiry, the knowledge generated was developed collaboratively, participants' voices were given space in the research report and/or program or policy-making arenas, and the capacity of the research to increase participants' control over their situations varied from study to study. All studies used qualitative research with one study drawing on quantitative data in addition to the qualitative component. The rigor of the quantitative and qualitative methods varied with the report of the qualitative design largely absent from one study, while another used a sophisticated qualitative method. All studies theorized about health care relationships from simple to sophisticated theorizing evident in the research report, thus closing the theory–practice gap. The relevance to nursing was discernible in all studies. Thus, this collection of studies, each of which used a participatory approach to generate knowledge for nursing practice, is a small window into new science pursued by nurses to address the theory–practice gap in nursing.

Participatory Action Research: state of the science

Participatory Action Research, and similar genres, deviate from historical, dominant discourses of science. As discussed previously, traditional scientific rationale is based on assumptions that shaped Western philosophical thought and science that separates theory from practice, subject from object, and mind from body and emotion, the origins of which are often attributed to the writings of the influential modernist authors Bacon, Descartes, and Locke (Maxwell, 1997). Bacon advocated for systematic inquiry to advance humankind's capacity to dominate and control nature. Descartes explicated a systematic method to advance Bacon's vision. And Locke fused the domination of nature and primacy of method with the sovereignty of the individual (Maxwell, 1997). Thus, the dominant discourse of scientific rationality was born, at the core of which are objectivity, prediction, and control. Gustavsen (2003) relates this paradigmatic turn to a class struggle that began in the seventeenth century when the middle class gained power and took steps to decouple reason from practice in the context of societies dominated by religious rules. AR, PAR, and PR, and their "offspring," are located within a postmodern paradigm where:

> the recognition of other people as subjects has paved the way for seeing research as a collaborative effort together with those concerned rather than as studies on them. A turn of this kind opens up new ways of conceptualizing the tasks of the social sciences but does not in itself solve all problems. A new agenda is set, but the various points on this agenda need considerable theoretical and practical development.
>
> *(Gustavsen, 1996, p. 90)*

Thus, participatory approaches to research are new forms of knowledge development that are in opposition to forms of logic and reasoning that have existed for about four centuries. It is no wonder then that conventional researchers view participatory forms of research as esoteric and difficult to relate to (Gustavsen, 2003).

With holistic ways of thinking about human nature and science reaching nursing in the late twentieth century, nurse researchers began to question the logic of dichotomizing subject/object, mind/body, theory and practice. Esteemed nursing theorists such as M. A. Newman and Rogers call for unifying theories of nursing with approaches to knowledge development in nursing. Newman (1997) notes that:

> Nursing claims to be a discipline dedicated to understanding and relating to the health of the whole person, not just the pathology that often brings the person to the attention of health care professionals. The preponderance of nursing research, however, fails to focus on this commitment. In an effort to be scientific, we have allowed our vision to be blurred by the paradigmatic demands of objectivity and control. In an attempt to be predictive, we have divided the person into parts.
>
> *(p. 34)*

Newman calls for "a break with a paradigm of health that focuses on power, manipulation, and control and move to one of reflective, compassionate consciousness" (p. 38). Newman notes that "we come to the meaning of the whole not by viewing the pattern from the outside but by entering into the evolving pattern as it unfolds" (p. 39). Newman posits that Participatory Research has the potential to unify nursing theory with research.

As mentioned previously, participatory approaches to research are challenging. Specific challenges facing researchers intent on using participatory approaches encompass attracting adequate funding, recruiting participants, developing and maintaining partnerships, ensuring that partners have the capacity and are ready for such engagement, extensive time requirements, addressing ethical considerations, reconciling research interests between academic and community partners, and generating rigorous research products (Fals Borda, 2001; Fox, Morford, Fine, & Gibbons, 2004; Gibbon, 2002; Green et al., 1995; Gustavsen, 2003; Minkler, Blackwell, Thompson, & Tamir, 2003; Salmon, Brown, & Pederson, 2010; Varcoe, 2006; Young, 2006; Young & Wharf-Higgins, 2010). Salmon, Brown, and Pederson (2010), Varcoe (2006), and Pavlish and Pharris (2012) point to the interpersonal tensions that participatory approaches elicit when working with marginalized groups. Here, co-researchers' priorities, life circumstances, and motivations may differ markedly from the academic researchers. Negotiating a level of participation that ensures a successful engagement has the potential to stretch the capacity of the research team.

From a scientific perspective, one of the most often cited criticisms of PAR relates to the perception that PAR is a "soft" method. Such critiques originate with those who hold to the idea of science as truth (Fals-Borda, 2001). Standards of research quality that apply to large quantitative studies do not translate well to smaller, more qualitative, participatory studies, thus compromising the potential for publication of these studies in quality journals (Seng, 1998). In the past decade, while peer-reviewed journals have become more attuned to the unique contributions of qualitative research, evidence-based practice remains a dominant discourse, with randomized controlled trials the gold standard. Adding to this challenge, there are differing perspectives on how the credibility/validity of participatory approaches should be judged. Greenwood and Levin (2007) make a strong claim that the credibility of such inquiries be "measured according to the actions that arise from it to solve problems" (p. 63). Given that participatory research is a process, I wonder how central processes such as empowerment and "finding voice" can be measured. Green et al. (1995) propose a more flexible way to evaluate the quality of such inquiries proposing that each inquiry should be ranked relative to its participatory elements (see Table 24.1).

PAR researchers understand science as a social construction and good science as inquiry that generates knowledge that is useful for worthy causes (Fals Borda, 2001). Because PAR focuses on voice and everyday experiences, qualitative methods are employed in PAR research to elicit participants' experiences, meanings, and interpretations. While the focus on experiences is salient to participatory approaches to research, because program-planners and policy-makers generally require numbers to argue for resources or policy changes, quantitative methods may be the most appropriate choice when working in these environments. Combining qualitative and quantitative research when using a participatory approach has the potential to influence program-planners and policy-makers while promoting community participation and individual empowerment (Young & Wharf-Higgins, 2010). Pavlish and Pharris (2012) emphasize the importance of using rigorous quantitative and/or qualitative methods to uncover patterns. They liken using rigorous research methods when carrying out participatory approach to research to the roots of a tree, that is, rigorous methods provide a solid foundation upon which the inquiry rests. However, there are challenges to research when using a combination of qualitative and quantitative methods in a PAR design. Since these methods are located within contrasting scientific paradigms, how does one philosophically, ontologically, and epistemologically locate the research? Further, to ensure a rigorous product, how the qualitative and quantitative methods were used or "blended" in the study must be clearly articulated.

Participatory approaches to inquiry such as PAR are new forms of generating knowledge. Therefore, PAR researchers face challenges and issues arising from deeply embedded historical views of science and the related influence of institutionalized scientific practices and processes on the development and sustainability of this new form of knowledge. Nurses who hold to a unitary view of nursing and who use participatory approaches contribute to closing the gap between theory and practice in nursing. However, PAR nurses are wise to attune to the challenges, issues, and debates that face those who use a new form of science and plan accordingly.

Future directions

Participatory Action Research (PAR), an offspring of Action Research and cousin to numerous, rapidly proliferating participatory approaches to research, holds promise for nursing research in terms of generating knowledge congruent with theories emanating from views of nursing located within a holistic paradigm. Given the synchronicity between holistic perspectives on nursing and PAR it is likely that we will see a proliferation of such research. It is notable that in 2010 the esteemed *Journal of Nursing Inquiry* devoted an entire issue to participatory health research, thus providing a significant toehold for this approach to research in the nursing academy and a powerful forum for discussion.

Is PAR a promising approach for nurse researchers? It depends. If the intended research focuses on inequities, injustices, and unsatisfactory or inefficient nursing practices, then PAR, with its capacity to surface issues and research questions relevant to both the academy and practitioners, may be the most promising approach. Given the challenges facing PAR researchers, nurse researchers undertaking PAR would be well advised to develop strategies to address the challenges. PAR is gaining recognition and acceptance as its applications demonstrate that it is an innovative and exciting form of knowledge development (Gustavsen, 2003; Khalou, 2010). PAR nurse researchers will contribute uniquely to clarifying and refining this innovative approach to nursing inquiry creating space for "theory and practice to interact in new ways" (Gustavsen, 2003, p. 147).

Notes

1   See Young and Hayes (2002).
2   Action Research (AR), Participatory Action Research (PAR) and Participatory Research (PR) as terms used to define a participatory approach to research are not clearly differentiated in the literature. There is currently a proliferation of labels used to describe participatory approaches to research. Gustavsen (1996) refers to the proliferation of participatory approaches to research as offsprings of AR. In this chapter, I use AR as an overarching term, strands of which are PAR, PR, and the newly emerging participatory approaches such as participatory health research, community-based collaborative research, Appreciative Inquiry, and so on.
3   Aboriginal in this study "refers to organic political and cultural entities that stem historically from the original Peoples in North America, rather than collections of individuals united by so-called 'racial' characteristics" (Erasmus & Dussault, 1996). First Nations, Inuit, and Métis Peoples of Canada are considered Aboriginal people" (Smith, Edwards, Martens, & Varcoe 2007, p. 321).

References

Adelman, C. (1993). Kurt Lewin and the origins of Action Research. *Educational Action Research*, 1, 7–24.
Barrett, E. A. M. (2010). Power as knowing participation in change what's new and what's next? *Nursing Science Quarterly*, 23, 47–54.
Bradbury, H. (2004). Doing work that matters despite the obstacles. *Action Research*, 2, 209–227.
Butcher, H. K. (2006/2008). Unitary pattern-based praxis: A nexus of Rogerian cosmology, philosophy,

and science [corrected] [published erratum appears in *VISIONS, The Journal of Rogerian Nursing Science, 15(1)*, 28]. *Visions: The Journal of Rogerian Nursing Science, 14(2)*, 8–33.

Choudhry, U. K., Jandu, J., Mahal, R., Singh, R., Sohi-Pabla, H., & Mutta, B. (2002). Health promotion and participatory action research with South Asian women. *Journal of Nursing Scholarship, 34*, 75–81.

Cooke, B., & Kothari, U. (2001). The case for participation as tyranny. In B. Cooke & U. Kothari (Eds.), *Participation: The New Tyranny?* (pp. 1–15). London: Zed.

Dick, B. (2006). Action research literature: 2004–2006: Themes and trends. *Action Research, 4*, 439–459.

Doane, G. H., Storch, J., & Pauly, B. (2009). Ethical nursing practice: Inquiry in action. *Nursing Inquiry, 16*, 232–240.

Doane, G. H., & Varcoe, C. (2005). Toward compassionate action: Pragmatism and the inseparability of theory/practice. *Advances in Nursing Science, 28*, 81–90.

Erasmus, G., & Dussault, R. (1996). *Report on the Royal Commission on Aboriginal peoples.* Ottawa, ON: The Commission.

Fals Borda, O. (2001). Participatory (action) research in social theory: Origins and challenges. In P. Reason & H. Bradbury (Eds.), *Handbook of action research: Participative inquiry and practice* (pp. 27–37). Thousand Oaks, CA: Sage.

Fox, C. E., Morford, T. G., Fine, A., & Gibbons, M. C. (2004). The Johns Hopkins Urban Health Institute: A collaborative response to urban health issues. *Academic Medicine, 79*, 1169–1174.

Freire, P. (1970). *Pedagogy of the oppressed.* New York: Herder & Herder.

Gibbon, M. (2002). Doing a doctorate using a participatory action framework in the context of community health. *Qualitative Health Research, 12*, 546–558.

Green, L. W., George, M. A., Daniels, M., Frankish, C. J., Herbert, C. J., Bowie, W. R., &, O'Neill, M. (1995). *Study of participatory research in health promotion.* Vancouver, BC: The Royal Society.

Greenwood, D. J., & Levin, M. (2007). *Introduction to action research* (2nd ed.). Thousand Oaks, CA: Sage.

Gustavsen, B. (1996). Action Research, democratic dialogue, and the issue of "critical mass" in change. *Qualitative Inquiry, 2*(1), 90–103.

Gustavsen, B. (2001). Theory and practice: The mediating discourse. In P. Reason & H. Bradbury (Eds.), *Handbook of action research: Participative inquiry and practice* (pp. 15–26). Thousand Oaks, CA: Sage.

Gustavsen, B. (2003). New forms of knowledge production and the role of action research. *Action Research, 1*, 153 153–164.

Kemmis, S., & McTaggart, R. (2003). Participatory action research. In N. K. Denzin & Y. S. Lincoln (Eds.), *Strategies of qualitative inquiry* (2nd ed., pp. 336–396). Thousand Oaks, CA: Sage.

Kesby, M. (2005). Retheorizing empowerment through participation as a performance in space: Beyond tyranny to transformation. *Signs, 30*, 2037–2065.

Khanlou, N. (2010). Editorial: Participatory health research. *Nursing Inquiry, 17*, 281.

Maguire, P. (1987). *Doing participatory research: A feminist approach.* Amherst: University of Massachusetts, Center for International Education.

Maxwell, L. (1997). Foundational thought in the development of knowledge for social change. In S. Thorne & V. Hayes (Eds.), *Nursing praxis: Knowledge and action*, (pp. 203–218), Thousand Oaks, CA: Sage.

Minkler, M., Blackwell, A. G., Thompson, M., & Tamir. H. (2003). Community-based participatory research: implications for public health funding. *American Journal of Public Health, 93*, 1210–1213.

Newman, M. A. (1997). Experiencing the whole. *Advances in Nursing Science, 20*, 34–39.

Pavlish, C. P., & Pharris, M. D. (2012). *Community-based collaborative action research: A nursing approach.* Sudbury, MA: Jones & Bartlett Learning.

Reason, P. (2006). Choice and quality in Action Research practice. *Journal of Management Inquiry, 15*, 187–203.

Reason, P., & Bradbury, H. (2001). Introduction: Inquiry and participation in search of a world worthy of human aspiration. In P. Reason & H. Bradbury (Eds.), *Handbook of action research: Participative inquiry and practice* (pp. 1–14). Thousand Oaks, CA: Sage.

Rogers, M. (1970). *An introduction to the theoretical basis of nursing.* Philadelphia, PA: F. A. Davis.

Salmon, A., Browne, A., & Pederson, A. (2010). "Now we call it research": participatory health research involving marginalized women who use drugs. *Nursing Inquiry, 17*, 336–345.

Seng, J.S. (1998). Praxis as a conceptual framework for participatory research in nursing. *Advances in Nursing Science, 20(4)*, 37–48.

Smith, D., Edwards, N., Martens, P., & Varcoe, C. (2007). "Making a difference": A new care paradigm for pregnant and parenting Aboriginal people. *Canadian Journal of Public Health, 98*, 321–325.

Stringer, E., & Genat, W. J. (2004). *Action research in health.* Columbus, OH: Pearson.

VANDU Women's Care Team (2009). *"Me I'm living it": The primary health care experiences of women who use drugs in Vancouver's Downtown Eastside.* Vancouver, BC: Author.

Varcoe, C. (2006). Doing Participatory Action Research in a racist world. *Western Journal of Nursing Research, 28,* 525–540.

Watkins, J. M., & B. J. Mohr (2001). *Appreciative inquiry.* San Francisco: Jossey-Bass.

Wheatley, M. (1994). *Leadership and the new science: Learning about organizations from an orderly universe.* San Francisco: Berrett-Koehler.

Williams, D. (1989). Political theory and individualistic health promotion. *Advances in Nursing Science, 12,* 14–25.

Yin, R. (2003). *Case study research: Design and methods* (2nd ed.). London: Sage.

Young, L. E. (2006). Participatory Action Research (PAR): A research strategy for nursing? *Western Journal of Nursing Research, 28(5),* 1–6. [Invited editorial.]

Young, L. E., & Hayes, V. E. (2002). *Transforming health promotion practice: Concepts, issues, and applications.* Philadelphia, PA: F. A. Davis.

Young, L. E., & Wharf-Higgins, J. (2010). Using participatory research to challenge the status quo for women's cardiovascular health. *Journal of Nursing Inquiry, 17,* 346–358.

25
Metasynthesis

Barbara Paterson

Nurse researchers have played a major role in the development and evolution of metasynthesis, a research approach entailing synthesizing findings of qualitative research studies (called "primary research") in order to generate new understandings and to suggest new directions for practice, theory development, research methodology, and/or policy development (Doyle, 2003; Sandelowski & Barroso, 2003; Thorne, Jensen, Kearney, Noblit, & Sandelowski, 2004). An example of the contributions of metasynthesis to nursing knowledge is a metasynthesis by Taverner and colleagues (2011). These researchers conducted a metasynthesis of neuropathic pain caused by leg ulceration. Synthesizing the findings from numerous studies resulted in the identification of symptoms of neuropathic pain associated with leg ulceration that had not previously been identified. Taverner et al. postulate that if neuropathic pain were effectively addressed in cases of leg ulceration, it is likely that sequelae of leg ulceration, such as chronic pain, depression and insomnia, might be prevented. A metasynthesis conducted by nurse researchers of qualitative studies regarding breastfeeding support (Schmied Beake, Sheehan, McCourt, & Dykes, 2011) revealed policy and practice directions to improve the support of breastfeeding mothers, particularly in regard to systems and services that foster continuity of caregiver support.

There has been a rapid proliferation in the past two decades of literature regarding metasynthesis as a research approach and distinct metasynthesis methods. Within this body of literature, there is considerable overlap, ambiguity and contradiction about what metasynthesis is and how it should be conducted. This often leaves novices with little direction about how to conduct metasynthesis research to best fit their research goals, available resources and ideological stance (Paterson, 2012). In this chapter, I will provide a historical and methodological overview of metasynthesis as a research approach, highlighting the major schools of thought in the field. I will present some of the most well-known metasynthesis methods, comparing and contrasting their epistemological and methodological underpinnings, as well as underscoring their distinctive features. I will also detail the critiques of metasynthesis that exist within relevant literature and the most common challenges that metasynthesists face when conducting such research. In conclusion, I will identify a number of best practices and directions for future development of metasynthesis, particularly in nursing research.

Historical overview

The evolution of metasynthesis is not entirely clear. Various authors provide different depictions of the earliest discussions of metasynthesis; however, there are a few authors who are known to have predicted the need for metasynthesis of qualitative research. For example, Glaser and Strauss (1967) suggested more than four decades ago that elements of grounded theory, such as theoretical sampling, might be applied to generate formal theory about the findings of grounded theory primary research studies; they did not, however, say how this would be accomplished. Grounded theory as a metasynthesis method was later developed by Kearney (1998).

The notion of metasynthesis was initially conceived in response to the inability to represent the findings of a body of qualitative research and to influence practice, theory or policy development beyond individual studies. Quantitative researchers used the techniques of meta-analysis to aggregate the findings of quantitative studies, but such approaches were regarded by many as antithetical to qualitative research. In addition, qualitative researchers were cautious about generalizing the findings of single studies to other sample populations, settings and contexts. This reluctance caused qualitative researchers to limit the applicability of their findings to one setting or with one sample population; generalizations drawn from a body of qualitative research about a specific phenomenon were not made. Paterson and colleagues (2001), for example, describe how they were aware that many qualitative researchers had determined that social support is critical to the experience of living with a chronic illness; however, most researchers concluded in their reports of such research that the reader could not generalize the findings beyond that particular study. Sandelowski, Docherty, and Emden (1997) cautioned that if qualitative researchers did not find a way to systematically synthesize qualitative research, while remaining true to the qualitative nature of the research, they would risk never contributing in a substantial way to the expansion and refinement of the body of knowledge in a particular field of study.

The first definitive text that instructed researchers about how to actually conduct a metasynthesis was authored by Noblit and Hare (1988). These authors introduced "meta-ethnography," a method for synthesizing ethnographic qualitative research studies. Noblit and Hare advocated three types of synthesis (reciprocal, refutational, and line-of-argument) in meta-ethnography; the selection of each type is dependent on whether the findings of primary research studies are similar or contradictory or whether the metasynthesis researcher wishes to look at different aspects of a particular phenomenon to develop an argument advocating for an alternate or a more comprehensive picture of the phenomenon. While this text was the first to provide guidelines to researchers about how to conduct metasynthesis research, it is vague or silent on many aspects, such as the selection and critical appraisal of primary research studies. The authors do not discuss the synthesis of qualitative research that is methodologically diverse. They referred to the metasynthesis of a small number of primary research studies (i.e., six or under) but do not explicate how the number of studies affects the metasynthesis process or outcomes.

Noblit and Hare's (1988) work was followed by some articles in refereed journals that explored why metasynthesis of qualitative research should occur and broad descriptions of how it might occur (e.g., Estabrooks, Field, & Morse, 1994; Jensen & Allen, 1996; Schreiber, Crooks, & Stern, 1997); however, these writings provided little direction to researchers about how to conduct metasynthesis. Later, Paterson and colleagues (2001) published a text about the method of "meta-study." They were the first authors to emphasize the need for systematic and transparent criteria and processes to select and appraise the primary research. Their text highlighted the way in which a large number of primary research studies with various interpretive methods could be synthesized to produce contextually based insights for researchers, theoreticians, and policy developers. The method "meta-study" is a complex one, involving four components (meta-data-analysis; meta-method; meta-theory; and metasynthesis) and because of its time-consuming processes, is not for the faint of heart (Paterson et al., 2001); however, the major contribution of the text was that it was the first to struggle in a practical and detailed way with both the processes and the challenges of metasynthesis, guiding metasynthesis researchers in the decisions that they must make in such research.

Although metasynthesis was originally conceived as a way of synthesizing qualitative research, some recent developments have included both qualitative and quantitative primary research. The phase of metasynthesis development that occurred following the introduction of meta-study is characterized by attempts to create metasynthesis in line with the systematic reviews in quantitative research. Researchers in the Joanna Briggs Institute of Australia were influential in revising the procedures of the Cochrane Collaboration to fit qualitative research (i.e., the qualitative systematic review). The emphasis of researchers in this phase is the need to enhance the rigor and credibility of metasynthesis research for funders and policy developers (Paterson, 2012; Pearson, 2004). At the same time, other researchers (Harden & Thomas, 2005; Oliver et al., 2008; Thomas et al., 2003) began to advocate for the integration of both qualitative and quantitative research in metasynthesis. These authors interpreted integration in metasynthesis as: (1) conducting a quantitative meta-analysis and a qualitative thematic analysis separately and then integrating the findings of each; (2) using qualitative methods to synthesize qualitative and quantitative primary research; or (3) using quantitative techniques to quantify the weight of evidence within the qualitative data within the body of primary research. Researchers who have conducted metasynthesis research within this phase have emphasized the need for quality control to provide evidence to funders and policy developers that the findings of the metasynthesis are grounded in systematic and credible approaches. Others have criticized these methods as positivistic and incongruent with the tenets of qualitative research.

Metasynthesis methods

Within the past two decades, over 20 distinct methods of metasynthesis have been developed. Some are formally recognized as a particular type of metasynthesis (e.g., formal grounded theory, realist review) and others are described as metasynthesis but not named as a specific method. Most have become associated with particular method developers (e.g., Paulson's realist review; Kearney's formal grounded theory), despite the fact that several methods overlap with one another and many recently developed methods are actually refined versions of earlier methods.

Table 25.1 highlights how some of the most well-known metasynthesis methods compare according to their structure/processes, intended outcome and defining attributes. The examples that are given are mainly written by nurse researchers or involve nurse researchers as a member of the research team. Some metasynthesis methods (i.e., Framework Analysis and Realist Review) that are gaining in popularity in the field have not been adopted by nurse researchers to date and therefore, the examples given for these methods are written by social scientists.

An overview of metasynthesis research reveals that many authors have adapted previous metasynthesis methods to develop a new method. For example, Finfgeld (1999) drew on Noblit and Hare's (1988) meta-ethnography to develop "meta-interpretation" and the origins of meta-study (Paterson et al., 2001) are in meta-ethnography and sociological meta-theory. Because of this, there are shared epistemological tenets among the many metasynthesis methods that have been developed since Noblit and Hare's (1988) seminal work in meta-ethnography (e.g., all involve the selection and synthesis of primary research, most involve a team of researchers); however, many metasynthesis method developers hold to different and often contradictory

Table 25.1 Metasynthesis methods

Method	Description	Defining attributes	Intended outcome(s)	Sources	Examples
Bayesian Synthesis	An adaptation of Bayesian meta-analysis that treats qualitative research as a resource equal to quantitative research. Using Bayesian statistics, the researcher attaches weight to the strength of evidence associated with those variables.	Realist High structure Low degree of iteration	Aggregated evidence to support a model for practice or policy	Voils et al., 2009 Crandell et al., 2011	HIV treatment adherence (Voils et al., 2009) Factors affecting child immunization (Roberts et al., 2002)
Critical interpretive synthesis	Involves researchers developing "synthetic constructs" that are then linked with constructs identified in a body of primary research. Can include quantitative, as well as qualitative, primary research. An adaptation of meta-ethnography and grounded theory. Must include a multidisciplinary team of researchers.	Idealist Moderate structure Low degree of iteration	A theoretical model that is shared with practitioners to determine its relevance to practice	Dixon-Woods et al., 2006	Use of morphine to treat cancer pain (Flemming & McInnes, 2012) Access to health care (Dixon-Woods et al., 2006)
Formal Grounded Theory	Synthesizes the findings of grounded theory primary research reports. Uses many of the procedures of grounded theory, such as constant comparative analysis.	Idealist Moderate degree of iteration Moderate structure	Middle-range theory that can be tested in future research	Kearney, 1998, 2001	Domestic violence (Kearney, 2001) Caring in nursing (Finfgeld-Connett, 2008)
Framework Analysis	Uses an *a priori* "framework" derived from background material and team discussions to determine which data to extract and synthesize. Involves organizing and analyzing data	Realist Low degree of iteration High structure	Theoretical models directly applicable to policy-makers, practitioners and designers of	Brunton et al., 2006 Oliver et al., 2008	Children's, young people's and parents' views of walking and cycling (Brunton et al., 2006) Public involvement in health services research (Oliver et al., 2008)

			interventions		
	(e.g., indexing using numerical codes, rearranging data into charts etc.).				
Meta-aggregation	Models the Cochrane process of systematic reviews in a pragmatist approach to metasynthesis.	Realist Low degree of iteration High structure	"Lines of action" on an individual and a community level to be tested in future research	Hannes & Lockwood, 2011 Pearson, 2004	Evidence-based practice in Belgian health care (Hannes & Pearson, 2012) Support for internationally educated nurses (Konno, 2006)
Meta-ethnography	An inductive and interpretive metasynthesis method that aims to translate qualitative primary research studies into each other by translating the findings and metaphors about the phenomenon under study across the different primary research studies. Although initially intended to synthesize ethnographies, the method is suitable for use with other qualitative methods.	Idealist Moderate degree of iteration Moderate structure	A conceptual model or theory about the phenomenon under study	Noblit & Hare, 1998	Medicine taking to treat asthma (Britten & Pope, 2012) Women's perceptions of breastfeeding support (Schmied et al., 2011)
Meta-study	Consists of three analytic components (meta-data-analysis, meta-method, meta-theory) and a synthesis component (metasynthesis).	Idealist High degree of iteration Low structure	Midrange theory about a phenomenon in order to provide insights for future research, policy or practice in the field of knowledge	Paterson et al., 2001	Meta-data-analysis: Balance and control in diabetes (Paterson et al., 1998) Meta-theory: Embedded assumptions about fatigue in chronic illness (Paterson et al., 2003) Meta-method: Influence of research frame on the understanding of living with chronic illness (Thorne et al., 2002) Metasynthesis: The shifting perspectives model of chronic illness (Paterson, 2001)

Table 25.1 Continued

Method	Description	Defining attributes	Intended outcome(s)	Sources	Examples
Narrative synthesis	A process of compiling qualitative data and narratives from primary research studies and building them into a mosaic or map. Must include a multidisciplinary team of researchers.	Idealist Low degree of iteration High structure	Theoretical models directly applicable to policy-makers, practitioners and designers of interventions Identification and explication of varying perspectives regarding complex or controversial issues Information to assist practitioners in identifying and practicing "best" practice Development of alternate perspectives on emerging issues	Popay et al., 2006	Hope interventions in mental health (Schrank et al., 2012) Patient-centered care of children with a chronic illness (Curtis-Tyler, 2011)
Qualitative meta-summary	Mixed method approach. Produces a map of the primary research findings by aggregating the data. Assumes that the more frequent a finding occurs, the more significant it is. Involves calculating 'effect sizes' for findings.	Realist Low degree of iteration High structure	Provides a basis for further synthesis Provides map of frequencies of findings	Sandelowski & Barroso, et al., 2003 Sandelowski et al., 2007	Factors that facilitate transition from child-centered to adult-centered health care (Lugasi et al., 2011) Antiretroviral adherence in HIV-positive women (Sandelowski et al., 2007)

Realist review	Assumes that complex social interventions are theories and act through various mechanisms. The method entails the researcher examining the program/intervention theory in a variety of contexts and then attempting to validate, refine or negate the theory by comparing it to the evidence within the body of primary research.	Realist Moderate structure High degree of iteration	Middle-range theory that explains how, why and in what circumstances complex interventions work	Pawson et al., 2005 Pawson, 2006	How and why internet-based medical education works and for whom (Wong et al., 2010) Efficacy of school feeding programs (Greenhalgh et al., 2007)
Thematic synthesis	Entails inductive coding and the identification of salient themes in the body of qualitative primary research. Uses techniques drawn from grounded theory and meta-ethnography, as well as computer software to code the findings of selected primary research studies line-by-line. Conclusions and hypotheses based on common elements across heterogeneous studies.	Critical realism Moderate structure Moderate degree of iteration	Theoretical models directly applicable to policy-makers, practitioners and designers of interventions	Harden et al., 2005 Thomas et al., 2003	Barriers to, and facilitators of, healthy eating among children (Thomas et al., 2003) Motivations to donate and experiences after donation of living kidney donors (Tong et al., in press)

interpretations of what metasynthesis is and what it entails. Paterson and colleagues (2001), for example, emphasize that the findings of qualitative research studies can only be truly understood in the light of the social, cultural, political and disciplinary contexts in which the primary research occurred, as well as in the context of the primary researcher's methodological and theoretical decisions and allegiances. Sandelowski (cited in Thorne et al., 2004) argues that metasynthesis interpreted in the way proposed by Paterson et al. will not address nurse researchers' need to have evidence-based conclusions to guide their clinical practice; she proposes methods of metasynthesis that are more systematic (i.e., less open to researcher interpretation) and only focused on the research findings.

Although the existing metasynthesis methods vary considerably in their epistemologies and processes, it is now widely recognized that synthesizing qualitative research can lead to a more generalizable and often more powerful explanations of the phenomenon under study than can be accomplished in a single research study (Walsh & Downe, 2005). For example, Paterson and colleagues (2001) were able to demonstrate through a metasynthesis of qualitative research about living with a chronic illness that the existing trajectory theories of how people perceived their disease did not reflect the evidence within the selected primary research. They developed an alternate model to mirror what they had discovered within the body of primary research (Paterson, 2001). Other outcomes of metasynthesis methods include: (1) identification of differences and similarities in understandings of the phenomenon under study across settings, sample populations, and researchers' disciplinary, methodological and/or theoretical perspectives (Paterson, Thorne, Canam, & Jillings, 2001); (2) operational models, theories or hypotheses to be tested later in other research (Paterson et al., 2001); (3) identification of directions for future research (Garrett & Thomas, 2006); (4) a historical overview of the development of theories or understandings of the phenomenon under study (Paterson et al., 2001); (5) a deeper understanding of the findings of quantitative systematic reviews (Russell, 2005); and (6) identification of significant attributes of a phenomenon to inform the development of interview guides or questionnaires/surveys (Russell, 2005).

Not all authors attribute the foundations of their method to others, e.g., the meta-theory component of meta-study is evident in critical interpretive synthesis, but the developers of this more recently developed method (Dixon-Woods et al., 2006) do not refer to the meta-study origins of their methods. Many metasynthesis method developers have changed their views about how metasynthesis should occur over time. Sandelowski (Sandelowski et al., 1997), for example, originally advocated for a metasynthesis method that would be true to the interpretive and reflexive nature of qualitative research. Her latest writing about metasynthesis (Crandell, Voils, Chang, & Sandelowski, 2011) espouses Bayesian statistical methods of synthesizing qualitative research data.

All metasynthesis methods are either mainly aggregative or mainly interpretive, but they contain elements of both aggregation and interpretation. For example, meta-ethnography is considered as mainly an interpretive method because it entails interpretive processes to generate a new model or theory; however, its procedural steps involve aggregating or combining the ideas, concepts or metaphors from different primary research studies.

The epistemological orientation of the various metasynthesis methods is idealism wherein the researcher assumes that "all knowledge is constructed" (Paterson, 2012, p. 6) or realism in "which researchers assume that they see the world as it is" (p. 6). Methods such as critical interpretive synthesis, narrative synthesis and meta-study have been influenced by an interpretive paradigm. They hold to a subjectivist idealist view of reality in which the aim of the metasynthesis is to develop conceptual and theoretical frameworks that contribute to a broad understanding of the phenomenon under study and how its defining elements connect and interact (Richardson &

Lindquist, 2010). Other methods, such as ecological triangulation and thematic synthesis proclaim a realist stance.

Metasynthesis methods also vary as to how iterative they are. Some (e.g., framework synthesis or thematic synthesis) are highly structured in regard to selecting primary research data and arriving at the metasynthesis findings. Others (e.g., formal grounded theory, thematic analysis) are iterative and circular in the way that they arrive at the metasynthesis findings; researchers who use these methods often change their research questions and their selection criteria as they locate new primary research or arrive at new understandings (Paterson, 2012).

Selecting a particular metasynthesis method has been challenging for many researchers because of the many variations among the methods. An additional challenge that relates to the selection of metasynthesis method is that some methods require specific expertise (e.g., it is not advisable to conduct formal grounded theory if there is no one on the team who is familiar with grounded theory). Also, some methods, such as meta-study and realist review, are by their very nature more time-consuming and intensive than others. These methods may not be feasible in the light of available resources.

Challenges in conducting a metasynthesis

Some authors (e.g., Light & Pillemer, 1984) have suggested that metasynthesis may compromise the integrity of primary research findings if it "pools" the primary research findings, blurring their individual contexts and meaning. They present metasynthesis as an interpretation of the primary researchers' interpretations, thus separating the metasynthesis findings from their origins within primary research studies. Consequently, metasynthesis researchers are charged with purposefully remaining true to the utmost of their ability to the primary researcher's interpretation. The significance of this concern varies across metasynthesis methods. For example, in methods where the ideal is to generate a nuanced understanding of the phenomenon under study, such as meta-ethnography, this is less of a concern than in methods where the researcher attempts to provide an in-depth portrayal of the phenomenon, such as in thematic synthesis.

A few authors (e.g., Hannes & Pearson, 2012; Jagosh et al., 2011) have recommended that metasynthesis researchers contact each primary researcher and ask whether the metasynthesis captures the primary research findings; however, others acknowledge that this impractical and problematic. In general, metasynthesis researchers address this by having more than one person read primary research reports several times, assess and interpret the primary research report and the discuss their interpretations until they reach consensus. Finfgeld (2003) suggests that dissertations provide the best source of primary research for metasynthesis because, in contrast to published articles, they present the primary research in full. Some recommend consulting experts in the field or key informants to garner their feedback about how well the metasynthesis captures the phenomenon under study (Britten et al., 2002; Wong, Greenhalgh, & Pawson, 2010). In this vein, Paterson (2007) took the findings of a metasynthesis of the self-disclosure of HIV experience to people with a chronic disease. Jensen and Allen (1994) recommend comparing the findings of the metasynthesis to theoretical literature.

A significant challenge in metasynthesis is determining which primary research reports should be included. This is a matter of some consequence because the metasynthesis findings are only as good as the relevance of the primary research that is selected for the metasynthesis. The number of relevant primary research studies to be included in metasynthesis a source of some controversy. Some authors (e.g., Sherwood, 1997, 1999) argue that to exclude pertinent primary research studies will compromise the integrity of the metasynthesis, but others (e.g., Sandelowski et al., 1997) argue that any more than ten primary research studies poses a threat to the trustworthiness of the metasynthesis findings because synthesizing a large number of studies blurs the uniqueness of each primary research report and constrains deep analysis. Paterson et al. (2001), on the other hand, advise that at least 12 discrete primary research studies be included in a metasynthesis to avoid the danger of excluding significant findings. The importance of including all studies that meet the inclusion criteria or a representative "some" depends upon the type of metasynthesis that is used and the research questions to be addressed. For example, when a single concept is being explored within a narrow context, such as the moral reasoning of social workers in a health care relationship (Varcoe et al., 2003), the sample of primary research may be less than five. However, in an investigation of a broad questions (e.g., "What is it like to live with a chronic illness?") with few contextual boundaries, the metasynthesis might involve several dozen primary research studies.

There is considerable debate within the field of metasynthesis about how much methodological variation should be included in the selected primary research studies. Some authors restrict the primary research to be synthesized according to a specific qualitative research method (e.g., Jensen & Allen, 1996; Noblit & Hare, 1988); they argue that grounded theory studies that focus on social processes are a very different entity than phenomenological studies that focus on phenomena. However, others (e.g., Paterson et al., 2001; Paterson, 2007; Sandelowski, Lambe, & Barroso, 2004) argue that there is benefit to including any qualitative research that contributes to understanding the phenomenon under study.

A challenge in metasynthesis is determining whether primary research reports represent discrete studies. Some metasynthesis researchers synthesize primary research reports that are actually derived from one study; they represent several primary research reports as discrete studies, when in actuality they are the same study. Finfgeld (1999), for example, used her dissertation and two articles derived from that dissertation in a metasynthesis of six primary research reports about courage in living with a chronic illness. The value or the danger of drawing on primary research reports that represent a single research study has not been widely debated as of yet. As well, the risks and the benefits of metasynthesis researchers including their own work in a metasynthesis have not been a topic of consideration in the literature.

In keeping with the debate regarding methodological variation in metasynthesis research, there exists a considerable body of literature about whether primary research that is of "poor quality" should be included in metasynthesis research. Some authors (e.g., Crandell et al., 2011; Sim & Madden, 2008, Thomas et al., 2003), particularly those leaning to the quantification and systematic review of primary research, believe that the credibility of metasynthesis will always be suspect unless metasynthesis researchers develop stringent measures of quality to assess the acceptability of primary research for inclusion in the metasynthesis and make these transparent in their writing about the metasynthesis findings. These researchers use appraisal tools designed for this purpose, such as the Qualitative Assessment and Review Instrument or the Critical Appraisal Skills Programme (Hannes, Lockwood, & Pearson, 2010), and exclude primary research that does not meet the establish cutoff score in the appraisal tool. Other authors advocate for primary research to be excluded if the researcher's "political agenda" (e.g., a theoretical allegiance) is evident throughout the primary research report (Paterson et al., 2001) or if the research is not truly qualitative (see Sandelowski et al., 2004, for criteria to assess primary research in this regard). Still others (e.g., Barroso et al., 2003; Paterson, 2007) state that excluding primary research on the basis of quality criteria is problematic because researchers do not always have space in journal articles to expound on the methodological details, editorial decisions may have limited what information is contained in published literature, standards of qualitative research have changed over time, and the contribution of the primary research report to the metasynthesis may be significant regardless of the quality of the research.

Another challenge in metasynthesis research is determining who should participate in the research. Different authors (e.g., Paterson et al., 2001; Dixon-Woods et al., 2006) advocate for multidisciplinary research team members, arguing that if primary research is to be selected from literature in several disciplines, the research team should be able to interpret the findings of particular studies in the primary researchers' disciplinary context. Some authors (e.g., Jagosh et al., 2011; Wong, 2012) stress the importance of including a librarian on the team. Paterson and colleagues (2009) note that including knowledge users and people with varying levels of experience with the phenomenon under study, including graduate students, will generate unique reflections that may be helpful in discerning the meaning and contextual factors influencing the primary research findings. They also recommend that before a research team is selected, the iterative and structural nature of the metasynthesis research be made clear to all potential team members. They note that one member of their team left the project because of the highly iterative and unstructured processes of meta-study; this individual preferred research that was more in keeping with quantitative and highly structured investigations.

Best practices in metasynthesis

There are a number of best practices that have been widely acknowledged as contributing to the rigor of metasynthesis research. These include that:

- Metasynthesis researchers should identify how the method(s) they use are grounded in or deviate from other metasynthesis methods, as well as why they selected the particular method they used.
- The selection of primary research should include both manual and electronic searches.
- Metasynthesis researchers should make clear what decisions they made throughout the research and their reasoning about the decisions. A metasynthesis report should include details about how the selection of primary research, data analysis and synthesis occurred, including how primary research studies were located and appraised and, when relevant, how data analysis integrated both qualitative and quantitative research data.
- Metasynthesis researchers should reflect upon and when possible, account for contradictory or outlier data within the primary research findings. Campbell et al. (2003) recommend that researchers acknowledge that the order in which they review primary research may affect the metasynthesis findings. Paterson and colleagues (2001) recommend in the analysis phase of metasynthesis the use of constant comparison (Noblit & Hare, 1988) and grouping the primary research studies in as many ways as possible (e.g., by setting, sample attributes, date). Other authors (Britten et al., 2002; Sandelowski et al., 2007) advise tabulation of the summarized findings to demonstrate that the findings are represented within the metasynthesis in order of frequency as they occur in the body of primary research.

Future directions

It is clear that the field of metasynthesis research is fraught with contradictory and often ambiguous claims. Nurses may question why they would be interested in metasynthesis when the evolution of this approach has not yet reached a state of clarity. They may also question its benefits to the profession. Regardless of its imperfections, the value of metasynthesis is found in the insights it generates, the broader questions it elicits and the contribution to theory that is relevant to nursing practice. For example, Duggleby and colleagues (2012) conducted a metasynthesis of hope among older adults. These researchers were able to illustrate how the meaning and realization of hope among older adults differ from that among youth who experience suffering in living with an illness. Their metasynthesis points to need for nurses to assist older adults to develop positive reappraisal as a strategy to be hopeful in living with an illness.

Despite the ever-growing body of metasynthesis research conducted by nurse researchers, there are some areas of nursing practice that have not been widely explored using metasynthesis approaches. Metasynthesis of studies that have evaluated the outcomes and processes of specific nursing interventions can offer new understanding of the efficacy of those interventions and substantiate nurses' articulation of how nursing interventions make important and unique contributions to the health and well-being of the people for whom they care.

Metasynthesis can also provide evidence of how interventions work, for whom and in what specific situations and contexts (Wong et al., 2012). Typically, research about the outcomes of nursing interventions, such as social support or patient teaching interventions, uses randomized controlled trials (RCTs) that do not readily reveal why someone chooses to participate or not participate in the intervention, or the fit of the intervention with users' real-world life. By drawing on a body of qualitative research, not a single study, metasynthesis can reveal who is likely to participate or not participate in an intervention and how, when and why it is likely to be effective.

Although there have been many advances in the field of metasynthesis research, there are several areas for future discussion, debate and study. For example, the majority of metasynthesis research has been published in English. While some metasynthesis proponents have included translation of articles written in languages other than English, there is a considerable body of literature (see review in Hubscher-Davidson, 2011) that questions the efficacy of translating research data and argues that translation offers another level of interpretation to any study (i.e., the translator interprets the data in the language in which the research report is written and then reinterprets the data to the research team in another language). As metasynthesis is already an interpretation of interpretations, it is likely that translation may threaten the integrity of metasynthesis research, particularly when the method that is used is highly iterative and unstructured. The impact of using translation in metasynthesis research is a topic for further investigation.

Similarly, there are a number of questions that remain unanswered about the nature of the research team in metasynthesis. For example, it is not known if the research team should include researchers within the national contexts of the primary research included in the metasynthesis. For example, can I as a Canadian researcher truly appreciate the context of research conducted within the Swedish health care system? What is the impact on the metasynthesis findings of me interpreting a Swedish study with a Canadian lens?

Some researchers (e.g., Paterson et al., 2001; Paterson, 2007) suggest that there are dangers in conducting metasynthesis as a sole researcher; however, others, such as Finfgeld (1999), have contributed metasynthesis findings to a field of knowledge but conducted this research alone. Currently, we do not know if specific metasynthesis methods are more malleable to being conducted by single researchers than others. Nurse researchers should provide evidence in a comparison of single and multiple researcher approaches to determine what, if any, the effects of single versus multiple members are on the duration, processes and outcomes of metasynthesis research.

The differences between metasynthesis methods are often subtle. As many methods share methodological and epistemological underpinnings, it is difficult to discern differences between some methods and what these differences contribute to the outcome of the metasynthesis research. This also makes it difficult to assert which methods works best for what kind of questions and for which researchers. Paterson (2012) recently attempted to provide a framework to assist researchers in such a decision. The framework includes considerations regarding whether (1) the method will result in the desired outcomes; (2) if the researchers have the appropriate skills, funds, time and expertise to conduct the method; and (3) if there is a fit between the researchers' need for structure, tolerance for ambiguity, or epistemological stance and the method. Although Paterson's (2012) method selection framework is a beginning in this regard, there is a need to develop definitive guidelines that will assist nurse researchers to determine which method will best achieve their research goals and fit with their expertise and available resources.

Conclusion

This chapter has presented an overview of metasynthesis, an approach to synthesize the findings of a body of qualitative (and at times, quantitative) research studies. The intent of metasynthesis in nursing is to provide insights that nurses can draw on in their practice, theory development and advocacy for policy revision or development. Metasynthesis, by its very nature, is not an exact science. It interprets interpretations of research (McCormick, Rodney, & Varcoe, 2003) to reveal patterns, processes and understandings that are relevant and fundamental to nursing practice (Richardson & Lindquist, 2012). This is more important than ever in the current context where nurses are struggling to consolidate their professional knowledge to articulate it to funders, the public and other disciplines. Although metasynthesis as a research approach presents its challenges, the contributions it offers to the nursing profession far outweigh these.

References

Barroso, J., Gollop, C. J., Sandelowski, M., Meynell, J., Pearce, P. F., & Collins, L. J. (2003). The challenges of searching for and retrieving qualitative studies. *Western Journal of Nursing Research, 25*(2), 153–178.

Britten, N., Campbell, R., Pope, C., Donovan, J., Morgan, M., & Pill, R. (2002). Using meta-ethnography to synthesize qualitative research: A worked example. *Journal of Health Services & Research Policy, 7*(4), 421–429.

Britten, N., & Pope, C. (2012). Medicine taking for asthma: A worked example of meta-ethnography. In K. Hannes, & C. Lockwood (Eds.), *Synthesizing qualitative research: Choosing the right approach* (pp. 41–58). Chichester: Wiley-Blackwell.

Brunton, G., Oliver, S., Oliver, K., & Lorenc, T. (2006). *A synthesis of research addressing children's, young people's and parents' views of walking and cycling for transport.* London: EPPI-Centre, Social Science Research Unit, Institute of Education, University of London.

Campbell, R., Pond, P., Pope, C., Britten, N., Pill, R., Morgan, M., & Donovan, J. (2003). Evaluating meta-ethnography: A synthesis of qualitative research on lay experiences of diabetes and diabetes care. *Social Science and Medicine, 56*(4), 671–684.

Crandell, J., Voils, C.I., Chang, Y., & Sandelowski, M. (2011). Bayesian data augmentation methods for the synthesis of qualitative and quantitative research findings. *Journal of Quality & Quantity, 45,* 653–669.

Curtis-Tyler, K. (2011). Levers and barriers to patient-centred care with children: Findings from a synthesis of studies of the experiences of children living with Type 1 diabetes or asthma. *Child: care, health and development, 37*(4), 540–550.

Dixon-Woods, M., Cavers, D., Agarwal, S., Annandale, E., Arthur, A., Harvey, J. et al. (2006). Conducting a critical interpretive synthesis of the literature on access to healthcare by vulnerable groups. *BMC Medical Research Methods, 6,* 35.

Doyle, L. H. (2003). Synthesis through meta-ethnography: Paradoxes, enhancements, and possibilities. *Qualitative Research, 3*(3), 321–344.

Duggleby, W., Hicks, D., Nekolaichuk, C., Holtslander, L., Williams, A., Chambers T., & Eby, J. (2010). Hope, older adults, and chronic illness: A metasynthesis of qualitative research. *Journal of Advanced Nursing, 68*(6), 1211–1223.

Estabrooks, C. A., Field, P. A., & Morse, J. M. (1994). Aggregating qualitative findings: An approach to theory development. *Qualitative Health Research, 4,* 503–511.

Finfgeld, D.L. (1999). Courage as a process of pushing beyond the struggle. *Qualitative Health Research, 9*(6), 803–814.

Finfgeld, D.L. (2003). Metasynthesis: the state of the art so far. *Qualitative Health Research, 137*, 893–904.

Finfgeld-Connett, D. (2008). Meta-synthesis of caring in nursing. *Journal of Clinical Nursing, 17*, 196–204.

Flemming, K., & McInnes, E. (2012) The use of morphine to treat cancer related pain: A worked example of critical interpretive synthesis. In K. Hannes & C. Lockwood (Eds.), *Synthesizing qualitative research: Choosing the right approach* (pp. 59–82). Chichester: Wiley-Blackwell.

Garrett, Z., & Thomas, J. (2006). Systematic reviews and their application to research in speech and language therapy: A response to T. R. Pring's "Ask a silly question: two decades of troublesome trials." *International Journal of Language Communication Disorders, 41*(1), 95–105.

Glaser, B. G., & Strauss, A. L. (1967). *The discovery of grounded theory: Strategies for qualitative research.* New York: Aldine de Gruyter.

Greenhalgh, T., Kristjansson, E., & Robinson, V. (2007). Realist review to understand the efficacy of school feeding programmes. *British Medical Journal, 335*(7625), 858–861.

Hannes, K., & Lockwood, C. (2011). Pragmatism as the philosophical foundation for the Joanna Briggs' meta-aggregative approach to qualitative evidence synthesis. *Journal of Advanced Nursing, 67*(7), 1632–1642.

Hannes, K., Lockwood, C., & Pearson, A. (2010). A comparative analysis of three online appraisal instruments' ability to assess validity in qualitative research. *Qualitative Health Research, 20*, 1736–1743.

Hannes, K., & Pearson, A. (2012). Obstacles to the implementation of evidence-based practice in Belgium: A worked example of meta-aggregation. In K. Hannes, & C. Lockwood (Eds.), *Synthesizing qualitative research: Choosing the right approach* (pp. 21–39). Chichester: Wiley-Blackwell.

Harden, A., & Thomas, J. (2005). Methodological issues in combining diverse study types in systematic reviews. *International Journal of Social Research Methodology, 8*(3), 257–271.

Hubscher-Davidson, S. (2011). Discussion of ethnographic research methods and their relevance for translation process research. *Across Languages and Cultures, 12*(1), 1–18.

Jagosh, J., Pluye, P., Macaulay, A. C., Salsberg, J., Henderson, J., Sirett, E., et al. (2011). Assessing the outcomes of participatory research: Protocol for identifying, selecting, appraising and synthesizing the literature for realist review. *Implementation Science, 6*, 24.

Jensen, L. A., & Allen, M. N. (1994). A synthesis of qualitative research on wellness-illness. *Qualitative Health Research, 4*, 349–369.

Jensen, L. A., & Allen, M. N. (1996). Meta-synthesis of qualitative findings. *Qualitative Health Research, 6*, 553–560.

Kearney, M. H. (1998). Ready-to-wear: Discovering grounded formal theory. *Research in Nursing and Health, 21*, 179–186.

Kearney, M. H. (2001) Enduring love: A grounded formal theory of women's experience of domestic violence. *Research in Nursing & Health, 24*, 270–282.

Konno, R. (2006) Support for overseas qualified nurses in adjusting to Australian nursing practice: A systematic review. *International Journal of Evidence-Based Healthcare, 4*(2), 83–100.

Light, R. J., & Pillemer, D. B. (1984). *Summing up: The science of reviewing research.* Cambridge, MA: Harvard University Press.

Lugasi, T., Achille, M., & Stevenson, M. (2011). Patients' perspective on factors that facilitate transition from child-centered to adult-centered health care: A theory integrated metasummary of quantitative and qualitative studies. *Journal of Adolescent Health, 48*, 429–440.

McCormick, J., Rodney, P., & Varcoe, C. (2003). Reinterpretations across studies: An approach to meta-analysis. *Qualitative Health Research, 13*, 933–944.

Noblit, G. W., & Hare, R. D. (1988). *Meta-ethnography: Synthesizing qualitative studies.* Newbury Park, CA: Sage.

Oliver, S., Rees, R., Clarke-Jones, L., Milne, R., Oakley, A., Gabbay, J., et al. (2008). A multidimensional conceptual framework for analysing public involvement in health services research. *Health Expectations, 11*, 72–84.

Paterson, B. L. (2001). The shifting perspectives model of chronic illness. *Journal of Nursing Scholarship, 33*(1), 21–26.

Paterson, B. L. (2007) Coming out as ill: Understanding self-disclosure in chronic illness. In C. Ebb & B. Roe (Eds.), *Reviewing research evidence for nursing practice: Systematic reviews* (pp. 73–87). Oxford: Blackwell.

Paterson, B. L. (2012). "It looks great but how do I know if it fits?": An introduction to meta-synthesis research. In K. Hannes & C. Lockwood (Eds.), *Synthesizing qualitative research: Choosing the right approach* (pp. 1–20). Chichester: Wiley-Blackwell.

Paterson, B. L., Canam, C., Joachim, G., & Thorne, S. (2003). Embedded assumptions in qualitative studies of fatigue. *Western Journal of Nursing Research*, *25*, 119–133.

Paterson, B. L., Dubouloz, C. J., Chevrier, J., Ashe, B., King, J., & Moldoveanu, M. (2009). Conducting qualitative metasynthesis research: Insights from a metasynthesis project. *International Journal of Qualitative Methods*, *8*, 22–33.

Paterson, B. L., Thorne, S. E., Canam, C., & Jillings, C. (2001). *Meta-study of qualitative health research: A practical guide to meta-analysis and metasynthesis*. Thousand Oaks, CA: Sage.

Paterson, B. L., Thorne, S., & Dewis, M. (1998). Adapting to and managing diabetes. *Image: Journal of Nursing Scholarship*, *30*, 57–62.

Pawson, R. (2006). *Evidence-based policy: A realist perspective*. London: Sage.

Pawson, R., Greenhalgh, T., Harvey, G., & Walshe, K. (2005). Realist review: A new method of systematic review designed for complex policy interventions. *Journal of Health Services Research Policy*, *10*(Suppl. 1), 21–34.

Pearson A. (2004*)*. Balancing the evidence: Incorporating the synthesis of qualitative data into systematic reviews. *Joanna Briggs Institute Report*, *2*, 45–64.

Popay, J., Roberts, H., Sowden, A., Petticrew, M., Arai, L., Rodgers, M. et al. (2006). *Guidance on the conduct of narrative synthesis in systematic reviews*. Retrieved on January 26, 2012 from http://tees.academia. edu/LisaArai/Papers/259152/Guidance_on_the_Conduct_of_Narrative_Synthesis_In_Systematic_ Reviews.

Richardson, B., & Lindquist, I. (2010). Metasynthesis of qualitative inquiry research studies in physiotherapy. *Physiotherapy Research International*, *15*, 111–117.

Roberts, K., Dixon-Woods, M., Fitzpatrick, R., Abrams, K., & Jones, D. R. (2002). Factors affecting uptake of childhood immunisation: An example of Bayesian synthesis of qualitative and quantitative evidence. *Lancet*, *360*, 1596–1599.

Russell, C.L. (2005). An overview of the integrative research review. *Progress in Transplantation*, *15*, 8–13.

Sandelowski, M., & Barroso, J. (2003) Classifying the findings in qualitative studies. *Qualitative Health Research*, *13*, 905–923.

Sandelowski, M., Barroso, J., & Voils, C. (2007). Using qualitative metasummary to synthesize qualitative and quantitative descriptive findings. *Research in Nursing & Health*, *30*, 99–111.

Sandelowski, M., Docherty, S., & Emden, C. (1997). Qualitative metasynthesis: Issues and techniques. *Research in Nursing & Health*, *20*, 365–371.

Sandelowski, M., Lambe, C., & Barroso, J. (2004). Stigma in HIV-positive women. *Journal of Nursing Scholarship*, *36*(2), 122–128.

Schmied, V., Beake, S., Sheehan, A., McCourt, C., & Dykes, F. (2011). Women's perceptions and experiences of breastfeeding support: A metasynthesis. *Birth*, *38*(1), 49–60.

Schrank, B., Bird, V., Rudnick, A., & Slade, M. (2012). Determinants, self-management strategies and interventions for hope in people with mental disorders: Systematic search and narrative review. *Social Science and Medicine*, *74*(4), 554–564.

Schreiber, R., Crooks, D., & Stern, P. N. (1997). Qualitative meta-analysis. In J. M. Morse (Ed.), *Completing a qualitative project: Details and dialogue* (pp. 311–326). Thousand Oaks, CA: Sage.

Sherwood, G. (1997). Meta-synthesis of qualitative analyses of caring: Defining a therapeutic model of nursing. *Advanced Practice Nursing Quarterly*, *3*, 32–42.

Sherwood, G. (1999). Meta-synthesis: Merging qualitative studies to develop nursing knowledge. *International Journal for Human Caring*, *3*, 37–42.

Sim, J., & Madden, S. (2008). Illness experience in fibromyalgia syndrome: A metasynthesis of qualitative studies. *Social Science and Medicine*, *67*, 57–67.

Taverner, T., Closs, J., & Briggs, M. (2011). A meta-synthesis of research on leg ulceration and neuropathic pain. *British Journal of Nursing*, *20*, S18–S27.

Thorne, S., Jensen, L., Kearney, M.H., Noblit, G., & Sandelowski, M. (2004). Qualitative metasynthesis: Reflections on methodological orientation and ideological agenda. *Qualitative Health Research*, *14*, 1342–1365.

Thorne, S. E., Joachim, G., Paterson, B., & Canam, C. (2002). Influence of the research frame on qualitatively derived health science knowledge. *International Journal of Qualitative Methods*. Retrieved on February 21, 2012 from http://www.ualbeta.ca/~ijqm/english/engframeset.html.

Thomas, J., Sutcliffe, K., Harden, A., Oakley, A., Oliver, S., Rees, R. et al. (2003) *Children and healthy eating: A systematic review of barriers and facilitators*. London: Evidence for Policy and Practice Information and Coordinating Centre, 2003. Retrieved on February 3, 2012 from http://eppi.ioe.ac.uk/EPPI Web/home.aspx?page=/hp/reports/ healthy_eating02/healthy_eating02.htm.

Varcoe, C., Rodney, P., & McCormick, J. (2003). Health care relationships in context: An analysis of three ethnographies. *Qualitative Health Research*, *13*, 957–973.

Voils, C. I., Hasselblad, V., Chang, Y., Crandell, J. L., Lee, E. J., & Sandelowski, M. (2009). A Bayesian method for the synthesis of evidence from qualitative and quantitative reports: An example from the literature on antiretroviral medication adherence. *Journal of Health Services Research and Policy*, *14*, 226–233.

Walsh, D., & Downe, S. (2005). Meta-synthesis method for qualitative research: A literature review. *Journal of Advanced Nursing*, *50*(2), 204–211.

Wong, G., Greenhalgh, T., & Pawson, R. (2010). Internet-based medical education: A realist review of what works, for whom and in what circumstances. *BMC Medical Education*, *10*, 12.

Wong, G., Greenhalgh, T., & Pawson, R. (2012). Realist methods in medical education research: What are they and what can they contribute? *Medical Education*, *46*, 89–96.

26

Synthesizing qualitative and quantitative research findings

Margarete Sandelowski, Corrine I. Voils,
Jamie L. Crandell, and Jennifer Leeman

Introduction

The rise of the evidence-based practice movement and the embrace of a more enlightened understanding of the contribution of diverse forms of evidence have led to a surge of interest in mixed research synthesis. Mixed research synthesis is the integration of findings from primary qualitative, quantitative, and mixed-methods studies in targeted domains of research (Pope, Mays, & Popay, 2007; Sandelowski, Voils, & Barroso, 2006). In this chapter, we provide an overview of the distinctive challenges of and approaches for conducting mixed research synthesis studies.

Challenges of mixed research synthesis

The primary challenge to conducting mixed research synthesis studies is how to manage the qualitative/quantitative divide that defines the "mix." The qualitative/quantitative binary is a familiar way to categorize research in the behavioral, social, and health sciences and it is useful as a shorthand communication of research practices. Yet this binary is also an obstacle to communication and methodological advancement as it reifies false distinctions; for example, between words and numbers, constructivist and positivist inquiry, and subjectivity and objectivity (Allwood, 2011; Sandelowski, Voils, & Knafl, 2009; Vogt, 2008), with the first word in each of these pairs aligned with qualitative and the second word with quantitative research.

Even as it reifies false distinctions, this binary blurs the line between prescribed research practice—what communities of scholars think qualitative and quantitative research should be and do—and actual research practice. Especially relevant to the mixed research synthesis enterprise is, for instance, the difference said to exist between qualitative and quantitative research findings in degree of interpretive complexity. An idealized notion of qualitative research findings is that they are more penetrating, nuanced, and thicker examinations of target phenomena than are quantitative research findings. Wholly glossed, however, is the relatively low interpretive complexity (i.e., closeness to data as given and thinness) of many qualitative research findings. For example, a large proportion of qualitative research findings presented in health sciences reports is in the form of surveys or topical or thematic summaries of data (Sandelowski & Barroso, 2007). Such findings are informative and worthy of inclusion in research synthesis studies, but they may in form be closer to quantitative survey findings in interpretive complexity than they are to findings in the form of grounded theories or phenomenological descriptions. Assuming that they address the same content, or aspects of the phenomena under investigation, both of these kinds of findings may therefore be amenable to the same synthesis-by-aggregation approaches described later in this chapter. Grounded theories or phenomenological descriptions are in turn more comparable in interpretive complexity to quantitative findings configured into structural equation models (Voils, Crandell, Chang, Leeman, & Sandelowski, 2011). Assuming they address the same content, both of these kinds of findings may therefore be amenable to the same synthesis-by-configuration approaches also featured later in this chapter. In short, differences between kinds of research findings addressing the same content may not rest on the qualitative/quantitative divide at all but rather in the actual degree of transformation of the data generated in the primary studies reviewed.

The differences that tend to lie on the qualitative/quantitative divide and present the greatest challenges to integrating qualitative and quantitative research findings are those related to sampling and data collection imperatives. We now address these differences and their implications for mixed research synthesis.

Differences in sampling imperatives in primary studies

One of the key challenges to integrating qualitative and quantitative research findings is the contrasting imperatives of the purposeful sampling associated with qualitative research and of the probability sampling associated with quantitative research. A purposeful sample is one that is informationally representative, "deliberately biased" (Wood & Christy, 1999, p. 189), and of sufficient size and composition to draw "illustrative inferences" regarding "possibility" (Wood & Christy, 1999, p. 185), support claims to informational redundancy or to theoretical or scene saturation (Sandelowski, 1995), and enable idiographic, analytic, or case-bound generalizations (Polit & Beck, 2010). A probability sample is one that is supposed to be representative of a target population on pre-selected factors, and of sufficient size and power to allow researchers to draw inferences regarding probability, minimize bias, support the use of inferential statistics, and allow nomothetic or formal generalizations from samples to populations.

Purposeful sampling is directed toward the intensive study of the single and singular case (e.g., individual, organization, moment, event) on a larger (than in probability sampling) range of dimensions with comparisons to other cases frequently only implied. Probability sampling is directed toward making explicit comparisons of a larger (than in purposeful sampling) number of cases on a smaller (than in purposeful sampling) range of variables. Although findings from probability samples will have a comparative reference point (e.g., in comparison to group A . . ., group B . . .), findings from purposeful samples may detail aspects of group A, but not necessarily in relation to any clearly expressed comparison group or common set of dimensions.

Probability sampling parameters (i.e., number and composition) are typically set in advance of data collection and analysis. In contrast, purposeful samples are by definition purposefully created in the course of the study to accommodate what researchers see as heuristic analytic lines. In addition, purposeful samples are not of persons *per se*, but rather of the experiences or events targeted for study. What is sampled may be elements of varying numbers of diversely conducted interviews with varying numbers of diverse participants, varying numbers and types of documents containing different kinds of information, and/or of varying numbers and types of field observations of different events conducted at different times. As Crouch and McKenzie (2006, p. 493) observed, "If anything is being 'sampled' [in purposeful sampling] it is not so much individual persons 'of a kind' but [rather] variants of a particular social setting . . . and of the experiences arising in it."

Findings from purposeful samples are therefore typically presented at the study level and focused on within-case or between-thematic lines. In contrast, findings from probability samples are typically presented at the subject level and focused on frequency counts and between- and cross-participant comparisons (Voils et al., 2009).

Differences in data collection imperatives in primary studies

Another challenge lies in differences in both the degree of structure (i.e., minimal to high) and endedness (i.e., open- versus closed-ended) of data collection. For example, a highly structured and closed-ended questionnaire will yield comparable information on the same dimensions of a target phenomenon. In contrast, a minimally structured and open-ended interview in which participants are asked to talk about anything they like with regards to that same target phenomenon will yield information on a wide array of dimensions, only some or none of which may overlap with each other or with closed-ended responses in the same domain.

Implications of these differences for mixed research synthesis

These differences compel researchers conducting mixed research synthesis studies to make decisions about a number of issues. One of these is how to determine the importance or prevalence of the findings appearing in research reports as the same percent frequency of a finding may be considered consequential in a purposefully selected sample but relatively inconsequential in a probability sample. For example, even if only 1 of 5 (20%) purposefully selected participants linked medication nonadherence to mistrust of providers, this finding would still be considered thematically significant as purposeful sampling mandates consideration of the range of possibilities pertaining to a target phenomenon regardless of sample size. In contrast, if mistrust was correlated with nonadherence in 20 of 100 randomly selected participants (also 20%), this finding might be statistically insignificant because, in probability sampling, statistical inference depends on the prevalence or frequency of observations, with infrequent observations considered outliers or even discarded.

The differences in both sampling imperatives and endedness of data collection matter even to decide whether a finding is present at all and, indeed, to decide on the very meaning of presence or absence. For example, a finding targeting a certain aspect of an experience may be present in a report of a study entailing open-ended data collection because it was deliberately elicited but may not necessarily be salient to the experience of participants. Or, an aspect of experience may be highly salient to these participants but absent as a finding because it was never elicited or because participants viewed it as so taken-for-granted it need not be mentioned or because the author of the report chose not to feature it (Sandelowski et al., 2009). Accordingly, researchers conducting mixed research synthesis studies must decide whether and when, for example, (1) absence is to be read as deliberate silence and therefore paradoxically as presence (MacLure, Holmes, Jones, & MacRae, 2010), as an artifact of the research process, or as the absence of relevance to the target phenomenon; and whether (2) presence is to be read as an artifact of the research process or as presence of relevance to the target phenomenon. Researchers must choose the metric by which presence or absence of a finding will be represented in reports of studies varying widely in sample size and composition and data collection techniques (Sandelowski et al., 2009). Because any such choice will entail advantages and disadvantages, researchers must decide on the metric that will best accommodate the studies under review and that will yield results deemed credible and meaningful by the audiences toward which the research synthesis study is directed.

Mapping the research synthesis field

An array of approaches has been developed to manage the consequences of differences in sampling and data collection mandates. What follows is a framework for organizing or mapping them.

Mapping research synthesis studies by mode and object of synthesis

As shown in Table 26.1, the mode of research synthesis studies may be mono-method or mixed-methods. Mono-method research synthesis studies entail the use of approaches to synthesis typically considered to be either qualitative (e.g., grounded theory) or quantitative (e.g., meta-analysis). Mixed-methods research synthesis studies entail the use of both qualitative and quantitative inquiry approaches. The object of research synthesis approaches may be findings in reports of primary qualitative studies alone, primary quantitative studies alone, or primary qualitative, quantitative, and mixed-methods studies. In this chapter, we feature mixed-methods (i.e., mixed-mode) mixed research (i.e., mixed-object) synthesis studies.

Mapping research synthesis studies by logics of research synthesis[1]

Regardless of the mode of research synthesis (i.e., mono- or mixed-methods) and of the object of synthesis (i.e., qualitative and/or quantitative findings), the defining logics of research synthesis studies are aggregation and configuration (Sandelowski, Voils, Leeman, & Crandell, in press). These logics do not lie on the qualitative/quantitative divide but rather on the nature of primary study findings, regardless of how they were produced. Although we separate them here, aggregation and configuration entail each other and may operate together in the same research synthesis study.

Aggregation

As summarized in Table 26.2, aggregation entails the assimilation of findings reviewers view as communicating the same thing about a target phenomenon or about the relationship between two or more aspects of that phenomenon. Synthesis by aggregation is essentially an exercise in convergent validation as it rests on what reviewers perceive as the repetition of the same finding across primary studies regardless of their methodological origins or characteristics.

Research synthesis by aggregation may be accomplished at the subject (participant) and/or study levels. Aggregation of quantitative findings at the subject level is the logic of meta-analysis in which the pooling of findings is dependent on sample size. Aggregation of qualitative findings

Table 26.1 Types of research synthesis studies by mode and object of synthesis

Research synthesis study types	Mode of synthesis	Object of synthesis
Mono-method/mono research	QL methods	QL findings
	QN methods	QN findings
Mono-method/mixed research	QL methods	QL & QN findings
	QN methods	QL & QN findings
Mixed-methods/mono research	QL & QN methods	QL findings
	QL & QN methods	QN findings
Mixed-methods/mixed research	QL & QN methods	QL & QN methods
	QL & QN methods	QL & QN methods

Note: QL = qualitative; QN = quantitative.

Table 26.2 Comparison of research synthesis logics

Logics	Aggregation	Configuration
Parameters		
Relationship between findings	Confirmatory (repetition of findings)	Complementary (coherent assembly of findings)
Point/direction of integration	Study-level Subject-level	Top-down Bottom-up
Process	Averaging, merging	Linking, meshing
Product	Pooled evidence summary	Theory, model
Examples of research synthesis methods	Meta-analysis (Bayesian, frequentist) Metasummary Vote counting	Grounded theory Meta-ethnography Realist synthesis Structural equation modeling
Examples of published reports	Voils, Hasselblad, Chang, Crandell, Lee, & Sandelowski, 2009 (subject-level Bayesian) Draucker, Martsolf, Ross, Cook, Stidham, & Mweemba, 2009 (study-level metasummary) Voils, Sandelowski, Barroso, & Hasselblad, 2008 (study-level vote counting) Crandell, Voils, Chang, & Sandelowski, 2011 (study-level Bayesian)	Kearney & O'Sullivan, 2003 (grounded theory) Malpass, Shaw, Sharp, Walter, Feder, Ridd, & Kessler, 2009 (meta-ethnography) O'Campo, Kirst, Schaefer-McDaniel, Firestone, Scott, & McShane, 2009 (realist synthesis) Cheung & Chan, 2009 (structural equation modeling)

alone or with quantitative findings at the subject level is an option only if the numbers of participants linked to findings in qualitative research reports are available from the reports themselves or from the authors, or if a reasonable range of values can be plausibly inferred from reports (Chang, Voils, Sandelowski, Hasselblad, & Crandell, 2009). A Bayesian approach to subject-level aggregation of qualitative and quantitative findings is described in Voils et al. (2009) and in Crandell, Voils, and Sandelowski (in press).

Because subject-level information is often not available or plausibly inferable from qualitative and sometimes quantitative reports, aggregation of qualitative and quantitative findings is typically possible only at the study level. In study-level aggregation, each study provides support for or against a finding regardless of sample size. For example, each study may be assigned a value indicating whether support was present (1) or absent (0). Presence may be assessed ordinally according to size of effect of quantitative findings and amount of space given over to a thematic line in qualitative studies (Onwuegbuzie & Teddlie, 2003). As we indicated previously, meaningful and consistently applied criteria for representing presence or absence of a finding must be carefully determined. Modes of research synthesis by study-level aggregation of qualitative findings include metasummary (Sandelowski & Barroso, 2007); of quantitative findings, vote counting (Bushman, 1994); and of qualitative and quantitative findings, adaptations of Bayesian meta-analysis (Berry & Stangl, 2000). Examples of published reports of research syntheses by study-level aggregation in which these methods were used are listed in Table 26.2.

Configuration

Research synthesis by configuration entails the arrangement of thematically diverse individual findings or sets of aggregated findings into a coherent theoretical rendering of them. In contrast to the thematic similarity of findings upon which aggregation depends, findings in configuration syntheses are conceived by reviewers as thematically diverse and therefore as not amenable to pooling. Instead of confirming each other, thematically diverse findings may contradict, extend, explain, or otherwise modify each other. In configuration synthesis, reviewers link as opposed to pool findings. An even greater degree of reviewer intervention is involved in configuration than in aggregation syntheses as the former entail "hindsight accounts of the connectedness of things" (Geertz, 1995, p. 2), that is, the "mesh(ing)" (Mason, 2006, p. 20) as opposed to merging of findings that may never have been placed together in the primary research reports reviewed.

Synthesis by configuration may be top-down and/or bottom-up. The top-down/bottom-up distinction does not lie wholly on the deductive/inductive divide as top-down approaches always entail hunches derived from the data that certain concepts or models might be useful and generative ways to configure findings, and bottom-up approaches always draw from prior understandings and theoretical leanings concerning which factors might belong together and their arrangement. Top-down configurations begin with a concept, conceptual framework, extant theory, or other shaping principle—drawn from the primary studies reviewed or from some other literature—by which individual or pooled sets of findings can be consolidated or mapped. Heretofore-unseen connections among findings may come into view by translating them into the language of the concept or constructs of a theory. Bottom-up configurations are data-derived, or accomplished from various novel assemblies of findings. Here a theoretical rendering is created from the findings to encompass and represent a particular assembly or arrangement of them.

Methods for both top-down and bottom-up configurations of qualitative and/or quantitative findings encompass variants of methods used in primary qualitative and quantitative research to develop and test theory, including grounded theory (Kearney, 2001, 2007), meta-ethnography (Noblit & Hare, 1988), realist synthesis (Pawson, 2006), and structural equation modeling (Cheung & Chan, 2005). Examples of published reports of research syntheses by configuration in which these methods were used are listed in Table 26.2.

Mapping mixed research synthesis studies by designs

As shown in Table 26.3, two basic designs are available for conducting mixed research synthesis studies: segregated and integrated (Sandelowski et al., 2006).

Segregated design

The defining attribute of the segregated design is adherence to the qualitative/quantitative binary. Regardless of whether researchers synthesize the findings from qualitative and quantitative studies concurrently or sequentially (in any order), they treat qualitative and quantitative findings as constituting different datasets tapping different aspects of experience targeted in the body of literature under review. In segregated designs, grouping by object of synthesis (qualitative or quantitative findings) is basic to all other groupings. Although reviewers adhering to the qualitative/quantitative binary will also likely use what they consider to be qualitative modes of synthesis to integrate qualitative findings and quantitative modes of synthesis to synthesize quantitative findings, they may use qualitative and/or quantitative modes of synthesis to integrate qualitative findings and qualitative and/or quantitative modes of synthesis to integrate quantitative findings. In any case, the two datasets are typically kept separate until the final phase of the study

Table 26.3 Comparison of designs for mixed research synthesis studies

Design	Segregated	Integrated
Features		
Stance toward QL/QN binary	Accepts	Transcends
Timing	Concurrent ↓↓ Sequential ↓ (QL or QN first) ↓	Concurrent
Mode and object of research synthesis	QL methods for QL findings QN methods for QN findings QL and/or QN methods for QL findings QL and/or QN methods for QN findings	QL and QN methods for QL and QN findings
Logic of synthesis	Aggregation Configuration	Aggregation Configuration

Note: QL = qualitative; QN = quantitative.

at which time researchers link these separately integrated products to create a metasynthesis of qualitative and quantitative findings.

Segregated designs may entail synthesis by both aggregation and configuration. For example, the qualitative findings may be integrated by metasummary (aggregation) and the quantitative findings by meta-analysis (aggregation). Yet the metasynthesis that links these sets of integrated findings will most likely be configurative with either the synthesized qualitative or quantitative findings serving as the comparative reference point, organizing framework, or placeholder for integrating the synthesized quantitative or qualitative findings, respectively (Sandelowski et al., 2009; Voils, Sandelowski, Barroso, & Hasselblad, 2008).

Segregated designs depend on clearly differentiating qualitative from quantitative studies and qualitative from quantitative approaches to research synthesis. Although segregated designs allow researchers to bypass the challenges of managing the differences in sampling and data collection mandates we outlined previously, the very differentiation of qualitative versus quantitative study by itself presents a challenge as certain studies will always defy simple categorization as qualitative, quantitative, or mixed-methods. Moreover, few qualitative research approaches escape quantitizing and no quantitative research approach escapes qualitizing. For example, the identification of themes in any kind of thematic analysis depends on enumeration and, although pushed to the background, all quantitative research rests on a series of subjective judgments made by researchers (Sandelowski et al., 2009). Metasummary may thus be conceived as a qualitative approach as it rests on a form of thematic analysis, but also as a quantitative approach as it entails the calculation of effect sizes (Sandelowski & Barroso, 2007).

Integrated design

The defining attribute of the integrated design is the transcendence of the qualitative/quantitative binary in every phase of the research synthesis study. In integrated designs, researchers treat qualitative and quantitative findings as potentially addressing the same aspects of an experience and as convertible. In contrast to segregated designs in which grouping by object of synthesis is foundational to all other groupings, in integrated designs, groupings based on the thematic similarity of the findings are foundational. Integrated designs may entail research synthesis by both aggregation and configuration.

Integrated designs allow reviewers to bypass the challenges of differentiating qualitative from quantitative modes and objects of synthesis. Yet they force reviewers to manage the differences in sampling and data collection mandates and therefore the challenges of data conversion, that is, of meaningfully transforming qualitative into quantitative and/or quantitative into qualitative findings in order to make them comparable in form and therefore combinable (Sandelowski, Voils, & Barroso, 2007; Sandelowski et al., 2009).

Conclusion

Conducting scientifically credible mixed research synthesis studies requires reviewers to have a good understanding of the implications of adhering to or transcending the qualitative/quantitative divide. Conducting research synthesis studies requires reviewers to show that the research problem toward which their study was directed can be addressed by the methodological choices they made. The research synthesis field and the mixed research synthesis field, in particular, are dynamic ones that call for methodological craftsmanship, flexibility, and a commitment to producing results that are credible and usable for practice.

Acknowledgments

This chapter was supported by a National Institute of Nursing Research, National Institutes of Health grant ("Integrating qualitative & quantitative research findings," 5R01NR004907, June 3, 2005–March 31, 2011), and with resources and facilities of the Veterans Affairs Medical Center in Durham, NC. Views expressed in this article are those of the authors and do not necessarily represent the Department of Veterans Affairs.

Note

1 This section, including Table 26.2, is an abbreviated version of material previously published in Sandelowski, M., Voils, C. I., Leeman, J., & Crandell, J. (2012). Mapping the mixed-methods mixed research synthesis terrain. *Journal of Mixed Methods Research, 6*(4), 317–331. (First published online 28 December 2011 by SAGE Publications.)

References

Allwood, C. M. (2011). The distinction between qualitative and quantitative research methods is problematic. *Quality & Quantity*. Published online March 2, 2011. doi: 10.1007/s11135-011-9455-8.
Berry, D. A., & Stangl, D. K. (Eds.). (2000). *Meta-analysis in medicine and health policy*. New York: Dekker.
Bushman, B. (1994). Vote-counting procedures in meta-analysis. In H. Cooper & L. V. Hedges (Eds.), *The handbook of research synthesis* (pp. 193–214). New York: Russell Sage Foundation.
Chang, Y., Voils, C. I., Sandelowski, M., Hasselblad, V., & Crandell, J. L. (2009). Transforming verbal counts in reports of qualitative descriptive studies into numbers. *Western Journal of Nursing Research, 31*(7), 837–852. doi: 10.1177/0193945909334434.
Cheung, M. W., & Chan, W. (2005). Meta-analytic structural equation modeling: A two-stage approach. *Psychological Methods, 10*(1), 40–64. doi: 10.1037/1082-989X.10.1.40.
Cheung, M. W., & Chan, W. (2009). A two-stage approach to synthesizing covariance matrices in meta-analytic structural equation modeling. *Structural Equation Modeling, 16*(1), 28–53. doi: 10.1080/1070551 0802561295.

Crandell, J. L., Voils, C. I., Chang, Y., & Sandelowski, M. (2011). Bayesian data augmentation methods for the synthesis of qualitative and quantitative research findings. *Quality & Quantity, 45*(3), 653–669. doi: 10.1007/s11135-010-9375-z.

Crandell, J. L., Voils, C. I., & Sandelowski, M. (in press). Bayesian approaches to the synthesis of qualitative and quantitative research findings. In K. Hannes (Ed.), *Worked examples of qualitative evidence synthesis.* Chichester: Wiley-Blackwell.

Crouch, M., & McKenzie, H. (2006). The logic of small samples in interview-based qualitative research. *Social Science Information, 45*(4), 483–499. doi: 10.1177/0539018406069584.

Draucker, C. B., Martsolf, D. S., Ross, R., Cook, C. B., Stidham, A. W., & Mweemba, P. (2009). The essence of healing from sexual violence: A qualitative metasynthesis. *Research in Nursing & Health, 32*(4), 366–378. doi: 10.1002/nur.20333.

Geertz, C. (1995). *After the fact: Two countries, four decades, one anthropologist.* Cambridge, MA: Harvard University Press.

Kearney, M. H. (2001). New directions in grounded formal theory. In R. Schreiber & P. N. Stern (Eds.), *Using grounded theory in nursing* (pp. 227–246). New York: Springer.

Kearney, M. H. (2007). From the sublime to the meticulous: The continuing evolution of grounded formal theory. In A. Bryant & K. Charmaz (Eds.), *The Sage handbook of grounded theory* (pp. 127–150). Los Angeles: Sage.

Kearney, M. H., & O'Sullivan, J. (2003). Identity shifts as turning points in health behavior change. *Western Journal of Nursing Research, 25*(2), 134–152. doi: 10.1177/0193945902250032

MacLure, M., Holmes, R., Jones, L., & MacRae, C. (2010). Silence as resistance to analysis: Or, on not opening one's mouth properly. *Qualitative Inquiry, 16(6)*, 492–500. doi: 10.1177/1077800410364349.

Malpass, A., Shaw, A., Sharp, D., Walter, F., Feder, G., Ridd, M., & Kessler, D. (2009). "Medication career" or "moral career"? The two sides of managing antidepressants: A meta-ethnography of patients' experience of antidepressants. *Social Science & Medicine, 68*(1), 154–168. doi: 10.1016/j.socscimed.2008.09.068.

Mason, J. (2006). Mixing methods in a qualitatively driven way. *Qualitative Research, 6*(1), 9–25. doi: 10.1177/1468794106058866.

Noblit, G. W., & Hare, R. D. (1988). *Meta-ethnography: Synthesizing qualitative studies.* Newbury Park, CA: Sage.

O'Campo, P., Kirst, M., Schaefer-McDaniel, N., Firestone, M., Scott, A., & McShane, K. (2009). Community-based services for homeless adults experiencing concurrent mental health and substance use disorders: A realist approach to synthesizing evidence. *Journal of Urban Health, 86*(6), 965–989. doi: 10.1007/s11524-009-9392-1.

Onwuegbuzie, A. J., & Teddlie, C. (2003). A framework for analyzing data in mixed methods research. In A. Tashakkori & C. Teddlie (Eds.), *Handbook of mixed methods in social and behavioral research* (pp. 351–383). Thousand Oaks, CA: Sage.

Pawson, R. (2006). *Evidence-based policy: A realist perspective.* London: Sage.

Polit, D. F., & Beck, C. T. (2010). Generalization in quantitative and qualitative research: Myths and strategies. *International Journal of Nursing Studies, 47*(11), 1451–1458. doi: 10.1016/j.ijnurstu.2010.06.004.

Pope, C., Mays, N., & Popay, J. (2007). *Synthesizing qualitative and quantitative health evidence.* Maidenhead: Open University Press.

Sandelowski, M. (1995). Sample size in qualitative research. *Research in Nursing & Health, 18*(2), 179–183. doi: 10.1002/nur.4770180211.

Sandelowski, M., & Barroso, J. (2007). *Handbook for synthesizing qualitative research.* New York: Springer.

Sandelowski, M., Voils, C. I., & Barroso, J. (2006). Defining and designing mixed research synthesis studies. *Research in the Schools, 13*(1), 29–40.

Sandelowski, M., Voils, C. I., & Barroso, J. (2007). Comparability work and the management of difference in research synthesis studies. *Social Science & Medicine, 64*(1), 236–247. doi: 10.1016/j.socscimed.2006.08.041.

Sandelowski, M., Voils, C. I., & Knafl, G. (2009). On quantitizing. *Journal of Mixed Methods Research, 3*(3), 208–222. doi: 10.1177/1558689809334210.

Sandelowski, M., Voils, C. I., Leeman, J., & Crandell, J. (2012). Mapping the mixed-methods mixed research synthesis terrain. *Journal of Mixed Methods Research, 6*(4), 317–331.

Vogt, W. P. (2008, August 27). Quantitative versus qualitative is a distraction: Variations on a theme by Brewer & Hunter (2006). *Methodological Innovations Online, 3*(1). Retrieved from http://erdt.plymouth.ac.uk/mionline/public_html/viewarticle.php?id=71.

Voils, C. I., Crandell, J. L., Chang, Y., Leeman, J., & Sandelowski, M. (2011). Combining adjusted and unadjusted findings in mixed research synthesis studies. *Journal of Evaluation in Clinical Practice, 17*(3), 429–434. doi: 10.1111/j.1365-2753.2010.01444.x.

Voils, C. I., Hasselblad, V., Chang, Y. K., Crandell, J., Lee, E. J., & Sandelowski, M. (2009). A Bayesian method for the synthesis of evidence from qualitative and quantitative reports: The example of antiretroviral medication adherence. *Journal of Health Services Research & Policy, 14*(4), 226–233. doi: 10.1258/jhsrp.2009.008186.

Voils, C. I., Sandelowski, M., Barroso, J., & Hasselblad, V. (2008). Making sense of qualitative and quantitative research findings in mixed research synthesis studies. *Field Methods, 20*(1), 3–25. doi: 10.1177/1525822X07307463.

Wood, M., & Christy, R. (1999). Sampling for possibilities. *Quality & Quantity, 33*(2), 185–202.

Part III
Contemporary issues in qualitative nursing research methods

Ethical issues in qualitative nursing research

Wendy Austin

Introduction

"Research is a step into the unknown" (CIHR et al., 2010, p. 7). This metaphor captures the need for all researchers to expect the unexpected and prepare for the ethical challenges that may arise in the quest for new knowledge. Striving to be an ethical researcher is an on-going process and involves sensitivity to values, norms, and relationships. It involves being competent, respectful, and worthy of trust. The discipline of nursing has similar demands. Nurse researchers' twofold fiduciary relationship with the public (as both nurses and scientists) is strengthened by the interdependence of their roles.

The ethical conduct of nursing research is of importance to all registered nurses: those caring for persons who are research participants; those involved in recruitment for research; those who are nurse research assistants; those on research ethics boards (REBs); and those preparing the next generation of nurse researchers. A very useful guide that speaks to nurses across research-related roles is the *Ethical Research Guidelines for Registered Nurses* (Canadian Nurses Association, 2002). This guide underscores the broad and deep involvement of nurses in research and the responsibilities that such involvement entails.

The aim of this chapter is to point to ethical issues that may arise for the nurse researcher undertaking a qualitative study. While the ethical conduct of science, including human science, is grounded in values that transcend all methods—values such as respect for human dignity, honesty, and justice—and which demand active attention on the part of both society and the scientist, qualitative research methods have distinct ethical issues. Certain benefits and risks to participants and to researchers are more prevalent in qualitative studies than in other types of research. Risks in qualitative research can be more subtle than those of clinical trials for instance. The risks to qualitative research participants are unlikely to be the life and death kind, but the emotional and social risks may be high. To date, the major scandals of science (often prompting new or revised codes of research conduct) have not involved qualitative studies. However, qualitative researchers must not be lulled into complacency. The question must be continually raised: Are we being ethical? Qualitative research designs are by nature dynamic and emergent; the particular ethical issues that will arise cannot be predicted with certainty. This means researchers using qualitative methods need to cultivate sensitivity and judgment in recognizing and addressing ethical issues as they arise (Vetlesen, 1994).

Although the issues addressed in this chapter are considered with regard to the current policies and practices of research ethics, it should be noted that the author's own approach is that of relational ethics. Relational ethics grounds ethical action in relationship and holds that the manner in which we engage with one another has moral significance. It recognizes that we live in the world as embodied beings, and that emotions are necessary to our rationality. It supports efforts to achieve mutual respect as we perceive one another's values, decisions, and circumstances. And it holds that, as we live in an interdependent world, context does matter when we consider what is and is not the fitting way to act. As a Canadian nurse researcher, the author follows the Canadian *Tri-Council Policy Statement: Ethical Conduct for Research Involving Humans* (CIHR et al., 2010), a key resource for this chapter. Considered in this chapter are researcher competence and relationships, as well as particular features of research projects (obtaining consent, privacy and confidentiality, benefits and risks related to participants and to researchers). The chapter concludes with further comments on the ethical qualitative researcher.

Researcher competence

A basic assumption in research ethics is that researchers will have competence in the methods used to answer their research questions. The notion that "bad science is bad ethics" is a valid one. (This is not to say that research ethics committees are the best arena for judging the quality of the science.) As the value of qualitative research is increasingly acknowledged and its repute (and funding) grow, more researchers are using qualitative methods, and some without the education or support necessary to do so. Qualitative methods can look "easy" to the uninitiated. Some researchers undertake activities inconsistent with their identified research methodology; others make claims that their qualitative results cannot support. With humor to reduce the sting of their call, Thorne and Darbyshire propose researchers "pay serious heed to what does and does not constitute rigorous, high-quality, empirical science within the qualitative tradition" (2005, p. 1105). That we do so is ultimately a matter of ethics.

Comprehensive training of all research team members is crucial to ethical research and key to minimizing risks to participants and researchers alike. Novice researchers need a planned, rather than a "watch and learn" approach to their training. They may not know what questions to ask or may suppress them in an effort to make a positive impression. Special training of all the team may be necessary depending on the project; team composition should reflect not only methodological expertise but also some knowledge of the research terrain ahead. For instance, a participant observation study in a clinic requires foresight of ethical and logistical challenges unique to the setting; the inclusion of someone with appropriate experience on the team (or as consultant) can accomplish this.

Researcher relationships

Researcher–participant relationships

In her reflection following a qualitative study, a nurse researcher noted: "The ethical commitments to these women [her participants] permeated my mind and actions throughout the study and still continue" (Bergum, 1989, p. 53). This researcher recognizes that the sharing of one's experience as a research participant may alter one's thinking about it. With publication of the research, further reflection may occur as one recognizes one's experience, now situated with that of others. This researcher knows too that using others' experiences for research purposes commits one ethically beyond procedural checks of informed consent or data handling and storage.

In qualitative research, the researcher–participant relationship is a particularly engaged one. It is physically situated not in the laboratory but often in the participant's home, workplace, or community. Researchers aim to build rapport and make participants comfortable enough to feel safe when revealing intimate life experiences or being observed going about their lives. The nature of rapport for participants can be glimpsed in the findings of a 20-study review which noted participant experiences in face-to-face interviews. Participants valued researchers' "empathy and respect, allowing space for sadness and upset, demonstrating interest, making the participant feel comfortable, non-judgemental active listening, warmth, caring, kindness, gentleness, and being able to cope with hearing painful accounts" (Graham, Lewis, & Nicolaas, 2006, p. 2). This type of interaction—given its confidential nature and the personal details shared within it—may prompt some participants to share far more than they had intended. It may lead some to believe a friendship is forming; others may confuse the researcher–participant relationship with a therapeutic one.

Nurse researchers may also be susceptible to the blurring of roles when interacting with participants. In a study of researchers' fieldwork experiences it was noted that researcher role issues were mainly raised by nurse researchers (Johnson & Clarke, 2003). This may be indicative of nurses' awareness of boundary issues, given their professional education in helping relationships; however, it may be that nurses' education to respond to those in need (especially when it is need of health information, of treatment and care, of assistance navigating the healthcare system) makes it particularly difficult to remain in the researcher role.

To mitigate role difficulties, orientation at the outset is required for participant and researcher to understand the purpose and limits of the research process. Disengagement ought to be acknowledged as a part of that process and strategies should be in place to facilitate it as the research comes to a close. This may be an area of research training in need of strengthening: a grounded theory study of the experiences of 30 qualitative health researchers found that the majority maintained some contact with their participants after study completion (e.g., correspondence, visiting) (Dickson-Swift, James, Kippen, & Liamputtong, 2006).

There is much variation in the researcher–participant relationship across methods (e.g., naturalistic observation to participatory action research) and research stages (recruitment to results dissemination). Power imbalances need to be considered throughout the research process (Karneieli-Miller, Strier, & Pessach, 2009). While it is commonly assumed that the greater power lies with the researcher, Corbin and Morse (2003) find that in qualitative research, particularly in unstructured interviews, it lies (or should lie) with the participant.

When a conflict of interest exists for the researcher (e.g., dual-role relationships, financial interests), not only does it skew the balance of power away from the participant, it jeopardizes the integrity of the research relationship. Transparency is required to reduce as much as possible the negative influence of such conflicts. Researchers need to identify and declare potential conflicts and act to avert or minimize them. Dual roles that are unavoidable due to a study's circumstances (e.g., the researcher is a participant's specialist caregiver, is a professor studying a student participant's skill acquisition, or is collecting narratives in his home community) should be identified and justified to the research ethics board (CIHR et al., 2010). Fundamentally, the greatest risks to participants in qualitative research lie within the researcher–participant relationship; researchers need to recognize this and act accordingly.

Research team relationships

The lone researcher has become a rarity: most qualitative projects involve at least co-investigators, research assistants (RAs), and transcriptionists. As with other types of teamwork, the research team is both a source of strength and support and the locus of power issues such as competing points of view and conflicting expectations. Working together ethically requires, from the outset, team building and negotiation of norms around responsibilities (e.g., training of RAs), potential issues (e.g., authorship) and practicalities (e.g., frequency of research meetings). It is important to acknowledge that emotion is part of the work of qualitative research and to develop strategies to assist team members (including interpreters and transcriptionists) to debrief and deal with the consequences of such work (Hubbard, Backett-Milburn, & Kemmer, 2001). A study of the impact of data collection on researchers studying sensitive topics found that some researchers may feel isolated within their team and need to go to family and friends for support (Johnson & Clarke, 2003). But the team should be a safe place to share issues and problems arising from the research (Hubbard et al., 2001). Novice team members, particularly students, may need encouragement to give voice to their concerns. Interpreters in cross-language studies may be treated as "ghostwriters—there, but generally unacknowledged" (Temple, 2002, p. 846), when it is more ethically sound if their contribution to the research process is recognized (Shklarov, 2007) and researchers offer preparation for it through initial briefing regarding research activities and debriefing after data collection (Adamson & Donovan, 2002). Keeping a reflexive journal during a research project can be a helpful strategy for all team members (Malacrida, 2007).

Obtaining consent

For the most part, it is standard (and required) procedure for researchers to secure and document the consent of research participants regarding their involvement in a particular study. To the uninitiated, obtaining consent can seem a simple, straightforward process. The ethical researcher knows it is not. For instance, in community-based research, engaging members of the community (e.g., Aboriginal elders) before beginning a project may be necessary to a successful and ethical consent process and study (CIHR et al., 2010; Ermine & Raven Browne, 2005). Ensuring that consent is voluntary, informed, and an on-going process can get complicated.

Voluntary consent

Genuine consent is inherently voluntary. No coercion may occur, even in the form of subtle pressures. Incentives to participate, financial or otherwise, are not to be such that they unduly influence consent so that any risks are considered "worth it." The circumstances (e.g., age, socioeconomic background) of the prospective participant must be taken into account when determining incentives. For instance, giving university students a course-credit option of research participation or submission of a scholarly paper may not be a real choice for some. (Note: Reimbursements (e.g., for travel time, babysitting) are not considered incentives.) Existing relationships may muddy the waters when it comes to voluntariness: how easy is it for a student to say no to a professor, patient to nurse, employee to manager, colleague to peer? Dependency within such relationships may decrease real choice. Other contextual elements can also be influential. For instance, if potential participants reside in an institutional setting where they have reduced opportunities for decision-making, saying no may be an unfamiliar act. Agreement may seem their only option or they may defer to another's decision (Thompson, 2002). It can happen, too, that intermediaries (e.g., clinic workers, cultural brokers, advocacy groups) involved in distributing information about a research project may give the impression that an individual should get involved. It must be made clear to potential participants that there can be no reprisal of any form for declining to participate in a study.

Informed consent

Prospective participants should know to what they are agreeing. The nature of qualitative research is such that it is not possible to predict everything that may occur, but prior to giving consent the participant needs to be aware of the steps involved in the project, its potential risks and benefits, measures taken to diminish risk and to ensure privacy and confidentiality, the limits on those measures, as well as plans for disseminating data. Providing this information involves several considerations. How should it be framed so that it is adequate, concise, cogent, and appropriate to the potential participant's level of comprehension? Will it need to be oral rather than written? Will it need to be translated into another language? Will pictures or diagrams help communicate the information more effectively?

A key component of consent is determining whether potential participants have the capacity to understand what is being asked of them and the ability to raise their own questions and concerns. If such is lacking, the decision regarding consent will need to be made by an authorized surrogate decision-maker. Persons unable to provide legal consent may be able to assent or dissent (in words or by actions) to their participation and this should be respected. Researchers involved with child health research have indicated a preference for a "family decision-making" model of consent that would allow child and family to jointly commit to a project, rather than the single person consent usually required by research ethics boards (Gibson, Stasiulis, Gutfreund, McDonald, & Dade, 2011, p. 504). Qualitative researchers have several means to document consent, including signed consent forms, consent logs, and audio- or videotaping.

In participant observation studies or fieldwork involving "non-participants," researchers will need to decide whether or not consent is sought. Although it is usually assumed to be unnecessary to acquire consent when using public spaces, where no privacy can be expected, researchers may choose to devise ways to address consent that are appropriate to their project circumstances. For example, Houghton and colleagues found solutions to non-participant (patients, staff, visitors) consent/assent in a clinical setting by acquiring consent from some patients, giving information sheets to staff, and strategically placing posters about the project to advise visitors (Houghton, Casey, Shaw, & Murphy, 2010).

Postponing consent

It is possible to postpone acquiring consent should the research design be such that prior consent is problematic to carrying it out (e.g., some form of deception is necessary to answer the research question). Ethics approval may be received for such studies that carry minimum risk to participants (and no interventions), but only if at some point participants will be debriefed and provided with information and the opportunity to refuse consent (CIHR et al., 2010, p. 37).

Consent as an on-going process

Consent is not a one-time act but an on-going process. Researchers need to keep the consent conversation open and be available to discuss participants' concerns, including their right to withdraw from the project at any time without untoward consequences. If and when participants withdraw from a study, it is for them to decide whether data they have contributed may be kept and used. They may request that it be entirely erased and discarded. When part of focus group data, participant data can be difficult to eliminate, yet discarding the contribution of other focus group members due to one's withdrawal is also problematic. Clearly understanding the participant's concerns and wishes may help resolve the situation, but the researcher may need the guidance of the research ethics board. Respecting consent involves supporting the participant in its control. In interview situations, it may be helpful to participants whose speech fluency may be impaired in some way or who are particularly vulnerable (e.g., children) to use visual cues (e.g., hand signal; stop sign) to indicate that they want to pause or stop.

Protecting privacy and confidentiality

Researchers have a responsibility to minimize threats to participants' privacy. "Privacy refers to an individual's right to be free from intrusion or interference by others" (CIHR et al., 2010, p. 55). Personal information and opinions are two of the privacy interests that may be put at risk for participants if researchers do not safeguard the information entrusted to them. Measures used to prevent unauthorized access need to be identified to participants and the research ethics board across the life of the data (collection, use, storage, retention/disposal). As the experiences of participants, essential to the presentation of qualitative results, may be recognizable to persons who know or know about them, promises of confidentiality to participants must be qualified (Morse, 2007). Researchers should outline to their participants the ways in which confidentiality will be protected. For instance, a broad scope for a study, in which both in-person and tele-interviews occur, reduces the risk of participant and third party (e.g., family members, community) identification. Changing or omitting potentially identifying details are useful strategies.

Threats to confidentiality may be unexpected. Examples include action research participants sharing results as next steps are planned; researchers being pressured to report back to a participant referral source and reluctant to refuse, as "then they might stop referring so many patients" (Johnson & Clarke, 2003, p. 426), and parents expecting that their children's data contributions will be shared with them (Allmark, 2002). Focus group participants need to be informed that the privacy of information shared in the group cannot be guaranteed. Strategies that support privacy can be used: pseudonyms for group members; agreement that "what is said in this group will stay in the group" except as research data; signed non-disclosure agreements. Some publicly available spaces (e.g., Internet chat rooms; open self-help groups, ceremonial space) may still offer reasonable expectations of privacy, and researchers need to take this into consideration if studying such spaces.

Disclosure of identity can be desirable and a matter of showing respect, such as with oral histories. A waiver of anonymity, however, must not compromise others. Researchers should be aware that the absence of privacy and confidentiality in oral histories can influence participants' comfort with results and their dissemination (Boschma, Yonge, & Mychajlunow, 2003). A further caution to researchers is that the nature of a research study may increase the likelihood that participants will disclose information that, ethically or legally, requires reporting (e.g., a child or elder is being abused; an inmate of a forensic facility is actively suicidal). Such limits on confidentiality need to be identified and discussed during the consent process. Nurse researchers have the advantage of being familiar with the limits on confidentiality in their role as nurses. They are aware that researchers, like nurses, can be subpoenaed to testify about crimes or other offences that may have been revealed to them.

Identifying benefits and risks to participants

Benefits

Although only *potential* benefits for participants can be named in qualitative research, many participants allow researchers to enter their lives due to a sense of altruism and the hope that others might learn from their experience. They wish to make a contribution to their society. Sharing experiences in a "safe" place (i.e., where their identity is to be protected) may be a benefit for some. Such sharing may provide a positive sense of catharsis (emotional release) or of empowerment and voice. A window into the way participants perceive the benefits of being involved with qualitative research is offered by Beck (2005). She completed a secondary, content analysis of women's volunteered descriptions of the benefits of being in an Internet study on birth trauma; the emerging themes were "experiencing caring by being listened to and acknowledged, sense of belonging, making sense of it all, letting go, being empowered, women helping women, and providing a voice" (p. 411). As Beck points out, such reactions show the powerful effects that research involvement can have on participants.

Risks

It is not possible to calculate a meaningful risk/benefit ratio for a qualitative research project, as the inherent unpredictability of this form of research applies to the risks involved. Emergent research design means that risks will also be emergent. For instance, achieving catharsis and gaining voice through research may be viewed as a benefit, but it may also be very risky. Participants may be shocked to find that in describing experiences, they are intensely reliving them or discovering new meaning. It may not be until some time after a project that participants know whether the experience was sufficiently worthwhile for them.

There are some concepts that are helpful to understanding risk related to research. One of these is "vulnerability." Vulnerability may be defined as a "diminished ability to fully safeguard one's own interests in the context of a specific research project. This may be caused by limited capacity or limited access to social goods, such as rights, opportunities and power" (CIHR et al., 2010, p. 197). For instance, children, persons with cognitive impairments or disability, prisoners, and residents in institutional settings can be vulnerable in the context of research participation. A qualitative study of parents' and children's perceptions of risk in research found that trust across interrelated relationships (e.g., parents, researchers, the institution) was involved in risk assessment; that it fluctuated across time; and that situations which eroded trust altered views of potential harms and benefits (Woodgate & Edwards, 2010).

Vulnerability can vary in degree at different times for the same person or group, depending on the circumstances (CIHR et al., 2010). Consider Morse's (2000) description of the vulnerability of patients in pain and her conclusion that these patients should be interviewed only post-pain. She reasons that persons in severe pain need to focus inwardly to have control of the pain and their emotional response to it; asking them to speak about it interferes with their control and thus to do so would be unethical. Note that Morse does not assume that research of persons who have pain should not be carried out because the participants are "vulnerable"; rather she looks to understand the way this vulnerability needs to be addressed within a study. She convincingly claims, "It is immoral not to conduct research with the critically ill or dying; they are the most disenfranchised members of our society and most in need of understanding" (p. 545).

Another important concept is that of the "sensitive topic." There has been much debate about what comprises a sensitive topic in research, but a useful definition is "one which potentially poses for those involved a substantial threat, the emergence of which renders problematic for the researcher and/or the researched the collection, holding, and/or dissemination of research data" (Lee & Renzetti, 1990, p. 512). How personal or sensitive the topic is can shape the experience of research more than the method of study. This was concluded in a study of participants' experience in both qualitative and quantitative social research (Graham, Grewal, & Lewis, 2007). Because qualitative studies often explore profound human experiences (e.g., rape, terminal illness, children's disfigurement, growing old), much of what is being explored meets the definition of "sensitive." However, it is also possible for issues which researchers assume to be banal can be distressing for a participant, for example, the collection of a particular type of demographic data can have a negative impact on an individual. The question "Do you have children?" can be distressing to a participant who has been diagnosed as infertile, and asking about employment can be distressing to someone who has lost his or her job. Researchers need sound reasons for their demographic questions.

In a web-based survey of qualitative researchers' perceptions of the risks inherent in qualitative interviews, researchers described low-risk research as that exploring topics that could be termed "impersonal," "mundane," "non-threatening": the kind of topic common to everyday social situations (Morse, Niehaus, Varnhagen, Austin, & McIntosh, 2008, p. 201). High-risk research involved vulnerable participants and inexperienced, unprepared researchers exploring highly sensational, controversial, or emotional topics. Researchers noted that risk is high when participants do not understand mandatory reporting requirements and disclose incriminating information. The authors of the research conclude, "It is this emotion that is the cardinal factor in shaping risk, is risk itself, and enables risk assessment" (p. 203).

New approaches to research bring new forms of risks. Cyberspace studies are carried out in environments in which researchers may be unable to verify age or identity, creating novel concerns regarding consent and protection from harm. Keller and Lee (2003) recommend that researchers do pilot studies to identify risk issues, which can include the absence of visual and auditory distress cues and participants going offline before debriefing can occur. Researchers can learn from one another's experiences: it is a responsible act to publish the issues faced and learning achieved when venturing into new territory. For instance, researchers who used an interactive website with a message board in studying the engagement of youth in health promotion describe their use of strategies such as setting "community standards" for the site. When posts were made that violated these standards, messages were edited or deleted and a replacement message left explaining the change. If a message appeared which indicated distress (e.g., a suicide threat), a reply was sent (direct if the email address was known) asking the person to seek help (Flicker, Haans, & Skinner, 2004). A risk unique to online studies is that of participants acting in ways they would not in the real world, like being offensive to others (rude, angry, or cruelly critical). Disconnect between actual and online conduct increases the complexity of cyberspace studies, including issues related to data accuracy (Haigh & Jones, 2007).

The dissemination phase of qualitative research may be the time of greatest risk for participants. This is when the risks to privacy and confidentiality heighten. Risk of identification emerges for third parties who had a role in participant experiences that have become data (Hadjistavropoulos & Smythe, 2001). Research findings and the products evolving from them (e.g., articles, presentations, books, plays) may be distressing for participants if they feel their experiences were ultimately misunderstood by the researcher or if they believe they have been negatively described (Morse et al., 2008). Offering participants information about the results of the qualitative studies to which they contributed is the common practice of most researchers. Research is lacking, however, on participants' views of the best way to receive study results and on the consequences for the participants of such disclosure (MacNeil & Fernandez, 2006).

Reducing risks to participants

There are principles that qualitative researchers can use to reduce risks to participants. Based on the results of their web survey of qualitative researchers' perspectives on risks, Morse and colleagues (2008) offer these: (1) risk assessment must be continuous during a project; (2) researchers need to have some familiarity with the topic's "emotional terrain" so they can anticipate risk more effectively; (3) in terms of privacy and confidentiality, the participant comes before the research goals; and (4) researchers need to recognize their own and their team's vulnerability. One of their principles, "Risk assessment, avoidance, and alleviation are the ongoing responsibility of the researcher" (p. 211), sums up the attitude that researchers must hold toward risks.

There are strategies for reducing risk related to qualitative interviews. Cowles' (1988) recommendations remain germane. One strategy is flexibility in planned interview time: more may be necessary if participants need to go slow, get distressed, or need to pause or take a break; less, if they get fatigued. Participants should control the pace. Cowles suggests brief counselling by the researcher at the end of an interview, if necessary. Brief counseling would in contemporary usage be termed "debriefing." Otherwise, any "counseling" is delimited by the participant and by the researcher's training (nursing education includes basic counseling skills), as well as the recognition that consent was acquired for research, not therapy. Information about local resources (e.g., support groups) and referrals should be made available and offered with discretion. Participants who cry during an interview, for instance, should not be made to feel their expression of emotion is somehow pathological. Many participants may need only to "come down" after the interview and should be given time to do so.

Risks to researchers

There are hazards to which qualitative researchers may be exposed, such as entrance into unstable situations, and even verbal or physical assault (Morse et al., 2008). Safety protocols, based on assessment of risk specifically related to a project, alert researchers and prepare them for appropriate responses. Paterson and colleagues (1999) offer a detailed protocol that addresses such items as equipment (e.g., alarms, cell phones), preparation (e.g., be accompanied by a colleague), appearance (e.g., dress for neighborhood), and visibility (e.g., do not share personal information). Other risk factors are related to the proximity and rapport of researcher and participant, which vary with method, study length, researcher personality and skill, and topic sensitivity. Researchers can pay an emotional toll studying human distress, tragedy, and injustice, with recurring intrusive thoughts about participants, anxiety, nightmares, and insomnia, especially when their own experiences resonate with those of their participants (McGarry, 2010). Morse (2000) cautions that researchers may "hear the participant's voice in [their] head many years after conducting a heart-wrenching interview" or when working with transcript or text data (p. 540). Data coding and analysis are periods that trigger researcher distress (Dickson-Swift et al., 2007) perhaps because, with participants absent, researchers are free to react (Woodby, Williams, Wittich, & Burgio, 2011). Those who do not react may worry they are desensitized, while those who think "this is really good stuff" may feel guilty (Dickson-Swift et al., 2007, p. 343). It is recommended that the researcher studying sensitive topics limit the number of interviews per week, allow time for processing/debriefing, and avoid evening interviews to prevent sleep disturbance (Cowles, 1988). Self-care for researchers, as with nurses, is a matter of ethics, as stress and fatigue increase the likelihood of poor communication, errors, and poor judgment.

The ethical qualitative researcher

Research in the twenty-first century is vastly complex and wide-ranging in its explorations. Researchers need to keep before them the broad ethical issues as well as those defined by their own research context. They need to ask: "What questions need to be studied and why? If not, why not? Is the diversity of society reflected in recruitment of participants? What processes are shaping dissemination of research results? How is research being used, for good and ill?" A particularly fundamental question is how fears about unethical research should be addressed. Whistleblowers may be perceived as "the enemy within" rather than being valued and respected for doing the right thing (Rhodes & Strain, 2004). Too often the systemic response is a call for increased oversight, stricter monitoring, and greater surveillance of research and researchers. Oversight as the dominant strategy for keeping research ethical is problematic. It may be ill-informed, as occurred when qualitative research began to evolve and its governance was guided by criteria developed for the natural sciences and based on an assumption that research designs can be fully specified in advance. Most importantly, however, a dichotomy is created in which researchers become the observed, and institutional controls (shaped by influences beyond the public good, such as corporate logic and concerns over legal liability) become omnipresent and all-powerful. A form of "ethics creep" can reach the point that rule-following trumps acting ethically (Haggerty, 2004, p. 391). The constantly monitored (thus controlled) researcher loses ownership of research integrity and becomes passive in awareness of threats to it.

To date, researcher misconduct has commonly been defined as consisting of deliberate fabrication (inventing data), falsification (deliberate distortion of data), and plagiarism (using others' ideas, words, or data without giving credit) in proposing, performing, or reviewing research—a definition that fails to account for questionable practices that may compromise or disserve research, researchers, and participants in subtler ways (such as practices having to do with how data are recorded and represented; how research is made accessible to peers; how research team members are treated, etc.) (National Academy of Sciences et al., 1992). When serious breaches of research ethics are examined and "How could this have happened?" is asked, the answer that seems most pertinent is that the persons who served as research "subjects" were not viewed as members of the researcher's own moral community. They were "other" in some way: female, old, psychiatric patient, dying, disabled, prisoner, Jewish, Roma, gay. The notion of the researcher as an impartial, objective, disengaged seeker after truth supports the distancing that makes such attitudes possible. Research does require intelligent governance and oversight, but the most pressing need is for researchers themselves to act with humility and vigilance about how they are with others: with participants, colleagues, communities.

A further need is for research environments to be places where it is safe to raise difficult, messy ethical questions, where dialogue about them is welcomed and expected. These questions need to be studied to deepen our understanding of them and to help us respond well. The cultivation of the moral imagination is an on-going demand for researchers; moral anxiety is never-ending and never resolved (Bauman, 1993). The territory of the qualitative researcher is always, in a sense, "uncharted" (Johnson & Clarke, 2003, p. 425). As one researcher in Johnson and Clarke's study noted, "I was just not prepared for some of the things that happened even though I thought I would be" (p. 425). These words can serve as a wise reminder to nurses embarking on a qualitative study.

References

Adamson, J., & Donovan, J. (2002). Research in black and white. *Qualitative Health Research, 12*(6), 816–825.
Allmark, P. (2002). The ethics of research with children. *Nurse Researcher, 10*(2), 7–19.

Bauman, Z. (1993). *Postmodern ethics*. Oxford: Blackwell.

Beck, C. T. (2005). Benefits of participating in Internet interviews: Women helping women. *Qualitative Health Research, 15*, 411–422.

Bergum, V. (1989). Being a phenomenological researcher. In J. Morse (Ed.), *Qualitative nursing research* (pp. 43–57). Rockville, MD: Aspen Publishers Inc.

Boschma, G., Yonge, O., & Mychajlunow, L. (2003). Consent in oral history interviews: Unique challenges. *Qualitative Health Research, 13*(1), 129–135.

Canadian Nurses Association. (2002). *Ethical research guidelines for registered nurses*. Ottawa: Author.

(CIHR) Canadian Institutes of Health Research, Natural Sciences and Engineering Research Council of Canada, and Social Sciences and Humanities Research Council of Canada. (December, 2010). *Tri-Council Policy Statement: Ethical Conduct for Research Involving Humans*. Retrieved on 24 February 2012 from http://www.pre.ethics.gc.ca/pdf/eng/tcps2/TCPS_2_FINAL_Web.pdf.

Corbin, J., & Morse, J. (2003). The unstructured interactive interview: Issues of reciprocity and risks when dealing with sensitive topics. *Qualitative Inquiry, 9*(3), 335–354.

Cowles, K. V. (1988). Issues in qualitative research on sensitive subjects. *Western Journal of Nursing Research, 10*(2), 163–179.

Dickson-Swift, V., James, E. L., Kippen, S., & Liamputtong, P. (2006). Blurring boundaries in qualitative research on sensitive topics. *Qualitative Health Research, 16*(6), 853–871.

Dickson-Swift, V., James, E. L., Kippen, S., & Liamputtong, P. (2007). Doing sensitive research: What challenges do qualitative researchers face? *Qualitative Research, 7*(3), 327–353.

Ermine, W. S., & Raven Browne, M. (2005). *Kwayask itôtamowin: Indigenous research ethics*. Regina, SK: Indigenous Peoples' Health Research Centre.

Flicker, S., Haans, D., & Skinner, H. (2004). Ethical dilemmas in research on internet communities. *Qualitative Health Research, 14*(1), 124–134.

Gibson, B. E., Stasiulis, E., Gutfreund, S., McDonald, M., & Dade, L. (2011). Assessment of children's capacity to consent for research: A descriptive qualitative study of researchers' practices. *Journal of Medical Ethics, 37*(8), 504–509.

Graham, J., Grewal, I., & Lewis, J. (2007). *Ethics in social research: The views of research participants*. Retrieved on 29 February 2012 from http://www.civilservice.gov.uk/wp-content/uploads/2011/09/ethics_participants_tech_ tcm6-5784.pdf.

Graham, J., Lewis, J., & Nicolaas, G. (2006). Ethical relations: A review of literature on empirical studies of ethical requirements and research participation. Economic & Social Research Council Research Methods Programme, Working Paper No. 30. Retrieved on 29 February 2012 from http://www.ccsr.ac.uk/methods/publications/documents/WP30.pdf.

Hadjistavropoulos, T., & Smythe, W. (2001). Elements of risk in qualitative research. *Ethics & Behavior, 11*(2), 163–174.

Haggerty, K.D. (2004). Ethics creep: Governing social science research in the name of ethics. *Qualitative Sociology, 27*(4), 391–414.

Haigh, C., & Jones, N. (2007). Techno-research and cyber ethics. In T. Long & M. Johnson (eds.) *Research ethics in the real world* (pp. 157–174). Edinburgh: Churchill Livingstone.

Houghton, C. E., Casey, D., Shaw, D., & Murphy K. (2010). Ethical challenges in qualitative research: Examples from practice. *Nurse Researcher, 18*(1), 15–25.

Hubbard, G., Backett-Milburn, K., & Kemmer, D. (2001). Working with emotion: Issues for the researcher in fieldwork and teamwork. *Social Research Methodology, 4*(2), 119–137.

Johnson, B., & Clarke, J. M. (2003). Collecting sensitive data: The impact on researchers. *Qualitative Health Research, 13*(3), 421–434.

Karnieli-Miller, O., Strier, R., & Pessach, L. (2009). Power relations in qualitative research. *Qualitative Health Research, 19*(2), 279–289.

Keller, H., & Lee, S. (2003). Ethical issues surrounding human participants research using the Internet. *Ethics & Behavior, 13*(3), 211–219.

Lee, R., & Renzetti, C. (1990). The problems of researching sensitive topics: An overview and introduction. *American Behavioral Scientist, 33*(5), 510–528.

MacNeil, S. D., & Fernandez, C.V. (2006). Informing research participants of research results: Analysis of Canadian university-based research ethics board policies. *Journal of Medical Ethics, 32*(1), 49–54.

Malacrida, C. (2007). Reflexive journaling on emotional research topics: Ethical issues for team researchers. *Qualitative Health Research, 17*(10), 1329–1339.

McGarry, J. (2010). Exploring the effect of conducting sensitive research. *Nurse Researcher, 18*(1), 8–14.

Morse, J. (2000). Researching illness and injury: Methodological considerations. *Qualitative Health Research*, *10*(4), 538–546.

Morse, J. (2007). Ethics in action: Ethical principles for doing qualitative health research. *Qualitative Health Research*, *17*(8), 1003–1005.

Morse, J., Niehaus, L., Varnhagen, S., Austin, W., & McIntosh, M. (2008). Qualitative researchers' conceptualizations of the risks inherent in qualitative interviews. *International Review of Qualitative Research*, *1*(2), 195–215.

National Academy of Sciences, National Academy of Engineering, Institute of Medicine: Panel on Scientific Responsibility and the Conduct of Research. (1992). *Responsible Science, Volume 1: Ensuring the Integrity of the Research Process*. Washington, DC: National Academy of Sciences. Retrieved on February 24, 2012 from: http://www.nap.edu/openbook.php?record_id= 1864&page=1.

Paterson, B., Gregory, D., & Thorne, S. (1999). A protocol for researcher safety. *Qualitative Health Research*, *9*(2), 259–269.

Rhodes, R., & Strain, J. (2004). Whistleblowing in academic medicine. *Journal of Medical Ethics*, *30*(1), 35–39.

Shklarov, S. (2007). Double vision uncertainty: The bilingual researcher and the ethics of cross-language research. *Qualitative Health Research*, *17*(4), 529–538.

Temple, B. (2002). Crossed wires: Interpreters, translators, and bilingual workers in cross-language research. *Qualitative Health Research*, *12*(6), 844–854.

Thompson, S. A. (2002). My research friend? My friend the researcher? My friend, my researcher?: Mis/informed consent and people with developmental disabilities. In W. C. van den Hoonaard (Ed.), *Walking the tightrope: Ethical issues for qualitative researchers* (pp. 137–151). Toronto: University of Toronto Press.

Thorne, S., & Darbyshire, P. (2005). Land mines in the field: A modest proposal for improving the craft of qualitative health research. *Qualitative Health Research*, *15*(8), 1105–1113.

Vetlesen, A. J. (1994). *Perception, empathy & judgement: An inquiry into the preconditions of moral performance*. University Park, PA: Pennsylvania State University Press.

Woodby, L., Williams, B., Wittich, A., & Burgio, K. (2011). Expanding the notion of researcher distress: The cumulative effects of coding. *Qualitative Health Research*, *21*(6), 830–838.

Woodgate, R., & Edwards, M. (2010). Children in health research: A matter of trust, *Journal of Medical Ethics*, *36*, 211–216.

28

Politics and qualitative nursing research

Joy L. Johnson

> Politics consists of ignoring facts.
> *(Henry Adams)*

While Henry Adams' claim about politics and facts runs counter to what many of us might hope would inform political decisions, too often we witness decisions being made either in the absence of evidence or contrary to the evidence. A Vice President of Research at a Canadian university was quoted as commenting, "The vast majority of policy in this country right now has been made for political reasons, not based on scientific evidence" (Peters, 2012, p. 19).

In this chapter we consider the overlapping spheres of politics and qualitative nursing research. The term "politics" is often narrowly applied to the science of running governmental or state affairs; its meaning, however, is much broader. Indeed, in its fullest sense, "politics" refers to the processes by which collective decisions are made and therefore applies to all institutions and interest groups. In this regard, a key element of politics is the process by which policy is formulated and applied and decisions made. Not surprisingly an essential component of politics is power, or the ability to influence others through decision-making, agenda-setting, and preference shaping. Power, however, is not simply possessed by individuals; our social structures influence our patterned social arrangements and norms. Humans (agents), in turn, reinforce social structures in a variety of ways. This reciprocal determinism reminds us that we are all part of political systems and therefore have the power to change them.

Politics and qualitative research intersect in a number of important ways. In this chapter we consider five related areas: the politics of evidence, the politics of research funding, the politics of grant writing and peer review, the politics of policy-making, and the politics of partnerships. In discussing the political spheres I draw on examples largely from the Canadian context, particularly my experiences in relation to my work with the Canadian Institutes of Health Research.

The politics of evidence

What counts as knowledge? The epistemological debates related to the value of qualitative research could fill this entire volume. The fact that such extensive dialogue has taken place is in itself worth commenting on, in that it points to a struggle to claim legitimacy for evidence that is grounded in everyday, subjective experience. Issues related to "generalizability" and the "control" of bias are often at the heart of these dialogues. Interestingly, it has largely been the proponents of qualitative approaches who have written extensively about the legitimacy of these approaches, with colleagues in the "hard sciences" remaining largely oblivious to the turmoil. This state of detente is perpetuated by the fact that certain research approaches, largely based in the bench and biomedical sciences remain the *sine qua non* of the "scientific method." The power associated with research that is purportedly directed at curing cancer, developing new vaccines, or determining the genetic basis of Alzheimer's disease is indisputable. This legitimacy is further reinforced with "top ranked" journals hailing from the life sciences (e.g. *Cell*, *Nature*, *Science*). This dynamic creates a politic in which certain types of research (i.e., bench science directed at curing disease) is seen as more valuable, more fundable, and indeed more important.

While some progress has been made in bolstering the epistemic legitimacy of qualitative approaches, and increasingly research funding bodies and scientific journals are recognizing the value and contributions of qualitative approaches, there are a number of factors that continue to reinforce the current dynamic in which qualitative approaches remain marginalized. First and foremost, there remains a perception that qualitative research is "easier" than other methods of research. This underselling and undervaluing of qualitative approaches undermine their legitimacy as valuable and rigorous forms of knowledge generation. Unfortunately, it is a group of methods that weak students and poorly trained researchers readily take up without a moment's thought. In addition, because of the inherent accessibility of the findings, researchers with no qualitative methodological expertise often feel they can legitimately comment on the quality of a qualitative research.

A related factor is the quality of qualitative research. While poor quality science is seen in all branches of research, there is a plethora of poorly conceptualized and executed qualitative studies that continue to unintentionally "make the case" that qualitative research has limited value. This is in part because of a lack of methodological rigor. Qualitative approaches are wrongly assumed by some to support an "anything goes" approach. In particular, qualitative researchers have not always been sufficiently transparent about how their analytic processes led to theoretical insights.

Another factor that shapes legitimacy is the perceived relevance of qualitative research. The past decade has witnessed a growing number of qualitative studies that focus on increasingly more idiosyncratic issues in more obscure populations. For example, we repeat studies on living with cancer in every possible ethnic group imaginable. To what end? While there are a number of pressing health issues that could benefit from intensive inquiry, we become caught up in repeating studies, or focusing on particular population niches.

Relatedly, the scale of qualitative research is another sticking point that continues to raise questions of epistemic legitimacy. Qualitative science, like all science, is easily compromised by insufficient data. Despite the fact that qualitative data are inherently "rich," too often we see studies conducted with very limited samples. While claims are made about "saturation," it is hard to imagine that no new insights can be gained after interviewing ten people. We have been reluctant to scale up our work, for example, by conducting team-based inquiries across a number of subpopulations.

The politics of evidence is ultimately about how qualitative research is positioned. While it is tempting for us as nurses to wring our hands and complain that qualitative research is not funded or published, we must also ask the question of how we might be unintentionally reinforcing the power of dominant science. Ironically, even the arguments regarding quality and relevance that are used above can be seen as a particular political maneuvering that relies on the "positivist rhetoric of rigorous research" and in turn reifies the qualitative–quantitative binary

(Dey & Nentwich, 2006). In the end, we must be mindful that the way we present our qualitative work may at times reinforce dominant views about what counts as knowledge.

The politics of research funding

"Follow the money" is the famous quote used by a source, Deep Throat, a journalist's anonymous source in the movie *All the President's Men*. This phrase has become a rallying cry for those trying to understand political decision-making. This directive is equally applicable to the politics of research funding. Nurses applying for research funds from funding organizations need to understand the political climate and the agendas that are driving funding decisions.

Funding for the majority of formal research in the world today is provided by governments and corporations. This means that most research follows government and corporate agendas. Examples of this agenda setting power abound. For example, in examining the funding of sex research, Udry (1993) provides an excellent example of how politics in the United States shaped the research agenda. Pointing to political interventions that blocked national sex surveys being funded by the National Institutes of Health in the United States, he argues that researchers must themselves become politically organized in order to shape the research agenda.

In 2007, the Canadian government, through its Science Technology and Innovation Council, announced key priorities for research (Government of Canada, 2007). The government of the day was concerned with enhancing Canada's "entrepreneurial advantage" by making Canada a world leader in science and technology. In an effort to focus strategically on research in the "national interest," a number of priority areas were identified and the national research-funding agencies receiving funding from the government were directed to "improve their responsiveness and accountability to the government." This agenda in turn shaped strategic funding opportunities being offered to researchers in Canada and spurred further discussions related to the commercialization of discoveries.

Not surprisingly one of the pressing issues facing all governments relates to the state of the economy. Research investments are increasingly framed as investments in innovation and commercialization. There is a growing interest in "big science," a term that implies big budgets, staffs, machines, and laboratories; a prime example is the Human Genome Project. These types of projects are framed as having high "rewards." Nursing's inability to scale up its research and frame its endeavors in relation to big science constitutes a major stumbling block in our progress. This is particularly the case for qualitative nursing research, where examples of international collaborations are the exception rather than the rule.

While much lip service continues to be paid to the notion of curiosity-driven or "pure" research that addresses the questions of the investigator, those who fund research are increasingly interested in "return on investment" (Panel on Return on Investment in Health Research, 2009). This concern arises because research-granting agencies like the National Institutes of Health and the Canadian Institutes of Health Research are accountable to those who hold the purse strings. Perhaps no better example of the link between the funding of research and the economy is the 2009 American Recovery and Reinvestment Act which directed funds to the NIH in order to "jump-start" the economy and create jobs.

In response to the challenge of demonstrating return on investment, funding agencies are asking questions about the benefits that are derived from research, and they are turning to models like the "payback model" to help track the value of research "investments." Categories of payback include knowledge; research benefits; political and administrative benefits, health sector benefits, and broader economic benefits (Buxton & Hanney, 1996). This pressure to produce is also felt by nongovernmental organizations such as the health charities that rely on donations from the public to fund research (Wooding, Hanney, Buxton, & Grant, 2005). Ultimately their continued existence relies on their ability to convince the public that they have made "wise" investments with their money.

Baylis (2012) argues that as a direct result of government funding philosophies that support "trickle-down" economics for science, science that does not support the "knowledge economy" is science that is not funded. As a counter-point to this mechanistic standpoint, organizations such as the Slow Science Academy (2010) argue that:

> We do need time to think. We do need time to digest. We do need time to misunderstand each other, especially when fostering lost dialogue between humanities and natural sciences. We cannot continuously tell you what our science means; what it will be good for; because we simply don't know yet. Science needs time.

What is the "payback" of qualitative nursing research? This research does not deal with cure, drug discovery, or nanotechnology. It will not result in the development of commercial projects that will stimulate the economy. Rather we concentrate our research on the day-to-day lives of the patients, families, health systems and communities. Through our research our intent is to develop new insights that will relieve suffering, improve health behavior and strengthen communities. Rose Kushner, an American physician, is quoted as remarking

> Few doctors in this country seem to be involved with the non-life threatening side effects of cancer . . . In the United States, baldness, nausea and vomiting, diarrhea, clogged veins, financial problems, loss of libido, loss of self-esteem, and body image are the nurses' turf.
> *(Mukherjee, 2010, p. 202)*

Politically, this is awkward turf to defend. It is much more appealing to hear about proposed research that will cure cancer and offer new hope than projects that help to illuminate the experience of suffering, Yet, this work is potentially life-changing and we need to continue to strive to make the case that qualitative nursing research can offer new insight and can improve patient care.

Those who conduct qualitative nursing research need to increasingly consider how their research provides "return on investment." This "return" includes how we improve nursing care, patient outcomes, and how we influence policy. We need to make the case that our work matters because it detects errors, leads to new insights about resilience, and heightens sensitivity of health professionals. More than that, we need to find ways to track these outcomes so that we can help funding agencies make the case that qualitative nursing research matters.

In order to advocate for qualitative nursing research, we must understand how the research agenda is shaped. Martin (1998) points out that a key element that structures the politics of research is hierarchy. Not everyone involved in the research enterprise is on an equal footing. He maintains that the more powerful researchers often have personal or professional links with powerful figures in funding organizations. They sit on boards, chair review committees, and provide advice on priorities. This hierarchy, he argues, keeps researchers in line, in that those that stray from conventional research topics or approaches are brought into line by the competition for funding. Benner and Sandström (2000) contend that research funding agencies play a particularly important role in maintaining this hierarchy. They maintain that granting agencies function as societal agents, structuring research performance and the institutional norms of academic research. As a result, the actions taking place within the academic system are dependent on and structured by the funding agencies.

Martin's observations regarding hierarchy provide two important insights regarding the politics of qualitative nursing research. On the one hand, it helps us understand how, generally speaking, qualitative nursing research may be marginalized. It also helps us understand how within the field of qualitative nursing research particular approaches are granted legitimacy and conversely how certain topics or approaches may be marginalized.

The politics of grant writing and peer review

The road to research funding still remains paved figuratively with quantitative cement.

(Leininger, 1994, p. 112)

While Leininger's remark was made close to two decades ago, the insight remains important, in that it recognizes there are politics involved in judging the credibility of research approaches. Indeed, it is naïve to assume that obtaining peer-reviewed funding is simply a matter of writing a methodologically strong grant. Given the arguments made above, one clear area for attention when writing qualitative research grant applications involves making the case that the proposed work is in line with the funding agency's mandate, and most importantly that the proposed research will make a difference. The way that one's work is positioned is extremely important. Indeed, the importance of the research is often cited as a key criterion for excellent qualitative research (Cohen & Crabtree, 2008).

Despite best efforts, some good research proposals do not get funded; research on the process of peer review suggests that errors of judgment do creep into the peer review process. Most of the errors can be traced to lack of clarity in the proposal itself, but external factors that can influence the outcome include biases introduced by the adjudication process, such as rules of order, group dynamics and adjudicator fatigue (Thorngate, Faregh, & Young, 2002). Thorngate et al. conducted a study of the peer review process undertaken by select peer review committees at the Canadian Institutes of Health Research (CIHR). At CIHR every proposal is assigned to a committee and it is initially reviewed and rated by two committee members. These two reviewers reveal their ratings and discuss their observations about the strengths and weaknesses of the grant and then the proposal is discussed by the committee as a whole. Thorngate et al.'s findings reveal some important insights related to the politics of peer review. In particular, disagreements about the merits of a study were common and this disagreement did not tend to be resolved through discussion. Indeed, the greater the initial disparity in a proposal's ratings, the more likely that in the end the grant would be poorly rated. This suggests that controversial applications were further downgraded through a discussion of the flaws of the application.

Thorngate et al. then compared the reviews of committees that considered biomedical applications with those committees considering broader issues related to the health system and the human health experience (i.e., committees more likely to consider proposals that utilized qualitative methods) and found there was more disagreement among the latter committees. These two types of committees also tended to use different criteria when judging proposals with the biomedical committees focusing on track record and logical derivation of the research ideas, while the broader health committees focused on specific issues related to design and methods. Indeed, the findings of this work suggested two separate subcultures when it comes to peer review.

The community of scientific peers exhibits far less solidarity than many people might think. While the focus of a peer review is on "good science," the push for resources and power inevitably shapes the process. As Chubin and Hackett (1990) point out, peer review simultaneously serves a set of values that are not entirely in harmony. These values include fairness, and expediency and these values are juxtaposed against the need to identify trustworthy, high quality and innovative knowledge. The process does not necessarily guarantee the product.

Cohen and Crabtree (2008) conducted a synthesis of published criteria for assessing qualitative research. They reviewed 45 book chapters and papers that offered explicit criteria for evaluating the quality of qualitative research. While they identified a number of "generic" categories for evaluation, they noted it was problematic to assume that there is agreement regarding a unified set of evaluative criteria, as it is based on the assumption that qualitative research is a unified field. They point out that one's ontological perspective shapes the values that drive research evaluation. Most importantly, they remind us that "it is important to understand that paradigms and debates about paradigms are political and used to argue for credibility and resources in the research community" (p. 338). They recognize that more innovative qualitative methods may be marginalized because they do not fit the evaluative criteria aligned with more traditional approaches. Similarly, Dey and Nentwich (2006) maintain that in the face of the irreducibly rich diversity of qualitative approaches, it is not possible to define "good" qualitative research by using fixed and transcendental quality criteria. These insights shed light on what happens in the peer review process and point to the importance of judging a research project within the context of the paradigm in which it has been proposed. To do otherwise is to not offer a true "peer" review. In the words of Richard Smith (2006), past editor of the *British Medical Journal*:

> So peer review is a flawed process, full of easily identified defects with little evidence that it works. Nevertheless, it is likely to remain central to science and journals because there is no obvious alternative, and scientists and editors have a continuing belief in peer review. How odd that science should be rooted in belief.

The politics of policy-making

> The shortest distance between two people is a story.
>
> *(Source unknown)*

An indisputable strength of qualitative research findings relates to the power of the narrative, and the ability of qualitative findings to be communicated in a compelling manner (Carey, 1997). Indeed, there is nothing as powerful as a good story. Qualitative nursing research findings can provide policy-makers with important insight into the complexity of a situation. For example, they can illuminate how contextual factors shape health and illness experiences, how current health systems do not meet the needs of particular groups, and can stimulate new insights into areas that are rife with preconceptions and assumptions. In addition, qualitative inquiry reveals nuanced understanding of policies that in turn can lead to more focused and in-depth investigations of policy implementation (Smit, 2003). This perspective recognizes the distinction between polices as they appear on paper, and policies as they are enacted.

One of the first authors to explicitly address qualitative research and policy-making was Rist (1994). Rist correctly noted that policy-making is multidimensional and multifaceted and that research is but one of the frequently contradictory and competing sources that can influence what is an ongoing process. When we think of policy-making, we often think of it as a singular event. Both the popular and the academic literature depict policy-making in a way that suggests a group of authorized decision-makers assemble at particular times and places, review an issue, consider alternative courses of action and then select a direction that seems well suited for achieving their purposes; the result is a decision. Unfortunately the process is much more complex. Policy-making is a process that involves many cycles and often choosing to *not* make a decision is an outcome of the policy process.

Research evidence is an important and necessary component in the policy-making process; but there is seldom enough evidence available in the policy arena. Researchers may be reluctant to share their findings with policy-makers because of limitations of the evidence they have uncovered. While ideally policy decisions should be based on evidence synthesized from multiple studies, we need to recognize that single studies can be used to help shape the policy process. This refocusing on the policy process (versus policy decisions) helps us to consider multiple ways that qualitative evidence can inform policy.

Rist (1994) argued that if researchers presume that their findings must be brought to bear upon a single event, a discrete act of decision-making, they will be missing those circumstances and processes where, in fact, research can be useful. However, the reorientation away from "event decision-making" and to "process decision-making" necessitates looking at research as serving an "enlightenment function" in contrast to an "engineering function."

Lavis and colleagues have written extensively about the ways that research evidence can be used to inform the policy *process*. For example, Lavis, Wilson, Oxman, Lewin, and Fretheim (2009) provide a number of suggestions related to how evidence can be used to clarify a policy problem. Policies are developed in response to the existence of a perceived problem or an opportunity; they never exist in a vacuum. The context is extremely important because it shapes the kinds of actions considered. Not all problems that are brought to a policy-maker's attention require action, and research evidence, particularly qualitative evidence, can provide an important source of insight into the experiences of those affected by the issue and the contextual factors that are driving the problem.

How else can qualitative nursing research help shape the *policy process*? First, we need to learn to share our findings with decision-makers. We cannot expect them to comb though the literature and so we must reproduce our findings in digestible one- to two-page briefing notes. Increasingly, I have witnessed the use of policy "decks" consisting of no more than ten printed PowerPoint slides being used effectively in face-to-face discussions with policy-makers. Second, we can enable the receptivity of policy-makers by influencing the policy cycle. This can be accomplished in a number of ways. For example, our research participants, particularly if they are part of the research process, are often willing to act as advocates and can marshal the citizenry to bring issues to policy-makers' attention. All media can serve as a powerful tool for awakening concern among policy-makers. In recent years we have seen a number of social media events that have gone "viral," the result being an increased receptiveness among policy-makers to reconsider decisions.

There are times, however, that a less confrontational approach is more effective. As discussed above, there are many factors that drive the policy process, research evidence is but one small piece and often researchers are unaware of the other contextual factors driving the process. For example, policy-makers may be aware of the evidence and want to act but be constrained by resources. Recognizing this, CIHR introduced a *Best Brains Exchange* in an attempt to deliver high-quality, timely and accessible evidence that is of immediate interest and use to senior government policy decision-makers. These one-day exchanges are driven by the needs of policy-makers and are conducted "in camera" so that a full exchange of concerns and ideas can take place. In this way policy-makers can freely explore options without feeling they are being boxed into a particular position.

The politics of partnership

There are a number of qualitative nursing researchers who do not conceptualize the policy process as one that takes place at the end of the grant once the findings are established. Rather, action is conceptualized as an integral part of the research process. This approach attempts to actively bridge the gap between science and practice. Drawing on the work of Habermas (1984), Freire (1970) and others, many nurses have underscored the importance of conducting research that is oriented to mutual understanding and change. Referred to as emancipatory enquiry, participatory action research, action science, critical research, and feminist methods, this approach is oriented to social change and praxis and are deeply political in that they are explicitly oriented to justice. At the core of this work is the need to work in partnership with community members.

In some circles, this partnered approach to research that is directed to ensuring that the knowledge is relevant to the community is known as integrated knowledge translation (iKT):

> Integrated knowledge translation is an approach to doing research that applies the principles of knowledge translation to the entire research process. The central premise of iKT is that involving knowledge users as equal partners alongside researchers will lead to research that is more relevant to and more likely to be useful to the knowledge users. Each stage in the research process is an opportunity for significant collaboration with knowledge users, including the development or refinement of the research questions, selection of the method-ology, data collection and tools development, selection of outcome measures, interpretation of the findings, crafting of the message and dissemination of the results.
>
> *(Canadian Institutes for Health Research, 2012)*

By their very nature, iKT projects seek to incorporate the expertise of knowledge users. Knowledge users will obviously be experts on their own knowledge needs, but they can also provide insight into the knowledge needs of other knowledge users in their sector.

A related model of partnership that is increasingly being used to support the use of evidence in policy and practice involves the explicit involvement of decision-makers in the research process. The rationale for this approach is that the relevance and utility of the research are assured by including decision-makers as members of the project team. Some research-funding organizations have developed programs that explicitly require the involvement of decision-makers. At CIHR, a funding program entitled "Partnership for Health System Improvement" supports teams of researchers and decision-makers interested in conducting applied and policy-relevant health systems and services research that responds to the needs of health care decision-makers and strengthens the health system.

Yet partnership in qualitative research has its own challenges. First, the funding timeline often tries the patience of the most dedicated partners. Once a partner has "signed on" to a project, the fact it is necessary to wait many months for peer review results to determine if funding is available seems unfathomable. Another timeline issue relates to the pace of research. Our partners have urgent needs, and the pace of research can be frustrating. Finally, and perhaps most importantly, it is extremely challenging to overcome the power dynamics inherent in the research process. In managing community partnerships it is difficult to overcome the power dynamics associated with competing agendas and varying levels of expertise and access to resources.

Negotiating and maintaining strong partnerships form a key element of the politics of qualitative nursing research. There are a number of principles that can be used as guideposts in this process. Key among them are the need to maintain open and frequent communication; recognize partnership takes time; and make trust and mutual respect the basis for the relationship.

The politics of qualitative research in action

Many nurses have mastered the politics of qualitative research. They have robust and thriving programs of research that are yielding important new knowledge that shapes health care policy and practice. The beginning chapters of this volume are a testament to these types of achievements. Nurses have built strong relationships with decision-makers and community members and are responding to real-world health concerns using qualitative methods. Indeed, in many research circles, nurses are seen to be in the vanguard of qualitative research. Understanding qualitative nursing research as a political endeavor enables nurses to carefully position their research as they apply for funding, understand the nuances of the peer review process, and ensure that their findings are used.

References

Baylis, F. (2012). Knowledge: The best return on investment. *The Mark*. First posted March 20, 2012. http://www.themarknews.com/articles/8299-knowledge-the-best-return-on-investment.

Benner, M., & Sandström, U. (2000). Institutionalizing the triple helix: Research funding and norms in the academic system. *Research Policy*, *29*, 291–301.

Buxton, M., & Hanney, S. (1996). How can payback from health services research be assessed? *Journal of Health Services Research and Policy*, *1*, 35–43.

Canadian Institutes for Health Research (2012). *CIHR guide to knowledge translation*. Ottawa: Canadian Institutes of Health Research.

Carey, M. A. (1997). Qualitative research in policy development. In J. M. Morse (Ed.), *Completing a qualitative project: Details and dialogue* (pp. 345–355). Thousand Oaks, CA: Sage.

Chubin, D. E., & Hackett, E. J. (1990). *Peer review and U.S. Science policy*. Albany, NY: SUNY Press.

Cohen, D. J., & Crabtree B. F. (2008). Evaluative criteria for qualitative research in health care: Controversies and recommendations. *Annals of Family Medicine*, *6*, 331–339. doi: 10.1370/afm.818.

Dey, P., & Nentwich, J. (2006). The identity politics of qualitative research: A discourse analytic inter-text. *Forum: Qualitative Social Research*, *7*(4), Art. 28. Retrieved from http://www.qualitative-research.net/index.php/fqs/article/view/173/387.

Freire, P. (1970). *Pedagogy of the oppressed*. New York: Continuum.

Government of Canada. (2007). *Mobilizing science and technology to Canada's advantage*. Ottawa: Publishing and Depository Services, Public Works and Government Services Canada.

Habermas. J. (1984). *The theory of communicative action*, Vol. 1, *Reason and rationalization of society*. Boston: Beacon.

Lavis, J. N., Wilson, M. G., Oxman, A., Lewin, S., & Fretheim, A. (2009). SUPPORT Tools for evidence-informed health Policymaking (STP) 4: Using research evidence to clarify a problem. *Health Research and Policy Systems*, *7*(Suppl. 1): S4. doi: 10.1186/1478-4505-7-S1-S4.

Leininger, M. (1994). Evaluation criteria and critique of qualitative research studies. In J. M. Morse (Ed.), *Critical issues in qualitative research methods* (pp. 95–115). Thousand Oaks, CA: Sage.

Martin, B. (1998). *Information liberation*. London: Freedom Press.

Mukherjee, S. (2010). *The emperor of all maladies: A biography of cancer*. New York: Scribner.

Panel on Return on Investment in Health Research (2009). *Making an impact: A preferred framework and indicators to measure returns on investment in health research*. Ottawa, ON: Canadian Academy of Health Sciences.

Peters, D. (2012). Research rising. *University Affairs*, *53*(1), 18–23.

Rist, R. C. (1994) Influencing the policy process with qualitative research. In N. K. Denzin & Y. S. Lincoln (Eds), *Handbook of qualitative research* (pp. 545–559). Thousand Oaks, CA: Sage.

Slow Science Academy (2010). The slow science manifesto. Retrieved from http://slow-science.org/.

Smit, B. (2003). Can qualitative research inform policy implementation? Evidence and arguments form a developing country. *Forum: Qualitative Social Research*, *4*(3), Art. 6.

Smith, R. (2006). Peer review: A flawed process at the heart of science and journal. *Journal of the Royal Society of Medicine*, *99*, 178–182. doi: 10.1258/jrsm.99.4.178.

Thorngate, W., Faregh, N., & Young, M. (2002). *Mining the archives: Analyses of CIHR research grant adjudications*. Ottawa, ON: Psychology Department, Carleton University.

Udry, J. R. (1993). The politics of sex research. *Journal of Sex Research*, *30*, 103–110.

Wooding, S., Hanney, S., Buxton, M., & Grant, J. (2005). Payback arising from research funding: Evaluation of the Arthritis Research Campaign, *Rheumatology*, *44*, 1145–1156. First published online July 27, 2005.

29

Internet qualitative research

Eun-Ok Im and Wonshik Chee

Introduction

There have been significant advances in nursing research during the past several decades, and an increasing number of nurses have been involved in research activities in some way (Havens, Stone, & Brewer, 2002). Furthermore, nurses have invested a great deal of time and effort in initiating and conducting research, including both quantitative and qualitative studies. With a recent emphasis on research funding in promotion and tenure process of the academia in general (Adderly-Kelly, 2003), nurses' research competence has become more important than ever before, and each research grant award plays an essential role in promotion and tenure process of a nurse researcher and her/his later research.

With a recent priority on innovativeness in research by major funding agencies and institutes, including the National Institutes of Health, researchers have tried to produce innovative and creative ideas in research methods, media, topics, and populations (Im & Chee, 2004). Nurse researchers have also tried to come up with and incorporate innovative research designs, recruitment strategies, delivery mechanisms of interventions, data collection procedures, and data analysis methods. Among them, one of the innovative aspects in nursing research that is arousing recent interest is the use of computer and Internet technologies in nursing research (Im, 2009).

Using computer and Internet technologies in nursing research, however, is not an easy job mainly because of non-face-to-face characteristics of the Internet as a research medium or method (McCormick, Cohen, Reed, Sparks, & Wasem, 1996). Indeed, computer and Internet technologies tend to be new in nursing research and have some methodological issues that have not been fully understood or investigated (Im & Chee, 2004). Recently, some researchers have begun to report methodological disadvantages in conducting studies using computer and Internet technologies (Hewson, Yule, Laurent, & Vogel, 2003; Mann & Stewart, 2000). However, these issues tend to focus on quantitative research methodology through the Internet, and few studies have discussed issues in Internet qualitative research. Because of paradigmatic differences between quantitative and qualitative research, the issues in conducting Internet quantitative research can be different from those in conducting Internet qualitative research (Hewson et al., 2003; Mann & Stewart, 2000). For example, in Internet quantitative research, interpersonal interactions are not as important as in Internet qualitative research. Rather, objective, neutral, and distant relationships between researchers and research participants are highly valued. Thus, a lack of interpersonal interactions is not an issue in Internet quantitative studies. However, in Internet qualitative research that emphasizes shortening the distance between researchers and research participants, a lack of interpersonal interactions could be a big challenge that needs to be overcome through various strategies.

With the recent interest in Internet qualitative studies, there is a definite need to discuss these issues which subsequently will provide researchers with some guidelines for future Internet qualitative research in nursing. In this chapter, issues in Internet qualitative research are discussed, and suggestions for future Internet qualitative research are made. First, the characteristics of Internet research are reviewed to provide background information on Internet qualitative research. Second, general types of Internet qualitative research are concisely described. Then, the method used to conduct the literature review to identify issues in Internet qualitative research in nursing is presented, and the identified issues in Internet qualitative nursing research are discussed. Finally, based on the discussions on the issues, suggestions for Internet qualitative research in nursing are made.

Characteristics of Internet research

Compared with traditional research, Internet research has its own unique characteristics that influence the relationships between researchers and research participants, and subsequently raise several issues in qualitative research (Im & Chee, 2004; Mann & Stewart, 2000). First of all, a prominent characteristic of Internet research is its non-face-to-face interactions. As mentioned above, because qualitative research usually emphasizes interactions between researchers and research participants, this unique characteristic could be problematic in most Internet qualitative research. Since research participants as well as researchers cannot see each other in person, it is difficult to establish trust between researchers and research participants. Internet interactions also make physical markers vague, and researchers cannot confirm social categories of research participants that often depend on their physical characteristics (e.g., race, ethnicity, gender) (Mann & Stewart, 2000). Subsequently, Internet research makes such markers as race, gender, status, and age inappropriate or invisible, and frequently raises a question on authenticity. However, some Internet researchers claim that the research participants' links to race, ethnicity, gender, and physical body are too strong to be undisclosed even in non-face-to-face Internet interactions (Burkhalter, 1999). They insist that the perspective or opinion of a person on racial/ethnic, socioeconomic, sexuality, and/or disability issues could show her/his identity as strongly as their physical characteristics could. Also, with recent advances in Internet interactions using cameras and microphones, these issues in Internet research could be resolved in the near future, or result in different issues that we could not envision at this point of technologies progress.

Internet research also has an issue with authenticity because many still view online space as the space that allows various fabricated roles (Johns, Hall, & Chen, 2003; O'Brien, 1999). Thus, researchers have struggled to establish ways to reliably distinguish "real authenticity" from "authentic fantasy" (Kollock & Smith, 1999; O'Brien, 1999). With advances in computer and Internet technologies, many ways to check authenticity of research participants have been developed. However, it is still difficult to differentiate authentic identities of research participants from those who fabricate, especially with an increasing number of spammers.

Researchers also point out that Internet space could be private or public depending on the characteristics and situations of the interactions occurring in the space (Kollock & Smith, 1999; Mann & Stewart, 2000). There are obvious public and private spaces that could be easily differentiated by visiting the sites. If data on identifiable private information are available and/or if its members perceive it to be private, the Internet interactions are private communication that should not be interrupted or observed. Also, if members of the Internet communities/groups perceive their Internet interactions as private, researchers need to respect that they are in a private domain. However, in reality, it is difficult for a researcher to determine if an Internet community/group is in a private or public domain because the boundary between private and public domains is frequently unclear from an outsider's perspective.

Despite recent changes in the characteristics of Internet users, Internet users still tend to be a selected sample of well-educated, literate, and articulate people who are skilled users of computers and have access to the Internet (Pew Internet & American Life Project, 2010). According to the Pew Internet Research on the Internet use (Fallows, 2005), over a half of the Internet users are female, but the online population still tends to be highly educated, predominantly white, younger participants. Thus, we can say that Internet users frequently do not represent the research populations that are targeted in nursing research. Therefore, generalizability is frequently an issue in Internet quantitative research, which is fortunately not an important issue for most of Internet qualitative research methodologies, however.

From a qualitative researcher's perspective, the Internet has at least one beneficial aspect: it provides a more immediate and prompt channel for communication between researchers and research participants. Researchers have reported that Internet users respond more promptly and that differences in time zones and geographic distance are not an issue in using the Internet (Kollock & Smith, 1999; Lakeman, 1997). Also, Internet researchers reported that research participants could more easily ask questions, get answers, and subsequently be informed (Im & Chee, 2001; Murray, 1995). Furthermore, the fact that the Internet allows both asynchronous and synchronous interactions (Kollock & Smith, 1999; Lakeman, 1997) is another beneficial aspect in Internet qualitative research. As indicated in the literature (Im & Chee, 2001), asynchronous Internet interactions can allow research participants on very different schedules or in distant time zones to participate in the study, and synchronous Internet interactions can allow research participants to communicate simultaneously, directly, and without time delay, if needed.

In the past, researchers emphasized financial cost saving in Internet research because it does not require physical travel and the expenses of paper, pencil, photocopying, and mailing fee (Frandsen, 1997; Kollock & Smith, 1999; Lakeman, 1997). However, Im and Chee (2001) pointed out a possible high cost of Internet research, including the expense for computer servers, computer software, maintenance and administrative operations for the servers, and sometimes expensive software development.

Finally, Internet research in general has unpredictable security issues as an important feature (Im & Chee, 2001; Kelly & McKenzie, 2002). Because virtually no Internet interaction is secure, Internet research frequently has an issue of intrusion by outsiders, especially when using a commercial web-hosting company to save the data collected through the Internet. For example, when a research participant registers with a website of an Internet study, the webmaster could keep track of what Internet users view or spend online, and the information can be easily passed on to third parties.

Types of Internet qualitative research

Data collection methods in general used by qualitative researchers could be roughly categorized into: (1) interviews; (2) observation; and (3) document analysis (Polit & Beck, 2008). In this chapter, Internet qualitative research methods broadly mean Internet methods that are used to collect qualitative data for interviews, observation, and document analysis. In other words, any specific types of Internet methods that are used for these three categories of data collection are considered Internet qualitative research methods. For example, emails could be used to conduct a simple structured interview, to observe group dynamics with or without interacting with the group, or to retrieve and analyze electronic documents related to specific topics. Thus, emails used for any of these three categories of data collection methods could be regarded as Internet qualitative research methods. Recently, netnography was suggested as a new branch of ethnography in marketing research (Kozinets, 2009); netnography is claimed to be ethnography on the Internet. According to Kozinets (2009), all the methods discussed above could be used for netnography if the methods are used for analyses of behavior of individuals on the Internet. Since netnography could be regarded as a type of participant observation that nurses have used in their studies, it could also be regarded as an Internet qualitative research method in nursing.

In general, there are various Internet methods that qualitative researchers could use to collect qualitative data: web-pages, online forums, email, chat groups, conferencing, focus group facilities, mailing lists, Usenet newsgroups, MU environments, multimedia environments, and search engines including Google, Yahoo!, and Bing. Web-pages contain electronic information that can be accessed through the Internet, and users can usually skip around web-pages by clicking web-links on the web-pages. Online forums are discussion sites on the Internet where Internet users can discuss specific topics through posting a series of messages. Emails are the most frequently used Internet methods. Emails refer to written documents that senders can write on the screen and electronically mail to target receivers. A chat group allows a synchronous electronic communication that participants can electronically communicate with each other simultaneously (real-time communication). Conferencing refers to asynchronous communication through which users can communicate with each other at a conference site (that is often limited only to the site). Focus group virtual facilities mean professional focus group companies and rooms through which focus groups can be conducted; these facilities recruit and screen their participants based on their databases. Mailing lists are lists of individual email addresses that can be reached by sending a single message to one designated email address. Like mailing lists, Usenet newsgroups can be reached by using one designated email address, but they are a little bit different from mailing lists because they take place only in a specific restricted computer server. MU environments refer to text-based descriptive environments with virtual environments (e.g., towns, buildings, rooms) that are similar to multimedia environments; multimedia environments have more multimedia functions (e.g., voice-based communication, video communication) than MU environments though. Search engines (e.g., Google, Yahoo!, Bing) also provide an important research method to find web-pages that contain important information that researchers want to retrieve. In this analysis, we included all the studies that used any types of Internet methods to collect qualitative data.

Methods

Through the PUBMED and CINAHL, the literature was searched using keywords of "Internet" or "online," "qualitative research," and "nursing," without a limit of time periods. A total of 274 articles were retrieved. Then, abstracts of all the retrieved articles were reviewed to identify if each article was related to Internet qualitative research. When the article was related to Internet qualitative research, the article was included in this review; a total of 44 articles were included in this review. Excluded were the articles that reported studies with a component of Internet methods, but without actual qualitative data collection through the Internet. Then, each article was reviewed in terms of issues in research process including specialty of authors, funding sources, aims and research questions, theoretical basis, study design, sample recruitment and retention, instruments, data collection procedures, data analysis process, major findings and discussion, and limitations of the studies. Then the identified issues were categorized to identify themes in the issues. The following section presents the themes of the issues identified in the analysis process. Table 29.1 summarizes a sample of ten studies that were reviewed for this chapter.

Table 29.1 Ten sample studies that were reviewed

Authors (year)	Purpose	Study design	Samples	Response and retention	Data collection methods	Internet research methods	Finding	Funding	Other issues
Adler and Zarchin (2002)	To examine a virtual focus group as an online peer support group	Focus group	7 women who at bed rest at home due to preterm labor	Not stated	Data collection through the Internet and sequential email questions for 4 weeks	Email loop (private communication system)	Three themes extracted: (a) "the effect of bed rest on participants' lives," (b) "the effect of bed rest on relationships with others," and (c) "the virtual focus group as an online peer support group."	Not stated	Selective participants (computer literate with access to home computers with Internet connections)
Beck (2004a)	To describe women's experience of birth trauma	Phenom-enology	40 mothers who had experienced birth trauma	Not stated	Data collection through the Internet or postal mail	Emails	Four themes extracted: (a) "to care for me: was that too much to ask?," (b) "to communicate with me : why was this neglected?," (c) "to provide safe care: you betrayed my trust and I felt powerless," and (d) "the end justifies the means: at whose expense?, at what price?"	Not stated	Two mothers used postal mail
Capitulo (2004)	To understand the culture of an online perinatal loss group	Ethnog-raphy	Over 447 emails from 80–87 online group members	Not stated	Participant observation using listserv and emails collected for 1 year	Listserv and emails (online support group)	A central theme of "shared metamorphosis" extracted (the women had transformed experience as the "mommy of an angel").	The AWHONN-Philips Medical Systems	Not stated

Author	Aim	Design	Sample	Response/Retention	Data collection	Intervention/tool	Findings	Funding	Limitations
Coulson et al. (2007)	To examine social support provided in messages posted in an online support group for Huntington Disease	Content analysis	1313 messages from online Huntington Disease bulletin board	N/A	All messages posted for 21 months	Bulletin board (online support group)	Five types of social support indentified: (a) informational support (56.2%), (b) emotional support (51.9%), (c) network support (48.4%), (d) esteem support (21.7%), and (e) tangible assistance (9.8%).	Not stated	Posted messages remained supportive in the manner they were intended
Davis et al. (2010)	To explore the research experience of using the Internet to conduct one-to-one online interviews about HIV risk	Triangu-lation	128 gay/bisexual men living in London	Not stated	Self-administered questionnaire on the Internet, online interviews and face-to-face interviews	Internet survey and private chatrooms	Online interviews emerge as a form of textual performances.	Medical Research Council	Not stated
Kenny (2005)	To explore engagement and group interaction in an online environment	Focus group study	38 nurses enrolled in a conversion program in a rural university	Retention rates: 95%	All posted messages and discussions using educational courseware for 2 months	Newly developed web-based program	Benefits of the online focus group (cost saving and convenience).	Not stated	Limited by computer access
Koch et al. (2009)	To explore the usages and perceptions of the benefit and value of a web-based intervention.	One-group post-test-only design	123 first year BSN students	Response rate: 22%	Web-based closed-ended questions and open-ended questions	Web-based intervention to support learning	Quantitative: 81% of participants perceived that the web-based activities enhanced their learning Qualitative: three themes extracted: (a) "enhances	Not stated	Despite the high value of interactive, multimedia learning, students did

Table 29.1 Continued

Authors (year)	Purpose	Study design	Samples	Response and retention	Data collection methods	Internet research methods	Finding	Funding	Other issues
							my learning," (b) "study at my own pace," and (c) "about the activities."		not want to completely abandon traditional learning
Mathew et al. (2008)	To explore the experience of Antiphospholipid Syndrome (APS) perinatal loss	Phenomenological study	38 women who experienced perinatal loss	Not stated	Email interviews for 4 months	In-depth, semi-structured email interviews	Two themes extracted: (a) "existence in bewilderment" and (b) "persistence in the quest for knowledge and information."	No funding	Women's visual cues could not be captured
Nahm et al. (2009)	To explore the influences of a web program on health behaviors	Exploratory qualitative study	116 older adults	Retention Rates: 77%	Four discussion forums (moderator-mediated)	The discussion board (online forum)	Three themes extracted: (a) "sharing current health behavior," (b) "having started or planned to start," and (c) "recognition of opportunity for improvement."	National Institute on Aging	Selective participants (with high levels of education and online experience)
Valaitis (2005)	To explore the use and perceptions of computers and the Internet as tools to support them among young students	Qualitative case study	19 students in grades seven and eight	Retention rates: 83%	Observations, field notes, youth interviews, facilitator interviews, and online surveys over 12 weeks	Computer-mediated communication	Four themes extracted: (a) "reduced social risk factors," (b) "increased community participation," (c) "increased opportunity for reflection," and (d) "increased recourses."	Social Sciences and Humanities Research Council	Online communication increased the feeling of powerlessness

Issues in Internet qualitative research

The issues in Internet qualitative research that were identified in this review included: (1) combined multiple methods; (2) specific specialty-related; (3) funding; (4) lack of theoretical bases; (5) lack of responses, low retention rates, and possible selection bias; and (6) lack of theoretical saturation. Each issue is discussed in detail as follows.

Combined multiple methods

Researchers tend to use multiple methods in one study: (1) both quantitative and qualitative methods; (2) both traditional and Internet methods; and (3) multiple qualitative methods. Many of the reviewed studies combined a qualitative research method with a quantitative research method rather than using a qualitative method only. Also, many of the articles combined traditional research method(s) and Internet research method(s). For example, Elford, Bolding, Davis, Sherr, and Hart (2004) used face-to-face or online interviews to consider if the Internet provides a new sexual risk environment for gay and bisexual men in London. In the same study, they have also used quantitative research method (online questionnaires) to provide comprehensive data for their research questions. Capitulo (2004) used multiple methods including online participant observation, a review of 447 emails, and participants' feedback on the study findings to explore the culture of an online perinatal loss group. Buckley and Toto (2001) combined multiple quantitative and qualitative methods including observations, surveys, tests, in-class discussions, and email communication analysis to explore how students learn in online learning environment. Considering that Internet research methods have not been fully developed yet, it would be natural for researchers to combine multiple methods in order to increase the rigor of the studies.

The major Internet methods used in Internet qualitative nursing research included online forums (discussion boards), Internet survey with open-ended questions, and online observations through Internet communities/groups. Among the reviewed articles, 17 studies used online forums (discussion boards), and 15 studies used emails and listservs. Three studies used private chat rooms (Blomberg et al., 2011; Davis, Bolding, Hart, Sherr, & Elford, 2010; Nolan et al., 2006), one used online observations (Capitulo, 2004), and another used observation, field notes, interviews, and an online survey (Valaitis, 2005). Also, the most frequently used qualitative data analysis methods were content analysis and thematic analysis. Only one ethnographical study (Capitulo, 2004), one grounded theory study (Green & Kodish, 2009), and six phenomenological studies (Beck, 2004a, 2004b, 2006; Beck & Watson, 2008, 2010; Mathew, Cesario, & Symes, 2008) were identified during the review. Also, except for two studies (Davis et al., 2010; Kenny, 2005), all studies reported themes as their findings regardless of their research methods. Considering the limitations of current Internet methods used to conduct a qualitative study, this small range of qualitative research methods and data analysis methods used in Internet qualitative research in nursing could be judged as reasonable.

Specific specialty-related

Nine of the retrieved articles were related to the specialty areas of oncology, and 19 articles were related to women's health (maternal or mid-life women's health issues). One article was related to HIV among gay/bisexual men living in London (Davis et al., 2010). Four retrieved articles were related to nursing education (Chen, Stocker, Wang, Chung, & Chen, 2009; Koch, Andrew, Salamonson, Everett, & Davidson, 2010; Sitzman & Leners, 2006; Oldenburg & Hung, 2009), and one article was related to community health, especially school health (Valaitis, 2005). This agrees with current trends in Internet qualitative research in general; Internet qualitative research has been reported to be effective in investigations on stigmatized conditions such as psychiatric diseases, HIV, infectious diseases, rare diseases, genetic diseases, and cancer (Miller & Sønderlund, 2010). Interestingly, only one of the reviewed articles was related to geriatric nursing (Nahm, Resnick, DeGrezia, & Brotemarkle, 2009), which may reflect age compositions of the Internet populations.

Funding

Nineteen retrieved articles (43%) reported a specific source of funding, and the major funding source was the National Institutes of Health. Even when considering differences in the calculation methods of funding rates in various funding agencies, this funding rate of Internet qualitative studies tends to be high; the general funding rate of the National Institutes of Health (NIH) was around 20% during the past ten years (NIH, 2011). Although there is the possibility that funded studies could be more likely to be published than those of non-funded studies, the innovative nature of Internet research could be a major reason for this finding. Indeed, the innovativeness of Internet research has frequently been pointed out as a strength of Internet studies, and the innovativeness could help result in successful funding because of a high funding priority on innovative studies. However, in reality, the use of the Internet can be sometimes viewed as a methodological major flaw because the Internet has been inadequately tested and evaluated as a research method/setting, and very few reviewers of funding agencies are experts in Internet research. Subsequently, reviewers can have stereotypes of Internet research (e.g., inherent selection bias) and limited knowledge of computer and Internet technologies. However, this finding may indicate that Internet research could be still attractive to many reviewers and funders because of its inherent innovativeness although the innovativeness could possibly diminish with an increasing usage of Internet research methods in nursing studies.

Lack of theoretical bases

Among the reviewed articles, 25 studies (57%) did not state the theoretical basis of their studies. Considering that specific qualitative research methods (e.g., grounded theory methods) do not require a theoretical basis to support their studies, this tends to be reasonable. Also, because Internet research itself tends to be new in the literature, there could be very few theoretical bases that could guide research phenomena occurring on the Internet. Indeed, even the studies that identified their theoretical bases tended to use traditional and/or conventional theoretical bases that have been used in qualitative research in general, rather than using a specific theoretical model/theory that aims at research phenomena on the Internet. The theoretical bases used in the reviewed studies included: feminism (East, Jackson, Peters, & O'Brien, 2009; East, Jackson, O'Brien, & Peters, 2011; Im et al., 2010a; Im, Lee, & Chee, 2010b; Im, Lee, Chee, Stuifbergen, & eMAPA Research Team, 2011), social cognitive theory (Nahm et al., 2009), Colazzi existential phenomenology (Beck, 2004a, 2004b, 2006; Beck & Watson, 2008, 2010), Friedemann's framework of systemic organization (Pierce, Seiner, Havens, & Tormoehlen, 2008), problem-based learning and the community of inquiry model (Oldendurg & Hung, 2009), and the information seeking process model (Legan, Sinclair, & Kernohan, 2011).

Lack of responses, low retention rates, and selective research participants

Twenty-five studies (57%) did not specify the response or retention rates. Only seven studies reported the response rate (Beck, 2006; Beck & Watson, 2008; Koch et al., 2009; Mackert, Stanforth, & Garcia, 2011; McClement, Fallis & Pereira, 2009; Parmelee, Bowen, Ross, Brown, & Huff, 2009; Sitzman & Leners, 2006), which ranged from 18.3% (Mackert et al., 2011) to 84.6% (Sitzman & Leners, 2006). Considering the low response rates reported in the literature on Internet research in general (Im & Chee, 2004), this response rate tends to be moderate. The retention rates reported in the remaining articles ranged from 44% to 95%. The highest retention rate (95%) was reported among nurses in Australia (Kenny, 2005), and the lowest retention rate was reported among Hispanic mid-life women in the US (Im et al., 2009). Considering general low retention rates even in studies using traditional research methods among ethnic minorities (Gilliss et al., 2001), these retention rates could also be considered moderate.

A frequently reported issue in Internet quantitative research is potential selection bias although recent statistical surveys on Internet users indicated changing demographics of Internet users (Pew Internet & American Life Project, 2010). In the Internet qualitative studies that we reviewed, selectiveness of research participants was also frequently reported. Im et al. (2010b) reported that the participants of their study were highly educated with high income. Nahm et al. (2009) also reported that their participants tended to be highly educated and have online experience. Kenny (2005) highlighted that computer access was a limiting factor in their study among nurses, and Adler and Zarchin (2002) also indicated that their participants tended to be computer-literate and have access to home computers with Internet connections. In Internet quantitative studies, the selection bias could be viewed as a major methodological flaw. However, in Internet qualitative research, this could be considered an important source of knowledge. Also, some Internet researchers claim that the potential bias will not be an issue even in Internet quantitative studies in the near future because of the changing demographics of Internet users (Im & Chee, 2001).

Lack of theoretical saturation

One of the important issues in Internet qualitative research is lack of theoretical saturation (Im & Chee, 2006). When synchronous interactions are used in data collection, this cannot be a significant issue because the interactions could be as prompt as in face-to-face interactions. However, when using asynchronous interactions in data collection, lack of theoretical saturation was reported as a major issue in Internet qualitative research because researchers could not promptly respond to research participants and/or get research participants' prompt responses or visual cues (Im et al., 2010a, 2011; Mathew et al., 2008). As mentioned above, the most frequently used data analysis methods in the reviewed studies were content analysis and thematic analysis, which do not require theoretical saturation. In other words, none of the reviewed studies used a qualitative research method that requires theoretical saturation. Also, none of the studies showed evidence to support that theoretical saturation was obtained in their studies.

Recommendations for future Internet qualitative research in nursing

Our literature review on Internet qualitative research in nursing indicated that many of the studies used combined multiple research methods; the studies tended to be limited to specific specialties; the studies tended to be highly funded; the studies lacked supporting theoretical bases; the studies tended to have low response and retention rates and selective research participants; and there existed no evidence of obtaining theoretical saturation in the studies. Based on the findings, we want to conclude this chapter with the following recommendations for future Internet qualitative research in nursing.

First of all, we suggest researchers continue to experiment with multiple methods of Internet qualitative research. As our review indicated, researchers actually combined multiple methods with a component of Internet qualitative research methods to investigate their research phenomena. Because the Internet research methods are still in their infancy, the trials with multiple qualitative methods are essential to further develop Internet qualitative research methodology. Until Internet qualitative research methods are refined and sophisticated with more trials and with advances in new computer and Internet technologies, researchers need to continue their efforts to experiment with new multiple methods.

Second, we suggest researchers use the unique characteristic of the Internet research that works well with people with stigmatized conditions, and incorporate this characteristic in their choices of research areas, study populations, and study designs. With the use of Internet research methods in diverse groups of research participants and in various areas of research phenomenon, the Internet research methods could be further developed and refined.

Third, researchers need to further develop theoretical bases that can guide studies on research phenomena occurring on the Internet. As the findings of the review indicated, there are few theoretical bases that can guide researchers to study research phenomena occurring on the Internet. Without proper and adequate guidance of theoretical bases, Internet qualitative research cannot be advanced with a concrete ground/basis.

Fourth, as discussed above, with a recent emphasis on innovation in research funding, the funding rate of Internet qualitative research tends to be high. As discussed above, in terms of the innovation criteria, Internet studies have high potential, but Internet studies can be low scoring in terms of other criteria such as low response rate, feasibility issues, and selectiveness of research participants. We suggest researchers develop creative strategies that could overcome the low response rate, feasibility issues, and selection bias while strengthening the innovative usage of the Internet in their qualitative studies. For example, researchers could adopt recruitment and retention strategies through both Internet and community settings to increase the response rate of potential and/or actual participants and to strengthen the feasibility of the recruitment and retention process.

Finally, researchers need to be creative to increase theoretical saturation through multiple methods. As discussed above, theoretical saturation could be difficult for most Internet qualitative studies because of asynchronous interactions during their data collection process. Thus, as mentioned earlier, adding synchronous interactions (e.g., chat groups) would be a way to increase theoretical saturation during the data collection process. Also, using specific email notification functions could possibly increase theoretical saturation in Internet qualitative research by alerting and motivating research participants to respond to the researchers' questions that aim to get in-depth data for theoretical saturation.

References

Adderly-Kelly, B. (2003). Promoting the scholarship of research for faculty and students. *Association of Black Nursing Faculty Journal, 14*(2), 41–44.

Adler, C. L., & Zarchin, Y. R. (2002). The "virtual focus group": Using the Internet to reach pregnant women on home bed rest. *Journal of Obstetric, Gynecologic, & Neonatal Nursing, 31*(4), 418–427.

Beck, C. T. (2004a). Birth trauma: In the eye of the beholder. *Nursing Research, 53*(1), 28–35.

Beck, C. T. (2004b). Post-traumatic stress disorder due to childbirth: The aftermath. *Nursing Research, 53*(4), 216–224.

Beck, C. T. (2006). The anniversary of birth trauma: Failure to rescue. *Nursing Research*, *55*(6), 381–390.

Beck, C. T., & Watson, S. (2008). Impact of birth trauma on breast-feeding. *Nursing Research*, *57*(4), 228–236.

Beck, C. T., & Watson, S. (2010). Subsequent childbirth after a previous traumatic birth. *Nursing Research*, *59*(4), 241–249.

Blomberg, K., Tishelman, C., Ternestedt, B. M., Törnberg, S., Levál, A., & Widmark, C. (2011). How can young women be encouraged to attend cervical cancer screening? Suggestions from face-to-face and Internet focus group discussions with 30-year-old women in Stockholm, Sweden. *Acta oncologica*, *50*(1), 112–120.

Buckley, J., & Toto, R. (2001). Assessment techniques for web-based instruction: Lessons learned from teaching a graduate course in instructional technology. *Seminars in Perioperative Nursing*, *10*(2), 97–103.

Burkhalter, B. (1999). Reading race online: discovering racial identity in Usenet discussions. In M. A. Smith & P. Kollock (Eds.), *Communities in cyberspace* (pp. 60–75). London: Routledge.

Capitulo, K. L. (2004). Perinatal grief online. *MCN: The American Journal of Maternal Child Nursing*, *29*(5), 305–311.

Chen, S. W., Stocker, J., Wang, R. H., Chung, Y. C., & Chen, M. F. (2009). Evaluation of self-regulatory online learning in a blended course for post-registration nursing students in Taiwan. *Nurse Education Today*, *29*(7), 704–709.

Coulson, N. S., Buchanan, H., & Aubeeluck, A. (2007). Social support in cyberspace: A content analysis of communication within a Huntington's disease online support group. *Patient Education and Counseling*, *68*(2), 173–178.

Davis, M., Boldling, G., Hart, G., Sherr, L., & Elford, J. (2010). Reflecting on the experience of interviewing online: Perspectives from the Internet and HIV study in London. *AIDS Care*, *16*(8), 944–952.

East, L., Jackson, D., O'Brien, L., & Peters, K. J. (2011). Condom negotiation: Experiences of sexually active young women. *Advances in Nursing Science*, *67*(1), 77–85.

East, L., Jackson, D., Peters, K., & O'Brien, L. (2009). Disrupted sense of self: Young women and sexually transmitted infections. *Journal of Clinical Nursing*, *19*(13–14), 1995–2003.

Elford, J., Bolding, G., Davis, M., Sherr, L., & Hart, G. (2004). The Internet and HIV study: Design and methods. *BMC Public Health*, *4*, 39.

Fallows, D. (2005). *How women and men use the Internet.* Retrieved on November 10, 2011 from http:// www.pewtrusts.org/uploadedFiles/wwwpewtrustsorg/Reports/Society_and_the_Internet/PIP_ Women_Men_122805.pdf.

Frandsen, J. L. (1997). The use of computers in cancer pain management. *Seminars in Oncology Nursing*, *13*, 49–56.

Gilliss, C. L., Lee, K., Gutierrez, Y., Taylor, D., Beyene, Y., Neuhaus, J., et al. (2001). Recruitment and retention of healthy minority women into community-based longitudinal research. *Journal of Women's Health & Gender-Based Medicine*, *10*(1), 77–85.

Green, R., & Kodish, S. (2009). Discussing a sensitive topic: Nurse practitioners' and physician assistants' communication strategies in managing patients with erectile dysfunction. *Journal of the American Academy of Nurse Practitioners*, *21*(12), 698–705.

Havens, D. S., Stone, P., & Brewer, C. S. (2002). Nursing and health services research: Building capacity and seizing opportunity. *Applied Nursing Research*, *15*(4), 261–263.

Hewson, C., Yule, P., Laurent, D., & Vogel, C. (2003). *Internet research methods: A practical guide for the social and behavioural sciences.* London: Sage.

Im, E. O. (2009). Computer technologies in nursing research: Editorial. *Nursing Research*, *58*(4), 227.

Im, E. O., & Chee, W. (2001). A feminist critique on the use of the Internet in nursing research. *Advances in Nursing Science*, *23*(4), 67–82.

Im, E. O., & Chee, W. (2004). Obtaining grants for Internet-based research projects. In J. J. Fitzpatrick & K. S. Montgomery (Eds.), *Internet for nursing research: A guide to strategies, skills, and resources.* New York: Springer.

Im, E. O., & Chee, W. (2006). An online forum as a qualitative research method: Practical issues. *Nursing Research*, *55*(4), 267–273.

Im, E. O., Lee, S. H., & Chee, W. (2010a). Black women in menopausal transition. *Journal of Obstetric, Gynecologic, & Neonatal Nursing*, *39*(4), 435–443.

Im, E. O., Lee, B., Chee, W., Stuifbergen, A., and eMAPA research team. (2011). Attitudes toward physical activity of white midlife women. *Journal of Obstetric, Gynecologic, & Neonatal Nursing*, *40*(3), 312–321.

Im, E. O., Lee, B., Hwang, H., Yoo, K. H., Chee, W., Stuifbergen, A., Walker, L., Brown, A., McPeek, C., Miro, M., & Chee, E. (2010b). "A waste of time": Hispanic women's attitudes toward physical activity. *Women and Health*, *50*(6), 563–579.

Im, E. O., Lim, H. J., Lee, S. H., Dormire, S., Chee, W., & Kresta, K. (2009). Menopausal symptom experience of Hispanic midlife women in the United States. *Health Care for Women International*, *30*(10), 919–934.

Johns, M. D., Hall, G. J., & Chen, S. S. (2003). *Online social research: Methods, issues, & ethics*. New York: Peter Lang Publishing.

Kelly, G., & McKenzie, B. (2002). Security, privacy, and confidentiality issues on the Internet. *Journal of Medical Internet Research*, *4*(2), e12.

Kenny, A. J. (2005). Interaction in cyberspace: An online focus group. *Journal of Advanced Nursing*, *49*(4), 414–422.

Koch, J., Andrew, S., Salamonson, Y., Everett, B., & Davidson, P. M. (2010). Nursing students' perception of a Web-based intervention to support learning. *Nurse Education Today*, *30*(6), 584–590.

Kollock, P. & Smith, M. A. (1999). Communities in cyberspace. In M. A. Smith & K. Peter (Eds.), *Communities in cyberspace*. London: Routledge.

Kozinets, R. V. (2009). *Netnography: Doing ethnographic research online*. London: Sage.

Lakeman, R. (1997). Using the Internet for data collection in nursing research. *Computers in Nursing*, *15*, 269–275.

Legan, B. M., Sinclair, M., & Kernohan, W. G. (2011). What is the impact of the Internet on decision-making in pregnancy? A global study. *Birth*, *38*(4), 336–345.

Mackert, M., Stanforth, D., & Garcia, A.A. (2011). Undermining of nutrition and exercise decisions: Experiencing negative social influence. *Public Health Nursing*, *28*(5), 402–410.

Mann, C., & Stewart, F. (2000). *Internet communication and qualitative research: A handbook for researching online*. London: Sage.

Mathew, S., Cesario, S., & Symes, L. (2008). Explaining "unexplained" perinatal loss: Experiences of women with antiphospholipid syndrome. *Journal of Perinatal and Neonatal Nursing*, *22*(4), 293–301.

McClement, S. E., Fallis, W. M., & Pereira, A. (2009). Family presence during resuscitation: Canadian critical care nurses' perspectives. *Journal of Nursing Scholarship*, *41*, 233–240.

McCormick, K. A., Cohen, E., Reed, M., Sparks, S., & Wasem, C. (1996). Funding nursing informatics activities: Internet access to announcements of government funding. *Computers in Nursing*, *14*(6), 315–322.

Miller, P. G., & Sønderlund, A. L. (2010). Using the Internet to research hidden populations of illicit drug users: A review. *Addiction*, *105*(9), 1557–1567.

Murray, P. J. (1995). Using the Internet for gathering data and conducting research: Faster than the mail and cheaper than the phone. *Computers in Nursing*, *13*, 206, 208–209.

Nahm, E. S., Resnick, B., DeGrezia, M., & Brotemarkle, R. (2009). Use of discussion boards in a theory-based health web site for older adults. *Nursing Research*, *58*(6), 419–426.

National Institutes of Health, Office of Extramural Research. (2011). *Paylines, percentiles and success rates*. Retrieved on November 10, 2011 from http://nexus.od.nih.gov/all/2011/02/15/paylines-percentiles-success-rates/.

Nolan, M. T., Hodgin, M. B., Olsen, S. J., Coleman, J., Sauter, P. K., et al. (2006). Spiritual issues of family members in a pancreatic cancer chat room. *Oncology Nursing Forum*, *33*(2), 239–244.

O'Brien, J. (1999). Writing in the body: Gender (re)production in online interaction. In M. A. Smith & K. Peter (Eds.), *Communities in cyberspace*. London: Routledge.

Oldenburg, N. L., & Hung, W. C. (2009). Problem solving strategies used by RN-to-BSN students in an online problem-based learning course. *Journal of Nursing Education*, *49*(4), 219–222.

Parmelee, P. A., Bowen, S. E., Ross, A., Brown, H., & Huff, J. (2009). Sometimes people don't fit in boxes: Attitudes toward the minimum data set among clinical leadership in VA nursing homes. *Journal of the American Medical Directors Association*, *10*(2), 98–106.

Pew Internet & American Life Project. (2010). *Pew studies Internet use and income levels*. Retrieved on November 17, 2011 from http://www.pewinternet.org/Media-Mentions/2010/Pew-Studies-Internet-Use-And-Income-Levels.aspx.

Pierce, L. L., Steiner, V., Havens, H., & Tormoehlen, K. (2008). Spirituality expressed by caregivers of stroke survivors. *Western Journal of Nursing Research*, *30*(5), 606–619.

Polit, D. F., & Beck, C. T. (2008). *Nursing research: Generating and assessing evidence for nursing practice* (8th ed.). Philadelphia, PA: Lippincott.

Sitzman, K., & Leners, D. W. (2006). Student perceptions of caring in online baccalaureate education. *Nursing Education Perspectives*, *27*(5), 254–259.

Valaitis, R. K. (2005). Computers and the Internet: Tools for youth empowerment. *Journal of Medical Internet Research*, *7*(5), e51.

30

Secondary qualitative data analysis

Sally Thorne

The allure of available data

All qualitative researchers appreciate the significant investments of time and resources that go into the creation of a typical qualitative data set. In the case of clinical qualitative studies, researchers also feel a commitment to the patients (caregivers, family members) who have committed their time and shared their experiences in the hopes that what they have lived through, rendered into an evidentiary format, may help in some way to ease the struggle of future patients. These practical and existential obligations have featured strongly in sparking an interest among nurse researchers to ensure that their hard-earned qualitative data is used to best advantage to advance the knowledge that supports the discipline in doing its work well. The appeal of fully capitalizing on all that a data set can offer has attracted lively methodological theorizing as well as considerable dialogue and debate (Sandelowski, 1997), all of which can inform nurses considering secondary approaches to their qualitative inquiries today. This chapter will describe secondary qualitative analysis as it is applied within nursing today.

History and tradition in the qualitative nursing research context

The history of secondary analysis as a legitimate qualitative inquiry form in nursing is actually relatively recent. When I first began writing about the approach (Thorne, 1994, 1998), there was limited available literature to draw upon (Lobo, 1986; McArt & McDougal, 1985; Woods, 1988), and what existed was primarily encouraging exploration of the possibilities, rather than providing guidance as to a rigorous methodological approach (Heaton, 2008). The notion of secondary analysis had been applied across the spectrum of methodological options wherever data may have subsequent purposes, and there had been a strong tradition of secondary statistical work. However, in the social science and qualitative health research fields, secondary approaches had primarily been used to describe a form of deductive analysis of subsidiary research questions within a program of research (Heaton, 1998, 2004). What nursing took up in a different way was a thoughtful consideration of the feasibility of inductively oriented and interpretive approaches to the analysis of textual data that had been generated for the explicit purposes of various kinds of original qualitative inquiries. In that this was still an era in which nursing scholars working within the qualitative modalities were highly self-conscious about challenges to the

393

integrity of their research methods (Sandelowski, 1986, 1993a), these early nursing contributions to the field (Hinds, Vogel, & Clarke-Steffen, 1997; Szabo & Strang, 1997) focused their attention on how we might work out the ethical, theoretical and methodological challenges toward a credible alternative form of qualitative inquiry. Since that time, although enthusiasm for exploiting extant qualitative databases to best capacity has attracted considerable attention across a wide range of disciplines, a coherent body of methodological guidance is just beginning to emerge (Gladstone, Volpe, & Boydell, 2007; Long-Sutehall, Sque, & Addington-Hall, 2011).

Overt and covert secondary analysis in qualitative nursing research

As Heaton (2004) points out, work that might be considered a form of qualitative secondary data analysis has been undertaken since at least the 1960s when Barney Glaser introduced the possibility of extending secondary analysis from quantitative to qualitative data (Glaser, 1962, 1963). However, having conducted a systematic review of all published qualitative secondary studies that was as comprehensive as possible under the circumstances in 2000 (Heaton, 2000), Heaton considered it to have remained "ill defined and underdeveloped as a qualitative methodology" for at least three decades (2004, p. v). Although some authors explicitly referenced their work as "secondary analysis," others used terms such as "*post hoc* analysis," "re-analysis" or "retrospective latent content analysis" to indicate the secondary nature of their analyses (p. 36). Most of these studies were conducted by researchers with direct knowledge of the databases, and drew upon a single data set. Heaton theorized that spectacular challenges to the original interpretations of scholars whose data were accessible for secondary review, such as Freeman's deconstruction of Margaret Mead's original Samoan data (Freeman, 1983), may have raised serious questions associated with truth claims in social theorizing and generated lively debates around the ethics of data sharing. More worrisome to Heaton was evidence of the existence of a subterranean layer of published research reports in which, although the methodological descriptions claimed the use of a primary approach, features of the samples or data sets across multiple publications suggested otherwise. This unreported form of secondary analysis, which becomes obvious to anyone conducting an in-depth review of these bodies of work, raises significant questions with regard to the integrity of the various methodological claims being made. For example, to position a research report as having faithfully been developed using the tenets of phenomenological methodology throughout would signal certain design assumptions and decisions that ought to preclude a second publication using the same database with the same study sample claiming a similarly faithful adherence to grounded theory. Thus, one of the key reasons to advance a solid body of methodological direction for secondary analysis as a distinct enterprise is to ensure that researchers have ample access to guidance that will ensure the integrity and credibility of their analytic processes and products.

Issues in the consideration of a secondary approach

As the secondary analysis methodological field has evolved in the qualitative context, it has become evident that there are significant issues to be wrestled through and worked out before the viability of a project can be assured. These pertain to various aspects of the available data set(s) as well as the kinds of claims that one hopes to be able to make on the basis of having reconsidered them.

Nature of existing data

In the conventional sense, it is important to distinguish naturalistic from non-naturalistic data. Naturalistic data, or data that exist outside of the research context but may be amenable to inductive forms of inquiry, are familiar to historians and documentary analysts in the social sciences. In the nursing research context, these might take the form of chart records, diaries, essays, photographs or autobiographies that pertain to certain health-related experiences and that might be available for analysis to discern various patterns or insights. Non-naturalistic data, in contrast, reveals the handprint of the researcher who has played a role in co-creating it. It has been shaped by the researcher in both overt ways (such as through the asking of certain questions and not others) and ways that are more covert and difficult to articulate (such as through the assumptive base that went into determining that a study was worth doing in the first place). Further complicating this issue is the reality that data forms can be either naturalistic or non-naturalistic (such as diaries generated spontaneously and those prompted by a researcher request), and analyses can be either primary or secondary (one author may explicitly tap a documentary source as a primary database for an inductive inquiry while another may capitalize upon it as a component of a secondary study).

Some key considerations in determining whether available data might be suitable for a secondary analysis are the fit between the data and the new question and the methods by which the original data set were constructed. Generally the greater the distance from the original question, the more problematic the secondary analysis will become. While such distance might not preclude all possibilities, it should increase the standard that the investigator will have to reach in order to convince a critical audience that the secondary results are a fair and reasonable interpretation of a phenomenon that is now significantly detached from its source.

Understanding the impact of the original methodological orientation is also necessary. Depending on the design of an interview, for example, certain themes may or may not have been prompted, explored, clarified or expanded, and therefore interpretations dependent on the qualitative equivalent of intensity or frequency of thematic material can be seriously confounded by misinterpretations of the design and implementation of the data collection process. And since we know that aspects of the form and substance of a qualitative study may be idiosyncratic to each individual researcher, team or study, assumptions based on general methodological claims by the original researcher may be somewhat misleading. Overall, understanding the implications of these important distinctions draws attention to the imperative that the secondary analyst has a deep and nuanced understanding of the nature of the data in the fullest sense—not only that it includes a certain volume of text pertaining to a particular health phenomenon, but the motivations and machinations that went into the generation of the text, a defensible position on what it likely privileges and what it obscures because of those elements, and an auditable and logical argument for how that text constitutes a legitimate and reasonable data source for the answering of the specific new question at hand.

Ethical and legal considerations

Among the most widely contested issues in qualitative secondary analysis is the recognition that it is fraught with ethical and legal complications that must be worked out in order to ensure the integrity of the process and product. First, and most obvious, is the issue of informed consent, or whether consent for reuse of data can be truly "informed" (Bishop, 2009). For the most part, the specific questions that lend themselves to the secondary study will not have revealed themselves prior to the development of the initial research. Thus, even with an explicit proviso embedded in an informed consent document that will permit secondary analysis into the future, it will be important to consider the range and scope of what that general consent can legitimately imply. If I have agreed to be interviewed for a study on how I construct hope in the presence of a serious illness, for example, have I implicitly agreed that my material could be used to demonstrate the inaccuracy with which patients estimate the probability of cure? While there may be conceptual similarities between two inquiry thrusts, and while a database may contain information pertinent to a second question, we still require an ethical framework to ensure that data are not collected for knowledge development in directions that the original participants would not have agreed to. Rather, there is a general acceptance that secondary studies toward somewhat similar motivations and reflective of refinements that advance as the science evolves are fine. Having one's data used in ways that feel manipulative or misleading would not. And yet this distinction becomes a very fine line, in most cases not subject to the kind of scrutiny that is enacted at the outset of an original study using human subjects.

Another ethical matter is confidentiality. While most qualitative researchers have a fairly sophisticated understanding of which kinds of data could potentially identify and/or create vulnerabilities for individuals or contexts, there may be an essential layer of insight and sensitivity lost when the data are reviewed by someone less intimately familiar with context. I know one nurse researcher who studied a particular immigrant group for many years, never including in her written reports what group members openly and frequently acknowledged as widespread community bending of certain legal requirements, as it was not relevant to her focus. A subsequent analyst might intentionally or unintentionally violate an implicit shared understanding of boundaries that had clearly characterized the earlier work.

As has been noted by colleagues in sociology (Hammersley, 2009; Parry & Mauthner, 2005) and anthropology (Manderson, Kelaher, & Woelz-Stirling, 2001), an expanding set of legal and ethical complexities is emerging in the consideration of data sharing, as qualitatively derived bodies of material become increasingly available within data archiving services. Although this issue seems not to have influenced nursing to any significant degree to this point, it likely looms on the horizon, presenting numerous technical and practical challenges, fueling polarities between enthusiasts and skeptics, and potentially raising the bar on what constitutes qualitative inquiry once large data sets and sample sizes become theoretically viable (Bishop, 2009).

Matters of voice and representation

Beyond these contextual and ethical sorts of issues, the limitations inherent in the secondary analytic study also include a number of intellectual and interpretive hazards that may jeopardize the quality of the study outcomes. As Sandelowski once pointed out, all interpretation, including scientific explanation, involves a certain degree of fabrication (Sandelowski, 1991, p. 165). The degree to which this fabrication can become problematic certainly increases when the rigorous grounding required to convincingly justify an original study becomes less onerous in the secondary situation. In other words, the fairly significant intellectual hurdles one must overcome to obtain both funding and ethical approval for an original piece of research do serve as something of a safeguard to the integrity of the reasoning. In the secondary study, which may not actually require separate ethical approval or funding, external scrutiny may not occur until the findings are considered for publication or presented to scholarly audiences. Thus, it makes sense that a high standard of credibility in the accounting for all aspects of the work ought to be an unequivocal expectation in the qualitative secondary analysis context.

Another set of complications arises when we consider matters of representation. In particular, we know that errors of interpretation on the basis of artifacts of frequency within smaller samples are not at all uncommon in qualitative health research (Thorne & Darbyshire, 2005). Secondary work deriving from data sets that may exaggerate or distort certain features of a phenomenon increase the likelihood of replicating and further complicating these misinterpretations or entrenching erroneous conclusions. A related issue is the matter of voice. Despite occasional lapses in the qualitative literature into the rhetorical claim that study participants "speak for themselves," the very nature of the research act is to render something that exists in its natural state into something that becomes a knowledge product (Alcoff, 2009). Thus, the risks of misappropriating voice through representing it in the form of research findings become more acute in the secondary context. For example, because the collective consciousness of a group may change as a result of such factors as a research process or a shifting sociopolitical context, interpretations that might have been acceptable to group members in the moment may no longer be acceptable in the fullness of time. Thus, what one appears to be saying on behalf of a particular kind of patient or situation may become increasingly problematic given time and distance beyond the original inquiry.

Despite these very real and important risks and limitations, secondary qualitative analysis still holds tremendous promise to the scholar seeking to do justice to the investments of original inquiries and to follow the logical threads of an investigative process. An emphasis on the complexities becomes helpful in ensuring that this kind of study is not taken lightly as a convenient and relatively effortless means by which to produce and publish a piece of research, but rather is understood as a highly complicated and necessarily rigorous enterprise that adds value to the extent that it is done well. And therefore a healthy respect for its perils becomes paramount.

Secondary research approaches

Despite considerable methodological work since the 1990s, the field has not coalesced around any dominant approach to secondary analysis in the qualitative spectrum, and the term continues to refer to a fairly wide array of study forms. In the style of an inductive analyst, I generated five categorical groupings to depict the various overall approaches within the field (Thorne, 1994) that still seem relevant today. A brief description of these approaches will set the stage for a more fulsome examination of the methodological opportunities that have been taken up by qualitative secondary analysts over time.

Analytic expansion

"Analytic expansion" is a term I used to refer to the kind of study in which a researcher makes further use of a primary data set in order to ask new or emerging questions that derive from having conducted the original analysis but were not envisioned within the original scope of the primary study aims. This kind of secondary analysis is the most common to date (Heaton, 2004). Examples within the nursing literature include Boehmeke and Dickerson's use of a database originally generated to address symptom experiences during adjuvant breast cancer chemotherapy to answer questions about how women transition from health to illness (Boehmke & Dickerson, 2006), and Bottorff and colleagues' extension upon a database constructed to consider couple interactions on women's tobacco reduction during pregnancy and postpartum to consider how dominant ideals of masculinity influence men's attitudes toward smoking (Bottorff, Oliffe, Kalaw, Carey, & Mroz, 2006).

Retrospective interpretation

This version of analytic expansion incorporates the temporal aspect of a program of inductive research, which typically continues long after the initial pass at the results has been written up and published. It involves re-entering the data to expand upon or further develop angles that were dealt with more superficially in the first instance, or perhaps in rare (but exciting) cases, to correct claims that were later seen to be a product of premature closure. Nursing examples of this version include Kavanagh and colleagues' study on social support based on two prior studies pertaining to experiences with perinatal loss (Kavanaugh, Trier, & Korzec, 2004), and Hsieh and colleagues' dialectic perspective analysis of descriptive accounts of communications in end-of-life family consultations to uncover and interpret dialogic tensions and contradictions in the communication of bad news to families (Hsieh, Shannon, & Curtis, 2006).

Armchair induction

I used the notion of armchair induction to reflect the contributions of those who engaged with fieldwork despite never having entered the field. Recognizing the significant investments and competencies that the development of qualitative databases typically entail, one can envision that the talents of some more theoretically inclined scholars might be better placed engaging with existing sets of text, and in fact might take advantage of perspectival distance from the human experience of text generation to produce different sorts of inquiry products than would primary investigators. It is perhaps characteristic of nurse scholars that this approach seems rather rare in our literature, with the vast majority of secondary studies being conducted by those who have played some role in the primary research or by their students. However, an example of this kind of inquiry can be seen in the work of Peters and colleagues, who capitalized on the availability of focus group data from a commissioned study of the impact of the working environment on the health of the Canadian nursing workforce in which some of the authors had been involved by bringing in an expert nurse ethicist to lead a secondary analysis on the question of the moral habitability of the working environment (Peters, Macfarlane, & O'Brien-Pallas, 2004).

Cross-validation

Consideration of thematic conclusions from a primary study across multiple distinct data sets can be of considerable value in confirming (or discounting) original interpretive directions and suggesting patterns that might have been invisible to the primary researcher prior to a more etic consideration. Since the aim of many qualitative inquirers includes a theoretical aspect, this approach provides a means by which to move beyond that which is limited to a distinct sample and context to that which may begin to represent a more general claim. Two examples of scholars with potentially comparable qualitative data sets for the purpose of validating, extending, and expanding their work are the studies by Yamashita and Forsyth, whose studies using different nursing theoretical frameworks and system contexts to study mental illness were combined in a secondary analysis of family coping (Yamashita & Forsyth, 1998), and Perry and O'Connor, who analyzed sets of data from independent studies on women who were caregiving to a husband with Alzheimer's disease and living with a memory-impaired spouse to develop conceptualizations on the preservation of personhood despite dementia (Perry & O'Connor, 2002).

Amplified sampling

Recognizing the limitations faced by qualitative approaches with regard to representation and generalization, this approach reflects the added value that may be obtained in considering the applicability of inductively derived claims across distinct and potentially quite different study contexts and populations. This form of approach could allow not only for considerations of confirmability, but also expansion upon meaning through the advantage of a wider lens. Although examples within the nursing literature seem few and far between, a study I was involved with might illustrate the idea. A colleague and I had been studying self-care in Type I diabetes (a socially legitimized chronic disease) in Canada and a colleague in Sweden had been studying the experience of persons with "environmental sensitivities" (a condition that was, and still is, discredited in many segments of the medical community). On the basis of secondary analysis of the combined work, we were able to tease out entrenched ideological positions about chronically ill patients that transcended evidence of a biological disease basis to distort health professional attitudes toward patient expertise, a finding that could not have arisen from the study of either clinical population alone (Thorne, Ternulf Nyhlin, & Paterson, 2000).

As is evident from the descriptions and examples, these categorizations do not reflect mutually exclusive categories, and there are variations in design within each. Naturally, each approach can also be employed as a component of ongoing inquiry. Thus secondary studies may be conducted as discrete and separate enterprises, or as a component of multi-pronged studies that use the secondary aspect to launch new primary data collection, or return to banked data in order to flesh out and develop newly generated themes. Thus, the general modality reflects quite a diversity of inquiry options, and a general discussion such as this cannot hope to do justice to all of the possible configurations that nurse researchers may dream up to answer their burning questions.

Methodological opportunities

Denzin and Lincoln used an often cited metaphor of the *bricoleur* to describe the adeptness of contemporary qualitative researchers at drawing from various methodological strategies in their endeavor to interpret the social world (Denzin & Lincoln, 1994). Drawing upon Lévi-Strauss' depiction of the working man creatively using the limited range of tools at hand to solve increasingly complex problems (Lévi-Strauss, 1966), and the more colloquial notion of jack-of-all-trades, this idea has come to reflect using any and all methods of inquiry to form better interpretations over time (Heaton, 2004). For the most part, this metaphor effectively characterizes the qualitative secondary analysis movement, in which scholars have been enthusiastic in capitalizing on analytic options at hand to answer their increasingly intricate questions within a line of scholarly inquiry. Thus, little by way of analytic convention has emerged, and the field reflects the full set of approaches that would be found across the range of primary studies.

It is generally accepted in the literature that a secondary study requires a well-defined and auditable analytic approach, and the product would be held to a standard of trustworthiness equivalent to that of primary research. For the most part, researchers have focused on the "fit" between primary studies and the secondary intention, with a general understanding that similarity of analytic approach advantages analytic integrity while too much difference may render eventual findings logically problematic. However, one might argue that the more important concern ought to be the ability of the secondary researcher to deeply examine the primary studies across a more comprehensive range of ingredients in order to deconstruct and interpretively explain not only where they went but also how they arrived at their destination. In other words, the nature of any database cannot really be appreciated outside of the context of an informed, critical appreciation for both its genesis and its offspring.

Understanding the methodological and theoretical context

Although there has been a long tradition of focusing on method as the central defining characteristic of a study (Janesick, 1994; Schwandt, 1996), one might convincingly argue that the more influential features shaping its scope and contours may reflect matters of theoretical (Sandelowski, 1993b) or disciplinary orientation (Thorne, Joachim, Paterson, & Canam, 2002). Thus, in order to understand what is and is not contained within any primary qualitative data set, one requires not only an understanding of what is explicitly claimed about such matters as methodological approach and study sample, but also what can be learned from available knowledge about researcher and context as well as discerned from a critical read of the primary text(s). Thus, generalizations about methodological fit" may not be all that helpful in justifying secondary work.

While some methodological fit problems might seem self-evident, others may be more covert. To illustrate, an explicit instance might include using findings generated using "narrative" methodology to support more generalized conclusions about actual events or experiences. Since narrative method inherently implies a socially mediated reconstruction of experienced realities, secondary claims would be inevitably limited to those that reflect a social constructivist positioning. However, the qualitative health literature is replete with cases in which the methodological justifications bear little relationship to what seems to have actually occurred, and may reflect more on the disciplinary and theoretical fashion of the time, the methodological identity of the scholarly community, or even the anticipated preference of reviewing audiences. In numerous instances, fancy language around methodological or theoretical positioning to launch a study evaporates into what is essentially a qualitative description (Sandelowski, 2000). Although an analysis of the evolving scientific and scholarly context within which the qualitative health world has emerged, particularly for nursing research, helps us attain some sympathy for discrepancies between what authors say they did and what actually seems to have happened (Thorne, 2008), these disjunctures create a climate within which deep interpretation of process and product becomes more important than apparent superficial fit. Without this kind of in-depth insight into the primary qualitative data sets, one cannot really do justice to a rigorous and fulsome secondary analysis.

Clarifying the interpretive lens

Beyond the methodological, disciplinary and theoretical groundings that may or may not have shaped the primary data set, it is important to understand for the purpose of any inductively derived analysis that the generation of any qualitative data set will have been shaped and guided by evolving interpretations within the constant comparative analytic process. Although we know that what differentiates an inductively generated data set from the more traditional qualitative data that may arise within a more deductively structured inquiry is to a large extent the engagement of the inquirer over time, it can be difficult in the secondary context to fully appreciate how the data have changed and evolved over time in alignment with the original analysis. While we recognize that thematic understandings emerging from the findings are supposed to influence subsequent interviewing technique, for example, it is quite challenging to view a primary data set from a perspective that accounts for the developmental process of the original researcher in making sense of it. Thus, the secondary analyst has to exert real caution with regard to interpretations that may be contingent on assumptions about matters of frequency or commonality.

Data sets are without doubt a product of numerous contextual features that are even more obscure than these matters of method, theory and disciplinary lens, and yet no less complex (van den Berg, 2005). Certainly the personal motivations, if we can grasp them, of the individual researcher may reveal a great deal about a data set, and sometimes unrecoverable features of context (such as coinciding public discourses, professional pressures) may have left their stamp on what exists (Rew, Koniak-Griffin, Lewis, Miles, & O'Sullivan, 2000). Thus, it becomes evident why the secondary researcher must be held to a particularly high standard of account-ability in making interpretive claims on the basis of what has been created through what must be acknowledged are complex primary processes.

Making your findings count

Despite variations in terminological preference between different qualitative research com-munities, questions of validity, generalizability, integrity and credibility are a challenge across the qualitative spectrum (Payne & Williams, 2005). In terms of secondary work, these are further complicated by problems that have been associated with findings deriving from all manner of studies drawing upon extant databases over which the researcher may have had no control (Windle, 2010). The key to a credible conclusion using qualitative secondary analysis approaches therefore will lie in the researcher's capacity to authentically account for the nature of the original data sets, to credibly justify the alignment of the question with the available material being used to answer it, and to effectively demonstrate a finely tuned sense of the limits and scope of conclusions that are warranted on the basis of the totality of these design decisions. Hollow rhetoric about inherent limitations followed by overly grandiose claims about the reach and general applicability of the findings will raise legitimate questions in the mind of readers and reviewers as to the credibility of the project throughout. Thus, while a clearly articulated and coherent line of reasoning from the beginning to the end is an essential quality criterion in any study, it seems especially indispensable in the secondary domain.

Issues in writing and reporting

Up to this point, we have been addressing mainly theoretical and conceptual issues associated with the secondary analysis project in qualitative nursing research. But it is also important to reflect on some of the more technical and practical issues that arise in writing up and reporting.

Aligning primary and secondary analysis

Recognizing the inherent complexities associated with translating original data sets into new interpretive frameworks and structures, a secondary study must provide readers with sufficient grounding in the primary works not only to justify the secondary analysis but also to build a foundation for the credibility of its outcomes. That said, we all recognize the severe length limits of most of the scholarly journals within which qualitative nurse researchers are likely to want to publish, and the confusing climate within which authors must respond to the beliefs and assumptions of reviewers who may not appreciate the intricate complexities of secondary work. At the very least one would hope that, beyond the obvious technical elements, descriptions of the primary work should allude to the disciplinary and interpretive lenses that may have influenced the enactment of the original studies insofar as this explains what exists for secondary consideration. Further, one would expect in the discussion of secondary findings evidence of serious and critical questioning as to the extent to which new interpretations reflect aspects of what went into the making of the primary studies. Further, where the conclusions of secondary studies reflect departures from those arising in the original works, one would hope for an explicit explanation of why that may be so. And in as much as it is necessary to critically reflect on the implications of the intellectual scaffolding that primary researchers may have brought into their studies, we also ought to be equally rigorous in our attempts to examine our own.

Citing and acknowledging

One important effect of an evolving body of scholarship in qualitative secondary analysis is that it provides us with language and method for clearly articulating what we are doing within the context of a community that better understands how to judge its quality. One hopes that the problem Heaton identified in relation to covert secondary analysis is rapidly disappearing, although with continuing perceived pressures for multiple publication, "salami slicing" into what are seemingly different versions of a single work is likely to continue (Norman & Griffiths, 2008). Thus, there is a clear need for an evolving culture of linkage and alignment, in which the ideas one is putting forth are explicitly and transparently placed in the context of what has come before, and in some instances, what is still to come. Given what we know of publication processes within our rapidly shifting information age, one can no longer expect the reader to guess at the chronology and derivation of ideas, and in the secondary context, one would expect the obligation of the researcher to be quite high in terms of laying out the history and trajectory of the various knowledge generation processes within which a secondary study is seeking to make a contribution.

Attending to potential threats to scholarly integrity

Although every credibility and integrity risk posed by primary qualitative research also applies in the secondary analysis context, with the exception perhaps of manipulating data during its construction phase, there are clearly additional threats to be considered here. One might be the overuse of specific data sets to squeeze out a diverse array of findings, such that different analyses linked to the same primary source bear little relationship to the original or to one another. One might envision, for example, disputes between primary researchers and secondary investigators who reframe their findings, potentially generating conflicting claims derived from the same data set (Irwin, Bornat, & Winterton, 2012). The apparent cost-effectiveness and ease of access of existing sources might well appeal to new researchers and trainees. However, given some of the complexities arising from the approach we have identified, one might want to discourage the impression that this kind of work is less complex than is primary inquiry.

Hammersley, who has been a leader in qualitative data analysis theorizing, discounts the argument put forth by authors that since all data are essentially constituted and reconstituted, the challenges posed by secondary studies are not overly significant (Hammersley, 2009). From his perspective, the issues of fit and context are matters that will require considerable ongoing methodological development to ensure that reused data produces meaningful knowledge.

Toward future developments in qualitative secondary analysis

Although qualitative secondary analysis is clearly becoming increasingly popular among nurse researchers, it seems fair to say that we are still evolving a shared theoretical and methodological framework within which we can confidently evaluate the quality of these research products. When I read examples in the literature, most of what I read seems fine scholarship, clearly developed beyond the confines of the original work, and making meaningful original contributions to our thinking. However, I also acknowledge that, for the most part, we readers have to take it on faith that the intricacies of ethics, context, and interpretive influence have been carefully and rigorously addressed, as space cannot permit the kind of in-depth excavation that would do justice to the underlying complexities that a fulsome qualitative secondary approach implies. However, my confidence in the creativity and integrity of my colleagues assures me that, as we expand beyond analysis of our own primary studies, engage more fully in data sharing and cross-comparisons, and even exploit our differences to advance the complexity of our inductively generated theorizing, we will find a language and a structure within which to advance a coherent methodological excellence for future generations. As Sandelowski once pointed out, "We have become inveterate data collectors, having been imbued with the idea that research means collecting new data" (Sandelowski, 1997, p. 129). Clearly there is a great deal more that we can do with what we already possess.

References

Alcoff, L. (2009). The problem of speaking for others. In A. Jackson & L. Mazzei (Eds.), *Voice in qualitative inquiry: Challenging conventional, interpretive and critical conceptions in qualitative research* (pp. 117–136). New York: Routledge.

Bishop, L. (2009). Ethical sharing and reuse of qualitative data. *Australian Journal of Social Issues, 44*(3), 255–272.

Boehmke, M., & Dickerson, S. (2006). The diagnosis of breast cancer: Transition from health to illness. *Oncology Nursing Forum, 33*(6), 1121–1127.

Bottorff, J. L., Oliffe, J., Kalaw, C., Carey, J., & Mroz, L. (2006). Men's constructions of smoking in the context of women's tobacco reduction during pregnancy and postpartum. *Social Science & Medicine, 62*, 3096–3108.

Denzin, N., & Lincoln, Y. (1994). Introduction: Entering the field of qualitative research. In N. Denzin & Y. Lincoln (Eds.), *Handbook of qualitative research* (pp. 1–17). Thousand Oaks, CA: Sage.

Freeman, D. (1983). *Margaret Mead and Samoa: The making and unmaking of an anthropological myth.* Cambridge, MA: Harvard University Press.

Gladstone, B., Volpe, T., & Boydell, K. (2007). Issues encountered in a qualitative secondary analysis of help-seeking in the prodrome to psychosis. *Journal of Behavioral Health Services & Research, 34*(4), 431–442.

Glaser, B. (1962). Secondary analysis: A strategy for the use of knowledge from research elsewhere. *Social Problems, 10*(1), 70–74.

Glaser, B. (1963). Retreading research materials: The use of secondary analysis by the independent researcher. *American Behavioral Scientist, 6*(10), 11–14.

Hammersley, M. (2009). Can we re-use qualitative data via secondary analysis? Notes on some terminological and substantive issues. *Sociological Research Online, 15*(1). Retrieved from http://www.socresonline.org.uk/15/11/15.html.

Heaton, J. (1998). Secondary analysis of qualitative data. *Social Research Update* 22. Retrieved on March 17, 2012 from http://sru.soc.surrey.ac.uk/SRU22.html.

Heaton, J. (2000). *Secondary analysis of qualitative data: A review of the literature.* York: Social Policy Research Unit, University of York.

Heaton, J. (2004). *Reworking qualitative data.* London: Sage.

Heaton, J. (2008). Secondary analysis of qualitative data: An overview. *Historical Social Research, 33*(3), 33–45.

Hinds, P. S., Vogel, R. J., & Clarke-Steffen, L. (1997). The possibilities and pitfalls of doing a secondary analysis of a qualitative data set. *Qualitative Health Research, 7*, 408–424.

Hsieh, H.-F., Shannon, S., & Curtis, J. (2006). Contradictions and communication strategies during end-of-life decision making in the intensive care unit. *Journal of Critical Care, 21*, 294–304.

Irwin, S., Bornat, J., & Winterton, M. (2012). Timescapes secondary analysis: Comparison, context and working across data sets. *Qualitative Research, 12*(1), 66–80.

Janesick, V. (1994). The dance of qualitative research design: Metaphor, methodolatry, and meaning. In N. K. Denzin & Y. S. Lincoln (Eds.), *Handbook of qualitative research* (pp. 209–219). Thousand Oaks, CA: Sage.

Kavanaugh, K., Trier, D., & Korzec, M. (2004). Social support following perinatal loss. *Journal of Family Nursing, 10*(1), 70–92.

Lévi-Strauss, C. (1966). *The savage mind.* Chicago: University of Chicago Press.

Lobo, M. (1986). Secondary analysis as a strategy for nursing research. In P. Chinn (Ed.), *Nursing research methodologies: Issues and implications* (pp. 295–304). Rockville, MD: Aspen.

Long-Sutehall, T., Sque, M., & Addington-Hall, J. (2011). Secondary analysis of qualitative data: A valuable method for exploring sensitive issues with an elusive population? *Journal of Research in Nursing, 16*(4), 335–344.

Manderson, L., Kelaher, M., & Woelz-Stirling, N. (2001). Developing qualitative databases for multiple users. *Qualitative Health Research, 11*(2), 149–160.

McArt, E., & McDougal, L. (1985). Secondary data analysis: A new approach to nursing research. *Image: Journal of Nursing Scholarship, 17*, 54–57.

Norman, I., & Griffiths, P. (2008). Duplicate publication and "salami slicing": Ethical issues and practical solutions. *International Journal of Nursing Studies, 45*, 1257–1260.

Parry, O., & Mauthner, N. (2005). Back to basics: Who re-uses qualitative data and why? *Sociology, 39*(2), 337–342.

Payne, G., & Williams, M. (2005). Generalization in qualitative research. *Sociology, 39*(2), 295–314.

Perry, J.-A., & O'Connor, D. (2002). Preserving personhood: (Re)membering the spouse with dementia. *Family Relations, 51*(1), 55–62.

Peters, E., Macfarlane, A., & O'Brien-Pallas, L. (2004). Analysis of the moral habitability of the nursing work environment. *Journal of Advanced Nursing, 47*(4), 256–367.

Rew, L., Koniak-Griffin, D., Lewis, M., Miles, M., & O'Sullivan, A. (2000). Secondary data analysis: A new perspective for adolescent research. *Nursing Outlook, 48*(5), 223–229.

Sandelowski, M. (1986). The problem of rigor in qualitative research. *Advances in Nursing Science, 3*, 27–37.

Sandelowski, M. (1991). Telling stories: Narrative approaches in qualitative research. *Image: The Journal of Nursing Scholarship, 23*, 161–166.

Sandelowski, M. (1993a). Rigor or rigor mortis: The problem of rigor in qualitative research revisited. *Advances in Nursing Science, 16*(2), 1–8.

Sandelowski, M. (1993b). Theory unmasked: The uses and guises of theory in qualitative research. *Research in Nursing & Health, 16*, 213–218.

Sandelowski, M. (1997). "To be of use:" Enhancing the utility of qualitative research. *Nursing Outlook, 45*(3), 125 132.

Sandelowski, M. (2000). Whatever happened to qualitative description? *Research in Nursing & Health, 23*, 334–340.

Schwandt, T. A. (1996). Farewell to criteriology. *Qualitative Inquiry, 2*, 58–72.

Szabo, V., & Strang, V. (1997). Secondary analysis of qualitative data. *Advances in Nursing Science, 20*(2), 66–74.

Thorne, S. (1994). Secondary analysis in qualitative research: Issues and implications. In J. M. Morse (Ed.), *Critical issues in qualitative research methods* (pp. 263–279). Thousand Oaks, CA: Sage.

Thorne, S. (1998). Ethical and representational issues in qualitative secondary analysis. *Qualitative Health Research, 8*, 547–555.

Thorne, S. (2008). *Interpretive description.* Walnut Creek, CA: Left Coast Press.

Thorne, S., & Darbyshire, P. (2005). Landmines in the field: A modest proposal for improving the craft of qualitative health research. *Qualitative Health Research, 15*, 1105–1113.

Thorne, S., Joachim, G., Paterson, B., & Canam, C. (2002). Influence of the research frame on qualitatively derived health science knowledge. *International Journal of Qualitative Methods, 1*(1) Retrieved on January 1, 2003 from http://www.ualberta.ca/~ijqm/.

Thorne, S., Ternulf Nyhlin, K., & Paterson, B. (2000). Attitudes toward patient expertise in chronic illness. *International Journal of Nursing Studies, 37*, 303–311.

van den Berg, H. (2005). Reanalyzing qualitative interviews from different angles: The risk of decontextualization and other problems of sharing qualitative data. *Forum Qualitative Sozialforschung / Forum: Qualitative Social Research, 6*(1), Art. 30. Retrieved from http://www.qualitative-research.net/index.php/fqs/article/view/499/1074.

Windle, P. (2010). Secondary data analysis: Is it useful and valid? *Journal of PeriAnesthesia Nursing, 25*(5), 322–324.

Woods, N. (1988). Using existing data sources: Primary and secondary analysis. In N. Woods & M. Catanzaro (Eds.), *Nursing research: Theory and practice* (pp. 334–347). St Louis, MO: C. V. Mosby.

Yamashita, M., & Forsyth, D. (1998). Family coping with mental illness: An aggregate from two studies, Canada and the United States. *Journal of the American Psychiatric Nurses Association, 4*(1), 1–8.

31

Evidence-based practice

Contributions and possibilities for qualitative research

Barbara Bowers

History and disciplinary influences of qualitative methodologies

This chapter invites nurse researchers to explore current approaches to qualitative research, with particular attention to developing an evidence base for practice. The aim of the chapter is to raise questions about what qualitative methodologies have to offer as we develop evidence to support practice. Embedded in and heavily influenced by the canons of "science," nurse researchers can gain much by looking beyond that domain, to recapture the tremendous potential found in the intellectual traditions that form the basis of qualitative methodologies.

Qualitative research methodologies have long histories and rich traditions in the humanities and social sciences (Hesse–Biber & Leavy, 2004). Sociology, anthropology, social psychology, political science, philosophy, education and literary theory, and more, have all contributed to the diversity of approaches used to understand the world, including a wide array of qualitative approaches. Most qualitative researchers are familiar with the pervasive discussions about paradigms, and the debates about the importance of ontology and epistemology in understanding, selecting and using a particular methodology (Kuhn, 1970; Guba & Lincoln, 1989, Holloway & Wheeler, 2010). However, questions about the disciplinary origins of methodologies, how a methodology is informed by the particular concerns of the discipline, and the implications of these differences for addressing questions relevant to nursing, are also important although infrequently acknowledged in nursing literature.

Considering the disciplinary origins of a methodology, the types of questions it was designed to address and the uses to which it has been employed, can help guide researchers in their selection of the most appropriate methodology for their study. Inconsistency between methodology and the study purpose or focus can weaken the quality of the study, and result in missed opportunities. While there are always multiple considerations when choosing a methodology, understanding what the methodology was designed for is relevant to making the choice and will influence the quality of the findings or evidence. Understanding the discipline that gave birth to a methodology is a part of this.

While greatly simplified here for heuristic purposes, considering the relationship of intellectual traditions to research methodologies is useful. For example, social psychologists generally focus on the social interactions and processes involved in meaning making, the interpretation of social symbols, and the intersection of individual and social. The form of grounded theory methodology developed and used by Strauss traces its origins to symbolic interaction (Blumer, 1969; Bowers & Schatzman, 2009; Strauss, 1987). Guided by the assumptions of symbolic interaction, this form of grounded theory allows researchers to probe how individuals interpret, engage in and respond to their social circumstances, and to identify and delineate the social processes those interpretations are embedded in (Maines, 1991). Hence, the methodology is well suited for studying the social processes involved in making meaning and the relationship between social process and human actions (Glaser & Strauss, 1967; Holloway & Wheeler, 2010). Many so-called "grounded theory" studies fail to explore social process, focusing only on individual meanings or perceptions, with no integration of social context or process; using "grounded theory" where phenomenology might be more appropriate. The common failure to appreciate this distinction between phenomenology and grounded theory, and the failure to integrate social process in a "grounded theory" study, can be traced to a lack of understanding about the link between grounded theory and the underlying social psychology, between source discipline and method.

Philosophy is concerned with logic, consciousness, and existential questions, about human experiences and "being-in-the-world." Although phenomenology, like grounded theory, comes in many forms, phenomenology is generally suited to questions about existential experiences and personal meanings. Philosophy (hence phenomenology) is less concerned with context and social processes than with individual meaning. Hence, phenomenology maximizes the use of first person accounts, and employs strategies that encourage introspection and deep reflection.

Infrequently used by nurse researchers, narrative analysis, in varying forms, is rooted in literary theory. Narrative analysis evolved, in part, to explore the structure of stories, the use and purpose of various story components and the meanings reflected in *how* a story is told as well as *what* is told (Ayres & Poirier, 2003; Parker & Wiltshire, 2003). Narrative analysis identifies the broader interpretive framework that people use to transform meaningless or disconnected events into meaningful episodes that comprise a story, giving the researcher access to the "textual interpretative world of the teller" (Cortazzi, 2002; Ezzy, 2002). As such, it is a useful methodology for examining how people construct their experiences over time, the consequences of attending to, and not attending to particular events. Narrative analysis reminds us about the importance of acknowledging and respecting the multiple versions or stories, and how limiting a single "correct" or objective view is for understanding human behavior.

Cultural anthropologists have attended to the organization of cultures, the rules and processes by which cultures operate and are passed on (Agar, 1980). Ethnography, while also comprising many distinct approaches and considerable ongoing debate, has generally been characterized by researcher immersion in a setting to observe and experience a culture from within, while also standing apart, maintaining a "marginal stance." Anthropology, and ethnography, encompass what is apparent and open to reflection as well as what is "back stage," not open to public view or, necessarily, to informant awareness. While there are certainly exceptions, most notably Kayser-Jones' (2002) work in nursing homes, ethnographies have not been common in nursing research.

Critical methodologies, influencing many disciplines, have directed scholars to raise questions about the values embedded in social structures, particularly how institutionalized values create and maintain inequalities across social spheres. These questions are certainly of interest to nurse scholars, many of whom are concerned with the consequences of social inequality for health (Cheek, 2000; Crowe, 2005; Powers, 2003; Smith, 2007). Critical discourse analysis (Traynor, 2003), a critical methodology, can be used to understand how the evolution of intellectual traditions, including nursing, shapes our understandings and determines possibilities, liberating us from the constraints of our current understandings and opening the way for transformations that create new ways of understanding and acting. Particularly in the US, nurse researchers have often not taken advantage of critical methodologies in conducting research.

This brief and highly simplified discussion of the relationship between disciplines and methodologies was intended as a heuristic, to demonstrate the relationship between disciplinary focus and the approaches that evolve to address questions of import to the disciplines. The purpose was to highlight the importance of understanding the assumptions and values embedded in research methodologies, informing the structure and substance of "findings" (Thorne, 2001) and bounding the possibilities for discovery. The evidence base needed for nursing practice is diverse, encompassing knowledge about populations, organizations, public policy, individual behavior, responses to individual, family and community circumstances. The quality of the evidence base is, at least to some extent, dependent on appropriate selection of methodology for the research question. This in turn, relies on the researcher's understanding of the methodologies available, including the history, assumptions and values inherent in the methodologies.

Qualitative research in nursing and health sciences

The widespread use of qualitative approaches for research is a relatively recent phenomenon in nursing and the health sciences (Hutchinson, 2001; Murphy et al., 1998; Parker & Wiltshire, 2003; Sandelowski, 1991; Speziale & Carpenter, 2007; Yardley, 2000). During the past few decades, the number and diversity of qualitative research reports in nursing and other health science journals have increased dramatically while nurse researchers using qualitative methodologies have also experienced a significant increase in funding success.

Grant proposal reviewers have lately been calling for *greater* use of qualitative methodologies, particularly for proposals submitted under person- or patient-centered initiatives, when proposing translational research projects and as an adjunct to clinical trials. To support this increased appreciation of qualitative research, the National Institutes of Health and National Science Foundation have recently developed guidelines for submitting proposals using qualitative methodologies (Office of Behavioral and Social Sciences Research, 2001; Ragin et al., 2004).

The surge in use of qualitative methodologies, however, has not always been accompanied by sufficient skill and understanding of qualitative methodologies. It is not uncommon for reviewers, as well as researchers conducting the research, to engage in methodological confusion or "muddling" (Caelli, Ray, & Mill, 2003; Holloway & Wheeler, 2010; Wuest & Stern, 1992). And research methodologies used by nurse researchers have been largely limited to a relatively narrow range of what is possible (Caelli et al., 2003; Mays & Pope, 2000; Shortell, 1999).

In the health sciences, nurse researchers have often led the way in proposing and conducting qualitative research. Nurse researchers, many who were mentored by researchers in the humanities and social sciences, have made important contributions to nursing knowledge and to the development of qualitative methods in nursing (Speziale & Carpenter, 2007). Nurse researchers have raised questions and engaged in sophisticated debates about the complexities and nuances of methodologies (Morse & Field, 1995; Latimer, 2003; Speziale & Carpenter, 2007) but these activities have remained at the margins of nursing scholarship. Despite these examples, a relatively narrow range of methodologies seem to predominate in the nursing literature.

Nurse researchers, particularly qualitative researchers, might consider, and seriously engage:

- Which qualitative methodologies have been predominant in nursing and which have been largely left behind?
- How thoughtfully have qualitative methodologies been adapted, used and developed in nursing research? Is the selection of methodology reasoned and well informed? Are the methodologies selected the ones most suitable to the purpose or have more suitable methodologies been missed?

- How has the context of nursing science influenced the use and evolution of qualitative methodologies? Has the environment within which nursing research is conducted discouraged the use of the fullest range of methodologies?
- Where is the yet-unrealized potential of qualitative methodologies for the development of nursing science? And how might nursing science benefit from more inclusive adoption of the range of qualitative methodologies that are not widely used? Are there important questions to which qualitative research has not been directed? And if so, what are these questions, how might qualitative research address them and to what end?

Nurses have adopted, adapted and developed qualitative methodologies, while making considerably more use of some methodologies than others. For example, phenomenology, grounded theory and thematic analysis have predominated in the qualitative studies conducted by nurse researchers. While examples of other qualitative methodologies are certainly represented in nursing literature, they are much less commonly used, particularly in the US. Nurses elsewhere, particularly in Europe and Australia, have made much greater use of critical methodologies, narrative analysis and ethnographies. This has afforded them opportunities to explore important questions that have been largely unaddressed by nurse researchers in the US (Crowe, 2005; Latimer, 2003).

Two important questions are suggested. First, does the predominance of this narrow range of methodologies in nursing research prevent nurse researchers from using the most appropriate methodologies for their studies? Second, does the predominance of these methodologies result in a failure to even consider some of the questions that are important to the discipline? For example, critical ethnography, a methodology not commonly used by nurse researchers in the US and rarely included in qualitative research courses in nursing programs (at least in the US), brings with it a rich intellectual tradition that would likely lead to questions that nurse researchers do not often consider or reflect on (Cheek, 2004; Cook, 2005). That is, learning about the methodology and its intellectual origins, understanding the purposes for which it has been used, the types of questions it is useful in addressing, could create possibilities for asking important questions that might not otherwise be asked. We are all aware of the wisdom about selecting a methodology only after deciding on your research question. However, it should also be obvious that exposure to intellectual traditions outside one's familiar or usual literature stimulates fresh ideas and perspectives and can be very useful in identifying "obvious" questions that have only become obvious in the context of a particular intellectual tradition.

Qualitative methodologies: to what use?

There is general acceptance that qualitative research methodologies are appropriate for generating knowledge about the "lived experience," understanding the perspective of the person experiencing the phenomenon, giving voice to the voiceless and that they can effectively serve as a corrective to the hegemony of researcher and practitioner assumptions about the nature of patient experiences. Qualitative methodologies are also selected for their effectiveness in sensitizing the reader to experiences of a particular group. That is, when well done, the reader is able to "enter" the experience of others, to feel their frustration or pain, to see the world from the perspective of the research participant.

However, restricting the rationale for conducting qualitative research to capturing the lived experience is problematic. It would be difficult to support the contention that quantitative research is unable to capture anything about lived experience. A more useful question might be "What do qualitative approaches capture about the lived experience that cannot be captured using more quantitative approaches?"

Sandelowski (2002) suggests caution in claiming that qualitative methodologies are necessary to capture the "voices of the voiceless," or to assume greater "truth telling" with interviews than with other forms of data collection, suggesting that qualitative researchers may well be "deluding themselves" about the greater access to "truth" when using qualitative methodologies. Significantly, the association between truth telling and methodology has never been substantiated. Indeed, while the "notoriously ambivalent relation of a researcher's text to the realities studied" (Alvesson & Sköldberg, 2000) has been accepted by many scholars, it has not been acknowledged or addressed in most qualitative (or quantitative) research reports. What many scholars have identified as the "interpretative, rhetorical and political nature of empirical research" should give any researcher, including those using qualitative approaches, pause in making claims about truth or correspondence to reality (p. vii). An important point here is that qualitative researchers would be wise to take care about the claims they make for their methodologies. These are important questions for qualitative researchers to address, debate and explore.

The same case can be made for suggesting that qualitative approaches are the most appropriate way to explore individual perspectives. This is not to question whether qualitative methodologies offer something unique. It is, however, to suggest that qualitative researchers would benefit from more thoughtful and critical reflection on just what each methodology has to offer, avoiding reliance on claims that are difficult to substantiate. Better to ask "What is it about the lived experience, or the lived experience in *this* instance that requires a qualitative methodology, and this particular qualitative methodology?"

Increasingly and pervasively, it is suggested that qualitative research is useful primarily as an adjunct or precursor to quantitative work, that it provides a starting place for the more advanced phase of work in an area and that it is a useful adjunct to clinical trials. Specifically, the evolution of qualitative research within the context of health sciences has encouraged a rather truncated, but widely accepted belief that the uses of qualitative research are specific to the following:

- Identifying variables to incorporate into quantitative designs. That is, it is preliminary or prior to more advanced quantitative studies (Morse et al., 2001; Noyes et al., 2008; Pope & Mays, 1995; Shortell, 1999; Sofaer, 1999).
- Building theory that can later be tested using more quantitative methodologies. Grounded theory in particular has been viewed as a methodology to use for developing theory in an area where there is none available for guiding theory testing research.
- Gaining insight into the relationships discovered between independent and dependent variables, particularly in RCTs. This use has gained considerable attention recently, as a way to make clinical trials more useful to both researchers and practitioners.

Qualitative methodologies are particularly well suited for exploring the processes of change that occur during or following clinical interventions in RCTs. Mixed methods intervention studies that reveal the mechanisms by which change occurs (as well as identifying conditions preventing change and how they operate) can provide the foundation for future intervention research and have much greater potential to guide practitioners as they attempt to use the findings of research (Morse, Penrod, & Hupcey, 2000). Effective use of mixed methods intervention research requires a sophisticated understanding of both methodologies and thoughtfully designed studies. Too often, the qualitative components are afterthoughts, tacked on awkwardly, undermining what the qualitative approach can offer.

The continuing perception that qualitative research is useful only prior to intervention studies, appropriate at an early stage in the development of knowledge, is supported by the frequent exclusion of qualitative studies from reviews used to develop the evidence base. While still generally seen as subordinate in value to RCTs, the Cochrane Qualitative Research Methods group has described qualitative research as particularly useful "alongside randomized trials" when searching for evidence of effectiveness in practice settings, for understanding the "experience of those involved in providing and receiving interventions, and . . . for evaluating factors that shape the implementation of interventions" (Noyes et al., 2008). However, the guidelines for Cochrane reviewers clearly specify the narrow parameters for inclusion of qualitative research, restricting use primarily to qualitative data reported in conjunction with intervention studies, in practice, narrowing the possibility of inclusion through resource, expertise and budget restrictions (Noyes et al., 2008). Reflecting on the uses of "qualitative" methodologies described above, it is clear that many widely accepted uses of qualitative research, possibly increasingly so, are consistent with the canons of science and fail to recognize the many other possibilities for qualitative methodologies.

Challenges and unrealized potential

Despite the increasing acceptance of qualitative research, these methodologies still do not enjoy the same autonomy, status, funding rates or educational resources that quantitative methodologies in nursing and health sciences experience. Qualitative researchers in nursing and health sciences continue to find themselves defending their choice of methodology and justifying the usefulness of their research, particularly when it is not in service of subsequent quantitative work. While preliminary work that captures subjects' perspectives, helps to build theory, contributes to the development of data collection tools for quantitative studies, and supplements clinical trials, all extremely important activities (Tripp-Reimer & Doebbeling, 2004), many other potential uses of qualitative research are at risk of being lost if qualitative researchers are enticed by the, likely temporary, benefits of aligning with these limited views. There is much to lose by inhabiting only the "contracted spaces" left to us if we accept these terms (Cheek, 2008).

The many missed opportunities that would result from this severe narrowing of options should be obvious. As Given has pointed out (2007), with the emphasis on evidence, narrowly construed, the rich traditions inherited from humanities and social sciences, and all they have to offer, are essentially precluded. It is indeed ironic that the increasing acceptance of qualitative method-ologies within nursing and the health sciences could actually decrease the opportunities for nurse researchers to benefit from the richness of qualitative research traditions available.

One obstacle to the development and use of qualitative research methodologies has been the widely held assumptions that reviewers of grant proposals and manuscripts (as well as academic mentors), and sometimes researchers themselves, hold concerning the nature, purposes, and quality of qualitative research. Assumptions about the nature and uses of qualitative methodologies continue to limit the diversity in qualitative methodologies used and the uses to which qualitative approaches are directed.

A possible antidote to this potential narrowing of methodological possibilities is a more thorough understanding and increasingly sophisticated rendering of qualitative methodologies, their uses and their origins. At the very least, it would mean failing to confirm the more narrow views of qualitative methodologies by providing much more robust rationales for and descriptions of qualitative methodologies in grant proposals and manuscripts. The often eclipsed nature of methods sections in qualitative research reports unfortunately perpetuates some of the misperceptions about qualitative methodologies. Negotiating with editors about maintaining the integrity of research reports is one strategy that many researchers have used successfully. Editors are often accepting of formats that do not conform to their templates when sufficient rationale has been provided. While reviewers and editors of journals such as *Qualitative Health Research* require no such convincing, many others do. Promoting the inclusion of methodologically sophisticated reviewers for journals is also an effective strategy (Hutchinson, 2001)

These strategies will only be effective if the researchers themselves have a sufficiently sophisticated understanding of the methodology they are using. This suggests the need for strong preparation, not a quick foray into qualitative methodologies. As Shortell (1999) pointed out, a common view of qualitative methodologies is that they are easy, that it's just about asking interesting questions. This view is likely perpetuated by the lack of required, or even available, courses in qualitative research methodologies, particularly courses beyond the introductory level.

Requiring only introductory coursework in qualitative methodologies, as opposed to the generally more robust requirements for quantitative work, leaves the impression that there is less to learn, that qualitative research expertise can be easily "picked up." The consequences of this are clear in what has been described as methodological slurring or muddling (Wuest & Stern, 1992.) While there are outstanding examples of methodological savvy, the literature is replete with examples of methodological confusion resulting from the failure of many nurse researchers to select the appropriate methodology or to understand the methodology they are using.

The heightened focus on evidence-based practice (Polit & Beck, 2010) and overemphasis on RCTs (DiCenso, Cullum, & Ciliska, 1998) also limits the creative and productive expansion of qualitative methodologies in nursing. As Grypdonck (2006) warns "there is a snake in the grass. There is a danger that the ideology of Evidence Based Health Care (EBHC) and quantitative research will affect qualitative research in its roots, which may endanger the quality of qualitative research" (p. 1373).

Beliefs about what constitutes "science" have exerted a strong influence on the selection of methodologies, and the way they have been used in nursing research (Hesse-Biber & Leavy, 2004). Alvesson and Sköldberg (2000, p. vii) note how the drive toward objectivity and researchers' fears of undermining any appearance of objectivity lead researchers to avoid debates about relationships between subject and object, standpoint, politics and ideology of research (Hesse-Biber & Leavy, 2004; Wilde, 1992). This drive toward appearing objective has also led to the upsurge in studies using triangulation to "confirm" the results of qualitative studies, perpetuating assumptions about their more tentative nature of qualitative research. Accepting these terms sidesteps questions about what each methodology has to offer and what is was designed to do.

Another challenge faced by qualitative researchers, including nurse researchers, is the tendency to confound data collection strategies with research methodologies. One of the earliest discussions on this topic was Harding's work on understanding and distinguishing between method and methodology, between the tools used to conduct a study and the overall design (Harding, 1987). That is, "interview" is not a methodology, it is a tool that is used in many methodologies. How it is developed and used is determined by the methodology it is serving. Interviews are used by phenomenologists, grounded theorists, ethnographers and others. But in each case, interviews are structured, timed and interpreted according to the methodology, or at least they should be. Failure to understand this, for example, contributes to the common muddling of phenomenology and grounded theory. Focus groups are also quite different in structure, implementation and interpretation depending on the methodology they are serving. Grypdonck (2006) warned against the tendency to confound methodologies and data collection methods, noting that "As qualitative researchers feel the hot breath of the EBHC movement on their neck," they may find it beneficial to focus on procedures and techniques at the expense of more reflective and creative extension of qualitative methodologies, undermining the rich traditions they are working in. C. W. Mills referred to this many decades ago, as methodological fetishism (Mills, 1959).

411

Further limiting the potential of qualitative approaches in nursing research is the failure to fully engage in the intellectual debates about qualitative research that are found in other disciplines. While some nurse researchers have written eloquently about and within these debates, reflecting on implications for the discipline, these debates have remained largely outside the mainstream of nursing, particularly in the US. As a consequence, the great potential of qualitative methodologies in nursing and the health sciences remains largely unrealized. For example, researchers in the social sciences have engaged in reflection, discussion and debate over the relationships between researcher and data, and between researcher and subject and the standpoint of the researcher.

Going back to the 1960s and the 1970s, researchers in the social sciences have written about how the standpoint, the perspective, the biography, the social history of the researcher influence the questions asked, and the interpretations generated from research projects. Few nurse researchers have addressed this issue or engaged in the ongoing debates about standpoint in relation to nursing research (Perry, 2011). Although there are important exceptions (Latimer, 2003; Morse, 1999; Morse et al., 2000; Sandelowksi, 2002; Sandelowski & Barroso, 2002; Streubert & Carpenter, 2011), these debates have remained largely on the margins. Nurse researchers could benefit from more consistently and deliberately engaging in the questions raised by these scholars and in considering the meaning these debates have for their own work. The papers included in these texts provide examples of how an intimate and sophisticated understanding of the origins, complexity and evolution of a methodology, with a carefully considered and creative adaptation to the questions central to nursing, can yield new and promising approaches for nurse researchers.

One such debate concerns the claims one makes about research "findings" and the widely accepted tentativeness of "facts." Embracing and engaging in these debates, much of which is relevant to any research methodology, would position nurse scientists well in discussions about the criteria to use when reviewing qualitative proposals or manuscripts and would do much to counter the impression that qualitative research is just about asking interesting questions. This is particularly the case in our current environment, where there is potential to reduce qualitative methodologies to "procedures and techniques" that are useful adjuncts to RCTs.

The promise of qualitative methodologies

Despite the caveats outlined above, there are exciting possibilities for qualitative researchers that nurse researchers have yet to take full advantage of. The growing interest in "patient-" and "person"-centered care has already expanded opportunities for qualitative researchers, as funders have come to accept the necessity for qualitative research. It will be important, however, for qualitative researchers be clear about what different qualitative methodologies have to offer; to expand beyond capturing under-represented perspectives, meanings and lived experiences.

The mainstream view of what constitutes evidence is based on a very narrow view of evidence. Morse et al. (2000) offer more complex and nuanced perspectives on what constitutes evidence, and the role qualitative research can play in building evidence for a discipline. One example is extending an area of research, building on prior work (quantitative or qualitative) by providing insights into the contexts and conditions under which prior findings are supported or not supported (Morse et al., 2001). Qualitative methodologies can effectively inform us about why something matters and to whom. That is, the perspectives captured by the study can be understood as they relate to context and condition. This type of insight is much more relevant to our practice colleagues than are "more generalizable" findings.

Using qualitative research methodologies in this way also highlights the usefulness of building qualitative studies on prior quantitative work, rather than the reverse. Using a quantitative study as the starting point, exploring the relationships between variables, identifying the social processes that account for positive or negative findings in prior work can contribute much to the development of the discipline.

Translational research offers a particularly fruitful opportunity for qualitative researchers to use a wide array of currently underutilized methodologies. Translational research arose from the recognition that findings from research conducted in controlled environments are not easily translated into "the real world." One of the most anticipated promises of translational research is discovering how social systems and organizations influence the adoption of healthier or more effective practices, how they support or undermine the adoption of health-promoting interventions, and finding ways to speed adoption of promising practices. When qualitative researchers engage in translational research, they would be wise to select methodologies that can inform them about systems and institutions, about how context and condition influence individual practices.

Continuing to focus on the individual perspectives and meanings (or using methodologies designed for that purpose), qualitative researchers could easily miss the opportunity to inform colleagues, particularly our practice colleagues, about the interaction between context and practice. This will require many qualitative researchers to refocus or expand their focus to encompass the context, to "enhance their peripheral vision" (Sofaer, 1999) and to expand beyond the currently predominant qualitative methodologies.

Qualitative research and generalizability

Despite decades of discussion about generalizability in qualitative research, the debate seems to have had very little impact on published reports of qualitative research in nursing (Chenail, 2010; Eisner, 1981; Firestone, 1993; Guba & Lincoln, 1985; Morse, 1999; Onwuegbuzie & Leech, 2010; Payne & Williams, 2005; Polit & Beck, 2010; Sandelowski, 1997; Schofield, 2002). For example, it has been and continues to be common for qualitative researchers to caution readers not to expect their findings to be generalizable, to proclaim the limits of their work for generalizing to anything or anyone beyond the sample or setting of the study. The claim that qualitative research is not generalizable also reinforces the common wisdom that qualitative research, by itself, is severely limited in its usefulness, and that larger, quantitative work is needed to confirm and position the findings from qualitative studies.

Sandelowski (1997) observed almost twenty years ago that "arguably, the single most important factor contributing to the failure to take the findings of qualitative studies seriously is the frequently cited charge that they are not generalizable" (p. 127). These claims are often made by qualitative researchers themselves, about their own work. Are we actually claiming that there is no possibility for application of our work beyond the specific site of the study itself? This would hardly justify the effort or expense involved in conducting research.

This truncated view of generalizability fails to acknowledge the significant literature proposing an expanded and more comprehensive understanding of generalizability than the widely accepted notion based exclusively on probability sampling theory (Chenail, 2010; Firestone, 1993; Lee & Baskerville, 2003; Lincoln & Guba, 1985; Morse, 1999; Polit & Beck, 2010; Sandelowski, 1997; Schofield, 2002). Schofield suggests that qualitative researchers' failure to concern themselves with generalizability can be traced to the influence of anthropology, with its early focus on exotic groups, making extrapolation to others irrelevant (Schofield, 2002).

The acceptance of probability sampling theory as the sole basis for generalizing also fails to integrate the important, and longstanding, discussions about responsibility for judging the extent to which research is useful beyond the site of the actual study. Quantitative research, with its underlying assumptions about generalizability, places the entire responsibility with the researcher. Contrary to this view, scholars of qualitative research have actively debated the appropriate locus of responsibility for judging the generalizability of qualitative research. Although grounded in findings sufficiently robust to make judgments about generalizability, some have argued that the responsibility for judging lies with the reader (Firestone, 1993) or with a complex interaction between the reader and the text (Sandelowski, 2004). When qualitative researchers claim their work is not "generalizable," they are either accepting the truncated view based on probability sampling or without understanding the significance and implications. The consequences of accepting such a restricted understanding of generalizability are particularly significant in the context of generating evidence for practice.

Conclusion

What role, if any, will qualitative research play in the development of an evidence base for nursing practice? In the pursuit of evidence, will qualitative researchers be equal partners or will their work become only a supplement to quantitative studies? Full engagement in developing an evidence base requires qualitative researchers to understand the intellectual traditions informing their methodologies, to match research questions to methodologies with the greatest potential to inform, to embrace and actively engage in the debates about fundamental issues such as standpoint, generalizability and the potential dangers of co-opting qualitative researchers into a narrowly conceived view of evidence.

References

Agar, M. H. (1980). *The professional stranger: An informational introduction to ethnography*. San Diego, CA: Academic Press.

Alvesson, M., & Sköldberg, K. (2000). *Reflexive methodology*. London: Sage Publications.

Ayres, L., & Poirier, S. (2003). Rational solutions and unreliable narrators: Content, structure, and voice in narrative research. In J. Latimer (Ed.), *Advanced qualitative research for nursing* (pp. 115–134). Oxford: Blackwell Science.

Blumer, H. (1969). *Symbolic interactionism: Perspective and method*. Englewood Cliffs, NJ: Prentice-Hall.

Bowers, B., & Schatzman, L. (2009). Dimensional analysis. In J. Morse, P. Stern, J. Corbin, B. Bowers, K. Charmaz, & A. Clarke (Eds.), *Developing grounded theory: The second generation*. Walnut Creek, CA: Left Coast Press.

Caelli, K., Ray, L., & Mill, J. (2003). "Clear as mud": Toward greater clarity in generic qualitative research. *International Journal of Qualitative Methods*, *2*(2), 1–13.

Cheek, J. (2000). *Postmodern and poststructural approaches to nursing research*. Thousand Oaks, CA: Sage.

Cheek, J. (2004). At the margins? Discourse analysis and qualitative research. *Qualitative Health Research*, *14*, 11–40.

Cheek, J. (2008). *Qualitative inquiry and the politics of evidence*. Walnut Creek, CA: Left Coast Press.

Chenail, R. J. (2010). Getting specific about qualitative research generalizability. *Journal of Ethnographic & Qualitative Research*, *5*(1), 1–11.

Cook, K. E. (2005). Using critical ethnography to explore issues in health promotion. *Qualitative Health Research*, *15*(1), 129–137.

Cortazzi, M. (2002). Narrative analysis in ethnography. In P. Atkinson, A. Coffey, S. Delamont, J. Lofland, & L. Lofland (Eds.), *Handbook of ethnography*. London: Sage.

Crowe, M. (2005). Discourse analysis: Towards an understanding of its place in nursing. *Journal of Advanced Nursing*, *51*(1), 55–63.

DiCenso, A., Cullum, N., & Ciliska, D. (1998). Implementation forum: Implementing evidence-based nursing: some misconceptions. *Evidence Based Nursing*, *2*(1), 38–39.

Eisner, E. (1981). On the differences between scientific and artistic approaches to qualitative research. *Educational Researchers*, *10*, 5–9.

Ezzy, D. (2002). *Qualitative analysis: Practice and innovation*. Crows Nest, NSW: Allen & Unwin.

Firestone, W. (1993). Alternative arguments for generalizing from data as applied to qualitative research. *Educational Researcher*, *22*, 16–23.

Given, L. (2007). Evidence-based practice and qualitative research: A primer for library and Information Professionals. *Evidence Based Library and Information Practice*, *2*(10), 15–22.

Glaser, B. G., & Strauss, A. L. (1967). *The discovery of grounded theory: Strategies for qualitative research*. New York: Aldine Publishing Company.

Grypdonck, M. (2006). Qualitative health research in the era of evidence-based practice. *Qualitative Health Research*, *16*(10), 1371–1385. doi: 10.1177/1049732306294089.

Guba, E. G., & Lincoln, Y. S. (1985). *Naturalistic inquiry*. Newbury Park, CA: Sage.

Guba, E. G., & Lincoln, Y. S. (1989). *Fourth generation evaluation*. Newbury Park, CA: Sage.

Harding, S. (1987). *Feminism and methodology*. Bloomington, IN: Indiana University Press.

Hesse-Biber, S. N., & Leavy, P. (Eds.). (2004). *The practice of qualitative research*. New York: Oxford University Press.

Holloway, I., & Wheeler, S. (2010). *Qualitative research in nursing and healthcare* (3rd ed.). Oxford: Wiley-Blackwell.

Hutchinson, S. (2001). The development of qualitative health research: Taking stock. *Qualitative Health Research*, *11*(4), 505–521.

Kayser-Jones, J. (2002). The experience of dying: An ethnographic nursing home study. *The Gerontologist*, *42* (Spec. No. 3), 11–19.

Kuhn, T. S. (1970). *The structure of scientific revolutions* (2nd ed.). Chicago: University of Chicago Press.

Latimer, J. (2003). *Advanced qualitative research for nursing*. Ames, IA: Blackwell Publishing Co.

Lee, A., & Baskerville, R. (2003). Generalizing generalizability in information systems research. *Information Systems Research*, *14*, 222–243.

Lincoln, Y., & Guba, E.(1985). *Naturalistic inquiry*. Newbury Park, CA: Sage.

Maines, D. (1991). *Social organization and social process: Essays in honor of Anselm Strauss*. Chicago: Aldine de Gruyter/New York: Hawthorne.

Mays, N., & Pope, C. (2000). Qualitative research in health care: Assessing quality in qualitative research. *British Medical Journal*, *320*(7226), 50–52.

Mills, C. W. (1959). *The sociological imagination*. New York: Oxford University Press.

Morse, J. (1999). Qualitative generalizability. *Qualitative Health Research*, *9*, 5–6.

Morse, J. M., & Field, P. A. (1995). *Qualitative research methods for health professionals*. Thousand Oaks, CA: Sage.

Morse, J., Penrod, J., & Hupcey, J. (2000). Qualitative outcomes analysis: Evaluating nursing interventions for complex clinical phenomena. *Journal of Nursing Scholarship*, *32*(2), 125–130.

Morse, J. M., Swanson, J. M., & Kuzel, A. J. (2001). *The nature of qualitative evidence*. London: Sage.

Murphy, E., Dingwall, R., Greatbatch, D., Parker, S., & Watson, P. (1998). Executive summary, qualitative research methods in health technology assessment: A review of the literature. *Health Technology Assessment*, *2*(16).

Noyes, J., Popay, J., Pearson, A., Hannes, K., & Booth, A. on behalf of the Cochrane Qualitative Research Methods Group. (2008). *The Cochrane Collaboration*. Chichester: John Wiley & Sons, Ltd.

Office of Behavioral and Social Sciences Research, National Institutes of Health. (2001). *Qualitative methods in health research: Opportunities and considerations in application and review*. NIH Publication No. 02-5046. Bethesda, MD: NIH.

Onwuegbuzie, A., & Leech, N. (2010). Generalization practices in qualitative research: A mixed methods case study. *Quality and Quantity*, *44*, 881–892.

Parker, J. M., & Wiltshire, J. (2003). Researching story and narrative in nursing: An object-relations approach. In J. Latimer (Ed.), *Advanced qualitative research for nursing* (pp. 97–114). Oxford: Blackwell Science.

Payne, G., & Williams, M. (2005). Generalization in qualitative research. *Sociology*, *39*(2), 295–314.

Perry, B. (2011). *Social research and reflexivity: Content, consequences, and context*. London: Sage.

Polit, D., & Beck, C. (2010). Generalization in quantitative and qualitative research: Myths and strategies. *International Journal of Nursing Studies*, *47*, 1451–1458.

Pope, C., & Mays, N. (1995). Reaching the parts other methods cannot reach: An introduction to qualitative methods in health and health services research. *British Medical Journal*, *311*, 42–45.

Powers, P. (2003). Empowerment as treatment and the role of health professions. *Advances in Nursing Science*, *26*(3), 227–237.

Ragin, C. C., Nagel, J., & White, P. (2004). *Workshop on scientific foundations of qualitative research.* National Science Foundation Report.

Sandelowski, M. (1991) Telling stories: Narrative approaches in qualitative research. *IMAGE: Journal of Nursing Scholarship, 23,* 161–166.

Sandelowski, M. (1997). "To be of use": Enhancing the utility of qualitative research. *Nursing Outlook, 45,* 125–132.

Sandelowski, M. (2002). Reembodying qualitative inquiry. *Qualitative Health Research, 12*(1), 104–115.

Sandelowski, M. (2004). Using qualitative research. *Qualitative Health Research, 14*(10), 1366–1386.

Sandelowski, M., & Barroso, J. (2002). Reading qualitative studies. *International Journal of Qualitative Methods, 1*(1), 74–108.

Schofield, J. W. (2002). Increasing the generalizability of qualitative research. In A. M. Huberman & M. B. Miles (Eds.), *The qualitative researcher's companion* (pp. 171–203). Thousand Oaks, CA: Sage.

Shortell, S. M. (1999). Editorial: The emergence of qualitative methods in health services research. *Health Services Research, 34*(5), Part II, 1083–1090.

Smith, J.L. (2007). Critical discourse analysis for nursing research. *Nursing Inquiry, 14*(1), 60–70.

Sofaer, S. (1999). Qualitative methods: What are they and why use them? *Health Services Research, 34*(5), Part II, 1101–1118.

Speziale, H. J. S., & Carpenter, D. R. (2007). *Qualitative research in nursing: Advancing the humanistic imperative* (4th ed.). Philadelphia, PA: Lippincott Williams & Wilkins.

Strauss, A. (1987). *Qualitative analysis for social scientists.* New York: Cambridge University Press.

Streubert, H. J., & Carpenter, D. R. (2011). *Qualitative research in nursing: Advancing the humanistic imperative* (5th ed.) Philadelphia, PA: Lippincott, Williams & Wilkins.

Thorne, S. E. (2001). The implications of disciplinary agenda on quality criteria for qualitative research. In J. M. Morse, J. M. Swanson, & A. J. Kuzel (Eds.), *The nature of qualitative evidence.* Thousand Oaks, CA: Sage.

Traynor, M. (2003). Discourse analysis: Ideology and professional practice. In J. Latimer (Ed.),*Advanced qualitative research for nursing* (pp. 137–154). Oxford: Blackwell Science,

Tripp-Reimer, T., & Doebbeling, B. (2004). Qualitative perspectives in translational research. *Worldviews on Evidence-Based Nursing, 1*(S1), S65–S72.

Wilde, V. (1992). Controversial hypotheses on the relationship between researcher and informant in qualitative research. *Journal of Advanced Nursing, 17,* 234–242.

Wuest, B. C., & Stern, P. N. (1992). Method slurring: The grounded theory/phenomenology example. *Journal of Advanced Nursing, 17,* 1355–1360.

Yardley, L. (2000). Dilemmas in qualitative health research. *Psychology and Health, 15,* 215–228.

Part IV

International qualitative nursing research

State of the science

International qualitative nursing research

State of the science in England, Wales and Scotland

Dawn Freshwater and Jane Cahill

Introduction

The title of this chapter is provocatively phrased in its reference to "Science." A review of this nature must take into account the vexed and even turbulent relationship that qualitative research methodologies have held with concepts of "Science" given that positivistic strongholds in nursing research and the overarching medical model impact not only on nursing research but on nursing as a profession. In our review of qualitative nursing research in England, Wales and Scotland we will, therefore, deconstruct popularly held concepts of Science when assessing its 'state' with regard to qualitative nursing research.

Before we do so, we believe it is helpful to provide a working definition of qualitative nursing research in the context of this chapter. We base our definition of qualitative health research on that supplied by Morse (2012), author of Chapter 2 in this handbook "The development of qualitative nursing research." We define qualitative nursing research as an inductive research approach for exploring health and illness in nursing, an approach which considers the perspectives of the people themselves rather than the researcher's perspective. Qualitative nurse researchers use qualitative inquiry in order to understand and make sense of participants' responses to health and illness and the meanings they construct from their experience.

We begin this chapter by providing the historical context of nursing research in England, Wales and Scotland against which we outline a framework by which we may critically review the significance of qualitative nursing research. Next based on our scoping review of qualitative nursing research in the three nations, we table the most frequent methods used in these countries by nurse researchers, supplying key references and outlining specific contributions of the methods to the nursing profession as a whole. A number of research centers of excellence focused on qualitative research approaches are currently operating in these countries and in this chapter we give a narrative overview of their profiles and critically review their contribution to the field, highlighting what we believe to be representative exemplars of cutting-edge qualitative nursing research. Finally, as we reflect on the future direction of travel for qualitative nursing research in these countries, we conclude the chapter with a deconstruction of the concept of Science as it impacts on qualitative nursing research.

The historical context of nursing research in England, Scotland and Wales: a brief overview

Although Florence Nightingale is often viewed as the first pioneering nurse researcher, the development of nursing research in the United Kingdom (UK) was brought about by the formation of the National Health Service (NHS) in 1948 (Kirby, 2004). Nevertheless in the 1950s it was still the trend for sociologists and psychologists to be undertaking research into nursing and nurses. In 1959, Marjorie Simpson set up a self-help group for nurse researchers which later became the Research Society of the Royal College of Nursing (RCN). This action was the beginning of establishing nursing research as a unique discipline with nurses being its proponents.

In 1972, the publication of the Briggs Report (DOHSS, 1972) recommended that nursing should become a research-based profession. This recommendation was instrumental in validating research as an integral part of a nurse's portfolio of activity, although subsequent to the publication of the Briggs Report the professional status of nursing and nursing research had suffered with claims that nursing had not become research-based (Hunt, 1981; Thomas, 1985; Webb & Mackenzie, 1993) and that nurses were not able to use research in practice. In response to such potentially damaging claims, the 1993 Report of the Task Group on the Strategy for Research in Nursing, Midwifery and Health Visiting (DoH, 1993) recommended that nurses should become proficient in research skills and methods, that is "research literature." In order for this to happen, changes needed to be effected with regard to both research infrastructure and nurse education. There have been some significant milestones which have furthered nurse education: first, research is now fully integrated into the pre-registration curricula (UKCC, 1986); second, nurse education was moved into higher education institutions (HEIs) in the 1990s, facilitating ongoing academic development at Master's and Doctoral levels. However, Rafferty et al. observed in 2003 a significant shortfall in research-literate nurses (Rafferty et al., 2003). This trend was linked to under-funding and led to two initiatives: (1) the HEFCE supporting capacity building for nurses and allied health professions dependent on RAE (Research Assessment Exercise) and REF (Research Excellence Framework) scores; and (2) the UK Clinical Research Collaboration's (UKCRC) report recommendation for the establishment of research training opportunities, career flexibility and information provision in support of career opportunities in nursing. More recently, the policy drivers supporting the development of clinical academic careers in nursing and allied health professions highlight the importance of research as a serious career option for nurses (DoH, 2006).

The furtherance of nursing research has been aided by organizations such as the RCN (which has an extensive Research and Development Resource, a Research Society, an Institute and funding for research projects), the Foundation of Nursing Studies and the Queen's Institute which all support nursing research. In addition, the DoH (Department of Health) has some specific funding streams available for nursing research as well as multi-disciplinary health research opportunities, for example, National Institute for Health Research (NIHR) and Research for Patient Benefit (RfPB). Funding for nursing research and, more specifically, nursing research itself, has been a long-standing problem in the three nations; one that has been debated widely (Freshwater, Cahill, Walsh, & Muncey, 2010). As such, these are significant developments and have influenced the way in which qualitative nursing research in the three countries has managed not only to survive, but also to grow from strength to strength.

The nature of nursing research is multi-faceted, complex and wide-ranging encompassing practice, care outcomes, effectiveness of interventions, education and management issues. In terms of how this impacts on the role of *qualitative* nursing research, there has been some debate both on what research questions qualitative research is most suited to answering and to its status as determined by the hierarchy of evidence. Qualitative research has been broadly placed within interpretivist or constructivist paradigms (Moule & Goodman, 2009) which are focused on the understanding of individual perspectives and experiences. Such an epistemological position places qualitative nursing research as the best method to examine patients' feelings and experiences concerning new NHS services and pathways of care or their experiences of medical conditions. However, the agenda of "fit for purpose" when matching research method with research question to build up the evidence base is not the only one. Evidence-based practice has become contentious because it has been underpinned by the *hierarchy of evidence* which places randomized controlled trials at the top with qualitative research designs being relegated to lower "supporting" positions. This view has been since challenged by Mantzoukas (2008) and later on in this chapter we deconstruct the concept of evidence using a postmodern lens and explicitly examine its role in the positioning of qualitative research (see Freshwater et al., 2010).

Although nursing research was previously carried out by psychologists, sociologists, historians as well as academics from social and welfare policy, the situation has changed over the past 30 years or so with nurses now designing, conducting and commissioning their own research (see, for example, Holloway & Wheeler, 2010; Todres, 2007). It is within this context of increasing autonomy and agency that qualitative nursing research is best reviewed. Owing to increases in the number of nurses educated to Master's and Doctoral level (Higher Education Statistics Agency, 2005), more nurses are taking research to a higher level and securing competitive funding from the DoH and major research councils. This ascendancy has had and continues to have a substantial impact on the nature of qualitative nursing research and its contribution to nursing research and the nursing profession. In the section that follows we review the range of research methods that figure prominently in nursing qualitative research in England, Scotland and Wales.

An overview of qualitative approaches used by nurse researchers in England, Scotland and Wales

Table 32.1 summarizes some of the most widely used qualitative research approaches used in England, Scotland and Wales. This is based on a scoping review of qualitative nursing research conducted in these countries and provides key pieces of research conducted using those methods. We recognize that other chapters in this text will provide specialist scholarship on prominent qualitative research methods in nursing research so the intention here is simply to give a snapshot of scholarly qualitative nursing research activity in these countries, highlighting their specific contribution to nursing research and the nursing profession.

All pieces of research referenced have been conducted in England, Scotland and Wales. In Table 32.1, methods of qualitative inquiry and data collection are included together for the following reasons. First, the distinction between qualitative analysis and data collection is not always easy to make in qualitative research; and second, some methods of qualitative analysis are predicated on a specific form of data collection so to separate the two is sometimes to impose an artificial distinction. Therefore, we prefer the term "qualitative approaches" within which the focus can be on collection or analysis.

Grounded theory

Gass (2008), in his study on mental health nurses who used electroconvulsive therapy, used purposive and then theoretical sampling based on previous findings and concepts that emerged. Gass' ideas about nurses' interactions were followed by theoretical sampling in the latter stages of his research as he added new participants, depending on the developing concepts. Turning to

Table 32.1 Qualitative approaches in nursing research

Qualitative approach	Exemplars of research using qualitative approach
Grounded theory	Newell (2008): Study of anorexia nervosa conducted by professional nurse from the perspectives of those who suffer from it: England
	Gass (2008): In research on the work of MH nurses in wards and ECT departments in Scotland, Gass observed and interviewed MH nurses who worked with patients using electroconvulsive therapy: Scotland
	Fenwick et al. (2009): Fenwick as the researcher explored women's experiences of having a Cesarean section in a setting in the southwest of England: England
Ethnography	Warren et al. (2000): A ward sister carried out an ethnographic study on female patients' perspective of fitting in during hospitalization on an acute medical ward in the south of England: England
	Cloherty et al. (2004): Reported on ethnographic research in the postnatal ward of a maternity unit in the south of England, involving observation and interviews with mothers and health professionals: England
	Fudge et al. (2008): The authors explored the understandings of user involvement in health service organizations and what influences them to put the involvement into practice. The setting was a multi-agency modernization program to improve stroke services in two London boroughs: England
Auto-ethnography	Muncey (2010): Episode from one of her stories as a vehicle for challenging the dominant discourse about teenage pregnancy and explored what tactics might be needed in order to present the story in different ways: England
	Muncey & Robinson (2007): Based on the second author's account of his psychosis. The authors demonstrate how the impact of evidence needs to be transformed by powerful personal endorsement rather than the patriarchy of psychiatry, offering a compelling case of how stories can provide the evidence: England
Narrative research	Carter (2004): Illustrates how children's narratives of pain can positively influence nursing practice, by requiring practitioners to be less distanced and passive: England
	Brown and Addington-Hall (2008): Explored through narrative inquiry how people with motor neuron disease talk about living and coping with their condition. The authors carried out longitudinal narrative interviews over 18 months with 13 patients recruited from four NHS primary care trusts: England
	Holloway, Sofaer-Bennett, and Walker (2007): In using narrative inquiry to explore the stigmatization of people with chronic pain, the authors give examples of a chaos narrative where participants report feeling trapped and imply their sense of having little control over their lives: England
Phenomenology	Todres et al. (2000): Story of "Anne" an intensive care nurse who was admitted to intensive care on three occasions when she experienced disseminated intravascular coagulation (DIC) and septic shock. The authors use a broadly phenomenological approach to explore her experiences using in-depth interviews and verbatim examples: England

Table 32.1 Continued

Qualitative approach	Exemplars of research using qualitative approach
	Fitzpatrick and Finlay (2008): The researcher Finlay reflected on her own personal experience of struggling with a severe shoulder injury and how this "sensitized" her to the impact of pain for patients undergoing rehabilitation phase following flexor tendon surgery: England
Action Research (AR)	Davies et al. (2008): The authors developed an AR project in which a research partnership was established between members of local communities in Wales and a professional researcher. The aim of the research was to work for positive change concerning disadvantaged groups: Wales
	Kilbride (2007): "Inside the Black Box: Creating excellence in stroke care through a community of practice": This study, based on setting up an in-patient stroke service in a London hospital, used a collaborative Action Research approach in order to achieve sustained service improvement in stroke services: London
Case study research	Clarke, Luce, Gibb, et al. (2004b); Clarke, Gibb, Luce, et al. (2009): In these studies exploring how people with dementia construct and manage risk, each of the 56 people with dementia who were interviewed twice over two months in turn nominated a family member and non-carer for interview, thus creating many case studies: England, Scotland Wales (Research carried out in three different UK countries)
	Walshe et al. (2008): This case study examined the impact of referral decisions in a community palliative care service. The case was the community care service in three primary care trusts in England. Interviews, observations and documentary analysis were used and the research highlighted core influences on referral services: England
Discourse analysis	Hui and Stickley (2007): The authors analyzed the discourses of the literature and health polices of the government and those of service users in the mental health arena using a Foucauldian DA. The authors highlight how different concepts take on different meaning among these two perspectives. Power in particular had varied connotations: England
	Benson et al. (2003): This study used a discourse analysis based on 16 semi-structured interviews on one mental health in-patient unit. The aim of the study was to explore how clients and staff understand the attributed meaning to aggressive situations: England
Performative Social Science	Jones (2006): The author gives examples of his own published narrative biography work, highlighting alternative ways to generate and present research, suggesting that the concept or research report/presentation is a dynamic vehicle: England
	Keen and Todres (2007): This paper gives several examples of dissemination through performance methods and includes a UK exemplar which uses the Internet to communicate qualitative data via DIPEx, a database of personal experiences of health and illness: England

the coding of the data, a prominent feature of grounded theory is theoretical coding whereby categories are related and linked to their sub-categories via their characteristics. These relationships lead to a core category, the basic social-psychological process in the research and around which all other categories are linked.

In Fenwick's (Fenwick et al., 2009) study on how women achieve normality after undergoing a Cesarean section, the author found that "achieving normality" was an important factor in the status passage to motherhood and hence this became a core category.

As an illustration of theoretical sensitivity (the researcher's ability to differentiate between significant and less important data and have insight into their meanings), Newell (2008), a specialist nurse and an expert in anorexia nervosa, explored the condition from the perspective of those who suffered from it. His expert knowledge and professional experience made him sensitive to patients' feelings and perceptions about their illness.

Ethnography

Warren (Warren et al., 2000) carried out research as a ward sister on the emotional experience of people in hospital. She assumed from her own theoretical perspective that fear would be the most dominant experience. However, Warren found that in the sample of older people embarrassment was a more strongly expressed emotion.

In Cloherty et al.'s (2004) micro-ethnography, the authors reported on ethnographic research in the postnatal ward of a maternity unit. The researchers used observations and interviews with mothers and health professionals with the aim of exploring beliefs, expectations and experiences of supplementation of breastfeeding.

In a macro-ethnography, Fudge et al. (2008) explored the understanding of user involvement in health organizations and what influenced them to put this involvement into practice. To achieve the study objectives, the authors used observation and interviews supplemented by documentary sources. The researchers also made judicial use of key informants with whom the researchers developed a sustained relationship throughout the study. The research resulted in an understanding that the interpretation of user involvement differs between health professionals and service users.

Auto-ethnography

Muncey (2010) includes an episode from one of her stories as a vehicle for challenging the dominant discourse about teenage pregnancy and explored what tactics might be needed in order to explore the story in different ways. In Muncey and Robinson (2007), based on an account of the second author's account of his psychosis, the authors demonstrate how the impact of evidence needs to be transformed by powerful personal endorsement rather than government hegemony or the patriarchy of psychiatry. What is required, as is demonstrated in this study, is the use of stories to provide the evidence. In terms of the study's contribution to mental health nursing, it provides compelling evidence of people's ability, including those who experience psychotic episodes, to maintain some sense of mental health. Nurse researchers might reflect that this is remarkable and what is interesting is that it is not studied in any great depth. Everyday and ordinary practice is often taken for granted in this way. Making the ordinary extraordinary is a timely and pressing challenge to all nurse practitioners and nurse researchers.

Narrative research

Carter (2004), in highlighting the value of children's narratives of pain, was able to directly impact clinical practice by allowing professionals to hear the children's experiences and experience empathy for them, i.e., to be "in-relation" with children. These two acts of "listening" and "empathy" have potential to inform innovative and patient-centered ways of pain management for children. Similarly Brown and Addington-Hall's (2008) study of the experiences of people with motor neuron disease led to the identification of "organizing threads"—these were living life as well as possible through keeping active and engaged, living in insurmountable situations, fear of the future and survival. These "threads" helped professionals to understand the patient and engage with them more effectively. This form of research was also therapeutic for patients in that, although their condition led to feelings of disempowerment, the construction of narrative, making sense of their conditions, led to feelings of agency and autonomy.

Phenomenology

Todres et al. (2000), in their study of "Anne," an intensive care nurse who was admitted to intensive care on three occasions when she experienced disseminated intravascular coagulation (DIC) and septic shock, were able to illustrate how in directly experiencing what it was like to be a patient, Anne had unique insight into the transition from dependence in critical care to developing independence and autonomy through recovery. Through gaining direct access to the lived experience of her patient through being a patient, and reflecting on her own reaction to being weaned from an incubator, "Anne" was able to use that knowledge, the ambivalence and tensions between the boundaries of dependence and independence, to inform her nursing practice.

Similarly, in the study by Fitzpatrick and Finlay (2008), the researcher (Finlay) reflected on her own personal experience of struggling with a severe shoulder injury and how this "sensitized" her to the impact of pain for patients undergoing rehabilitation phase following flexor tendon surgery. As in the previous example, this empathy, generated from direct experience of what the patient goes through, can lead to nursing practice that is empathic, patient-centric and ethically informed. In addition, empathy has the potential to lead to increased technical competence: the researcher recounted how having a first-hand insight into what it was like being a patient helped her to "see" the pain in patients' movements during rehabilitation.

Action Research (AR)

In Davies et al. (2008), the authors developed an AR project in which a research partnership was established between members of local communities in Wales and a professional researcher. The aim of the research was to work for positive change concerning disadvantaged groups. Although the research was not wholly qualitative, it illustrates the main hallmarks of AR, these being the democratization of the ongoing consultation and the negotiation process, and the iterative and responsive process of "feedback, reflection and adjustment." The findings of this project were implemented immediately—free exercise classes were set up in local communities and the intervention also led to a reduction in depression and an increase in quality of life (Davies et al., 2008).

Kilbride (2007): "Inside the Black Box: Creating excellence in stroke care through a community of practice" was based on setting up an in-patient stroke service in a London hospital, and used a collaborative action research approach in order to achieve sustained service improvement in stroke services. Prior to the study, there had been no specialist stroke service for the 325 patients who were admitted to the Trust each year, and care was fractured and uncoordinated. So this was an ideal question for Action Research in that the existing service indicated ineffectiveness and gaps in service provision. This study's success was down to the researchers undertaking a systematic monitoring of the emerging processes in the study around consultation and negotiation and being appropriately responsive to these. The study also benefited from a mixed methods approach to data collection (focus groups, in-depth interviews, documentary analysis, audits and participant observation) which yielded rich data and effected a multi-faceted solution to the problem from the viewpoint of multiple stakeholders. The impact of this project was startling: from being placed in the bottom 5% in the country, the stroke service became placed in the top 5% in the National Sentinel Stroke Audits (Clinical Effectiveness & Evaluation Unit, 2002, 2004, 2006). This reversal of fortune led to the unit receiving a national award for service redesign in 2005.

Case study research

In the case study research reported by Walshe et al. (2008), the researchers examined the impact of referral decisions in a community palliative care service. The "case" was the community care service in three primary care trusts in England. Interviews, observations and documentary analysis were used from a range of perspectives (general and palliative care professionals, patients, managers and commissioners) and the research highlighted core influences on referral services. In keeping with the tenets of case study research, data collection and analysis recurred iteratively and the refinements to the theoretical propositions were responsive to the diversity of the situations (that is, the way that community palliative care was provided in each of the three Trusts). The core influences identified concerned the way that personal, interpersonal and interprofessional factors shaped referral practices. The authors called for policy-makers to take into account these multi-layered influences on decision-making processes in referrals.

While flexibility and responsiveness are the hallmark of case study research, these features can also cause problems at the data analysis stage. First, there is the issue of generalizability—the relevance of each case to its neighbouring cases. Second, there is the issue of structure and design. Flexibility contingent upon the unique features of the case can lead to ad hoc design and the original research questions may become obscured in vast amounts of data. For example, in studies exploring how people with dementia construct and manage risk (Clarke, Luce, Gibb, & Cook, 2004; Clarke et al., 2009), 56 people with dementia who were interviewed twice over two months each in turn nominated a family member and non-carer for interview, thus creating many case studies. The large numbers were driven by the need to uphold context dependency by creating the necessary local knowledge. This case study is an important exemplar in that it outlines the significant challenges at the data analysis point.

Discourse analysis (DA)

Benson et al. (2003) used a discourse analysis based on 16 semi-structured interviews on one mental health in-patient unit. The aim of the study was to explore how clients and staff understand the attributed meaning to aggressive situations. Discourse analysis in this study revealed that client and staff discourses surrounding aggressive situations were startlingly similar, focusing on a central concern which was the attribution of blame. These findings, although context-bound, have implications for the professional discourse of mental health care, including the current policy agenda which is predicated on a discourse in turn constructed with the primary function of exoneration from and attribution of blame. Awareness of how such discourses sculpt professional practice, particularly with vulnerable or challenging client groups, has far-reaching significance for nursing and other health professionals.

McHoul and Grace (1995) distinguish between Foucauldian and non-Foucauldian discourse. In Foucault's works, specialist discourses are linked to power. In Foucauldian DA, DA reveals the language that operates within the particular discourse under study. For instance, within nursing and health care, professionals use particular types of discourse to impose their own reality or the reality of the system upon their clients. For example, in the study reported by Hui and Stickley (2007), the authors analyzed the discourses of the literature and health polices of the government and those of service users in the mental health arena using a Foucauldian DA applied to literature and health policies published by the UK government and service users. The authors highlight how different concepts take on different meaning among these two perspectives. Power in particular had varied connotations, with issues of power and knowledge being more flexibly and innovatively explicated by service users. In particular, service users held ideas of *power sharing* as well as *power shifting*, with the former holding connotations of power being divided, allocated and distributed. In terms of the impact on nursing practice, the authors recommend that a greater awareness of the significance of language should inform nursing practice, namely how the rhetorical language of policies can affect how involvement is configured with regard to service users. DA is one way of encouraging nurses to reflect on the tensions and conflicts in their day-to-day practice.

Qualitative research centers in England, Scotland and Wales

What follows in this section is a brief overview of three institutions (one from each country) in which qualitative nursing research is undertaken. The first two institutions support designated qualitative research centers, while in the last example a sustained program of qualitative research is undertaken in the institution although not associated with a designated qualitative center. We do not intend to give an exhaustive account of all the research that has taken place in the center; rather to give a representative profile of the center's activity, highlighting what we believe to be key contributions to nursing research and to the nursing profession.

Bournemouth Centre for Qualitative Research

This Centre has considerable expertise in research approaches and programmes that seek to improve the everyday lives of health and social care service users and citizens. Scholarly activity in the Centre emphasizes "insider views" of lives lived within their social, environmental and systemic contexts with the aim of generating the kind of knowledge that is able to integrate evidence with unique life histories and social contexts. A brief description of the three research programs of the Centre is given below but readers are referred to the following link to gain a more comprehensive insight into the Centre's activity: http://www.bournemouth.ac.uk/cqr/index.html.

The Centre specializes in three main areas, *Humanizing Health and Social Care*, *Novel and Innovative Research Methodologies* and *Performative Social Science*.

Humanizing Health and Social Care

This program of the Centre's research aims to focus on reintroducing the human dimension of care which has become increasingly obscured by an excessively technological and specialized approach to treatment. The program is allied to the newly emergent *Global Institute for Research in Humanizing Care Contexts*, represented by partners in ten countries from all continents.

The program focuses on a range of theoretical, methodological and empirical projects, including: the development of a new theory of well-being; the development of research projects that humanize the public understanding of research findings by utilizing tools from the arts and humanities; and the pursuit of research projects that focus on living with health-related technology such as insulin delivery technology in diabetes.

Novel and Innovative Research Methodologies

This program focuses on the creative ways of approaching the human and social realms. Such a move into new territory has been in part motivated by a scientific concern with "truth." The program's activities seek to incorporate insights, not just from the philosophy of science but from the philosophies of art, literature, ethics and aesthetics. Alongside traditional qualitative methodologies such as grounded theory, ethnography and narrative analysis, this program pursues novel and innovative methodologies that draw upon multiple influences and epistemologies from philosophy, the arts and the humanities. The program highlights a number of innovations for which it has a demonstrated track record. These include Performative Social Science, Embodied Enquiry, the Biographic Narrative Interpretive Method, the cut-up technique, Unitary Appreciative Inquiry, and integrative approaches to "mixing" qualitative research methods.

Performative Social Science

This program arose from a dissatisfaction with limitations in three publications and presentation of Jones's (2006) own narrative data (such as reciting papers to audiences or reading text from PowerPoint presentations to them). The program therefore focuses on the arts and humanities as possible tools for disseminating material, viewing qualitative researchers as natural allies of the arts and humanities. Possibilities include, but are not limited to, performance, film, video, audio, graphic arts, new media (CD-ROM, DVD, and web-based production), and poetry, and so forth (Jones, 2006). A key tenet of this program is that text and audience come together and inform one another in a relational way. As such, research methods in the social sciences do not simply describe the world as it is, but also enact it. Performative Social Science thus has effects; makes differences; enact realities; and helps to bring into being what they also discover.

Qualitative Health Research Unit (QUARU): Swansea University

QUARU is part of the Centre for Health Information, Research and Evaluation (CHIRAL). This center is committed to "hands-on" research that makes a difference, at the point of health care delivery, to patient and population health and well-being.

A range of qualitative methodologies is used by the unit, including Phenomenology, Ethnography, Case Study, leading to methods use in: Interviewing, Focus Group, Consultation Workshops, Bio-Photographic Elicitation Interviews, Bio-photographic data collection, Summative Analysis, Content Analysis, Visual Analysis and Thematic Analysis. Within the unit there is a program of work focused on "Nursing Studies." Readers are referred to the following link to gain a comprehensive overview of the range of the center's academic activity in qualitative nursing research: http://www.swan.ac.uk/ils/research/chiral/methodologies/observational studies/quaru/.

To provide an exemplar, a nursing study is underway which is in line with a program of research funded by the General Nursing Council (GNC) Trust for England and Wales to explore what "patient-centered professionalism" means to a wide range of registered nurses working in the community, including Health Visitors and District Nurses, a range of stakeholder groups supporting those nurses, and the general public. The study employs consultation with six workshop groups of professionals and the public to examine the concept in detail. Tri-sessional workshops are strongly facilitated by four members of the team who work in a cross-disciplinary manner, using mixed methods to elicit in-depth, rich and thick descriptions of the concept. A final list of ten themes will be produced that define patient-centered professionalism for these mixed groups. Outputs will include learning materials that could be incorporated into Continuing Professional Education (CPE) documentation for on-going nurse training or documentation to support newly qualified nurses.

School of Health in Social Science, University of Edinburgh

Within the School of Health in Social Science, the Nursing Studies program has evidenced a substantive portfolio of qualitative nursing research. Within Nursing Studies, the research falls into two main areas: Experience of Health and Illness and Healthcare: Organization and Policy. Below we outline key pieces of qualitative nursing research which have been undertaken in these areas. However, interested readers are referred to the link below to access more detail on the range of qualitative nursing research undertaken in the Nursing Studies program: http://www.ed.ac.uk/schools-departments/health/nursing-studies/home.

Experience of Health and Illness

- RELinQuiSh: REcovery following critical illness is a longitudinal qualitative exploration of perceived health care and support needs among survivors: developing timely interventions following hospital discharge.
- DTRF: An exploratory study of patients suffering from severe and enduring pain in surgical wards.
- An analysis of the experience of parenthood and of the health visiting service, from the perspectives of Pakistani and Chinese mothers of young children.

Healthcare Organization and Policy

Below is listed a suite of qualitative research projects based on tobacco control in the community and smoke-free homes:

- Qualitative Study of Changes in Smoking (and Drinking) Behavior Following Implementation of the Prohibition of Smoking in Enclosed Public Places.
- Qualitative Study Smoking in Homes, NHS Health Scotland.

Future directions of qualitative nursing research in England, Scotland and Wales

A useful way to reflect and speculate on the future directions of qualitative nursing research in England, Wales and Scotland is in a sense to take a step back from the evidence we have presented; that is, to deconstruct and refine the concept of Science as it impacts on qualitative research. In our reading and reframing of the concept of "State of the Science" we draw on Thomas Kuhn's (1962) concept of paradigm as a "set of practices that define a scientific discipline at any particular period in time." We maintain that paradigms have a key role in sculpting scientific practice while being mindful that the concept of paradigms has suffered from a series of slippery and imprecise definitions leading to uncritical, unmindful overuse (and abuse) of the term (see Holloway's critique in Holloway & Biley, 2011). In order to arrive at a more informed assessment of the role of paradigms in positioning qualitative research, we draw on the notion of paradigmatic frame (see

Madill & Gough, 2008; Morgan, 2007) which differentiates understandings of paradigms on a continuum of specificity and paradigm differentiation. An awareness of how different understandings of what constitutes a paradigm will allow us to give a more considered approach of how qualitative research may be positioned within nursing research and nursing science.

We have selected two exemplars of paradigms that have impacted on qualitative research—"Evidence-based practice" and "mixed methods"—paying particular attention to how specific discourses have underpinned the formation of these paradigms. The purpose of these exemplars is to illustrate how the understanding and positioning of qualitative research as a science have been sculpted by various paradigmatic formulations and practices.

Evidence-based practice

The paradigm of evidence-based practice (EBP) has become the cornerstone of contemporary health care, and is underpinned by the hierarchy of evidence model in which randomized controlled trials are explicitly prized and determine what best evidence is. Within this paradigm supported by the hierarchy of evidence, qualitative research, despite improvements to its status, still struggles to achieve the equivalent standing of its quantitative counterpart. What we wish to highlight is that the question of what constitutes evidence is still open to debate (Freshwater & Rolfe, 2004; Rolfe, 2010) and, given EBP's wide-ranging influence in terms of epistemological dominance in policy, the academy, industry and commerce, the status of qualitative nursing research as evidence cannot be eschewed.

One way of answering this question with regard to the future of qualitative research is by recourse to the conceptual map of discourse development (Cahill, 2010; Freshwater & Cahill, 2009; Freshwater, Cahill, & Essen, in press; Freshwater, Cahill et al., 2010) which has itself been derived from a conceptual map of the therapeutic relationship (Hardy, Cahill, & Barkham, 2007; Cahill et al., 2008). We wish to highlight that we understand discourse development as the formation of a relationship and posit that discourses directly underpin paradigm development. This conceptual map may be used as a heuristic device to describe how discourses of evidence are created, developed and maintained. We contend that discourses of evidence have directly underpinned and perpetuated the paradigm of evidence-based practice in which qualitative research has been delegated a secondary and subservient role.

Understanding discourse development as a relational activity is crucial for impacting the future direction of qualitative research. If we concede that paradigm development and its supporting discourses are relational activity, then we are able to unpack the processes through which the discourses surrounding evidence and the status of evidence in evidence hierarchies are established and perpetuated. This conceptual framework also allows the recipient of any given research paradigm to assume a more active stance, in so far as they can position themselves within the discourse and have an impact on its course and development. Development of this conceptual map concerns issues of knowledge generation and production; that is, epistemology. We believe it is important to cultivate an awareness of how discourses surrounding evidence are produced and perpetuated as it enables critical reflection on the validity of evidence and how such evidence is used, or indeed manipulated within policy and practice. Moreover, the ability to stand outside a research paradigm and observe its development enables one to have an impact on its direction. Using the conceptual map as a guide in the section that follows, we suggest how qualitative research has been situated within the context of an evidence-based culture and hypothesize how it might develop (Figure 32.1).

Considering the development of qualitative research with recourse to the conceptual map, we may attribute the development to external factors such as consumers (practitioners/researchers)

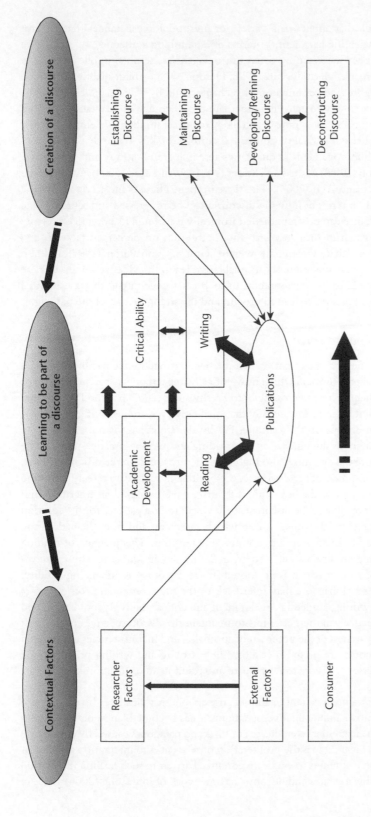

Figure 32.1 Conceptual map of discourse development

seeking meaningful research that applies to a variety of methodological stances that are not necessarily defined by the scientific paradigm. In terms of establishing a discourse of qualitative research, this has, in part, been activated by dated but nevertheless seminal publications (e.g. Denzin & Lincoln, 2005; Greenhalgh & Hurwitz, 1998; Heron, 1998) by high-quality qualitative research (of which we have provided examples in this chapter) and by a dedicated readership.

In the maintenance phase, a way to actively perpetuate the discourse of qualitative research is to ensure that research outputs are high impact and likely to attract funding. To ensure impact, it is essential to include checks on quality control. Examples of key research publications concerning methodological improvements in qualitative research are Holloway and Freshwater (2007), Koch and Harrington (1998), Manias and Street (2001), Whitehead (2004), Whittemore et al. (2001) and Freshwater and Avis (2004). The development phase is most critical for the future of qualitative research in terms of how the discourse can be progressed and refined. One of the ways in which a discourse can be strengthened ironically is through its potential to create and provoke dissonance, which in turn serves to focus attention on perceived factures and anomalies stimulating further debate which adds weight. Gournay and Ritter (1997) and also Griffiths (2005) have in their reactive responses to qualitative research evidence served to raise its profile and subsequently add to its development. In such cases we contend that these initial points of dissonance have the potential to lead to growth and the strengthening of the paradigm.

Paradigm of mixed methods research

Next we turn to the mixed methods paradigm, which has been birthed by the paradigm wars of quantitative and qualitative approaches and which now critically impacts on its "parent" paradigm of qualitative research. It is helpful here to cross-refer to Freshwater's (2007) postmodern critique of the discourse as this has implications for the way that qualitative research is configured vis-à-vis mixed methods research designs. In this critique, Freshwater's emphasis is not so much on the content of the mixed methods discourse as in the reading and writing practices that, while they have served to perpetuate the discourse, also highlight fracture points in the discourse. First, Freshwater deals with the consumers of the discourse, the health and social care researchers, who in their eagerness to become part of the academic discourse, have displayed an uncritical and unquestioning stance in their reading of the discourse, believing it to be a panacea for the solution of the unsolvable, interpreting the discourse as one which integrates and fuses dialectical and opposing paradigms as a way of overcoming uncomfortable tensions. This practice of reading the discourse has, according to Freshwater, led to a flatness in its quest for unity across methodological approaches, a unity which is promoted in the discourse as enhancing validity. With recourse to the conceptual map, we may refer back to the four components of *learning to be part of a discourse*: reading, writing, academic development and critical ability. It could be argued that reading and writing practices, in their attempts to maintain the discourse, have lost sight of critical ability, a reflexive awareness of the potential of anomalies and inconsistencies as potential building blocks for the discourse of mixed methods. Such reading and writing practices will ultimately stymie the discourse they serve to perpetuate and result in an ossification of academic development.

Freshwater points to a particularly salient example, an example that illustrates how in its aim to innovatively mix quantitative and qualitative paradigms it has become bland due to its focus on integration and fusion, in an attempt to eradicate conflicts and paradoxes caused by conflicting methodological approaches. First, there is the proliferation of references to integration and fusion in mixed methods research and attempts to eradicate potential barriers to such healing integration (Bryman, 2007, 2008). Freshwater cites and deconstructs the work of Johnstone (2004) who, in her quest to promote her work in the health sciences as an exemplar of integration, actually presents a protocol for mixed methods research that emerges as bland through its efforts to remove contradictions and is uncritical in its unquestioning application of works of other authors on integration, such as Creswell's (1994) five reasons for integrating mixed methods research. Second, there is the trend in mixed methods research of pinning down its internal and competing components in order to present a coherent and comprehensive map of the area. Creswell notes this tension in his (2009) editorial on mapping the field of mixed methods research: while recognizing that a mapping exercise may be interpreted as an attempt to fix the field and provide a template to which new components must be assimilated, Creswell also argues that the map is simply the beginning of a conversation rather than an attempt to impose determinacy. Similarly in assessing the impact of these paradigms on qualitative research as a "Science," we too are wishing to contribute to the conversation through writing, research and practice.

Conclusion

In this chapter we have reviewed the state of the science of qualitative nursing research in England, Wales and Scotland and in doing so we have also attempted to deconstruct popularly held concepts of Science. We began this chapter by providing a brief historical overview of nursing research in England, Wales and Scotland, against which we critically reviewed the significance of qualitative nursing research. Based on our scoping review of qualitative nursing research in the three nations, we tabled the most frequent methods used in these countries by nurse researcher, outlining the specific contributions of the methods to the nursing profession as a whole. We identified three centers of excellence focusing on qualitative research currently operating in these countries, which we supplemented with our narrative overview of their profiles. Finally, we reflected on the future direction for qualitative nursing research in these countries, closing the chapter with a deconstruction of the concept of Science as it impacts on qualitative nursing research.

References

Benson, A., Secker, J., Balfe, E., Lipsedge, M., Robinson, S., & Walker, J. (2003). Discourses of blame: Accounting for aggression and violence on an acute mental health inpatient unit. *Social Science & Medicine*, *57*(5), 917–926.

Brown, J., & Addington-Hall, J. (2008). How people with motor neurone disease talk about living with their illness: A narrative study. *Journal of Advanced Nursing, 62*(2), 200–208. doi: 10.1111/j.1365-2648.2007.04588.x.

Bryman, A. (2007). Barriers to integrating quantitative and qualitative research. *Journal of Mixed Methods Research, 1*(1), 8–22. doi: 10.1177/2345678906290531.

Bryman, A. (2008). *Social research methods* (3rd ed.). Oxford: University Press.

Cahill, J. (2010). Clinically representative research: An emerging paradigm. Unpublished doctoral thesis, University of Leeds.

Cahill, J., Barkham, M., Hardy, G., Gilbody, S., Richards, D., Bower, P., et al. (2008). A review and critical appraisal of measures of therapist–patient interactions in mental health settings. *Health Technology Assessment, 12*(24), iii–x.

Carter, B. (2004). Pain narratives and narrative practitioners: A way of working "in-relation" with children experiencing pain. *Journal of Nursing Management, 12*(3), 210–216. doi: 10.1046/j.1365-2834.2003.00440.x.

Clarke, C. L., Gibb, C. E., Keady, J., Luce, A., Wilkinson, H., Williams, L., & Cook, A. (2009). Risk management dilemmas in dementia care: An organizational survey in three UK countries. *International Journal of Older People in Nursing, 4*(2), 89–96. doi: 10.1111/j.1748-3743.2008.00149.x.

Clarke, C., Luce, A., Gibb, C., Williams, L., & Cook, A. (2004). Contemporary risk management in dementia: An organizational survey of practices and inclusion of people with dementia. *Signpost, 9*(1), 27–31.

Clinical Effectiveness and Evaluation Unit. (2002). *National Sentinel audit of stroke, 2001/2*. Report for site code 175. Prepared on behalf of the Intercollegiate Stroke Group by Clinical Effectiveness and Evaluation Unit. London: Royal College of Physicians.

Clinical Effectiveness and Evaluation Unit. (2004). *National Sentinel audit of stroke, 2004*. Report for site code 230. Prepared on behalf of the Intercollegiate Stroke Group by Clinical Effectiveness and Evaluation Unit. London: Royal College of Physicians.

Clinical Effectiveness and Evaluation Unit. (2006). *National Sentinel audit of stroke, 2006*. Report for site code 230. Prepared on behalf of the Intercollegiate Stroke Group by Clinical Effectiveness and Evaluation Unit. London: Royal College of Physicians.

Cloherty, M., Alexander, J., & Holloway, I. (2004). Supplementing breast-fed babies in the UK to protect their mothers from tiredness or distress [Research Support, Non-US Government]. *Midwifery, 20*(2), 194–204. doi: 10.1016/j.midw.2003.09.002.

Creswell, J. W. (1994). *Research design: Qualitative and quantitative approaches*. Thousand Oaks, CA: Sage.

Creswell, J. W. (2009). Mapping the field of mixed methods research. *Journal of Mixed Methods Research, 3*(2), 95–108.

Davies, J., Lester, C., O'Neill, M., & Williams, G. (2008). Sustainable participation in regular exercise amongst older people: Developing an action research approach. *Health Education Journal, 67*(1), 45–55. doi: 10.1177/0017896907086157.

Denzin, N. K., & Lincoln, Y. S (Eds.). (2005). *The SAGE handbook of qualitative research* (3rd ed.). Thousand Oaks, CA: Sage.

Department of Health. (1993). *Report of the Taskforce on the strategy for research in nursing, midwifery and health visiting*. London: Department of Health.

Department of Health. (2006). *Modernising nursing careers: Setting the direction*. London: Department of Health.

Department of Health and Social Security. (1972). *Report of the Committee on Nursing*. London: HMSO.

Fenwick, S., Holloway, I., & Alexander, J. (2009). Achieving normality: The key to status passage to motherhood after a caesarean section [Research Support, Non-US Government]. *Midwifery, 25*(5), 554–563. doi: 10.1016/j.midw.2007.10.002.

Fitzpatrick, N., & Finlay, L. (2008). "Frustrating disability": The lived experience of coping with the rehabilitation phase following flexor tendon surgery. *International Journal of Qualitative Studies in Health and Well-being, 3*(3), 143–154. doi: http://dx.doi.org/10.1080/17482620802130407.

Freshwater, D. (2007). Reading mixed methods research contexts for criticism. *Journal of Mixed Methods Research, 1*(2), 134–146. doi: 10.1177/1558689806298578.

Freshwater, D., & Avis, M. (2004). Analyzing interpretation and reinterpreting analysis: Exploring the logic of critical reflection. *Nursing Philosophy, 5*(1), 4–11. doi: 10.1111/j.1466-769X.2004.00151.x.

Freshwater, D., Cahill, J., Walsh, E., & Muncey, T. (2010). Qualitative research as evidence: Criteria for rigour and relevance. *Journal of Research in Nursing, 15*(6), 497–508. doi: http://dx.doi.org/10.1177/1744987110385278.

Freshwater, D., & Cahill, J. (2009). Practice of mixed methodologies in mental health nursing research. In 5th International Mixed Methods Conference, Harrogate, UK, 8–10 July 2009.

Freshwater, D., Cahill, J., & Essen, C. (in press). Narratives of collaborative failure: Identity, role, and discourse in an interdisciplinary world. *Nursing Inquiry*.

Freshwater, D., & Rolfe, G. (2004). *Deconstructing evidence based practice*. London: Taylor & Francis.

Fudge, N., Wolfe, C. D., & McKevitt, C. (2008). Assessing the promise of user involvement in health service development: ethnographic study [Research Support, Non-US Government]. *British Medical Journal, 336*(7639), 313–317. doi: 10.1136/bmj.39456.552257.BE.

Gass, J. (2008). Electroconvulsive therapy and the work of mental health nurses: A grounded theory study. *International Journal of Nursing Studies, 45*(2), 191–202. doi: 10.1016/j.ijnurstu.2006.08.011.

Gournay, K., & Ritter, S. (1997). What future for research in mental health nursing? *Journal of Psychiatric Mental Health Nursing, 4*(6), 441–442; discussion 443–446.

Greenhalgh, T., & Hurwitz, B. (1998). *Narrative based medicine*. London: BMJ Books.

Griffiths, P. (2005). Evidence-based practice: A deconstruction and postmodern critique: Book review article. *International Journal of Nursing Studies, 42*(3), 355–361. doi: 10.1016/j.ijnurstu.2004.11.004.

Hardy, G., Cahill, J., & Barkham, B. (2007). Active ingredients of the therapeutic relationship that promote client change: A research perspective. In P. Gilbert & R. L. Leahy (Eds.), *The therapeutic relationship in the cognitive behavioral psychotherapies*. New York: Routledge.

Heron, J. (1998). *Sacred science: Person centred inquiry into the spiritual and the subtle*. Ross on Wye: PCCS Books.

Higher Education Statistics Agency. (2005). *Developing the best research professionals. Qualified graduate nurses:*

Recommendations for preparing and supporting clinical academic nurses of the future. London: UK Clinical Research Collaboration.

Holloway, I., & Biley, F. C. (2011). Being a qualitative researcher. *Qualitative Health Research, 21*(7), 968–975. doi: 10.1177/1049732310395607.

Holloway, I., & Freshwater, D. (2007). *Narrative research in nursing*. Oxford: Blackwell Publishing.

Holloway, I., Sofaer-Bennett, B., & Walker, J. (2007). The stigmatisation of people with chronic back pain. *Disability and Rehabilitation, 29*(18), 1456–1464. doi: 10.1080/09638280601107260.

Holloway, I., & Wheeler, S. (2010). *Qualitative research in nursing and healthcare* (3rd ed.). Oxford: Wiley-Blackwell.

Hui, A., & Stickley, T. (2007). Mental health policy and mental health service user perspectives on involvement: A discourse analysis. *Journal of Advanced Nursing, 59*(4), 416–426. doi: 10.1111/j.1365-2648.2007.04341.x.

Hunt, J. (1981). Indicators for nursing practice: The use of research findings. *Journal of Advanced Nursing, 6*(3), 189–194.

Johnstone, P. L. (2004). Mixed methods, mixed methodology health services research in practice [Research Support, Non-US Government]. *Qualitative Health Research, 14*(2), 259–271. doi: 10.1177/1049732303260610.

Jones, K. (2006). A biographic researcher in pursuit of an aesthetic: The use of arts-based (re)presentations in "performative" dissemination of life stories. *Qualitative Sociology Review, 2*(1), 66–85.

Keen, S., & Todres, L. (2007). Strategies for dissemination of qualitative research findings: Three exemplars. *Forum: Qualitative Social Research, 8*(3), Art. 17. Retrieved from http://nbn-resolving.de/urn:de:0114-fqs0703174.

Kilbride, C. (2007). Inside the Black Box: Creating excellence in stroke care through a community of practice. Unpublished doctoral thesis, City University, London.

Kirby, S. (2004). A historical perspective on the contrasting experiences of nurses as research subjects and research activists. *International Journal of Nursing Practice, 10*(6), 272–279.

Koch, T., & Harrington, A. (1998). Reconceptualizing rigour: The case for reflexivity. *Journal of Advanced Nursing, 28*(4), 882–890.

Kuhn, T. S. (1962). Historical structure of scientific discovery. *Science, 136*(3518), 760–764.

Madill, A., & Gough, B. (2008). Qualitative research and its place in psychological science. *Psychological Methods, 13*(3), 254–271. doi: 10.1037/A0013220.

Manias, E., & Street, A. (2001). Rethinking ethnography: Reconstructing nursing relationships [Research Support, Non-US Government]. *Journal of Advanced Nursing, 33*(2), 234–242.

Mantzoukas, S. (2008). A review of evidence-based practice, nursing research and reflection: Levelling the hierarchy. *Journal of Clinical Nursing, 17*(2), 214–223. doi: 10.1111/j.1365-2702.2006.01912.x.

McHoul, A., & Grace, W. (1995). *A Foucault primer: Discourse, power and the subject*. Melbourne: Melbourne University Press.

Morgan, D. (2007). Paradigms lost and pragmatism regained. *Journal of Mixed Methods Research, 1*(1), 48–76. doi: 10.1177/2345678906292462.

Morse, J. M. (2012). Introducing the first Global Congress for Qualitative Health Research: What are we? What will we do—and why? *Qualitative Health Research, 22*(2), 147–156. doi: http://dx.doi.org/10.1177/1049732311422707.

Moule, P., & Goodman, M. (2009). *Nursing research: An introduction*. London: Sage.

Muncey, T. (2010). Review: Conceding and concealing judgment in termination of pregnancy: A grounded theory study. *Journal of Research in Nursing, 15*(4), 379–380.

Muncey, T., & Robinson, R. (2007). Extinguishing the voices: Living with the ghost of the disenfranchised. *Journal of Psychiatric and Mental Health Nursing, 14*(1), 79–84.

Newell, C. (2008). *Recovery in anorexia nervosa*. Bournemouth: Bournemouth University.

Rafferty, A., Bond, S., & Traynor, M. (2003). Does nursing, midwifery and health visiting need a research council? *Nursing Times Research, 5*(5), 325–335.

Rolfe, G. (2010). Back to the future: Challenging hard science approaches to care. In T. Warne & S. McAndrew (Eds.), *Creative approaches to health and social care education*. Basingstoke: Palgrave.

Thomas, E. (1985). Attitudes towards nursing research among trained nurses. *Nurse Education Today, 5*(1), 18–21.

Todres, L. (2007). *Embodied enquiry: Phenomenological touchstones for research, psychotherapy and spirituality*. Basingstoke: Palgrave Macmillan.

Todres, L., Fulbrook, P., & Albarran, J. (2000). On the receiving end: A hermeneutic-phenomenological analysis of a patient's struggle to cope while going through intensive care. *Nursing in Critical Care*, 5(6), 277–287.

United Kingdom Central Council. (1986). *Project 2000: A new preparation for practice.* London: United Kingdom Central Council for Nursing, Midwifery and Health Visiting.

Walshe, C., Chew-Graham, C., Todd, C., & Caress, A. (2008). What influences referrals within community palliative care services? A qualitative case study. *Social Science & Medicine*, 67(1), 137–146. doi: 10.1016/j.socscimed.2008.03.027.

Warren, J., Holloway, I., & Smith, P. (2000). Fitting in: Maintaining a sense of self during hospitalization. *International Journal of Nursing Studies*, 37(3), 229–235.

Webb, C., & MacKenzie, J. (1993). Where are we now? Research-mindedness in the 1990s. *Journal of Clinical Nursing*, 2, 129–133.

Whitehead, L. (2004). Enhancing the quality of hermeneutic research: Decision trail. *Journal of Advanced Nursing*, 45(5), 512–518.

Whittemore, R., Chase, S. K., & Mandle, C. L. (2001). Validity in qualitative research. *Qualitative Health Research*, 11(4), 522–537.

33

Qualitative nursing research in Ireland

An overview of the journey to date

Carolyn L. Tobin

Introduction

This chapter includes an overview of qualitative nursing and midwifery research undertaken in the Irish Republic over the past 20 years. The Republic of Ireland includes the 26 counties of Ireland and does not include the six counties of Northern Ireland which are governed by the United Kingdom. It is worth noting that midwifery is considered a distinct discipline in Ireland and it is therefore necessary to include it as a separate search in order to capture midwifery research in the literature review of qualitative nursing and midwifery research undertaken in Ireland over the past 20 years, which is included in this chapter. Nursing research in Ireland is still comparatively new, with little nursing research activity evident in the country prior to the early 1990s. However, pioneers of nursing research worked hard to establish nursing inquiry from the 1970s and saw the fruition of their vision in the development and rapid growth of nursing research production over the past 15 years. Despite the impact of the global recession on Ireland, Irish nursing research is well placed to contribute to nursing science in the coming decades.

In order to understand the journey Irish qualitative nursing research has taken, this chapter provides an overview of the history of Irish nursing research, describing the fundamental innovations that have provided the building blocks for the increased research productivity evident in the past 15 years. A literature review of qualitative nursing research over that time was undertaken as the basis for the discussion of research productivity, trends and focus over the past 15 years. Exemplars of some of the work undertaken in Ireland are provided, and the chapter concludes with a view towards the future of Irish qualitative nursing research.

An overview of the history of qualitative nursing research in Ireland

Sources suggest that during the 1970s and 1980s there was little nursing and midwifery research activity occurring in the Irish Republic (Condell, 2004; McCarthy, Savage, & Lehane, 2006). The Irish Nursing Research Interest Group (INRIG) was formed in 1976 with the aim of facilitating the discussion and dissemination of research findings. The activities of INRIG are credited with promoting research awareness and encouraging early research activity through guidance, supervision and financial support and as such it was the forerunner to the far-reaching restructuring that resulted from the Commission on Nursing (Government of Ireland, 1998).

McCarthy and Lehane (2004) provide a history of INRIG from its inception in 1976 to its dissolution in 2004 and suggest that INRIG's focus in its latter years on policy development and lobbying for the importance of nursing research to the future of Irish nursing education and practice included several submissions to key committees concerned with the development of Irish nursing. These included submissions to the Irish Nursing Board: An Bord Altranais, *The Future of Nurse Education and Training in Ireland* (An Bord Altranais, 1994), the *Report of the Commission on Nursing* (Government of Ireland, 1998) and *A Research Strategy for Nursing and Midwifery in Ireland* (Department of Health and Children, 2003). The vision of the group to promote nursing research and evidence-based practice provided the context and background for the diverse and widespread nursing and midwifery research production and utilization that are currently enjoyed by Irish nurses and midwives (McCarthy & Lehane, 2004). Therefore, the work of INRIG provided a framework for the development of the contemporary nursing and midwifery profession in Ireland that is situated within a context of nursing knowledge production, dissemination, evaluation and application to practice. Other key institutions credited with fostering research awareness and development during this period are the Irish Nursing Board, An Bord Altranais, and two academic institutions that provided advanced education opportunities to nurses, primarily in the preparation of nurse teachers, the Royal College of Surgeons in Ireland and the Department of Nursing at University College Dublin (Treacy & Hyde, 1999). While the period from the late 1970s to mid-1990s was a time of sparse research production in Ireland (Condell, 2004), the past 15 years have been unprecedented in terms of the increase in the production of quality nursing and midwifery research that has occurred there (Condell, 2008). This increase in research production can be understood in terms of the broader changes to the structure of nurse education that occurred in the same time frame.

Fundamental changes to the structure of nurse education and practice emanated from the Report of Commission on Nursing (Government of Ireland, 1998). As a result of this comprehensive consultative process with key stakeholders in nursing and midwifery research, practice and education, several innovations paved the way for the professional development of nursing and midwifery in Ireland. Among the most radical changes was the proposed transfer of nurse education to university or higher level education, with entry to the nursing profession in Ireland via a four-year honors degree program. The formation of a National Council for the Professional Development of Nursing and Midwifery (NCPDNM) was also proposed along with clinical career pathways for advanced clinical specialists, and nurse and midwife practitioners were developed, and these roles had an explicit research agenda (Condell, 2004). The nursing policy division of the Department of Health and Children was also charged with drawing up a national strategy for nursing and midwifery research (Government of Ireland, 1998). Another significant development was the establishment of nursing and midwifery clinical research fellowships within the structure of the existing Irish Health Research Board. While the process of securing research fellowships was highly competitive, these fellowships offered nurses an opportunity to study at doctoral level on a fully funded basis, which was crucially important as the mean age of doctoral students who received Health Research Board (HRB) funding in years 1999–2008 was 39 years (Condell, 2008). This funding provided the possibility of undertaking doctoral level research for individuals with financial responsibilities. The transfer to university-level education was put into effect in 2002 for general nurse education, followed by post-registration education in midwifery and children's nursing in 2006. The effect of this transfer was far-reaching as nurse educators now had access and in many cases were required to undertake doctoral-level education in order to attain career progression. Integration into academic institutions provided new career paths for nurses within academia, where scholarship and research activity were valued and rewarded. Nursing students were benefiting from research education at undergraduate level, and opportunities for further studies at Master's, MPhil and doctoral levels were fast developing within the context of the academy. Qualified nurses already on the register also had the opportunity to complete their bachelor's degree as government funding was made available for them to complete their education to honors degree level.

The publication in 2003 of *A Research Strategy for Nursing and Midwifery in Ireland 2003–2008* (Department of Health and Children, 2003) marked the drive towards consolidation of research activity with a goal of capacity building and focused research that would propel the future of nursing and midwifery research and practice in Ireland. The strategy outlined 21 recommendations to this end. These included a research and development for health division, within the Health Research Board and the appointment of nursing research advisor which was a joint appointment between the Health Research Board and the National Council for the Professional Development of Nursing and Midwifery. The explicit role of the nursing research advisor was to focus on building research capacity for nursing and midwifery research while ensuring that nursing had a voice and an executive function within the broader health research community (Condell, 2008). During this time, the NCPDNM also undertook a national baseline survey of research activity in Irish nursing and midwifery, the findings of which were published in a report (National Council for the Professional Development of Nursing and Midwifery, 2006). This report outlined the increased research productivity of nursing and midwifery researchers in Ireland but highlighted that much work was "fragmented, uncoordinated and under-reported" (p. 9).

When the *Research Strategy for Nursing and Midwifery in Ireland 2003–2008: Review of Attainments* (Condell, 2008) was published, Ireland was still experiencing an economic growth period. Funding for nursing and midwifery research had increased and the nursing research advisor reported that 19 of the 21 recommendations made in the initial report had been met or were in progress (Condell, 2008). In 2009, the year the decline in the Irish economy began to take hold, the Department of Health published its *Action Plan for Health Research, 2009–2013* (Department of Health and Children, 2009), which highlighted the value of health research as central to the broader national socioeconomic goals. The Health Research Board's *Strategic Business Plan, 2010–2014: The Future of Irish Research* (Health Research Board, 2010), also reiterated the importance of continued support for health research; however, the report also acknowledged that funding had been reduced overall by 16% since 2008 and was falling further behind the Organisation for Economic Co-operation and Development (OECD) average.

Review of the literature on qualitative Irish nursing and midwifery research

A literature review was conducted in order to gain an accurate picture of the qualitative nursing and midwifery research that has been undertaken in Ireland over the past 20 years. Databases used to access qualitative work included CINAHL and Medline. Key words used included "nursing," "midwifery," "qualitative," "research," "Ireland," and "Irish." Only original qualitative or mixed methods studies published in international peer-reviewed journals in the previous 20 years (1992–2012) were included. Studies had to be undertaken by Irish nurse or midwife researchers either as principal investigator or part of the research team. Nursing and midwifery qualifications of authors and stated affiliations to academic or health care institutions in the Irish Republic were required. A detailed search of Irish nursing and midwifery academic institution websites was also undertaken to ensure an accurate picture of qualitative research activity in Ireland was represented. A total of 510 full text articles were retrieved, of which 216 met the inclusion criteria. This work spanned the years 1996 to 2012. Although references were found for a small number of qualitative studies that preceded this, full text of the articles could not be

439

accessed as the Irish journals in which these articles were published were no longer in production and the relevant articles were not readily accessible online. Articles were read and data entered into an Excel spreadsheet, including the full reference, details of funding, sample size, nursing discipline, for example, mental health, midwifery, etc., number of authors, research approach used, for example, grounded theory, phenomenology, aim and purpose of the study, the research focus; identifying the specific clinical issue, education or professional nursing issues, and key findings. Data were then analyzed using descriptive statistics to identify trends in Irish qualitative nursing and midwifery research over the past 16 years.

Qualitative research output

Just one published qualitative study was included from this search in 1996 and was undertaken by Hyde (1996), entitled "Unmarried pregnant women's accounts of their contraceptive practices: a qualitative analysis." The study used a descriptive qualitative approach with a sample group of 51 women and findings included seven categories constructed from the data to capture the ways in which the women became pregnant, namely "fertility denial," "destiny dependence," "progressive remissness," "occasional or intermittent risk-taking," "calculated risk-taking," "proactive fertility management," and "contraceptive failure or misuse." There were no qualitative studies accessed for 1997 and a further one was located for 1998 again by Hyde (1998) entitled "Single pregnant women's encounters in public: changing norms or performing roles." A grounded theory approach was used to gather and analyze data. The sample group was 51 women, and findings from the study suggested that

> while dominant public discourses on non-marital childbearing within the culture were negative (albeit challenged) at the time data were being collected, responses from others whom participants interacted with in verbal face to face encounters in public were generally (though certainly not exclusively) experienced as positive in tone.
>
> *(p. 84)*

In concurrence with the preceding discussion, research activity in Ireland began to increase in the mid- to late 1990s, but the real explosion in research activity did not occur until after nurse education was transferred into third-level (university-level) institutions in 2002, followed by midwifery and children's nursing in 2006. Data from this search reveal a steady increase of research outputs from 1999 onwards. A total of five published qualitative studies were retrieved from that year, three of which were funded. In 2001, this increased to double that with 10 published studies, 4 of which were funded, and by 2007 this number had tripled to 30 studies, 12 of which were funded. Qualitative research outputs then appear to have stabilized with published research productivity continuing through 2011 at the mid- to upper 20s per year, achieving 30 published studies for years 2007 and 2008. The upward trend in productivity then dipped in 2009 to 24 published studies. This slight reversal in research output may have been due to the fact that the global recession hit Ireland badly in 2009, with subsequent far-reaching effects on every aspect of Irish economic life (O'Connor, 2010). The impact can also be seen on funding opportunities, for while research productivity increased sharply from 2005 to 2011 the ratio of research funding did not improve in tandem with research output (Figure 33.1). However, the overall trend of Irish qualitative nursing research toward increased productivity, despite the challenges of a global recession, is in keeping with international trends (Polit & Beck, 2009).

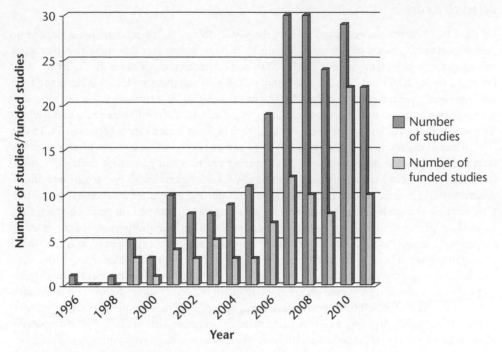

Figure 33.1 Research output and funding

Working in research teams

All studies undertaken from 1996 to 2000 that were accessed in this review appear to have been conducted by single research investigators. From 2000 onwards, the trend of working in research teams began to emerge. This trend was first evident in the work of Murphy et al. (2000) in a study entitled "The Roper, Logan and Tierney (1996) model: perceptions and operationalization of the model in psychiatric nursing within a health board in Ireland." The study aimed to determine whether the Roper, Logan and Tierney model was an appropriate model for planning nursing care for clients with mental illness. It had a sample group of 20 participants, and a research team of six. It was found that there was little evidence that the Roper, Logan and Tierney model guided care planning and that goals and nursing interventions were frequently not explicitly documented. The second multi-author study published that year was Hyde et al. (2000), entitled "Young people's perceptions of and experiences with drugs: Findings from an Irish study." The aim of the study was to determine Irish children's perceptions and experiences in relation to illicit drugs as they approached adolescence. Findings suggested that most participants had a high level of exposure to a drug culture, yet had little direct experiences with actually being offered or using drugs. Most children who participated in the study expressed anti-drug attitudes. The sample included 78 children and there were seven investigators. Both studies used a descriptive design and both were externally funded. This trend toward team-based research continues, along with the trend toward multi-authored studies being more successful at gaining funding, trends which again are in line with other international findings (Polit & Beck, 2009). Fifty of the 216 studies included here were conducted by research teams of 4–10, of which 50% were funded studies, as compared to the 39% funded in the total number of studies included in the review, suggesting that studies that have four or more in the research team are more likely to be funded.

Research focus

Of the 216 studies included in the review, the vast majority, at 106 studies, were focused on professional nursing issues or education (Figure 33.2). This finding is consistent with earlier work carried out nationally (Higgins & Farrelly, 2007) and internationally (Polit & Beck, 2009). Both Polit and Beck (2009) and Higgins and Farrelly (2007) discuss this trend, highlighting the term "endogenous" research that was coined by Traynor et al. (2001) and refers to researchers focusing on their own profession as opposed to conducting clinically focused research, a trend which Traynor et al. argued is more prevalent in nurses than in other health care professions. This trend is born out in the results of this review, but perhaps may also be understood in terms of the far-reaching, radical changes occurring in Irish nursing practice and education during this time. Research on professional nursing and education was undertaken by all five major disciplines, general nursing, mental health, midwifery, children's nursing and intellectual disability nursing. Care of the older adult and palliative/oncology nursing also accounted for research specifically focused on professional nursing practice and education. The aim and purpose of the research focused on a broad range of topics that reflected the changes being experienced in Irish nursing during that time. These were predominantly related to the move into higher level education and all the changes that emerged as a result of that, but also the demands of Ireland as a new multicultural society that had an impact on every discipline of nursing. Inquiry focused on issues such as the evaluation of new curricula, research capacity building, and scope of practice, cultural awareness and sensitivity; also, evaluating new roles, for example, that of clinical practice coordinator, student preceptors' experiences, students' experiences of university education, and faculty experiences of becoming academics with all the concomitant expectations that transition involved.

The remaining 110 studies were fairly evenly divided between the main nursing disciplines. General nursing, which is the largest discipline, had a total of 23 studies on a wide variety of clinically focused topics, such as cardiac care, diabetes, emergency and intensive care, infection prevention, sexual health, stroke care and women's health. Twenty-three studies focused on children's nursing. Mental health and midwifery both had 13 studies published in this time, while intellectual disability nursing had the smallest number of qualitative studies published at two.

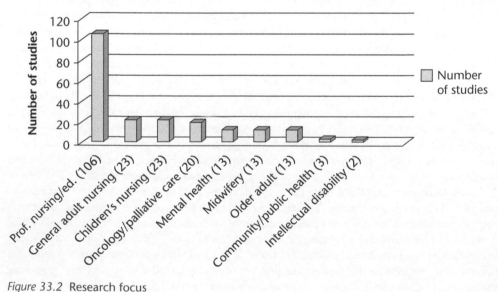

Figure 33.2 Research focus

Oncology and care of the older adult, while not distinct nursing disciplines, produced impressive numbers of qualitative studies relative to the overall findings, with oncology and palliative care being second only to general nursing in terms of productivity with 20 studies, and care of the older adult producing 13 studies. Community and public health nursing had three qualitative studies included.

Trends in research design

The most commonly occurring research designs were descriptive (132), mixed methods (36), grounded theory (22), and phenomenology (20); much less common, ethnography was used three times, with action research, person-centred research and discourse analysis all being used just once (Figure 33.3).

Descriptive research designs were by far the most common, being used in 61% of studies, across all nursing disciplines. The descriptive design was more likely to be adopted by larger research teams of four or more. It was the approach adopted in 72% of the multi-authored studies. Although not always explicitly stated, it appears that more complex research designs are employed primarily in doctoral studies, with non-doctoral work accounting for more of the descriptive designs. This may be due to the demands for more complex theoretical work to be demonstrated at doctoral level along with the expectations of a more innovative approach to the subject under inquiry.

Mixed methods studies comprised the second largest group at 17%. Mixed method studies were carried out across the disciplines. The predominant combination of mixed method design appeared to be combinations of quantitative data collection, usually a survey, combined with a descriptive qualitative approach, usually follow-up interviews with a subset of the sample from the larger study.

Grounded theory and phenomenology were the two other most commonly used designs. Grounded theory accounted for 10% of the published studies. Grounded theory was employed in professional nursing issues, mental health, midwifery, general and children's nursing research. Of the 22 studies that used grounded theory, 36% were funded studies, of which 88% were

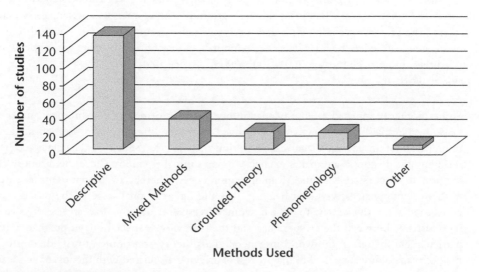

Figure 33.3 Research approach

doctoral studies. Phenomenology was the design of choice in 9% of included studies, of which 45% were funded. It was not possible to determine how many of these were doctoral studies. Phenomenology appears to have been used from the very early work in Irish research and continues to be a popular research design as indicated by current trends. There were six studies that were categorized as "other." These included three ethnographic studies, one that was described as a person-centered approach and one utilizing discourse analysis.

Exemplars of work undertaken

The body of qualitative work represented in this review covers a wide variety of topics relevant to different nursing disciplines, practice, and education. All have contributed to the development of nursing and midwifery knowledge in unique and innovative ways, however, due to space and time limitations it is not feasible to provide an overview of individual studies. In this section, however, I want to offer exemplars of studies that employed the three most common qualitative research designs.

In a study funded by the Irish Health Research Board as part of their Clinical Nursing and Midwifery Fellowships, Lalor, Begley and Galavan (2009) explored 41 women's experiences of ultrasound diagnosis of fetal abnormality up to and beyond the birth in the Republic of Ireland, using a grounded theory design. Lalor et al. argued that while ultrasound had revolutionized the management of pregnancy and its possible complications, little consideration had been given to the psychosocial consequences of mass screening resulting in fetal anomaly detection in low-risk populations, particularly in contexts where termination of pregnancy services are not readily accessible, such as the Irish Republic. From the sample group, 31 women chose to continue the pregnancy and ten women accessed termination of pregnancy services outside the Republic. Researchers collected data from repeated in-depth individual interviews pre- and post-birth and analyzed transcripts using the constant comparative method. Using Glaser's (1978) classic approach to grounded theory, researchers explored women's experiences in relation to the following: being informed that their baby had an abnormality, concerns that emerged as the pregnancy continued and the birth approached, and key issues that emerged following the birth up to 12 weeks postnatal, whether or not the woman had a live baby. Researchers constructed a theoretical framework of "Recasting Hope," grounded in women's experiences, which represented the process of coping with and surviving such a traumatic event. Four sub-core variables were identified each with a linear and temporal construction, in keeping with the classic grounded theory approach (Glaser, 2001, 2003, 2005) (Figure 33.4).

Lalor et al. stated:

> Some mothers expressed a sense of incredulity when informed of the anomaly and the "Assume Normal" phase provides an improved understanding as to why women remain unprepared for an adverse diagnosis. Transition to phase 2, "Shock", is characterized by receiving the diagnosis and makes explicit women's initial reactions. Once the diagnosis is confirmed, a process of "Gaining Meaning" commences, whereby an attempt to make sense of this ostensibly negative event begins. "Rebuilding", the final stage in the process, is concerned with the extent to which women recover from the loss and resolve the inconsistency between their experience and their previous expectations of pregnancy in particular and beliefs in the world in general. This theory contributed to the theoretical field of thanatology as applied to the process of grieving associated with the loss of an ideal child. The framework of Recasting Hope was intended for use as a tool to assist health

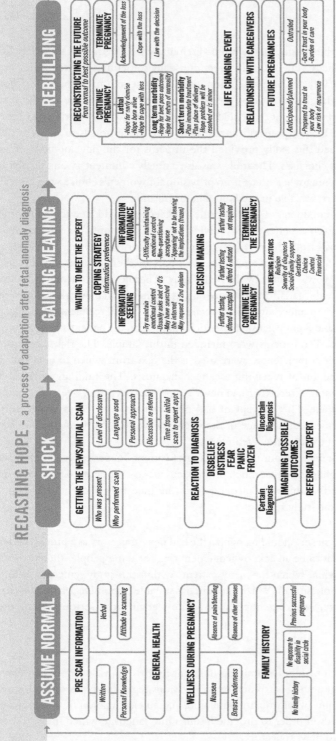

RECASTING HOPE – a process of adaptation after fetal anomaly diagnosis

ASSUME NORMAL

PRE SCAN INFORMATION
- Written
- Verbal
- Personal Knowledge
- Attitude to scanning

GENERAL HEALTH

WELLNESS DURING PREGNANCY
- Nausea
- Breast Tenderness
- Absence of pain/bleeding
- Absence of other illnesses

FAMILY HISTORY
- No family history
- No exposure to disability in social circle
- Previous successful pregnancy

SHOCK

GETTING THE NEWS/INITIAL SCAN
- Who was present
- Who performed scan
- Level of disclosure
- Language used
- Personal approach
- Discussion re referral
- Time from initial scan to expert appt

REACTION TO DIAGNOSIS
- DISBELIEF
- DISTRESS
- FEAR
- PANIC
- FROZEN

IMAGINING POSSIBLE OUTCOMES
- Certain Diagnosis
- Uncertain Diagnosis

REFERRAL TO EXPERT

GAINING MEANING

WAITING TO MEET THE EXPERT

COPING STRATEGY
information preference

INFORMATION SEEKING
- Try maintain emotional control
- Usually asks alot of Q's
- May have searched the internet
- May request a 2nd opinion

INFORMATION AVOIDANCE
- Difficulty maintaining emotional control
- Non-questioning acceptance
- 'Appearing' not to be hearing the implications (frozen)

DECISION MAKING
- Further testing offered & accepted
- Further testing offered & refused
- Further testing not required

CONTINUE THE PREGNANCY

TERMINATE THE PREGNANCY

INFLUENCING FACTORS
- Religion
- Severity of diagnosis
- Social/Family support
- Gestation
- Choice
- Control
- Financial

REBUILDING

RECONSTRUCTING THE FUTURE
from normal to best possible outcome

CONTINUE PREGNANCY
- Lethal
  - Hope for early demise
  - Hope born alive
  - Hope to cope with loss
- Long term morbidity
  - Hope for best poss outcome
  - Hope for return of normality
- Short term morbidity
  - Plan immediate treatment
  - Hope problem will be resolved or is minor

TERMINATE PREGNANCY
- Acknowledgement of the loss
- Cope with the decision
- Live with the decision

LIFE CHANGING EVENT

RELATIONSHIP WITH CAREGIVERS

FUTURE PREGNANCIES
- Anticipated/planned
  - Prepared for trust in your body
  - Low risk of recurrence
- Outruled
  - Don't trust in your body
  - Burden of care

WOMAN CENTRED SUPPORTIVE INTERVENTION

- Availability and content of scan information leaflet
- Focus on normality
- Option to access additional information ie websites
- Individual discussion re risk
- Space on reverse of leaflet to write questions for discussion at next appointment

- Written information on the specific condition for the parents and can be utilised to inform family members
- Set up link support person
- Honesty regarding the initial diagnosis
- Set ideal and maximum time frame from initial scan to referral
- Acknowledgement of personal impact of diagnosis/the loss of the healthy baby that was hoped for
- Contact number for health professional for support and opportunity to ask further questions before planned visit

- Continuity of caregiver
- Recognise and match information with preference
  INFORMATION SEEKING
- Guide and support with multiple information sources ie discuss scientific literature, websites & referral to other experts
  INFORMATION AVOIDANCE
- Allow the woman to 'opt-in' to information ie provide written information that they can read when they are ready
- Midwife role (home visits)
- Planning antenatal visits
- Planning ahead (packing bag/info re birth/funeral)
- Planning place of birth

- Plan of care for remainder of pregnancy and birth
- Plan neonatal care if survival is likely
- Postnatal examination and consultation
  outstanding test results given
- appropriate risk assessment for future pregnancies
  referral for genetic counselling if appropriate
  pre pregnancy counselling
- Assessment of emotional wellbeing
- Acknowledgement of experience
- Support groups
- Ongoing access to designated 'link support' person and also to provide access to support in future pregnancies

Figure 33.4 Recasting hope

Source: Reprinted with permission from Lalor et al. (2009), p. 466.

professionals through offering simple yet effective interventions grounded in women's experiences of this event.

(2009, p. 462)

This work provided an invaluable insight for the multi-disciplinary team caring for women who are diagnosed with a fetal anomaly. The anomaly screen is usually something women anticipate with excitement seeing it primarily as a happy occasion where they get to "meet their baby" for the first time. Lalor et al. highlight the lack of preparedness most women have for the first ultrasound scan as a major screening event that could possibly have negative consequences. The work also brings to light the lack of preparation of health care professionals to manage the situations optimally, and indeed this study provided the impetus for the development of an education program for relevant clinicians. The study was also a timely commentary on the ethical ramifications of providing screening where there is no provision for women's choice with respect to termination of the pregnancy available in the Republic of Ireland.

Tobin and Begley (2008) conducted a study entitled "Receiving bad news: a phenomenological exploration of the lived experience of receiving a cancer diagnosis," which explored the impact of a cancer diagnosis from the perspectives of the patient, nurse, and doctor. The study was funded by the Irish Health Research Board as part of their clinical nursing and midwifery fellowships. The study was guided by the philosophy of hermeneutic phenomenology, and used an application of a Heideggerian and Gadamerian hermeneutic framework. Data were collected via unstructured in-depth interviews, with a total sample of 38 (10 recipients of a cancer diagnosis, 20 registered nurses and 8 physicians). This article focused on the patient's perspectives of receiving a cancer diagnosis. Ten patients were included in this sample. The rich, phenomenological data, viewed in their completeness, were used as the text from which to develop an interpretation of the phenomenon of receiving a cancer diagnosis. The findings offered an interpretation of the phenomenon of receiving bad news as a process occurring over a period of time rather than a one-off event. The concept of bad news was interpreted as a trajectory represented through three themes: "disturbance of the everyday world," "surfacing within the lived world," and "embodiment within the lived world."

The contribution this study made to our understanding of patients' experiences of receiving a cancer diagnosis included highlighting that much of the focus was on the actual delivery of the diagnosis, without cognizance that this was but one part in the trajectory of bad news. Tobin and Begley (2008) argue that the study findings

suggest that nurses and physicians should recognize the bad news trajectory as a process rather than an event. There needs to be an acknowledgement that for some people, there exists a period of suspected-knowing, which for many patients within this study, emerged before contact with healthcare professionals. What is required is suitable responsive techniques that balance managing anxiety, ensuring hope, and acknowledging the seriousness of the recipients' concerns.

(p. 38)

Suggestions for further research includes examining different models of disclosure of bad news across and within differing care settings, exploration of decisions regarding types of disclosure, timing of disclosure, and amounts of information disclosed, and an examination of the language used by health care professionals in order to provide insights into language which may assist or hinder the recipient on the bad news trajectory.

In a multi-disciplinary and multi-center collaboration, Mac Neela, Scott, Treacy and Hyde (2007) explored mental health nurses' use of psychological language in practice. Entitled "Lost in translation, or true text: mental health nursing representations of psychology," the inquiry focused on exploring the ways in which psychological knowledge influenced practitioners' talk about their nursing practice. This article focused on a secondary analysis of data undertaken by the research team in a larger study which was funded by the Irish Health Research Board as part of its research program in nursing decision-making, and was carried out to identify the nursing contribution to care. The aim of this secondary analysis of transcripts was to identify and analyze how nurses talk about psychological concepts and techniques. The current debate within mental health nursing around models of care, with the divergent views between the traditional and dominant biomedical model "psychiatric nursing," and the psychosocial model of "mental health" nursing provided the impetus for this inquiry. Researchers conducted 10 focus groups, involving 59 mental health nurses to explore the relationship between mental health nursing and psychology, as they argued psychological concepts are a key to the psychosocial model of mental health nursing and an intrinsic part of mental health nursing practice. Questions posed to focus groups included, "How do nurses conceptualize care?" "What problems do clients present with?" "How do nurses perceive their contribution to care?" and "How do nurses organize their care?" Formal psychological terms were identified in the transcripts and followed by a close re-reading of the transcripts to identify references to psychological concepts or techniques. The extracts related to psychological work were clustered in themes and linked to three categories. These were analyzed in relation to literature on nursing empowerment and representation of knowledge within a social context. Researchers found that psychological talk was organized into three categories: "psychological concepts" which related directly to psychological work with clients, from which two sub-categories emerged: "psychological phenomena" and "attributable causes." Another category of organizational context was seen as a contextual category affecting all of the psychological work performed by the participants (Figure 33.5).

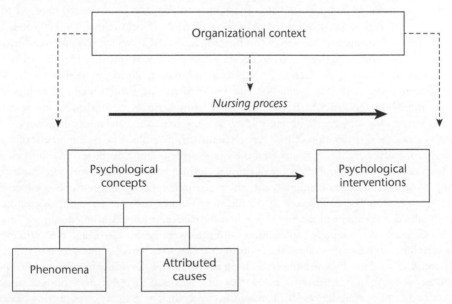

Figure 33.5 Interrelationship of proposed categories

Source: Reprinted with permssion from Mac Neela et al. (2007), p. 503.

Authors argued that empowerment perspectives help to explain the patterns found in the use of psychological knowledge by nurses. Discussion emphasized the ambiguity nurses expressed toward psychological knowledge, seeing it partly as the language of oppression where it represented a disempowering influence, as nurses associated it with the formal rule-based system. The less formal "everyday" language used by nurses was conceptualized as a form of resistance, leading to a separate form of clinical knowledge for everyday decision-making. In this way nurses used a combination of formal psychological concepts and informal explanations to describe patient problems and nursing care. Mac Neela et al. (2007) argued that this conflict was indicative of the disempowerment and invisibility of nurses' contribution and suggested that nurses' appropriate psychological language and use it to support and explain nursing knowledge, utilizing it as a tool for articulating formal nursing discourse with a potential empowering influence. The value of this work in making mental health nursing visible, while revealing a potentially inhibiting ambivalence toward psychological concepts, is of importance to mental health nurses as they strive to establish an alternate psychosocial model of mental health nursing that more comprehensively describes the unique contribution mental health nurses make to the health and well-being of their clients. It is also interesting in that it highlights issues that resonate with other nursing disciplines in Ireland, for example, midwifery and intellectual disability nursing as those disciplines strive to embrace viable alternatives to the biomedical model of care.

Future of Irish qualitative research

The global recession has undoubtedly affected the production of nursing research in Ireland as funding has been significantly reduced as part of the overall austerity measures experienced in the country (Department of Health and Children, 2009), The Irish Nurses and Midwives Act 2011 was signed into legislation on December 21, 2011. The full scope of changes that will proceed from this new legislation is yet to be seen, however, as of January 1, 2012 Parts 1, 2, and 12 of the Act had been signed into effect. Part 2 of the Act requires that all nurses and midwives demonstrate continued competency. The details of how this is to be measured have yet to be worked out, and Part 12 pertained to the dissolution of the National Council for the Professional Development of Nursing and Midwifery (An Bord Alranais, 2012), which was subsumed into the Nursing Board as part of the rationalization of state agencies (Department of Health, 2010).

However, Irish nursing research is firmly placed on building blocks put in place by the work of the Commission on Nursing, the National Council for the Professional Development of Nursing and Midwifery, and An Bord Altranais. Nursing is firmly established within academia and is growing at a fast pace. With entry-level nursing established at honors degree level, the emergence of a new generation of Irish nurse scientists is possible. The establishment of career pathways for nurses within academia, and the options for integration of research into clinical roles with advanced nurse and midwife practitioner appointments, together with a graduate-level nursing workforce, ensures continued growth in research capacity and research productivity. However, we cannot be complacent, as the future growth of Irish nurse research is contingent upon sustained investment in nursing research and practice, with a continued journey toward raising awareness of the unique contribution nurses make to health care outcomes. While Irish nurse researchers have always valued the contribution that qualitative methods have to offer, the global trend toward funding quantitative nursing research, and the utility and benefits of multi-disciplinary work must be balanced to ensure that future Irish nurse researchers continue to value the production of nursing knowledge that informs both the art and science of nursing practice. Despite these challenges Irish nurse researchers are poised to make a significant contribution to the production of nursing and midwifery knowledge in the twenty-first century and beyond.

References

An Bord Altranais. (1994). *The future of nurse education and training in Ireland*. Dublin: An Bord Altranais.

An Bord Altranais. (2012). Nurses and Midwives Act 2011. Available at: http://www.nursingboard.ie/en/nurses-midwives-act-2011.aspx.

Condell, S.L. (2004). Journeying to professionalism: The case of Irish nursing and midwifery research. *International Journal of Nursing Practice, 10*(4), 145–149. Retrieved from http://search.ebscohost.com/login.aspx?direct=true&db=rzh&AN=2004206484&site=ehost-live.

Condell, S.L. (2008). *Research strategy for nursing and midwifery in Ireland, 2003–2008: Review of attainments*. Dublin: Children, DOHA.

Department of Health. (2010). Nurses and Midwives Bill 2010: A further step in assuring patient safety and modernises the regulation of nursing and midwifery professions. Retrieved from http://www.dohc.ie/press/releases/2010/20100422.html.

Department of Health and Children. (2003). *A research strategy for nursing and midwifery in Ireland*. Dublin: Children, DOHA.

Department of Health and Children. (2009). *Action plan for health research, 2009–13*. Dublin: Children, DOHA.

Glaser, B. (1978). *Theoretical sensitivity*. Mill Valley, CA: Sociology Press.

Glaser, B. (2001). *The grounded theory perspective: Conceptualization constrasted with description*. Mill Valley, CA: Sociology Press.

Glaser, B. (2003). *The grounded theory perspective II: Descriptions remodeling of grounded theory methodology*. Mill Valley, CA: Sociology Press.

Glaser, B. (2005). *The grounded theory perspective III: Theoretical coding*. Mill Valley, CA: Sociology Press.

Government of Ireland. (1998). *Report of the Commission on Nursing: A blueprint for the future*. Dublin: The Stationery Office.

Health Research Board. (2010). *Strategic business plan, 2010–2014: The future of Irish research*. Dublin: Health Research Board.

Higgins, A., & Farrelly, M. (2007). Peer-reviewed publication output of psychiatric nurses in the Republic of Ireland. *Journal of Psychiatric & Mental Health Nursing, 14*(5), 495–502. Retrieved from http://search.ebscohost.com/login.aspx?direct=true&db=rzh&AN=2009640833&site=ehost-live.

Hyde, A. (1996). Unmarried pregnant women's accounts of their contraceptive practices: A qualitative analysis. *Irish Journal of Sociology, 6*, 179–211.

Hyde, A. (1998). Single pregnant women's encounters in public: Changing norms or performing roles. *Irish Journal of Applied Social Sciences, 2*(2), 84–105.

Hyde, A., Treacy, M., Whitaker, T., Abaunza, P. S., & Knox, B. (2000). Young people's perceptions of and experiences with drugs: Findings from an Irish study. *Health Education Journal, 59*, 180–188.

Lalor, J., Begley, C. M., & Galavan, E. (2009). Recasting hope: A process of adaptation following fetal anomaly diagnosis. *Social Science and Medicine, 68*, 462–472.

Mac Neela, P. M., Scott, P. A., Treacy, M. P., & Hyde, A. (2007). Lost in translation, or the true text: Mental health nursing representations of psychology. *Qualitative Health Research, 17*(4), 501–509. Retrieved from http://search.ebscohost.com/login.aspx?direct=true&db=rzh&AN=2009558211&site=ehost-live.

Mccarthy, G., & Lehane, E. (2004). *The history of the Irish Nursing Research Interest Group (INRIG), 1976–2004*. Dublin: INRIG.

Mccarthy, G., Savage, E., & Lehane, E. (2006). Research priorities for nursing and midwifery in Southern Ireland. *International Nursing Review, 53*(2), 123–128. Retrieved from: http://search.ebscohost.com/login.aspx?direct=true&db=rzh&AN=2009212500&site=ehost-live.

Murphy, K., Cooney, A., Cooney, D., Connor, M., O'Connor, J., & Dineen, B. (2000). The Roper, Logan and Tierney (1996) model: Perceptions and operationalization of the model in psychiatric nursing within a health board in Ireland. *Journal of Advanced Nursing, 31*(6), 1333–1341.

National Council for the Professional Development of Nursing and Midwifery. (2006). *Report on the baseline survey of research activity in Irish nursing and midwifery*. Dublin: Midwifery, NCFTPDONA.

O'Connor, T. (2010). The structural failure of Irish economic development and employment policy. *Irish Journal of Public Policy, 2*(1). Retrieved from http://publish.ucc.ie/ijpp/2010/01/tomoconnor/03/en.

Polit, D. F., & Beck, C. T. (2009). International differences in nursing research, 2005–2006. *Journal of Nursing Scholarship, 41*(1), 44–53. Retrieved from http://search.ebscohost.com/login.aspx?direct=true&db=rzh&AN=2010284366&site=ehost-live.

Tobin, G. A., & Begley, C. (2008). Receiving bad news: A phenomenological exploration of the lived experience of receiving a cancer diagnosis. *Cancer Nursing, 31*(5), E31–9. Retrieved from http://search.ebscohost.com/login.aspx?direct=true&db=rzh&AN=2010030262&site=ehost-live.

Traynor, M., Rafferty, A. M,. & Lewison, G. (2001). Endogenous and exogenous research? Findings from a bibliometric study of UK nursing research. *Journal of Advanced Nursing, 34*(2), 212–222. Retrieved from: http://search.ebscohost.com/login.aspx?direct=true&db=rzh&AN=2001066184&site=ehost-live.

Treacy, M., & Hyde, A. (1999). *Nursing research design and practice*. Dublin: University College Dublin Press.

34

Qualitative nursing research in Canada

State of the science

Joan M. Anderson with Sheryl Reimer-Kirkham,
Patricia Rodney, and Heather McDonald

Introduction

I am honored by Professor Cheryl Beck's invitation to write the chapter on the state of the science of qualitative nursing research in Canada. The contents of this book reflect the diverse qualitative research methodologies that have found a niche in the Canadian landscape of nursing research. A theoretical perspective informs each approach, and provides direction for action to scholars, practitioners and policy-makers in the discipline and profession of nursing. Our profession does not allow us the luxury of theorizing without action; as a practice discipline we grapple with complex issues in health, health care, human suffering and healing that intersect with the wider social, economic, political and cultural processes within our society. Indeed, a colleague of mine—a sociologist—drew my attention to a recent article by Roy Romanow (2012), the former Premier of Saskatchewan and Commissioner on the Future of Health Care in Canada. Romanow reminds us of the narrative of this nation—one of a "shared destiny" and organizing collectively around shared values—but he is concerned that

> In recent years . . . the soil has been tilled for the sprouting of views at odds with this narrative. We now feel a palpable momentum toward individualism, decentralization, and privatization . . . all sorts of dubious and unfair policies are being inflicted on Canadians . . . that . . . often . . . ignore the difference between equality and equity; policies that pretend there is a level playing field in Canada in terms of access to opportunity, and that those who are disadvantaged . . . are solely responsible for their own fate. As though living on the margins, or suffering from poor health, mental illness or addiction is somehow a conscious lifestyle choice.
>
> *(Romanow, 2012, pp. 1, 6)*

One might ask, "What does qualitative research have to do with this?" My reply—"A great deal!"

Qualitative research, as I understand it, is a descriptive, interpretive, and analytic science. Some genres of qualitative research, underpinned by critical theoretical perspectives, require that we question that which is taken-for-granted, including the theories that are often taken as "the facts" in the practice of nursing. The methods some of us employ in our science direct us to examine the context of individual lives and experiences, and the issues that Romanow so eloquently documents, and engage in dialogue about how we might collectively address them. At the same time, the narrative of the Canadian nation as a "shared destiny," and organizing collectively around shared values should be contested, as it unwittingly erases the history of the colonization of Indigenous peoples in Canada, a history that has shaped their health (Anderson & Reimer-Kirkham, 1998) An understanding of this history and its consequences should be at the very core of nursing practice, research and policy.

Nursing scholars in this country have been—and remain—powerful voices not only in the practice and policy domains, but also in the direction of health research at the local and national levels. As I have argued elsewhere:

> The giant steps forward within the fairly short time span of 10 years [2000–2010] have been made possible, in part, by the synergies created through the resources that became available to the nursing research community, enhanced research training, interdisciplinary collaboration, and a climate that has fostered the communication of nursing research. One of the milestones in Canadian health research has been the launching of the Canadian Institutes of Health Research (CIHR) in the year 2000.
>
> *(Anderson, 2009, p. 47)*

It is within this climate that qualitative research developed in Canada. As we reflect on our history, we can take pride in knowing that nurses were among the architects in the new transformative arrangement for conducting health research in Canada, and brought to the table the multiple ways in which research can be conducted. Qualitative research had to be interpreted to those skeptical of this science, but sound and convincing arguments paved the way for a thriving qualitative, well-funded, nursing research community in Canada. As we look to the future, we know that the scholars who are now taking the leadership in qualitative research will face many challenges as they engage with the pressing issues in health and health care in Canada and globally. Not least among these challenges are the inequities in health of different population groups, such as the Indigenous peoples in Canada; and the widening income disparities between rich and poor. Furthermore, as Bottorff and her colleagues (2011), who are Fellows of the Canadian Academy of Health Sciences, have pointed out, we now face challenges to research funding. To ensure the success of the next generation of researchers in nursing "we require a national strategy that will bolster training and career opportunities" (p. 14). Despite the multiple challenges we face, there will be opportunities to share nursing knowledge to address the issues of equity, ethics and social justice, which have underpinned the research discourse in nursing in this country. Other disciplines now look to nursing for leadership not only in qualitative research, but also in the discourse on ethics and social justice. Indeed, nursing scholars have generated knowledge that allows them to continue to provide direction in health care ethics (see, for example, Storch, Rodney, & Starzomski, 2013). Furthermore, we have now reached the level of maturity both in the discipline of nursing and in qualitative research that many of us no longer subscribe to the qualitative/quantitative divide. Evolving epistemologies provide a lens for seeing the world in multiple and complex ways that are complementary rather than competing, and in so doing, allow us to move into new frontiers of knowledge development in the discipline of nursing. I will have more to say about this later in the chapter.

But how did we get to this point? In this chapter, I begin by discussing *the context of the development of qualitative research* in this country. Second, I present my interpretation of the *intersecting factors influencing the development of qualitative nursing research*, using exemplars from scholars who have conducted qualitative research from different qualitative perspectives. I should stress that this is *not* meant to be a review of qualitative studies conducted in Canada—such is not the intent of this chapter. Rather, I draw on exemplars in an attempt to show the breadth of the theories and methodologies that are being used. Readers will note that I have drawn heavily on the *Canadian Journal of Nursing Research*, the oldest peer-reviewed academic nursing journal in this country. This is not the only nursing research journal in Canada, nor is it the only journal in which Canadian nurses publish their work. But this journal publishes research conducted from varied methodological perspectives, and has opened up a space for addressing issues that are central to nursing, health, and health care in Canada. Founded in the 1960s as *Nursing Papers* by Professor Moyra Allen of McGill University, and now led by Professor Laurie Gottlieb as Editor-in-Chief, this journal has provided—and continues to provide—a crucial forum for dialogue among Canadian scholars and practitioners, and is therefore an excellent resource for tracking issues within the purview of nursing, and the research methodologies that Canadian nurses have used to address them. Third, I examine *the state of the science in qualitative research in Canada*, and draw attention to some methodologies which, though finding a niche in Canada, may not have moved into the "mainstream" of the qualitative research discourse. Following this, I open up a dialogue with three nursing scholars about the future of qualitative research in Canada: Drs. Reimer-Kirkham and Rodney, both third-generation qualitative researchers, who have taken up their careers within the university, and Dr. Heather McDonald, a fourth-generation qualitative researcher, who had a third-generation qualitative researcher supervise the writing of her doctoral dissertation.[1] Dr. McDonald is now pursuing a research and policy career within Indigenous communities. These three scholars were not selected at random. As readers will see, each brings a particular perspective, which I believe will be central in the future development of qualitative research not only in Canada, but also within the international nursing community. I conclude the chapter by reflecting on some broader questions based on my experience in conducting qualitative research over the past 30 years. I add my thoughts on the future of qualitative research in Canada and beyond.

I turn now to the context of the development of qualitative research in Canada, but with a caveat! Every scholar who subscribes to critical, analytic interpretation recognizes that her positionality shapes her narrative in profound ways. I situate myself as one who has received her education in the disciplines of nursing and sociology—with ties to critical medical anthropology—an "inter-disciplinarian" perhaps, who sits in an "in-between space." As an immigrant woman from the Global South who has sought "home" in Canada, my location in the Canadian nation cannot be glossed over. This positionality has provided me with a view "from the margins" which, paradoxically, has made me more attuned to how nursing knowledge is constructed "at the centre," and by whom, in the Global North. Given my positionality, I recognize that my narrative about the development of the science of qualitative research in Canada may quite likely differ from those of other scholars. I do not see this as "a problem." Rather, I believe that this acknowledges one of the fundamental premises of a qualitative science—the primacy of interpretation, but also the obligation to show how we arrive at our interpretations.

The context of the development of qualitative research in Canada

I am privileged to have been a member of the academic community for well over 30 years, and as I look back on the challenges we faced, and the opportunities that became available, I am struck by the giant steps that have been made in the development of qualitative nursing research in this country. This is, in no small measure, due to the philosophy of nursing, and outstanding nursing leadership. Early leaders paved the way for exploring multiple methods in nursing research, including qualitative research. Professor Elizabeth Logan, an early nursing leader who joined McGill University in the 1940s, had this to say about the art, science, and practice of nursing:

> Get the information from the patient and not from a textbook . . . Open your eyes and ears . . . Don't tell but ask . . . Write what you observe or hear, think about it, and then go back and observe some more . . . Return again and again to the patient . . . Understand the context of the patient . . . Use your sciences to understand what you are seeing and hearing . . . Keep developing your knowledge . . . Nursing is nursing—it is specific to the patient—so know the context, but, more importantly, know the patient.
>
> *(French, 2010, p. 15)*

This quote reflects awareness of the importance of listening; *using one's knowledge as an interpretive framework for what one is hearing*; and, understanding that nursing knowledge is constructed within complex socio-political and economic contexts of patients' lives. As such, this quote from Professor Logan is foundational to qualitative inquiry. As researching the profession back in the 1960s (see, for example, Gilchrist, 1969) gave way to examining the kinds of questions that nurses need to investigate if they are to develop the knowledge base for nursing practice, the need to incorporate qualitative approaches into nursing science became more evident. This is not to say that nurses were not engaged in addressing clinical problems at the time. In fact, in that same issue of *Nursing Papers* (1969) in which questions about the profession were being asked, another paper appeared on nursing in chronic illness, demonstrating the ways of assisting "students to acquire depth in understanding the patient's universe" (Hooton, 1969, p. 12). Scholars at McGill University School of Nursing, including Dr. Moyra Allen, developed "A model for nursing"—a plan for research and development. Dr. Allen spoke to this model at an International Conference, "Research — A Base for the Future?" hosted by the University of Edinburgh, Department of Nursing Studies in 1981. She described the model as one that gave a full role to nursing in the health care field, stating that "The evolution and development of this model of nursing has stimulated two thrusts of inquiry, one basic nursing research and the other applied nursing research" (Allen, 1982, p. 320). Dr. Allen described the research plan and its implementation as being pursued through description, measurement, practice and evaluation.

It could be argued that "qualitative" research, in the 1960s, 1970s, and early 1980s, was viewed through a "descriptive" lens, and conceptualized on a continuum with quantitative studies. As such, it was seen as a way to begin the study of a particular phenomenon within the paradigm of quantitative research. But other perspectives were being put forward for exploring two distinctive research paradigms—qualitative and quantitative—each having different epistemological underpinnings. Quantitative studies, within this discourse, were conceptualized within a "positivist paradigm." I will return to this point later. I turn, now, to my interpretation of the intersecting factors influencing the development of a qualitative science in Canada, with exemplars of qualitative studies.

Intersecting factors influencing the development of qualitative nursing research and exemplars of qualitative studies

The realities of nursing education in Canada in the 1960s, 1970s, and 1980s created the necessity for nurses to seek doctoral education in other disciplines. With no PhD programs in nursing in this country, many early nursing scholars sought out doctoral education in the United States—some in nursing, and others in disciplines such as education, psychology, anthropology, and sociology. Those remaining in Canada pursued their doctoral education in disciplines other than nursing. The synergies created between nursing and other complementary disciplines, far from diminishing nursing, enriched it, as nurses drew on methodologies such as Glaser and Strauss' *The Discovery of Grounded Theory* (1967). Grounded theory was a milepost for qualitative nursing research not only in the United States, but also in Canada. It set the stage for a new genre of nursing research, and remains an important and widely used qualitative research method, as exemplified in the works of scholars in Canada, such as Baker and Stern (1993); King, LeBlanc, Sanguins, and Mather (2006); Wuest (2000); Wuest, Malcolm, and Merritt-Gray (2010); and Johnson, Kalaw, Lovato et al. (2004), among many others. In addition to grounded theory, the writings of Leininger (e.g., 1970), a highly respected nurse anthropologist from the United States, were influential in Canada. Along with her, scholars such as Diers (1979) opened up different ways of thinking about investigating clinical problems. As well, those nurses who sought out doctoral education in the social science disciplines in the 1970s and 1980s became exposed to the questioning of positivism as the only scientific approach to the study of the social sciences.

While many Canadian nursing scholars were by now familiar with grounded theory, the writings of social scientists such as Richard Bernstein (1978) made their way into the social sciences discourse in the 1970s and early 1980s, and became influential in nursing. Quentin Skinner (1978), in a review essay of Bernstein's book, opened his essay with a remark from the English sociologist Anthony Giddens, that "it has come to be widely agreed that 'those who still wait for a Newton' of the social sciences 'are not only waiting for a train that won't arrive, they're in the wrong station altogether'" (Skinner, 1978, p. 26). Such perspectives heightened the "paradigm" debate in nursing circles, and had a significant impact on the shaping of nursing scholarship. At the same time, the works of phenomenologists such as Alfred Schutz (1973) had an enormous influence on the social sciences, and opened up a philosophical discourse on the nature of knowledge, and questioning of the epistemic claims we make about the social production of knowledge. Nurse researchers in the United States and Canada took up phenomenology as a methodology, and still do. For example, Rose (1985) examined the responses of families to the treatment setting, and stated the objective of her study as "to elicit the families' perspectives of their experiences of mental illness and its treatment" (p. 73).

As these methodological advances progressed, the challenges of conducting qualitative research were also recognized. For example, Canadian scholar Ogden Burke (1985), in observing the major shifts and evolution "from more hard-nosed, purely quantitative approaches toward more context-embedded, qualitative methods of enquiry" (p. 69), pointed out the issues many qualitative researchers were grappling with, for example, qualitative reporting conventions. She noted that:

> For quantitative data collection and analysis, the terrain is well marked, and indeed we have developed almost a shorthand to communicate this to each other. In qualitative studies, the procedures and thought processes used must be made more explicit.
>
> *(Ogden Burke, 1985, p. 70)*

While grounded theory, phenomenology and other qualitative methods may have found fertile ground in nursing, a number of intersecting factors within Canada prompted us to respond to the issues Burke and other critics raised, and to develop qualitative research as a rigorous science. There was increasing demand for doctoral education in nursing in Canada, so that nurses could engage, through nursing research, practice and policy, with the complex issues in health and health care that we faced as a nation. The planning for and launching of research-intensive doctoral programs in nursing, and the availability of research funding for qualitative studies, opened up a new dialogue among nurse researchers in Canada, and between Canada and the

United States. Dr. Janice Morse, who was at the University of Alberta, and Director of the International Institute for Qualitative Methodology, University of Alberta, and Editor of *Qualitative Health Research*, must be given credit for her efforts in promoting a dialogue for exploring different qualitative approaches, not only through the journal *Qualitative Health Research*, but also in ongoing dialogue with scholars across the country and internationally. In the 1980s she brought several nursing scholars together—first- and second-generation qualitative researchers from both Canada and the United States—to engage with different approaches in qualitative research. This resulted in a book, *Qualitative Nursing Research: A Contemporary Dialogue* (1989, 1991). This kind of respectful dialogue contributed to rigorous qualitative inquiry in Canada, which did not privilege one methodology over the other. The book itself covered a wide range of qualitative methodologies and issues in qualitative research by scholars at various stages of career. For example, Dr. Pamela Brink, a leader in qualitative research in Canada, contributed a chapter on issues of reliability and validity (Brink, 1991).

Coupled with dialogue and collegiality among nurse researchers, and the launching of PhD programs in Canada, there was a growing awareness of the health and health care inequities among different population groups. The health and health care issues of the Indigenous peoples of this country that are rooted in Canadian history and the White Settler narrative came to the forefront. Increasing diversity of the Canadian population and a growing awareness of the health issues of different population groups, including women; an aging population and chronic illness management; health care restructuring with a focus on efficiency to address rising health care costs; and the movement to homecare management—all focused attention on the complexity of the issues that are within the domain of nursing research and practice. This all happened at a time of increasing understanding of the social determinants of health; a focus on ethics in health and health care; and a call for social justice among different groups of citizens, scholars, and practitioners. Governments were paying attention to the research on the social determinants of health. In fact, as early as the 1970s "The Lalonde Report" (Canada, 1974), *A New Perspective on the Health of Canadians* was published; and, in 1986, "The Epp Report," *Achieving Health for All* (Canada, 1986) recognized that one of the challenges we face is to find ways of *reducing health inequities* in different population groups.

All these factors coalesced to open up a new set of research questions within the profession of nursing, and an exploration of different methodologies that would be nimble enough to address them. As one looks back on different publications in the *Canadian Journal of Nursing Research*, these issues are documented, along with the methodologies used to study them. With a thriving qualitative research environment in Canada, conferences were hosted, including the Fourth Multidisciplinary Qualitative Health Research Conference in 1998. The School of Nursing at the University of British Columbia (UBC) sponsored this conference, and Dr. Joan Bottorff from the UBC School of Nursing chaired the Planning Committee.

The state of the science

The 1990s, and into the twenty-first century, saw ongoing "fine-tuning" of different qualitative methodologies. For example, distinctions were being made between different phenomenological approaches. Paterson, Tschikota, Crawford, et al.'s (1996) study on gender issues for male nursing students was "guided by the tenets of interpretive phenomenology . . . The goal of interpretive phenomenology is to reveal similarities and differences in the participants' lived experience" (p. 27). McIntyre, Anderson, and McDonald (2001) drew on hermeneutic phenomenology in their study of women's abortion experiences, and stated, "In hermeneutic phenomenology a particular phenomenon is opened up for questioning. This type of examination considers how meanings are created in and through language and why we speak, think, and act as we do" (p. 51).

Researchers continued to draw on other methodologies; among them, Participatory Action Research was used to study women with heart disease (Arthur, Wright, & Smith, 2001) as well as the quality of health care workplaces (Rodney, Doane, Storch, & Varcoe, 2006). Tiwari, Wong, and Ip (2001) used narrative inquiry to provide a cultural interpretation of Chinese women's response to battering, and Stajduhar, Martin, Barwick, and Fyles (2008) used an interpretive descriptive research design to study the factors influencing family caregivers' ability to cope with providing end-of-life cancer care at home. Johnson, Kalaw, Lovato, et al. (2004) used a grounded theory approach to study adolescents' experiences of controlling their tobacco use. Bottorff, Kelly, Oliffe, et al. (2010) also used grounded theory methods and a gender relations framework to study tobacco use patterns in traditional and shared parenting families. Gastaldo, Gooden, and Massaquoi (2005) used a qualitative poststructuralist perspective to address trans-nationalism in the intersection of migration, gender and health promotion studies. In a similar vein, Perron and Holmes (2011) used a Foucauldian perspective and poststructural ethnography to explore the ways in which forensic psychiatric nurses construct the subjectivity of mentally ill inmates; and Lynam and Cowley (2007) used Bourdieu's theory of social relations to study marginalization as a social determinant of health. Baumbusch (2010) drew on critical ethnography in a study in long-term care; and, Ronquillo, Boschma, Wong, and Quiney (2011) used oral history to explore the contexts surrounding Filipino nurse migration in Canada. Hyman, Mason, Guruge, et al. (2011) used focus groups to study the perceptions of factors contributing to intimate partner violence among Sri Lankan Tamil immigrant women in Canada; and an ethnographic approach, using observation and interview data collection methods, was used to study the connections between prostate cancer support groups and men's health literacy and consumer orientation to health services (Oliffe, Bottorff, McKenzie, et al., 2011).

Canadian scholars (e.g., Thorne, Reimer-Kirkham, & MacDonald-Emes, 1997; Thorne, Reimer-Kirkham, & O'Flynn-Magee, 2004; Thorne, 2008) continue to examine methodologies "capable of generating new insights about clinically relevant human phenomena" (Thorne, 2008, p. 17). In discussing the origins of interpretive description and how her book on the topic is organized, Thorne (2008) notes:

> Drawing thoughtfully upon some of the best analytic maneuvers that phenomenology, ethnography, grounded theory, naturalistic inquiry, and other classic approaches have to offer, [this book] attempts to illustrate how an interpretive description logic model guides researchers through the intricate sequence of study design and implementation to generate research products that hold true to their inherent limitations as well as being meaningful and applicable to disciplinary and professional audiences.
>
> *(p. 17)*

Thorne has elaborated on interpretive description in Chapter 22 in this volume.

Feminist philosophical thought and critical feminist perspectives have also been taken up by Canadian researchers in nursing, and have guided the research of scholars such as C. McDonald, McIntyre, and Merryfeather (2011) who used "Gadamerian hermeneutics as a methodology and feminist philosophical thought as an analytic framework" to explore "understandings of experiences of disclosure of sexual orientation for older 'lesbian' women" (p. 50). Other scholars such as MacDonnell (2011) explored "how a critical feminist lens was a crucial element in creating a participatory policy study which used a qualitative design and comparative life history methodology" (p. 313). Kinch and Jakubec (2004) conducted a feminist phenomenological study to explore the meaning of older women's experiences as they negotiated health care. And Ward-Griffin, Bol, and Oudshoorn's (2006) study on the perspectives of women with dementia receiving care from their adult daughters was guided by socialist-feminist theory and a life course perspective. Institutional ethnography, coined by Canadian sociologist Dorothy Smith (e.g., 1987, 1999), provided the theoretical and methodological tools to address questions germane to nursing practice. For example, Angus (2001) designed an institutional ethnography to follow the experiences of 18 women on their return home after aortocoronary bypass surgery; and Rankin (2003) used institutional ethnography to critically analyze information about "patient satisfaction" as it was generated through a patient survey.

In addition to drawing on theoretical perspectives in the European tradition, some Canadian nursing scholars have been influenced by Black feminist scholars, such as Patricia Hill Collins (1990), who have provided insights into the social construction of Black feminist thought and epistemology. This discourse has opened up a new knowledge base for teasing out the complex social relations and the intersecting oppressions that organize human experience. Collins' compelling arguments, along with scholars such as Brah and Phoenix (2004), about how the intersectionalities of gender, race, class, and other social relations work in producing inequalities have resonated well with the discourse on the social determinants of health in Canada. With increasing emphasis on health care inequities and the social determinants of health (e.g., Reutter & Kushner, 2010), and a deeper understanding of how different social relations intersect to organize the human experience of health, illness, suffering and healing (see, for example, Ponic, Reid, & Frisby, 2010; Reimer-Kirkham & Sharma, 2011; Salmon, Browne, & Peterson, 2010; Young & Higgins, 2010), a growing number of Canadian scholars have integrated an inter-sectionality paradigm into their research (e.g., Guruge & Kanlou, 2004; McPherson & McGibbon, 2010; Van Herk, Smith, & Andrew, 2011).

In a similar vein, postcolonial and Indigenous scholars have provided an understanding of the processes of colonization, and how *history* has shaped our lives. Nursing scholars have drawn on the writings of postcolonial scholars such as Said (1979, 1994), Bhabha (1994), Spivak (1999), and Gandhi (1998), among others, as they have brought subaltern voices into the nursing discourse. Homi Bhabha reminds us that:

> a range of contemporary critical theories suggest that it is from those who have suffered the sentence of history—subjugation, domination, diaspora, displacement—that we learn our most enduring lessons for living and thinking. There is even a growing conviction that the affective experience of social marginality—as it emerges in non-canonical cultural forms— transforms our critical strategies.
>
> *(Bhabha, 1994, p. 172)*

Racine (2003), a third-generation qualitative researcher, gives her interpretation of how postcolonialism can be articulated in nursing research: "Postcolonialism challenges Western science as the unique source of knowledge production and uncovers health care inequities related to gender, race, and class resulting from the process of colonization and postcolonization" (p. 95). The writings of Indigenous scholars such as Irihapeti Ramsden (1993) in New Zealand, noting that "[h]istorians will describe this period in the Pacific as post-colonial [and a] time of redefinition of identity" (p. 5), have become highly influential in Canadian nursing research. The changes in the health care system that were being called for in New Zealand resonated with the discourse among the Indigenous peoples of Canada, and nursing scholars committed to working with Indigenous communities. Tuhiwai Smith's (1999) work has outlined a decolonizing methodology which some Canadian nurse-researchers are now drawing on (see, for example,

H. McDonald, 2011). These critical approaches—Indigenous epistemologies, postcolonial epistemologies, and Black feminist epistemologies—have informed the methodological approaches in the research of scholars such as Anderson (2000, 2002); Anderson and Reimer-Kirkham (1998); Browne (2009); Browne and Smye (2002); Browne, Smye, Rodney, Tang, Mussell, and O'Neil (2011); Donnelly (2002); Guruge and Khanlou (2004); Holmes, Roy, and Perron (2008); H. McDonald (2011); Poudrier and Mac-Lean (2009); Racine (2003); Racine and Petrucka (2011); Reimer-Kirkham and Anderson (2002); Reimer-Kirkham and Browne (2006); Smye and Browne (2002); Tang and Anderson (1999); Tang and Browne (2008); Van Herk, Smith and Andrew (2011); and Varcoe (1996, 2006) among others. This angle on knowledge development has given us an historical perspective from which to produce *critical, contextual, knowledge* that can become embodied in nursing *practice, praxis,* and *policy* with *all populations,* not only those of the Global South, or people of Indigenous descent, or those who are positioned at the margins.

The above lists of studies and methodological perspectives are not meant to be exhaustive. There are many more excellent examples. Suffice to say that my reporting is a heuristic device to show the range of studies and methodological perspectives that are being taken up in Canada. I should also point out that in interpreting the perspectives of the authors whose work I have drawn on, it is not my intention to put their research into "neat categories." I recognize that some authors bring various perspectives to their work.

It is evident from the foregoing discussion that multiple approaches are being used in qualitative research in Canada. In fact, nine of the 15 Landmark Articles (reprints from the *Canadian Journal of Nursing Research*) selected for publication in the *40th Anniversary Issue 1969–2009: A Ten-Year Retrospective of the Canadian Journal of Nursing Research* (2009) used a qualitative approach; two used both qualitative and quantitative approaches. Among the qualitative methods used was the "ethnographic tradition" of qualitative research (Beagan & Ells, 2009) in which qualitative interviews were conducted with 20 nurses to explore the moral experience of nurses in their working lives. Baker, Varma, and Tanaka's (2009) use of a constructivist research paradigm allowed them to address how adolescents experience and respond to perceived racist incidents in a Canadian province. In a similar vein, Browne (2009) used an ethnographic design to examine the discourses that influence nurses' knowledge and assumptions about First Nations patients, and highlighted the need for strategies to help nurses to think more critically about the perspectives that they bring to patient care. Berman, Giron, and Marroquin (2009) used a narrative study to examine the experiences of refugee women who had experienced violence in the context of war; and Duggleby and Wright (2009) used grounded theory to describe the processes by which palliative patients live with hope. C. McDonald (2009) used interpretive inquiry, relying on Gadamerian hermeneutic and feminist philosophical thought, to generate understandings about the experience of lesbian disclosure; and Rodney, Varcoe, Storch, and their colleagues (2009) used constructivist (naturalistic) inquiry to explore the meaning of ethics, and the enactment of ethical practice. Weiss, Malone, Merighi, and Benner (2009), American contributors to this volume, used an interpretive phenomenological approach to study skill acquisition and clinical and ethical reasoning among nurses caring for critically ill patients in the United States. And Werezak and Stewart (2009) used a grounded theory approach to explore the process of learning to live with early-stage dementia. Hilton, Thompson, and Moore-Dempsey (2009) used both qualitative and quantitative methods in a participatory evaluation to describe the impact of nurses' work on an AIDS prevention street nurse program. Similarly, Miranda (2009) used both qualitative and quantitative methods to investigate the extent to which participants are willing to be randomized, and the factors that affect their treatment preferences. It is clear from examining the research that has been conducted over the past 20 or so years, that no one qualitative methodology is privileged. Various approaches are being used with scientific rigor. As demonstrated in two of the studies cited above, nurses are also using both qualitative and quantitative methods in the same study to illuminate different aspects of social reality, putting into question the "distinct" "paradigm" debate of some 30 years ago. I will say more about this later. I turn now to a dialogue with third- and fourth-generation Canadian nurse researchers—nurses who obtained their PhD degrees in Canada in the discipline of nursing, and who are among those who are mapping the terrain of qualitative nursing research in this country.

In dialogue with Drs. Reimer-Kirkham, Rodney, and McDonald

Anderson: Thank you, Sheryl, Paddy and Heather, for participating in this dialogue session. Let us start by considering the questions: How have you engaged with qualitative nursing research? And, given your understanding of the issues nurses will be addressing as they provide care to diverse client populations (along the axes of gender, race, class, sexual orientation, religion, age, and other social relations), how do you conceptualize the future of qualitative research in Canada?

Rodney: My earliest work for my Master's thesis was a small phenomenological study—this helped me to better appreciate the unique subjectivities of nurses' experiences nursing dying patients in a critical care setting, and opened up a rich view for ethical inquiry, which has informed all of my ethical work ever since. I completed a critical ethnographic study for my PhD research in order to understand nurses' enactment of their moral agency in often constraining organizational contexts, followed by two small ethnographic studies (using focus groups) to explore end-of-life policy challenges and nurses' ethical concerns across diverse practice contexts. From there I became interested in *action* to address the problems earlier studies have uncovered, and so I have embarked on co-leading programs of Participatory Action Research (PAR). I have also had the opportunity to learn from communities by serving as a co-investigator on several qualitative studies led by other colleagues related to inequities in health care for groups who have been marginalized.

Anderson: Paddy, how do you see the future of qualitative research?

Rodney: I believe that it is crucial that such research be well housed in critical paradigms of inquiry so that we can attend to widespread inequities in the resources for health and health care. Further, I believe that we need to purposefully move toward interventions through methodologies such as PAR, including subsequent policy action. We should actively involve care providers, patients, families and communities as well as administrators and policy-makers in all of our actions.

Reimer-Kirkham: Qualitative research methods have offered me an excellent *entrée* into a research program dedicated to addressing issues of equity and the negotiation of diversity in health care. The interconnectedness of globalizing societies, tied together with historical imperialisms and current-day economic systems, has researchers investigating not single foci, but rather intersecting factors that result in health and social inequities. Increasingly, we are recognizing that such complexities are best addressed through interdisciplinary teams, often employing mixed methods with democratizing, decolonizing ideals. Qualitative nurse researchers cannot operate in isolation, siloed apart from other disciplines, nor without grounding one's method in fertile theoretical or philosophic traditions. Other disciplines benefit from our "first-hand" sensibilities, particularly in relation to the embodiment of social suffering and health inequities.

McDonald: I was first exposed to the reality of multiple epistemologies and partial knowledge during my Master's education. This ground-shattering understanding was furthered during my doctoral research (employing decolonizing methodologies) as I internalized how the axiom *knowledge is power* has served to perpetuate disadvantage within Canada's Indigenous peoples. These were transformative processes. A necessary step in moving toward a more equitable Canada is to acknowledge that we all are subject to the insidious influences of (neo–)colonial discourses. Nursing science has the ability to counter popular discourses and to highlight the transformative potential of efforts to decolonize our minds. Further, research that contributes to Indigenous decolonization is needed. Such research engages Indigenous peoples and Indigenous epistemologies. This is a call to do more than include Indigenous voices; it pushes for research based on Indigenous understandings and the need for self-determination.

Anderson: Heather, how might Indigenous epistemologies inform research for all populations?

McDonald: Indigenous epistemologies have underscored the foundational link between self-determination (meaning the ability to articulate one's own reality and map one's own future) and health. Hence, any population that experiences health inequities could benefit from research that contributes to self-determination. Further, powerful societal discourses can erode the self-determination of groups through their pervasiveness. For example, Holmes, Roy, and Perron (2008) write a compelling argument about how the discourse of "evidence-based practice" has colonized and thus weakened nursing's agenda to attend to multiple sources of knowledge for our necessarily broad knowledge base for practice. In this context, decolonizing methodologies could be applied to research with nurses.

Anderson: Sheryl, you have taken up the concepts of spirituality and religion in your research. Speak to me about how you see these concepts being taken up in the future.

Reimer-Kirkham: After several decades of predicting the increasing irrelevance of spirituality and religion in both individual lives and public spheres, social commentators now name religion as one of the most salient features of society today, surpassing race/ethnicity as an organizing social classification (Modood, 2005). Nursing too is undergoing a significant shift in this regard, with the recognition that our discourses of generic spiritualities must be broadened to account for today's pluralistic societies, where citizens may be very religious, somewhat religious, or non-religious, across a full range of organized, creedal religions and emergent spiritualities (Fowler et al., 2011; Pesut et al., 2009). This shift views religion in the context of other intersecting social structures to shape individual identities and responses to health and illness, and as both oppressor and oppressed. Critical qualitative inquiry has allowed a new approach to this field of study, focusing on religion and spirituality as pathways to social exclusion and/or inclusion, and complicated by gender, imperialisms, nationalisms, and class.

Anderson: (*To everyone*) As we look to the future of nursing research in Canada, how might spirituality, ethics and social justice intersect in the social production of knowledge that can inform nursing practice, praxis and policy, and the practice/policy/research dialectic?

Rodney: I think that the first element of your questions is "should." Yes, I believe that spirituality, ethics and social justice *should* intersect in the social production of knowledge that can inform nursing practice, praxis and policy, and the practice/policy/research dialectic. The *how* is more difficult. I think that progressing forward in this manner means accepting an explicit ethical mandate in our work that is linked to social justice. And I think that we will need to engage collaborative teams to work together from various areas of expertise—for instance, using mixed methods that include various forms of qualitative and post-positivist inquiry. Further, I think that we will need to have access to policy expertise and democratic political engagement to *actualize* our goals (Rodney, Harrigan, Jiwani, et al., 2013).

Reimer-Kirkham: I suspect qualitative inquiry will continue as a popular choice for Canadian nurse researchers, not all of whom will necessarily take up critical approaches explicitly orientated toward social justice. I am optimistic about the widening international influence of contemporary trends in Canadian nursing research that clearly align knowledge production with emancipatory ends. As one resource for such efforts, religions and spiritualities may contribute to the moral grounding and fortitude that will be required to sustain momentum toward these ends (Fowler & Reimer-Kirkham, 2011).

McDonald: Today's health and health care issues are not neutral. They are embedded in complex power arrangements, reproduced through dominant discourses and persistent social structures that benefit some more than others. Improvements in health and health care require knowledge that can reset the power balance between social groups in the areas of policy, practice and research. Such knowledge is produced using an explicitly ethical methodology that is underpinned by an awareness of how tightly woven and complex is the web that shapes knowledge, health and movement towards social justice. Indeed, the "how" of knowledge production must move to a position of central importance in order to shift towards a healthier Canadian society.

Anderson: My thanks to you, Sheryl, Paddy and Heather, for participating in this dialogue.

Reflections and conclusion

Three scholars who are among those setting the agenda for nursing research in Canada give a similar message: all recognize the complex intersections that result in health and health care inequities; the need for theories and research methodologies to address them; and the need for ongoing interdisciplinary dialogue. Nursing's contribution to this interdisciplinary discourse enriches the body of knowledge and methodologies that scholars from other disciplines draw on.

Earlier in the chapter I questioned whether the current use by some researchers of qualitative and quantitative methods in the same study would put into question the "distinct" "paradigm" debate of some 30 years ago. The notion, prevalent in the 1980s, that quantitative research was "positivist" and qualitative research was not, sidestepped the issue that qualitative research can be positivist if the intent is to treat findings as value-free "facts" (see for example, Breda in Chapter 17 in this volume). I would now argue that quantitative methods used critically and interpretively, might well represent a "flight from positivism." For example, in a recent article by Canadian researchers Bungay, Halpin, Halpin, et al. (2012) in which "129 Canadian-born and immigrant women's experiences of violence and associated structural and interpersonal factors within indoor commercial sex venues" (p. 262) were examined and contrasted, both qualitative and quantitative methods were used not only to highlight women's experiencing of violence, but also the structural inequalities that organized women's experiences. As we discuss issues of social inequalities and health inequities in Canada and in other parts of the world, it would seem that quantitative measures are also needed to underscore these inequalities. This does not negate a rigorous critical analysis, for example, a postcolonial or feminist analysis (see, for example, Reimer-Kirkham & Anderson, 2010) to tease out the genesis of such inequalities, and to show how they are expressed in people's everyday lives. In fact, drawing on actual numbers helps us to more fully explicate the contrasts between different social groups (for example, income disparities), and how these disparities influence health outcomes. So, the paradigm debate should not simply be about whether we draw on numerical or narrative data in our studies, but rather the *epistemological underpinnings* of our research and the lens through which our data are interpreted, recognizing that different kinds of data illuminate different aspects of social reality.

Those of us engaged in critical scholarship (e.g., postcolonial scholarship, feminist scholarship, and other critical perspectives) may well see the work we do as "critical inquiry" which embraces both quantitative and qualitative methods, as we grapple with the complex issues that people who seek nursing care confront in their everyday lives. But whether or not we wish to embrace a mode of inquiry that is inclusive of qualitative and quantitative methods, what is clear from looking back over the past 20 to 30 years is that rigorous qualitative nursing research and good science are thriving in Canada; scholars are employing innovative approaches to engage with different research questions to address the complex issues in nursing and health care at the level of practice, praxis and policy. Partnerships and collaborations among community partners, researchers, clinicians, and policy-makers, now so evident in nursing research, mean that nurses are not doing research "on" people, but in partnership "with" them (see, for example, Varcoe, Brown, Calam, et al., 2011).

Although ontologies and epistemologies located within the dominant European tradition remain center-stage in our theorizing about methodologies and methods, there is a discernible shift in the nursing research discourse in this country to include ontologies and epistemologies grounded in the voices of Indigenous peoples, those of the Global South, and the subaltern within our society. As we engage with the participants in our research studies, and listen to their narratives, what we learn from them often opens up new ways of understanding the context of suffering, and why people who seek health care make the decisions they do. We now recognize that including people from different communities as participants in our research studies, and then analyzing our data through lenses derived solely from European perspectives, disregards the systems of knowledge of those who are not part of these traditions. Therefore, "inclusion" deserves no less than positioning our work in the ontologies and epistemologies that reflect different ways of being-in-the-world and the histories that have shaped different lives. Such inclusion is imperative as we address issues of equity and social justice in nursing not only as discourse, but also as praxis and practice. The shift to a more inclusive discourse in nursing will gain ground, I think, through the recognition of the genesis of inequities in health and health care, and the will to grapple with the dialectics of neo-colonial processes as we embrace the decolonization of the mind as an ongoing project for all of us.

Note

1   In tracing the history of the development of qualitative research in Canada, I have used the terms first-, second-, third- and fourth-generation qualitative researchers. I see the first generation as including scholars such as Dr. Moyra Allen and Professor Elizabeth Logan who were both at McGill University; Professor Helen Elfert at McGill, and then at UBC; Dr. Peggy Ann Field and Dr. Pamela Brink, both from the University of Alberta. They were among the prominent scholars in Canada in the 1960s, 1970s, and early 1980s, who laid the groundwork for qualitative research, and mentored second-generation researchers such as myself. Drs. Reimer-Kirkham and Rodney could be seen as third-generation, and Dr. McDonald fourth-generation qualitative researchers, who obtained their PhD degrees in nursing in Canada.

Acknowledgments

I thank Dr. Cheryl Beck for inviting me to write this chapter. I also thank Drs. Sheryl Reimer-Kirkham, Patricia Rodney and Heather McDonald, who are among the scholars charting the course of qualitative research in this country, for entering into a dialogue about the future of qualitative research in Canada, and for commenting on the chapter.

To the authors whose works I have cited, I recognize that I may have interpreted your work in ways that you may not have anticipated, even though I tried to remain true to what I think you intended. Furthermore, it is not my intent to position your research into "neat categories," as some authors bring various perspectives to their work.

I should also stress that this is *not* meant to be a review of qualitative studies conducted in Canada—such is not the intent of this chapter. Rather, I draw on exemplars in an attempt to show the breadth of the theories and methodologies that have been taken up in this country over the past 20 or so years.

References

Allen, M. (1982). A model of nursing: A plan for research and development. In *"Research—A Base for the Future?" International Conference Proceedings* (pp. 315–330), University of Edinburgh: Nursing Studies Research Unit.

Anderson, J. M. (2000). Gender, "race," poverty, health and discourses of health reform in the context of globalization: A postcolonial feminist perspective in policy research. *Nursing Inquiry, 7*, 220–229.

Anderson, J. M. (2002). Toward a post-colonial feminist methodology in nursing research: Exploring the convergence of post-colonial and black feminist scholarship. *Nurse Researcher: The International Journal of Research Methodology in Nursing and Health Care, 9*(3), 7–27.

Anderson, J. M. (2009). Discourse: Looking back, looking forward: Conceptual and methodological trends in nursing research in Canada over the past decade. *Canadian Journal of Nursing Research, 41*(1), 47–55.

Anderson, J. M., & Reimer-Kirkham, S. (1998). Constructing nation: The gendering and racializing of the Canadian health care system. In V. Strong-Boag, S. Grace, A. Eisenberg, & J. Anderson (Eds.), *Painting the maple: Essays on race, gender, and the construction of Canada* (pp. 242–261). Vancouver: UBC Press.

Angus, J. (2001). The material and social predicaments of home: Women's experiences after aortocoronary bypass surgery. *Canadian Journal of Nursing Research, 33*(2), 27–42.

Arthur, H. M., Wright, D. M., & Smith, K. M. (2001). Women and heart disease: The treatment may end but the suffering continues. *Canadian Journal of Nursing Research, 33*(3), 17–19.

Baker, C., & Stern, P. N. (1993). Finding meaning in chronic illness as the key to self-care. *Canadian Journal of Nursing Research, 25*(2), 23–36.

Baker, C., Varma, M., & Tanaka, C. (2009). Sticks and stones: Racism as experienced by adolescents in New Brunswick. *Canadian Journal of Nursing Research, 41*(1), 108–126.

Baumbusch. J. (2010). Conducting critical ethnography in long-term residential care. *Journal of Advanced Nursing, 67*(1), 184–192.

Beagan, B., & Ells, C. (2009).Values that matter, barriers that interfere: The struggle of Canadian nurses to enact their values. *Canadian Journal of Nursing Research, 41*(1), 86–107.

Berman, H., Giron, E. R. I., & Marroquin, A. P. (2009). A narrative study of refugee women who have experienced violence in the context of war. *Canadian Journal of Nursing Research, 41*(1), 144–165.

Bernstein, R. (1978). *The restructuring of social and political theory*. Philadelphia, PA: University of Pennsylvania Press.

Bhabha, H. (1994). *The location of culture*. London: Routledge.

Bottorff, J., DiCenso, A., Doran, D., Estabrooks, C., Johnson, J., Johnson, C., et al. (2011). Commentary: Does nursing research have a future? *Canadian Nurse, 107*(4), 14.

Bottorff, J., Kelly, M. T., Oliffe, J., Johnson, J., Greaves. L., & Chan, A. (2010). Tobacco use patterns in traditional and shared parenting families: A gender perspective. *BMC Public Health, 10*, 239. Retrieved from http://www.ncbi.nlm.nih.gov/pmc/articles/PMC2881096/?tool=pubmed.

Brah, A., & Phoenix, A. (2004). Ain't I a woman? Revisiting intersectionality. *Journal of International Women's Studies, 5*(3), 75–86.

Brink, P. (1991). Issues of reliability and validity. In J. M. Morse (Ed.), *Qualitative nursing research: A contemporary dialogue* (pp. 164–186). Newbury Park, CA: Sage.

Browne, A. J. (2009). Discourses influencing nurses' perceptions of First Nations women. *Canadian Journal of Nursing Research, 41*(1), 166–191.

Browne, A. J., & Smye, V. (2002). A post-colonial analysis of health care discourses addressing Aboriginal women. *Nurse Researcher: The International Journal of Research Methodology in Nursing and Health Care, 9*(3), 28–41.

Browne, A. J., Smye, V. L., Rodney, P., Tang, S. Y., Mussell, B., & O'Neil, J. (2011). Access to primary care from the perspective of Aboriginal patients at an urban emergency department. *Qualitative Health Research, 21*(3), 333–348.

Bungay, V., Halpin, M., Halpin, P., Johnson, C., & Patrick, D. M. (2012). Violence in the massage parlor industry: Experiences of Canadian-born and immigrant women. *Health Care for Women International, 33*(3), 262–284.

Canada, Government of Canada (1974). *A new perspective on the health of Canadians: A working document, Marc Lalonde, Minister of National Health and Welfare*. R.B.W: Owen Sound—02KXH1011- P-4081. Ottawa.

Canada, Health and Welfare Canada (1986). *Achieving health for all: A framework for health promotion: The Honourable Jake Epp Minister of National Health and Welfare, Minister of Supply and Services*. Ottawa.

Collins, P. H. (1990). *Black feminist thought: Knowledge, consciousness and the politics of empowerment*. Cambridge, MA: Unwin Hyman.

Diers, D. (1979). *Research in nursing practice*. Philadelphia, PA: J. P. Lippincott Company.

Donnelly, T. T. (2002). Representing "Others": Avoiding the reproduction of unequal social relations in research. *Nurse Researcher: The International Journal of Research Methodology in Nursing and Health Care*, *9*(3), 57–67.

Duggleby, W., & Wright, K. (2009). Transforming hope: How elderly palliative patients live with hope. *Canadian Journal of Nursing Research*, *41*(1), 204–217.

Fowler, M., & Reimer-Kirkham, S. (2011). Religious ethics, religious social ethics, and nursing. In M. Fowler, S. Reimer-Kirkham, R. Sawatzky, & E. Johnston Taylor (Eds.), *Religion, religious ethics, and nursing* (pp. 27–60). New York: Springer.

Fowler, M., Reimer-Kirkham, S., Sawatzky, R., & Johnston Taylor, E. (Eds.). (2011). *Religion, religious ethics, and nursing*. New York: Springer.

French, S. (Autumn 2010). Elizabeth Logan: Spotlight on an illustrious career (pp. 15–17). *McGill in Focus: Nursing Building on Strengths: An Annual Publication for the McGill School of Nursing Alumnae Community*. McGill School of Nursing, Montreal.

Gandhi, L (1998). *Postcolonial theory: A critical introduction*. New York: Columbia University Press.

Gastaldo, D., Gooden, A., & Massaquoi, N. (2005). Transnational health promotion: Social well-being across borders and immigrant women's subjectivities. *Wagadu*, *2*, 1–16.

Gilchrist, J. (1969). Profession or union: Who will call the shots? *Nursing Papers* [now the *Canadian Journal of Nursing Research*], *1*(2), 4–10.

Glaser, B. G., & Strauss, A. L. (1967). *The discovery of grounded theory*. New York: Aldine.

Guruge, S., & Khanlou, N. (2004). Intersectionalities of influence: Researching the health of immigrant and refugee women. *Canadian Journal of Nursing Research*, *36*(3), 32–47.

Hilton, B. A., Thompson, R., & Moore-Dempsey, L. (2009). Evaluation of the AIDS prevention Street Nurse Program: One step at a time. *Canadian Journal of Nursing Research*, *41*(1), 238–258.

Holmes, D., Roy, B., & Perron, A. (2008). The use of postcolonialism in the nursing domain: Colonial patronage, conversion, and resistance. *Advances in Nursing Science*, *31*(1), 42–51.

Hooton, M. (1969). Learning the concept: Nursing in chronic illness. *Nursing Papers* [now *Canadian Journal of Nursing Research*], *1*(2), 11–16.

Hyman, I., Mason, R., Guruge, S., Berman, H., Kanagaratnam, P., & Manuel, L. (2011). Perceptions of factors contributing to intimate partner violence among Sri Lankan Tamil immigrant women in Canada. *Health Care for Women International*, *32*, 779–794.

Johnson, J. L., Kalaw, C., Lovato, C. Y., Baillie, L., & Chambers, N. A. (2004). Crossing the line: Adolescents' experiences of controlling their tobacco use. *Qualitative Health Research*, *14*(9), 1276–1291.

Kinch, J. L., & Jakubec, S. (2004). Out of the multiple margins: Older women managing their health care. *Canadian Journal of Nursing Research*, *36*(4), 90–108.

King, K., LeBlanc, P., Sanguins, J., & Mather, C. (2006). Gender-based challenges faced by older Sikh women as immigrants: Recognizing and acting on the risk of coronary artery disease. *Canadian Journal of Nursing Research*, *38*(1), 16–40.

Leininger, M. (1970). *Nursing and anthropology: Two worlds to blend*. New York: John Wiley.

Lynam, J., & Cowley, S. (2007). Understanding marginalization as a social determinant of health. *Critical Public Health*, *17*, 137–149.

MacDonnell, J. A. (2011). Gender, sexuality and the participatory dimensions of a comparative life history policy study. *Nursing Inquiry*, *18*(4), 313–324.

McDonald, C. (2009). Lesbian disclosure: Disrupting the taken for granted. *Canadian Journal of Nursing Research*, *41*(1), 260–275.

McDonald, C., McIntyre, M., & Merryfeather, L. (2011). Bringing ourselves into view: Disclosure as epistemological and ontological production of a lesbian subject. *Nursing Inquiry*, *18*(1), 50–54.

McDonald, H. (2011). Arthritis, aches and pains, and arthritis services: Experiences from within an urban First Nations community. Unpublished doctoral dissertation, University of British Columbia.

McIntyre, M., Anderson, B., & McDonald, C. (2001). The intersection of relational and cultural narratives: Women's abortion experiences. *Canadian Journal of Nursing Research*, *33*(3), 47–62.

McPherson, C. M., & McGibbon, E. A. (2010). Addressing the determinants of child mental health: Intersectionality as a guide to primary health care renewal. *Canadian Journal of Nursing Research*, *42*(3), 50–64.

Miranda, J. (2009). An exploration of participants' treatment preferences in a partial RCT. *Canadian Journal of Nursing Research*, *41*(1), 276–290.

Modood, T. (2005). *Multicultural politics: Racism, ethnicity, and Muslims in Britain*. Minneapolis: University of Minnesota Press.

Morse, J. (Ed.). (1991). *Qualitative nursing research: A contemporary dialogue* (2nd ed.). Newbury Park, CA: Sage.

Ogden Burke, S. (1985). Reporting on qualitative and quantitative research: Evolving issues and criteria. *Nursing Papers* [now *Canadian Journal of Nursing Research*], *17*(2), 69–71.

Oliffe, J. L., Bottorff, J. L., McKenzie, M. M., Hislop, T. G., Gerbrandt, J. S., & Oglov, V. (2011). Prostate cancer support groups, health literacy and consumerism: Are community-based volunteers re-defining older men's health? *Health: An Interdisciplinary Journal for the Social Study of Health, Illness and Medicine, 15*(6), 555–570.

Paterson, B. L., Tschikota, S., Crawford, M., Saydak, M., Venkatesh, P., & Aronowitz, T. (1996). Learning to care: Gender issues for male nursing students. *Canadian Journal of Nursing Research, 28*(1), 25–39.

Perron, A., & Holmes, D. (2011). Constructing mentally ill inmates: Nurses' discursive practices in corrections. *Nursing Inquiry, 18*(3), 191–204.

Pesut, B., Fowler, M., Reimer-Kirkham, S., Johnson Taylor, E., & Sawatzky, R. (2009). Particularizing spirituality in points of tension: Enriching the discourse. *Nursing Inquiry, 16*(4), 337–346.

Ponic, P., Reid, C., & Frisby, W. (2010). Cultivating the power of partnerships in feminist participatory action research in women's health. *Nursing Inquiry, 17*(4), 324–335.

Poudrier, J., & Mac-Lean, R.T. (2009). "We've fallen into the cracks": Aboriginal women's experiences with breast cancer through photovoice. *Nursing Inquiry, 16*(4), 306–317.

Racine, L. (2003). Implementing a postcolonial feminist perspective in nursing research related to non-Western populations. *Nursing Inquiry, 10*(2), 91–102.

Racine, L., & Petrucka, P. (2011). Enhancing decolonization and knowledge transfer in nursing with non-western populations: Examining the congruence between primary health care and postcolonial feminist approaches. *Nursing Inquiry, 18*(1), 12–20.

Ramsden, I. (1993). Kawa Whakaruruhau cultural safety in nursing education in Aotearoa (New Zealand). *Nursing Praxis in New Zealand, 8*(3), 4–10.

Rankin, J. (2003). "Patient satisfaction": Knowledge for ruling hospital reform—an institutional ethnography. *Nursing Inquiry, 10*(1), 57–65.

Reimer-Kirkham, S., & Anderson, J. M. (2002). Postcolonial nursing scholarship: From epistemology to method. *Advances in Nursing Sciences, 25*(1), 1–17.

Reimer-Kirkham, S., & Anderson, J. M. (2010). The advocate-analyst dialectic in critical and postcolonial feminist research: Reconciling tensions around scientific integrity. *Advances in Nursing Science, 33*(3), 196–205.

Reimer-Kirkham, S., & Browne, A. J. (2006). Toward a critical theoretical interpretation of social justice discourses in nursing. *Advances in Nursing Science, 29*(4), 324–339.

Reimer-Kirkham, S., & Sharma, S. (2011). Adding religion to gender, race, and class: Seeking new insights on intersectionality in health care contexts. In O. Hankivsky (Ed.), *Health inequities in Canada: Intersectional frameworks and practices* (pp. 112–127). Vancouver, BC: UBC Press.

Reutter, L., & Kushner, K. E. (2010). "Health equity through action on the social determinants of health": Taking up the challenge in nursing. *Nursing Inquiry, 17*(3), 269–280.

Rodney, P., Doane, G. H., Storch, J., & Varcoe, C. (2006). Workplaces: Toward a safer moral climate. *Canadian Nurse, 102*(8), 24–27.

Rodney, P., Harrigan, M. L., Jiwani. B., Burgess, M., & Phillips, J. C. (2013). A further landscape: Ethics in health care organizations and health/health care policy. In J. Storch, P. Rodney, & R. Starzomski (Eds.), *Toward a moral horizon: Nursing ethics for leadership and practice* (2nd ed., pp. 358–383). Toronto: Pearson-Prentice Hall.

Rodney, P., Varcoe, C., Storch, J., McPherson, G., Mahoney, K., Brown, H., et al. (2009). Navigating towards a moral horizon: A multisite qualitative study of ethical practice in nursing. *Canadian Journal of Nursing Research, 41*(1), 292–319.

Romanow, R. (2012). The future of health care: Medicare must be preserved and made truly comprehensive. *CCPA Monitor: Economic, Social, and Environmental Perspectives, 18*(8), 1, 6–7.

Ronquillo, C., Boschma, G., Wong, S., & Quiney, L. (2011). Beyond greener pastures: Exploring contexts surrounding Filipino nurse migration in Canada through oral history. *Nursing Inquiry, 18*(3), 262–275.

Rose, L. (1985). Responses of families to the treatment setting. *Nursing Papers* [now the *Canadian Journal of Nursing Research*], *17*(2), 72–84.

Said, E. (1979). *Orientalism*. New York: Vintage Books.

Said, E. (1994). *Culture and imperialism*. New York: Vintage Books.

Salmon, A., Browne, A. J., & Pederson, A. (2010). "Now we call it research": Participatory health research involving marginalized women who use drugs. *Nursing Inquiry, 17*(4), 336–345.

Schutz, A. (1973). *Collected papers 1: The problem of social reality.* The Hague: Martinus Nijhoff.

Skinner, Q. (1978). The flight from positivism: The restructuring of social and political theory by Richard J. Bernstein. *New York Review of Books, 25*(10), 26–28.

Smith, D. E. (1987). *The everyday world as problematic: A feminist sociology.* Toronto: University of Toronto Press.

Smith, D. E. (1999). *Writing the social: Critique, theory, and investigations.* Toronto: University of Toronto Press.

Smye, V., & Browne, A. J. (2002). "Cultural safety" and the analysis of health policy affecting Aboriginal people. *Nurse Researcher: The International Journal of Research Methodology in Nursing and Health Care, 9*(3), 42–56.

Spivak, G. C. (1999). *A critique of postcolonial reason: Toward a history of the vanishing present.* Cambridge, MA: Harvard University Press.

Stajduhar, K. I., Martin, W. L., Barwick, D., & Fyles, G. (2008). Factors influencing family caregivers' ability to cope with providing end-of-life cancer care at home. *Cancer Nursing, 31*, 77–85.

Storch, J. L., Rodney, P., & Starzomski, R. (Eds.) (2013). *Toward a moral horizon: Nursing ethics for leadership and practice* (2nd ed.). Toronto: Pearson-Prentice Hall.

Tang, S., & Anderson, J. (1999). Human agency and the process of healing: Lessons learned from women living with a chronic illness—"rewriting the expert." *Nursing Inquiry, 6*(2), 83–93.

Tang, S., & Browne, A. J. (2008). "Race" matters: Racialization and egalitarian discourses involving Aboriginal people in the Canadian health care context. *Ethnicity & Health, 13*(2), 109–127.

Thorne, S. (2008). *Interpretive description.* Walnut Creek, CA: Left Coast Press.

Thorne, S., Reimer-Kirkham, S., & Macdonald-Emes, J. (1997). Interpretive description: A noncategorical qualitative alternative for developing nursing knowledge. *Research in Nursing and Health, 20*, 169–177.

Thorne, S., Reimer-Kirkham, S., & O'Flynn-Magee, K. (2004). The analytic challenge in interpretive description. *International Journal of Qualitative Methods, 3*(1), 1–11. Retrieved from http://ejournals.library.ualberta.ca/index.php/IJQM/article/viewFile/4481/3619.

Tiwari, A., Wong, M., & Ip, H. (2001). *Ren* and *Yuan*: A cultural interpretation of Chinese women's responses to battering. *Canadian Journal of Nursing Research, 33*(3), 63–79.

Tuhiwai Smith, L. (1999). *Decolonizing methodologies, research and Indigenous peoples.* London: Zen Books Ltd.

Van Herk, K. A., Smith, D., & Andrew, C. (2011). Examining our privileges and oppressions: Incorporating an intersectionality paradigm into nursing. *Nursing Inquiry, 18*(1), 29–39.

Varcoe, C. (1996). Theorizing oppression: Implications for nursing research on violence against women. *Canadian Journal of Nursing Research, 28*(1), 61–78.

Varcoe, C. (2006). Doing participatory action research in a racist world. *Western Journal of Nursing Research, 28*(5), 1–16.

Varcoe, C., Brown, H., Calam, B., Buchanan, M. J., & Newman, V. (2011). Capacity building is a two-way street: Learning from doing research within Aboriginal communities. In G. Creese & W. Frisby (Eds.), *Feminist community research: Case studies and methodologies* (pp. 210–231). Vancouver: UBC Press.

Ward-Griffin, C., Bol, N., & Oudshoorn, A. (2006). Perspectives of women with dementia receiving care from their adult daughters. *Canadian Journal of Nursing Research, 38*(1), 120–146.

Weiss, S. M., Malone, R. E., Merighi, J. R., & Benner, P. (2009). Economism, efficiency, and the moral ecology of good nursing practice. *Canadian Journal of Nursing Research, 41*(1), 340–364.

Werezak, L., & Stewart, N. (2009). Learning to live with early dementia. *Canadian Journal of Nursing Research, 41*(1), 366–384.

Wuest, J. (2000). Negotiating with helping systems: An example of grounded theory evolving through emergent fit. *Qualitative Health Research, 10*, 51–70.

Wuest, J., Malcolm, J., & Merritt-Gray, M. (2010). Daughters' obligation to care in the context of past abuse. *Health Care for Women International, 31*, 1047–1067.

Young, L., & Higgins, J. W. (2010). Using participatory research to challenge the status quo for women's cardiovascular health. *Nursing Inquiry, 17*(4), 346–358.

35

Australia and New Zealand qualitative nursing research

Jennieffer Barr

Introduction

Nurses and midwives in Australasia are cognizant that they are responsible for providing the best possible standard of patient care. They are increasingly called upon to justify their clinical decisions and outcomes to peers, colleagues, government organizations and health care clients. To meet these expectations, research activity has increased and evidence-based practice is promoted as the best way to ensure quality of nursing care.

History of research development of Australasian nurses

The Australian and New Zealand history of research development differs significantly to some other developed countries. Unlike the United States of America, Canada and the United Kingdom, there has been no dedicated funding from governments to build a critical mass of nurse researchers. Like Europe, Australasian nursing research is underfunded (Gledhill, Mannix, MacDonald, & Poulton, 2011; Traynor, Rafferty, & Lewison, 2001). Therefore, to build research capacity, nurses and midwives in Australasia have used higher degree programs and competitive funding sources.

National competitive funding is challenging at best but even less funding is awarded to qualitative research. However, specific nursing organizations have tried to address this deficit by funding qualitative research. For example the Queensland Nursing Council administered a research grant program from 1996 to 2010. Overall this funding body provided almost 2 million Australian dollars to nurse and midwifery researchers. A survey (Gledhill et al., 2011) was undertaken to profile this research. Of the research applications presented for consideration 39% pursued quantitative design funding, while 37% were proposing to conduct qualitative research. In New Zealand some funding is provided specifically for nurses. For example, two organizations that provide nurse research funds are the Nursing Education Research Foundation and the College of Nurses Aotearoa. However, while lack of designated funding and minimal organizational research positions lead to slow development of research, Australian and New Zealand nurses have risen to this challenge undertaking significant research and arguing for the need increased research to inform practice, policy, workforce decision and education.

Professional and regulation bodies have played a key role in advocating and expecting the use and implementation of nursing and midwifery research. This has led to change in education and more detailed regulation and accreditation. In the first half of the twentieth century nurses engaged in scholarly activity focusing on the knowledge required for nurses. Professional development was closely aligned with changes in the education of registered nurses from the hospital to the university setting. In turn, nursing and midwifery research developed from these educational changes, particularly as nurses engaged in postgraduate degrees. Specifically, doctoral degrees highlighted the need to use and engage in research (Usher & Mills, 2012); however, at first education about research did not flourish in nursing delivered programs but rather was dependent on other disciplines such as sociology, psychology and education due to the lack of expertise in research understandings and skills. Many Australian and New Zealand nurses engaged in nursing doctoral programs provided in the United States of America and to some degree the United Kingdom. This has led to close alliances and engagement with international organizations such as the Royal College of Nurses Australia and New Zealand Nursing Organisation linked to the International Council of Nurses (ICN). Table 35.1 provides examples of professional bodies working towards increased research.

It is worthy to note that all professional groups in Australasia believe that all nurses and midwives are accountable for the quality of care they deliver and that research is an important component to achieving this overall goal. The core arguments presented from such groups and organizations are that providing quality care can only happen if first the nurse is knowledgeable and able to be a research consumer. Ideally, the term "research consumer" refers to a health care professional who acknowledges the merit and usefulness of research, has skills in critically appraising research findings, and who can translate research findings into practice. Another area of interest for the research consumer is how to manage the nursing workforce, including the ongoing urgent need for recruitment and retention of nurses. However, while these professional bodies seek to support and encourage the use of research, there has not been a significant increase in implementing nursing research through these organizations. As most have limited money, there have only been token gestures of financial support for undertaking nursing research.

Another key factor in the development of nursing and midwifery research in Australia was national shared goals of competency standards for the registration of all nurses and midwives implemented through the Australian Nursing and Midwifery Council (ANMC). ANMC acknowledges the use of research to promote excellence in practice, thus creating a core

Table 35.1 A brief outline of the contribution of key professional bodies

Professional body	Contribution
Royal College of Nursing Australia (RCNA)	Declared that all nurses be committed to research (either conducting and/or using research)
New Zealand Nurses Organization	Declared that all nurses be committed to research (either conducting and/or using research)
Australian College of Midwives	Declared that all midwives be committed to research (either conducting and/or using research)
Australian and New Zealand College of Mental Health Nurses	Created a Research Board
Australian College of Critical Care Nurses (ACCCN)	Created a Research Advisory Panel

competency for registered nurses to incorporate research findings into nursing practice (Australian Nursing and Midwifery Council, 2006). The Australian Nursing and Midwifery Council (2006) national competency standards for registered nurses are available at: www.anmc.org.au/ userfiles/file/competency_standards/competency_standards_RN.pdf.

Australian accreditation for educational programs includes the expectation that staff delivering nursing or midwifery tertiary education will be research active and skilled at embedding research findings into the curriculum to inform clinical practice. Also research and research infrastructure have increased in health care settings in both Australia and New Zealand. Nurse researchers, ranging from clinical professors who are directors of research centers through to research assistants working in research teams are now common within tertiary, clinical and government sites in Australasia.

The Nursing Council of New Zealand (NCNZ) through its Health Practitioners Competence Assurance Act (2003) also legislated for nurse registration to be aligned to professional competency and development audit. Therefore, registration bodies in both Australia and New Zealand require nurses and midwives to maintain continuing competency with the view that evidence-based practice is pivotal to engaging in effective health care. This has provided an important political argument for increased focus on research which is likely to need more nursing research roles and increased funding that is available for research in Australia and New Zealand.

Research approaches and methods used most frequently

Qualitative research has been embraced in Australasia. This has been reflected in a study undertaken by Borbasi and others (2002), who analyzed 509 published nursing research articles in 11 Australian and United Kingdom nursing journals between 1995 and 2000. In this period, qualitative approaches were more popular (47%) compared to quantitative research (41%). This has changed in the recent years with increased attention turning towards quantitative research with nurses and midwives applying for national competitive grants, who favor positivistic research designs. However, qualitative research approaches continue to be valued. Table 35.2 presents one study implemented in Australia that shows the types of qualitative studies that have been funded through the Queensland Nursing Council.

Table 35.2 Types of qualitative methodologies and methods in Queensland Nursing Council applications, 1996–2000

Types of research approaches/methods	Percentage of all qualitative projects
Focus groups	36.6
Action Research	24.4
Phenomenology	22
Participatory Action Research	17.1
Grounded theory	12.2
Ethnography	5
Thematic analysis	2
Phenomenography	1
Combined interviews/focus groups	1
Hermeneutics	1
Narrative	1
Constructivism	1

Source: Gledhill et al. (2011).

The interpretive paradigm has been a favored approach to inform nursing research in Australia and New Zealand. Phenomenology and hermeneutics have been commonly applied, particularly by those undertaking higher degree research programs. Phenomenology considers perception, representation and purpose or intention within people's actions in everyday lives. Historically, phenomenology commenced as an exploration of one's consciousness and an attempt was made to explain how one perceives meaning. For Husserl, the founder of phenomenology, this research approach was formed as the study of mental representation and intentionality. Basically, phenomenological inquiry leads to awareness of living an experience from first-hand; that is, from those who live the actual experience. It is a study on reflection; on becoming consciously aware of what matters to those living or who have lived that particular experience. Globally nurses and midwives have become aware of the importance of seeking out those who live with the experience as a way to build understanding. Nurses and midwives have also become conscious of the need to examine human experiences that previously have not been central to inquiry, and yet such daily living and engaging in typical regular activity need exploring for heightened understanding for the delivery of health care. Heidegger's work arguing the need for awareness of taken-for-granted daily experiences is deemed important to understanding and that meanings within such experiences should be shared with others. An example of this was the seminal work of Taylor (1993a, 1993b) who looked at the ordinariness of nursing; the caring activities and meaningful nurse–patient engagement which leads to the facilitation of patient well-being.

Hermeneutics is also interested in experiences as recollected by those who live through the activity or event. Specifically, hermeneutics focuses on the development of interpretation and the understanding of texts; text being more than written material but also images, symbols and spoken words. Such interpretation is useful for the development of theories about phenomena under study. In particular, Gadamer's approach to hermeneutics in focusing on the procedure or technique of interpretation with the view to represent the intended meaning from those who live the experience has been important in developing suitable methods, in particular, the hermeneutic circle. Language is seen as the vehicle of sharing meaning and therefore the everyday living of others can be highlighted and known. One of the many examples is the study that examined the daily experiences of new mothers with postpartum depression (Barr, 2008). Here the meaning that was uncovered revolved around surviving the day as one struggles with the impact of mental illness, while trying to adapt to a new social role, that of mothering.

Other research approaches have contributed significantly to research including postmodern and post-structural research approaches. "Truth" is seen as possibilities of multiple truths rather than a single entity. This recognizes multiple realities for humans, however, compared to the interpretive paradigm, these research approaches question assumptions embedded in modern thought. Language is seen as a significant feature and as such the examination of discourse is paramount to these research approaches. A great deal of research has been undertaken to examine and challenge the status quo of many situations related to nursing and health conditions and only through deconstruction can one then facilitate emergence of a new way of thinking or practicing. For example, the thesis undertaken by Wilkinson (2007) in New Zealand is a good example. Studying the development of nurse practitioners in New Zealand, Wilkinson used Foucault's argument that interconnection between knowledge, discourse and power has influenced the development of nurse practitioners in New Zealand. Wilkinson set out to show that developing roles of advanced nursing roles (known in Australia and New Zealand as Nurse Practitioner) need to be aware of the historical discourse of control by medical professionals. She argues for the need for an independent autonomous scope of practice, which is only limited by imagination of possibilities of an advanced practice nurse role in contemporary health care.

Methods used have been diverse but favored qualitative methods, as would be expected, have included interviews and focus groups. A significant number of qualitative research projects have been undertaken in Australasia as nurse researchers responding to local and national needs for greater understanding of a health issue, event or nursing process or workforce issue. A common method used has been focus groups to create an interactive dialogue between people within limited time.

Contribution to nursing

This section will now focus on the contribution that Australasian research has made to nursing.

The Australian and New Zealand context of research

Australia is a large geographical country with significant distances between rural and remote towns in most states. Not only is the country harsh and dangerous from both heat and cold in desert areas, the relatively small population of Australia places an economic challenge to providing sound and effective health care across the country. The complexity of health care provision in contemporary society with aging populations and increasing co-morbidity of chronic illnesses means that health care costs are escalating. Like the international trend, the Australian population is also moving towards urban living and there is a decline in rural residents. This means less available rural workforce and disintegrating rural infrastructure. Effective health care provision in rural and remote Australia is further compounded by limited access to services, higher costs in delivering these services, and transport problems (Allan, Ball, & Alston, 2007).

The impact this has had on Australian rural nurses is evident. In one study by T. Kidd, Kenny, and Meehan-Andrews (2012), it was found that emergency nurses encountering violence in accident and emergency departments of rural hospitals did not feel safe when the nearest police station was four hours' drive away. It is typical to find minimal staff onsite, such as three nurses providing care and a doctor on call (available to come in when a nurse contacts this person). Generalist nurses in rural hospital settings lack confidence about the diversity of health care issues encountered, particularly in emergency departments. In these focus groups, nurses reported feeling isolated; being concerned about lack of frequency of exposure to specific health care issues; feeling unprepared for providing care for those with mental illness; and not feeling safe with drug- and alcohol-associated violence (T. Kidd et al., 2012).

Both New Zealand and Australia need to provide culturally appropriate nursing and midwifery care due to their multicultural societies. Therefore, recent research is focusing on specific cultural groups. An example is a study undertaken in South Eastern Sydney, New South Wales in Australia by Davidson and others (2011). This study aimed to describe the experiences of Chinese Australians with heart disease following discharge from hospital following an acute cardiac event. The research team was particularly interested in health-seeking beliefs of this particular cultural group. Both focus groups and interviews were used to obtain descriptions and then apply thematic analysis to elicit key themes of the need to link traditional values and beliefs with Western medicine and how traditional beliefs can inhibit risk factor modification. Risk factor modification has become an important component to cardiac rehabilitation and re-occurrence of cardiac events, and yet this project highlights the complexity and need to work with traditional beliefs and evidence-based nursing and medicine practices.

Of particular significance is appropriate indigenous health care. Indigenous populations from both Australia and New Zealand have a great burden of disease and have a lower life expectancy than non-indigenous people in these countries. The key is for services to be appropriate and accessible. Many studies have been undertaken to determine how to enhance service provision to indigenous people, such as the study undertaken in Western Australia by DiGiacomo and others (2010). One approach to such health care is to educate and employ indigenous health workers. However, recruiting and retaining indigenous nursing students has been a significant issue. Creating cultural safety in indigenous health education is one way to address this issue. An additional approach is to understand the types of care provided by indigenous nurses to indigenous patients (Simon, Willis, Smye, & Rameka, 2006). A qualitative study was undertaken that asked what might constitute Maori nursing practice. Maori registered nurses described the promotion of cultural awareness and identity, which was reported as being comforting to patients of Maori descent. The use of Western scientific models on Maori health care was seen as in conflict at times to traditional healing, which was deemed as important by Maori patients. There is a great deal more research being undertaken to look at indigenous health care and the related contribution that nurses and midwives can make. This is true of other cultures as well and the need for culturally and linguistically diverse nursing and midwifery students is acknowledged as important in Australia and New Zealand to address multicultural societies (Jeong et al., 2011).

A focus on education for nurses and midwives has been a key research area. A specific area pertinent to Australia has been the exploration of the transition from Enrolled Nurse (Diploma) to a Registered Nurse (Bachelor of Nursing student). Moving from a diploma level of education to a Bachelor of Nursing program has been identified as challenging for these nurses (Hutchinson, Mitchell, & St John, 2011). These adaption challenges continue for clinically registered nurses who have a history of previous practice as Enrolled Nurses. The need for support as a new graduate when first employed as a registered nurse is seen as vital by those nurses who have previously practiced as Enrolled Nurses, and yet qualitative research findings report their perception of being unsupported in comparison to their peers who were not previously enrolled nurses (Cubit & Lopez, 2012).

Australasia has been active in examining clinical education of nurses. Evaluating student exposure to specific areas of clinical experience has been an important research inquiry and has included students engaging with the elderly (Clendon, 2011), in the perioperative environment (Callaghan, 2011), and in acute care (James & Chapman, 2009–2010). In addition to specific clinical opportunities, how to enhance student learning has been a major focus. The ability of final-year nursing students to assess, detect and act on clinical cues of deterioration in a simulated environment has been evaluated (Endacott et al., 2010). Using mannequins and critical care case scenarios, students were observed and interviewed to ascertain their ability to systematically determine through health assessment when health conditions deteriorate. This research concluded that nursing curricula should provide opportunities to practice synthesizing information such as linking pathophysiology with patient assessment and identifying patterns of symptoms and signs displayed in patients' current health status rather than seeing these elements of health assessment as separate pieces of information. Finally, exposing student nurses to clinical areas has also been found to impact on their decisions for career pathways. A qualitative study found that clinical exposure did influence career decisions about types of specialist areas and work location (McKenna, McCall, & Wray, 2010). In Table 35.3 can be found examples of additional qualitative studies.

Nursing's contribution to global nursing

Across the world longevity and poor lifestyle choices are leading to increased chronic illness. Nursing research has embraced a primary health care approach with the view to prevent or minimize the impact of illness. Often such programs addressing chronic illness involve multidisciplinary teams where community or practice nurses play a key role. Qualitative research has identified that it is essential when working in a multidisciplinary team to delineate the various

Table 35.3 Examples of additional studies

Authors	Methodology	Description
Clarke et al. (2012)	Semi-structured interviews with qualitative data analysis	A Unit Manager's leadership program was reported favorably as being useful and building the confidence of Nursing Unit Managers.
Cleary et al. (2011)	Interview questions following a structured questionnaire	Mental health nurses desired continuing professional development (this response was common among senior staff too).
Kapp & Annells (2010)	Hermeneutic phenomenology	Home-bound patients with pressure ulcers experience social isolation. Therefore, nurses should routinely assess for risk of social isolation. Another significant finding was that some health care professionals had not perceived the pressure ulcers as a priority.
Walthew & Scott (2011)	Qualitative data collection in the form of focus groups	Student nurses had difficulty articulating the difference between health education and health promotion. However, they did consider health promotion part of their professional responsibilities.
Wellard, Cox, & Bhujoharry (2007)	Qualitative interpretive design using interviews to gain rich data	Those undergoing cardiac surgery who also had diabetes are concerned about the care they received for their diabetes. Alternatively, nurses providing the care did not feel competent at providing care for diabetes. This highlights the need for education about diabetes in cardiac health services.
Winters & Neville (2012)	Qualitative descriptive study	The finding that "moral distress" was felt when nurses missed or delayed care was a key concept identified.

roles to ensure the team functions efficiently, the team has healthy peer relationships which complement each discipline's health care delivery and in turn optimize health outcomes (Cioffi, Wilkes, Cummings, Warne, & Harrison, 2010).

Care of the aged is a commonly explored area in nursing. Qualitative research is a commonly applied approach with the view to improve residential living and optimize nurses' educational needs in this area. Some examples of research are presented. Bland (2007) implemented critical ethnography to examine nursing home residents' comfort. Findings included: task–orientated and routine care while providing comfort to residents, also made them feel uncomfortable. Such a contradiction requires change to optimize comfort. Chang and others (2009) implemented Action Research to address the challenges of caring for a resident with advanced dementia. Findings included: staff require education and training about palliative care to care for those with advanced dementia.

Nurses are an aging population and as such will also be vulnerable to chronic illness. Focusing on nurses and their well-being is not a new topic with many exploring bullying but recent focus on mental illness among nurses is a welcome initiative by J. D. Kidd and Finlayson (2010).

Recommendations for future research

With the ever changing nature of practice it will be essential for research to keep abreast of the impact of change. For example, a change in practice leading to early discharge following the birth of a baby means a reduced time for the provision of postnatal education. Shortened postnatal care has required changes to midwifery expectations of the type of care that can be provided. Breastfeeding mothers are now typically at home when their milk comes in, rather than as an in-patient, which involves easy access to guidance and support. Changes like this require a process of transition from staff engaging in practice in a traditional manner to adapting to a new way of practice (McKellar, Pincombe, & Henderson, 2009). McKellar and others (2009) introduced an educational intervention to optimize positive education experiences of parents during the shortened duration of hospital-based postnatal care through an Action Research project. A surprising finding was that some ward midwives were reluctant to embrace and use the educational resource for education in the way it was designed, which was engaging with mothers. Rather, these staff reported placing the brochure into the discharge package for self-select use by parents. This particular finding highlights the complexity when practice changes, requiring workforce change and adaptation. In the future, as change occurs, research should be immediately implemented as a standard way of operating. Qualitative research could explore and examine the following:

- explore the impact of change;
- propose new ways of practice;
- provide rich detail to develop conceptual and theoretical frameworks;
- define variables useful for quantitative research for measuring the effectiveness of change strategies.

With an increasing expectation for increased use of research to inform practice, as research users become knowledgeable and critical in the evaluation of current practice, identification of gaps in nursing knowledge is likely to increase. Local requests for research to be implemented and then the findings used at the same clinical site, appear to be increasing.

Specific areas of likely inquiry for Australasia are developing. The first obvious need is for increased understandings about health care needs and nursing those with refugee status due to the increasing numbers of refugees from countries experiencing war and significant internal political conflict. An additional inquiry area is related to the increasing concerns about infections. Globally the world is concerned about antibiotic-resistant bacterial organisms but new infections are occurring. A specific infection in Australia of concern is the Hendra virus, a virus that passes between horses to humans with most resulting in fatalities. While a priority research strategy was to develop a vaccination, most recent cases of this infection led to the first survivors from the Hendra virus. Admittedly this infection is most rare; however, it is an example of future possibilities of other evolving infections, as well as new autoimmune health states that are developing. Nurses can take a leading role to research the impact on people's lives of those developing and surviving these rare conditions, as such conditions appear to be increasing and lead to reduced quality of health.

Conclusion

Active researchers will need to foster new generations of nursing researchers in order to expand and build nursing knowledge. While doctoral degrees are contributing to this expansion, the recent increase in the number of positions created in the clinical environment investing money and time to nursing research has been an important development in both Australia and New Zealand. Finally, the number of active researchers will grow as the accreditation bodies in Australasia have developed research-focused competencies and as registered nurses and midwives engage as consumers of research. The absence of evidence in so many areas of clinical practice is likely to stimulate their need to become involved in the implementation of research. Therefore, it is expected that there will be an increase of partnerships between universities, health services, government and non-government organizations.

References

Allan, J., Ball, P., & Alston, M. (2007). Developing sustainable models of rural health care: A community development approach. *Rural and Remote Health*, 7, 818–830.

Australian Nursing and Midwifery Council. (2006). National competency standards for registered nurses. Retrieved on 13 February, 2012 from www.anmc.org.au/userfiles/file/competency_standards/competency_standards_RN.pdf.

Barr, J. (2008). Postpartum depression, delayed maternal adaptation, and mechanical infant caring: A phenomenological hermeneutic study. *International Journal of Nursing Studies*, 45, 362–369.

Bland, B. (2007). Betwixt and between: A critical ethnography of comfort in New Zealand residential aged care. *Journal of Clinical Nursing*, 16(5), 937–944.

Borbasi, S., Hawes, C., Wilkes, L., Stewart, M., & May, D. (2002). Measuring the outputs of Australian nursing research published 1995–2000. *Journal of Advanced Nursing*, 38(5), 489–497.

Callaghan, A. (2011). Student nurses' perceptions of learning in a perioperative placement. *Journal of Advanced Nursing*, 67(4), 854–864.

Chang, E., Daly, J., Johnson, A., Harrison, K., Easterbrook, S., Bidewell, J., Stewart, H., Noel, M., & Hancock, K. (2009). Challenges for professional care of advanced dementia. *International Journal of Nursing Practice*, 15, 41–47.

Cioffi, J., Wilkes, L., Cummings, J., Warne, B., & Harrison, K. (2010). Multidisciplinary teams caring for clients with chronic conditions: Experiences of community nurses and allied health professionals. *Contemporary Nurse*, 36(1–2), 61–70.

Clarke, C., Diers, D., Kunisch, J., Duffield, C., Thoms, D., Hawew, S., Stasa, H., & Fry, M. (2012). Strengthening the nursing and midwifery unit manager role: An interim programme evaluation. *Journal of Nursing Management*, 20, 120–129.

Cleary, M., Horsfall, J., O'Hara-Aasons, M., Jackson, D., & Hunt, G. (2011). The views of mental health nurses on continuing professional development. *Journal of Clinical Nursing*, 20, 3561–3566.

Clendon, J. (2011). Enhancing preparation of undergraduate students for practice in older adult settings. *Contemporary Nurse*, 38(1–2), 94–105.

Cubit, K., & Lopez, V. (2012). Qualitative study of Enrolled Nurses' transition to Registered Nurses. *Journal of Advanced Nursing*, 68(1), 206–211.

Davidson, P. M., Daly, J., Leung, D., Ang, E., Paul, G., DiGiacomo, M., Hancock, K., Cao, Y., Du, H. Y., & Thompson, D. R. (2011). Health-seeking beliefs of cardiovascular patients: A qualitative study. *International Journal of Nursing Studies*, 48, 1367– 1375.

DiGiacomo, M., Davidson, P. M., Taylor, K. B., Smith, J. S., Dimer, L., Ali, M., et al. (2010). Health information system linkage and coordination are critical for increasing access to secondary prevention in Aboriginal health: a qualitative study. *Quality in Primary Care 18*, 17–26.

Endacott, R., Scholes, J., Buykx, P., Cooper, S., Kinsman, L., & McConnell-Henry, T. (2010). Final-year nursing students' ability to assess, detect, and act on clinical cues of deterioration in a simulated environment. *Journal of Advanced Nursing*, 66(12), 2722–2731.

Gledhill, S., Mannix, J., MacDonald, R., & Poulton, G. (2011). Nursing and midwifery research grants: Profiling the outcomes. *Australian Journal of Advanced Nursing*, 28(3), 14– 21.

Halcomb, E., & Peters, K. (2009). Nursing student feedback on undergraduate research education: Implications for teaching and learning. *Contemporary Nurse*, 33(1), 59– 68.

Hutchinson, L., Mitchell, C., & St-John, W. (2011). The transition experience of enrolled nurses to a Bachelor of Nursing at an Australian university. *Contemporary Nurse*, 38(1–2), 191–200.

James, A., & Chapman, Y. (2009–2010). Preceptors and patients—the power of two: Nursing student experiences on their first acute clinical placement. *Contemporary Nurse, 34*(1), 34–47.

Jeong, S., Hickey, N., Levett-Jones, T., Pitt, V., Hoffman, K., Norton, C., & Ohr, S. (2011). Understanding and enhancing the learning experiences of culturally and linguistically diverse nursing students in an Australian Bachelor of Nursing program. *Nurse Education Today, 31*, 238–244.

Kapp, S., & Annells, M. (2010). Pressure ulcers: Home-based nursing. *British Journal of Community Nursing, 15*(suppl.) S6–S13.

Kidd, J. D., & Finlayson, M. P. (2010). Mental illness in the nursing workplace: A collective autoethnography. *Contemporary Nurse, 36*(1–2), 21–33.

Kidd, T., Kenny, A., & Meehan-Andrews, T. (2012). The experience of general nurses in rural Australian emergency departments. *Nurse Education in Practice, 12*, 11–15.

McKellar, L., Pincombe, J., & Henderson, A. (2009). Encountering the culture of midwifery practice on the postnatal ward during Action Research: An impediment to change, *Women and Birth 22*, 112–118.

McKenna, L., McCall, L., & Wray, N. (2010). Clinical placements and nursing students' career planning: A qualitative exploration. *International Journal of Nursing Practice, 16*, 176–182.

Simon, V., Willis, E., Smye, B., & Rameka, M. (2006). Characterising Maori nursing practice. *Contemporary Nurse, 22*, 203–213.

Taylor, B. (1993a). Ordinariness in nursing: a study, part 1. *Nursing Standard, 7*(39), 35–38.

Taylor, B. (1993b). Ordinariness in nursing: a study, part 2. *Nursing Standard 7*(40), 37–40.

Traynor, M., Rafferty, A. M., & Lewison, G. (2001). Endogenous and exogenous research? Findings from a bibliometric study of UK nursing research. *Journal of Advanced Nursing, 34*(2), 212–222.

Usher, K., & Mills, J. (2012). Introduction to nursing and midwifery research. In S. Borbasi & D. Jackson (Eds.), *Navigating the maze of research: Enhancing nursing and midwifery practice.* Chatswood, NSW: Mosby, Elsevier.

Walthew, P., & Scott, H. (2011). Conceptions of health promotion held by pre-registration student nurses in four schools of nursing in New Zealand. *Nurse Education Today, 32*, 229–234.

Wellard, S.J., Cox, H., & Bhujoharry, C. (2007). Issues in the provision of nursing care to people undergoing cardiac surgery who also have type 2 diabetes. *International Journal of Nursing Practice, 13*, 222–228.

Wilkinson, L. (2007). The New Zealand Nurse practitioner polemic: A discourse analysis. Unpublished doctoral dissertation, Massey University, Wellington, New Zealand.

Winters, R., & Neville, S. (2012). Registered nurses' perspectives on delayed or missed nursing cares in a New Zealand hospital. *Nursing Praxis in New Zealand, 28*(1), 19–28.

36

Qualitative nursing research in Latin America

The cases of Brazil, Chile, Colombia, and Mexico[1]

María Claudia Duque-Páramo, Maria Itayra Padilha, Olivia Inés Sanhueza-Alvarado, María Magdalena Alonso Castillo, Fabiola Castellanos Soriano, Karla Selene López-García, and Yolanda Flores-Peña[2]

Introduction

Since the 1980s, qualitative nursing research in Latin America has been gradually on the increase. This expansion has been reflected in the growing number of qualitative studies, with a wide range of theoretical and methodological approaches, and on many different topics and subject areas, which have been published in journals in various countries. Qualitative research has thus had an impact on both clinical and academic practice, and contributed reflections on the development of nursing as a profession. The Pan American Health Organization (PAHO) has had an important influence on these advances, by promoting professional development (Prado et al., 2008), recognizing nursing as a key component of the process of change in the health sector in various countries in the region, and developing technical cooperation in research, particularly through the Pan American Nursing Research Colloquia, conferences, and publications.

Bearing in mind that these developments have not been uniformly in evidence across the region, we focus this chapter on Latin America on an analysis of four countries which reflect different processes and characteristics, but which are all highly advanced in nursing research: Brazil, Chile, Colombia, and Mexico (Mendoza-Parra et al., 2009). In each case, the analysis was carried out by nurses with a background in research, and specifically qualitative research, in each of the four countries in question, which we have supplemented with interviews of researchers, and with analysis of documents found both on international databases and in national and local publications.

This approach allows us to present an analysis that is focused at a national level, to recognize the efforts of research nurses within those countries, and to suggest interpretations that differ from the homogenizing and hegemonic view presented by authors who have based their analysis on international databases (Gastaldo et al., 2002; Mendoza-Parra et al., 2009).

There were four key factors in the origin and development of qualitative research in these countries: (1) the contribution of Master's and doctoral programs at postgraduate level; (2) the empowering of research nurses; (3) the consolidation of research groups; and (4) the recognition of nursing as a social science. In Brazil and Colombia, qualitative nursing research has primarily developed from theoretical, critical positions in the social sciences, and from studies and experience of Action Research, and Participatory Action Research. Another point of origin, which is common to the four countries considered here, has been seen in global developments in qualitative nursing research, as well as in the influence of schools of thought such as phenomenology and ethnography, and of thinkers such as Michel Foucault, Orlando Fals Borda, Paulo Freire, and the humanist Humberto Maturana.

However, the tendency to take a qualitative approach is also suggested by various other factors. These include: criticism of the positivist paradigm and the biomedical model; the influence of social sciences on the practice of nursing; conceptual developments in the field of nursing care; the training of research nurses in other countries; the influence of North American ideas about nursing; and, in some cases, individual efforts and interest in the existential dimension—in people's voices, experiences, and suffering.

We begin with the case of Brazil. In a Latin American context, Brazil has been the pioneer in nursing research and was the first country in the region to have a nursing doctoral program (Ailinger et al., 2005). Brazilian nurses have also been a guiding light, acting as teachers and encouraging the spread of qualitative research throughout Latin America, by contributing to the training of nurses from Mexico, Chile, and Colombia, who have found in Brazil a country culturally similar to their own, but with high academic standards, where they can pursue their postgraduate studies. Those nurses have since developed doctoral programs in their own countries, in which training in qualitative research has been given a privileged position.

Brazil

Historical context

Throughout its history, nursing research has largely been linked to Brazilian postgraduate programs, influencing and being influenced by their trends and perspectives, shifting from a more positivist tradition linked to the biomedical model, to a perspective more closely tied to the human sciences and bearing the qualitative brand. Strictly speaking, postgraduate studies in nursing began in Brazil in 1972, when the Anna Nery School of Nursing of the Federal University of Rio de Janeiro began to offer a Master's degree in basic nursing. In 1982, the School of Nursing of the University of São Paulo began a doctoral program in nursing (Barreira & Baptista, 2000; Padilha & Nelson, 2009). In 1998, there were 14 postgraduate courses in nursing, a number which grew to 51 in 2011, an increase of 364.28%. This is of enormous significance for the development of the nursing profession in terms of professional qualification.

Discussion of the production, dissemination, and socialization of knowledge in Brazilian nursing must also include the Brazilian Nursing Association (ABEn), which has established itself in the 86 years since its foundation as the vital organ responsible for a large proportion of the production and dissemination of knowledge in Brazilian nursing. It achieves this though its national and regional events, as well as through the *Brazilian Nursing Journal* (*Revista Brasileira de Enfermagem*), the official means of distribution for the ABEn.

Influenced by the American model, the first scientific studies in nursing, up to the end of the 1970s, followed the classic positivist method as their only frame of reference in their research. They took objects of study directed towards the biological component of nursing care, analyses of administrative activities developed by nurses in health institutions on practical grounds, standardization and testing of skills, and studies of normal biological parameters (Boemer & Rocha, 1996).

Following these first steps in research, and in accordance with scientific advances in the 1980s, nurses became conscious of new and unexplored areas of potential study, such as power relationships in institutions, the working process, social class, gender, health history, etc. Nursing came to be discussed and understood as a social practice, and historical materialism became the favored theoretical viewpoint. On the other hand, nurses concerned with the subject to whom care is provided, with the subjectivity of this relationship, with communication, and with the intersubjectivity of this production of knowledge, produced new research, this time of a phenomenological sort. Qualitative phenomenological research then manifests itself as the way of getting closer to understanding the existential dimension of professionals and patients, with research carried out on suffering, loss, and conflict.

The international movement which recognizes the non-neutrality of science (Japiassu, 1983) also gained ground in Brazil, and nursing then incorporated new objects of study, including: questions of gender and female health; health and lifestyle; health promotion; communication in nursing; health and citizenship; human resources; health of the worker; the deinstitutionalization of psychiatric patients; the hospital as a diagnostic and therapeutic tool, and as the scene of domination and subordination; the history of nurses' work; the difficult relationships between members of a health team in situations of serious illness and death; education in nursing; and the labor market.

Until the end of the 1980s, quantitative and qualitative studies in the field of nursing were produced in parallel, in accordance with the philosophy of postgraduate studies. However, the following decade saw the beginning of a new trend, where the production of knowledge showed a clear tendency to scorn quantitative approaches (Silva, 2009).

Current aims and contributions

Just over three decades have passed since Brazilian nurses began their studies, taking a qualitative approach. A key role in strengthening and increasing the production of knowledge in postgraduate nursing programs is played by research groups. There are currently 410 such research groups in the Research Directory of the National Counsel of Technological and Scientific Development (CNPq) (Brasil, 2011). These groups are made up of teaching researchers, together with undergraduates, and Master's and doctoral students in nursing. We believe that the potential of an area of knowledge can be seen as a global public good, to contribute to the refinement of activities relating to education, health care, and policies, and the improvement of personal and public health (Pang et al., 2003).

Despite scientific production in nursing knowledge being largely restricted to universities and postgraduate programs, there is broader discussion on research and its interface with practice, with teaching, and with the process of nursing work. One of the studies carried out on Brazilian scientific production identified that the past ten years have seen the prioritization of studies on the subject of assistance, including those that treat the process of care and the determining factors in quality of life and health/illness. A second priority has been studies relating to the management of services, including studies on the politics and practice of health and nursing, education and nursing, organization of work, management, and communication in nursing. The third priority has been studies labeled "professional," which include research relating to the fundamentals of care, theoretical and philosophical concepts, technologies, professional ethics, and the history of nursing (De la Cuesta Benjumea, 2010; Prado & Gelbcke, 2001).

Methods, perspectives, approaches, tools

Over the years, Brazilian researchers have brought to bear various techniques and styles of qualitative research in the area of nursing. Here we opt to draw attention to some of the most common modes of qualitative design in Brazilian studies. Among the most frequently applied are: phenomenology; ethnography; grounded theory; dialectics and historical materialism; historical research; and convergent-care research.

Phenomenology is a descriptive, rigorous, and practical science, which shows and explains "Being" in itself, and is concerned with the essence of lived experience. In its approach of attempting to understand the Other on its own terms, it resembles that of nursing, which takes a holistic view, seeing man as a whole (Capalbo, 1994). In a bibliometric study carried out between 1982 and 2002 at the Center for Nursing Studies and Research of ABEn, 217 studies with a phenomenological approach were identified, 70% of which were drawn from Master's dissertations. This research showed that the majority of those studies were produced from 1990 onwards, in the Federal Universities of Santa Catarina and Rio de Janeiro, and the University of São Paulo, in Ribeirão Preto. The most common areas of study were adults, women, and child health (Merighi, Gonçalves, & Ferreira, 2007).

Ethnography took root in Brazil in the 1990s. It focuses on culture and social practice, and its theoretical basis is in anthropology. It is a methodology well suited to discovering people's lifestyles and experiences—their worldview, emotions, ceremonies, habits, meanings, attitudes, behavior, and actions. In ethnography's early days, there was a concern to give a detailed description of its findings, since it was thought that the voices of the subjects of the research would thus be secured. Nowadays we see that, as the relationship between theory and research is better articulated and understood, as well as describing their findings in detail, ethnographic studies in nursing also set out a descriptive process with interpretation of those findings in the light of anthropological theories or theories of nursing, which comes to constitute a new kind of knowledge (Elsen & Monticelli, 2003).

The use of *grounded theory* in Brazil began slowly from 1989, with only six studies. Nonetheless, the following decade saw studies multiply to around 150. Its methodology is a complex process of data analysis, and opens up new pathways for the researcher as a methodological framework for interactionist studies. Most of the studies which have employed it are the products of postgraduate courses. It is a framework which demands the close involvement of the researcher at all stages, presenting problems for the involvement of research assistants, and which also requires, as other methodologies do, a considerable input of time and energy, especially when it is the first example of such research (Cassiani, Caliri, & Pelá, 1996).

The methods of *dialectics and historical materialism* very often have been used when dealing with health/illness phenomena and health institutions, since it is necessary to set these phenomena in the dual context of the wider social picture and of each individual example within the particular historical period of its occurrence (Gelbcke, Peña, & Gallo, 2008). In Brazil, it is worth noting the contribution of studies made since the 1980s, when nursing began to be seen as a social practice and important studies were undertaken on the working process in nursing and the use of health care technology. The patient, the nurse, and the nursing team are seen as social subjects whose final aim is to attend to the social needs in the area of health, the individual's recovery, or health control over the population as a whole.

Historical research appeared on the Brazilian horizon in 1990, and is of particular interest to nurses in certain areas. Padilha et al. (2007) analyze the bibliography relating to historical studies that are linked with Brazilian postgraduate studies in nursing in the period 1972–2004. They identified 126 studies with this historical perspective, and divided them according to the following categories: professional identity and institutionalization of nursing; schools; specialisms; and organizing bodies. Another study by the same authors (2012) on the scientific production of Brazilian research groups in the history of nursing from 1999 to 2009 identifies 34 such research groups, with a total production of 2206 articles, 230 books, 745 book chapters, and 1603 full-length works, or extended abstracts. The conclusion to be drawn is that the dissemination and socialization of knowledge show that this area is already well established.

The final methodological slant suggested here is *converging assistance research*, put forward by the Brazilian researchers Mercedes Trentini and Lygia Paim (2004) as a new research modality, which focuses its research on the scene of nursing care, combining theory and practice. Its approach is inspired by Action Research in its explicit interrelation with nursing assistance practice, and its specialism is in the area of application, that is, the area of health. The choice of this method as a research approach obliges the researcher to go into the field and participate in some form in the practice of nursing, becoming directly involved with the object of the research. Nevertheless, the independence of the research process is respected, as the principles of scientific research are kept in mind at all times. This research modality permits the health professional/ researcher to reflect on the context of his or her own practice, and to carry out research at the same time as delivering health care. A bibliometric study (Reibnitz, Prado, Lima, & Klock, 2012) gives evidence that convergent-care research has been employed in theses and dissertations at postgraduate level, both in nursing and in other subject areas, such as public health, phono-audiology, and biomedical gerontology. It has been used in a number of different settings and with various participants.

Challenges and limitations

In recent decades, developmental initiatives in nursing research, whether individual, collaborative, or cross-institutional, have multiplied on a global scale, with the aim of improving the quality of care provided and patient confidence, while also seeking to promote more efficacious health policies. Evidence-based research, clinical research, systematic reviews, convergent-care research, phenomenological and socially representative studies have all had the same objective: to provide answers to questions of professional practice. However, despite all the advances in knowledge, the funding of such research and the involvement of researchers, there is a great chasm between the production of this research and the implementation of its conclusions in public health services or hospitals. The chasm that still needs to be bridged, in my view, is the promotion of studies whose objective is really one of transformation and integration between the scientific and nursing communities. To achieve this, partnerships between schools, community organizations, health services, and scientists are essential, as their roles change from being producers of knowledge or those who apply the knowledge produced (Padilha, 2011).

Future directions

In sum, the advances in scientific production in Brazilian nursing from its inception to the present day are remarkable, and particularly so during the past two decades. In this respect, it is important to emphasize the decisive contribution of postgraduate programs as support spaces that encourage reflection, analysis, and criticism of the relationship between theory and practice in the field of nursing. This process also allows further light to be shed on an area in search of its own independence and professional identity, by making more available to society the various ways of understanding nursing, and of knowing, being, and doing nursing (Rodrigues & Bagnato, 2003).

What is apparent in the first decade of the twenty-first century is that qualitative and quanti-tative approaches are no longer mutually opposed, following the realization that they are not necessarily aligned with different paradigms or worldviews. What is important is that both are kept in mind while carrying out research, especially when the respective focus, techniques, and procedures of both are adopted as fitting the present context and leading to a contribution to knowledge, and therefore contributing to resolving the problems of the society in which we live (Silva, 2009).

Chile[3]

Historical context

At the beginning of the twentieth century, the overall state of Chilean health was marked by a high rate of mortality, the result of the cholera epidemic of 1886–1888 and the influenza epidemic of 1892–1893. When coupled with the civil war of 1891 and the 1896 economic crisis, this led to the capital city, Santiago, having the highest death rate of any in the developed world. The levels of infant mortality, again high in comparison to other countries of the Americas, were attributed to the poor education of their mothers, to the alcoholism of their fathers, and to a life of unhealthy habits (Murillo, 1899).

This led to an attempt to seek health solutions in foreign countries (Salgado-Paris & Sanhueza-Alvarado, 2010), and the University of Chile, founded in 1843 (www.memoriachilena.cl), sent the doctor Eduardo Moore to Europe, to investigate its health care practices. In England, he discovered the work of lay nurses, trained according to the guidelines laid down by Florence Nightingale (Salgado-Paris & Sanhueza-Alvarado, 2010). Thus began in 1902 the first three-year course in nursing in the San Francisco de Borja Hospital, followed in June 1906 by the State Nurses' School, part of the University of Chile (www.med.uchile.cl). The section that was under the remit of Public Hygiene (now the Ministry of Health) was integrated into the Ministry of the Interior in 1907 (Murillo, 1899).

The second degree in nursing was created in Valparaíso University in 1933 (www.uv.cl), and southern Chile saw the third in 1948, at the School of Nursing of Concepción University. There are now around 80 in existence.

The university reform that took place during the 1960s gave rise to a process of questioning the character and social role of education, which brought change to the universities, taking them from a markedly professionalizing outlook to a preoccupation with a university's social role, and seeing a university's intake broaden, along with the funds earmarked for education, while greater emphasis was placed on research and associated sectors (Agüero, 1987). In terms of nursing, this had the effect of confirming it as a degree course with the same rights and responsibilities as any other academic course. The role played by teachers was strengthened in the 1970s by Kellogg Scholarships, which allowed students to apply for Master's degrees in the United States, thus beginning the study of theories and models, the basis of the nursing process; this gave the teacher's role a broader scope, which now included extension work and research, and formally established a teaching care agreement (www.uv.cl). The 1970s and 1980s saw the creation of Master's programs in nursing both in the capital and in the regions; there were Master's programs in mental health, community health, and medical and surgical health, and there are currently six academic nursing Master's programs.

Current aims and contributions

It is clear that the development in Chilean nursing before the 1970s supported its social consolidation as a profession and discipline, broadening its view of the various knowledge paradigms in order to investigate the reality of the situation and thus make a contribution as a discipline to the country's social reality. But this progressive development was abruptly halted, and a key factor in limiting the range of its influence was the imposition of a military regime from 1973 to 1989. This period brought an end to the independence of nursing among the health services, leaving it, as it had been originally, under the direction of doctors, and it also saw the end of the university degree devoted to nursing. This led to complex and lengthy pay claims by both professionals and unions, for which purpose both the Chilean Nurses Association and the Chilean Association of Nursing Education (ACHIEEN) joined forces. In hindsight, the delay that this caused to the development of the discipline as a social science is most regrettable.

The development of research in Chilean nursing is principally linked to the positivist paradigm, the dominant strand in the country's research and technology policies, which had come out of the National Commission for Scientific and Technological Research (CONICYT) since 1967. The start of Master's programs in Chile saw an increase in scientific production in nursing; however, the approach that was taken followed the quantitative paradigm. An attempt to explain the dominance of this approach must consider it from the perspective of gender, because of its important role in determining the social division of work and the education that men and women received in Chilean society. Nursing has not been immune to the binary division of disciplines which associates "the feminine" with social aspects, with caring for others and with the arts, and "the masculine" with science, numbers, and sport (Berríos-Cortez, 2007; Velásquez et al., 1999).

In reference to the beginnings of qualitative research in Chile, María Figueroa F. indicates that she introduced some qualitative research at Concepción University during the 1980s, at least in two nursing Master's programs, as well as in specialization programs, based on her study of Rosemarie Rizzo Parse in *Nursing Science*.

Methods, perspectives, approaches, tools

Mendoza-Parra and Paravic-Klijn (2004) have studied the state of the art of Chilean nursing and its tendencies during the period 1965–2003, identifying the subjects of study on which nurses focused: from 1965–1969, it was the nursing professional; from 1970–1989, the focus was on the child and adolescent at risk of illness; 1990–1999 saw it shift to the hospitalized adult; and 2000–2003 saw a tendency to study the health needs of adults at risk of falling ill. In terms of publications, the same study found that 93.5% (n = 200) of those published by Chilean nurses exhibited the quantitative paradigm, in a descriptive mode. In their 2004 study of South American publications from 2002 to 2005, Alarcón-Muñoz and Astudillo-Díaz (2007) found that of 151 articles published in three Latin American journals (one Chilean, one Cuban, and one Colombian), the vast majority (80.8%) were quantitative studies; 17.3% were qualitative studies, and 1.3% showed a mixed approach, with both qualitative and quantitative features. The Chilean journal supplied most of the qualitative studies. In terms of authorship, 78.8% of the publications were by academic nurses with clinical or administrative professionals or students, with just 21.2% being authored by professionals from the clinical field, i.e., alone. Of all the 151 articles published, 26.5% came from the Chilean journal, 55% from the Cuban, and 18.5% from the Colombian. The Chilean journal was the Iberoamerican research journal *Ciencia y Enfermería* (*Science and Nursing*), first published in 1995 by the Nursing Department of Concepción University, which has contributed to the transmission of knowledge in nursing with both quantitative and qualitative approaches. Mendoza-Parra et al. (2009) state that during the 1990s qualitative studies began to appear in indexed journals, the first such Chilean study being that of Muñoz (1995a), on the ethnographic model, and the second being Sanhueza's, which followed the interactionist line (Sanhueza-Alvarado & Villela-Mamede, 2000).

Changes in the health situation of Chile in the last decades of the twentieth century show health indicators that require greater care on the part of the adult population, due to the damage caused by chronic diseases. As professionals from hospitals and universities united, nursing research took as its key subject the adults who were hospitalized during the 1990s (Mendoza-Parra et al., 2009). The country's nurses expressed their concern over interpersonal relationships in a hospital context, as well as interference produced by technology concerning the patient, since the perspective of the subject who was in care required consideration, recognizing intersubjective language as a vital component that needed to be researched. The interpretative slant is therefore presented as a point of reference relevant to nursing's everyday tasks, especially in situations of suffering, pain, and conflict—in sum, wherever there are important significant issues that should be recognized.

Recent decades have seen a growing concern to disseminate knowledge acquired through research at scientific events. Prominent among these are the National Nursing Research Days, organized by the Chilean Association of Nursing Education (ACHIEEN), and National Nursing Conferences, organized by the Chilean Nurses Association. There are three journals in circulation in Chile, confirming the advances made in nursing's scientific production (Jara-Concha et al., 2009).

Doctoral programs, which prepare paradigms of various types for the production of independent researchers, did not appear in Chile until the 2000s. The two programs currently in existence in Chile as of 2012 have played an important role in promoting qualitative research in the country. The first was inaugurated in 2004 at Concepción University and included the special subject "Qualitative Nursing Research," which deals with phenomenological, ethnographical, and interactionist approaches. The second has been offered since 2006 in Andrés Bello University, Santiago, and, in collaboration with the University of São Paulo, it includes a compulsory subject which treats in detail the philosophical frameworks of Heidegger, Merleau-Ponty, Husserl, and Schultz. Qualitative research has also been included in the various nursing Master's programs offered in the country.

Luz Angélica Muñoz González, a pioneer of qualitative research in Chile who studied the ethnographic modality in depth, using Spradley's ethnographic model, indicated in 1995 how necessary it was to include the study and foundations of qualitative research in the nursing curriculum from the undergraduate level, since this is "the understanding of phenomena experienced by those involved in nursing" (Muñoz, 1995b). At the undergraduate level in most current curricula, the vast majority of academic courses include only the methodology of quantitative research. On this matter, a study by Flores-Montiel (2009) of undergraduate theses at the School of Nursing of Chile's Southern University between 1999 and 2007 found that of the 297 theses, 66.7% were quantitative, being predominantly cross-sectional studies, and qualitative studies comprised 33.3% of the theses, preferably with a phenomenological approach.

Professor Muñoz, having graduated from the doctoral program in nursing of São Paulo University in 1993, says: "My interest in training in qualitative research arose in the course of my professional and academic life [in the Southern University of Valdivia, Chile], in the context of the experiences that people and their families had of the health care services" (pers. comm., 2011). Her conviction that "qualitative research was the future for the professional discipline" found support there, as she explored different paradigms, and theoretical and philosophical frameworks, while sharing her inquiries with peers, professors, and groups that were interested in this research approach. This allowed her not only "to look at the phenomena in a new light, but also to select new ways forward to produce the research that fit most closely" with her own worldview. On this point, Muñoz and Lorenzini (2008) declare that "when a researcher is interested in the relationship with the human dimension, it is necessary to undertake qualitative research." Referring to its development in Chile, Muñoz says: "It began when nursing schools saw the need to learn the paradigm and its various pathways; many universities in the country also ran courses and seminars [during the 1990s and part of 2000]" (pers. comm., 2011).

485

Magali Boemer, Professor in the School of Nursing of São Paulo University in Ribeirão Preto, was the first foreign academic to begin qualitative research in the Chilean context. In 1993, Professor Boemer visited the Nursing Department of Concepción University to give a course entitled "Research Methodology: *Phenomenology*." The students were enrolled on the Master's program in nursing, some of them teachers from that same university's Nursing Department, along with students who came from Peru, Venezuela, Argentina, and Panama. She says: 'The Master's program only looked at the classical method of research, that is, quantitative research; qualitative research and the phenomenological modality were unknown, so the challenge was to present it as a new research horizon." This visit also helped facilitate the necessary conversations to open a new doctoral program in nursing run jointly by the University of São Paulo at Ribeirão Preto and Concepción University. Further collaboration has also made possible the development of courses in qualitative research, and the inclusion of students and teachers in research centers, as well as allowing students to make visits to deepen their knowledge of qualitative methodology.

Challenges and limitations

Every year, students on Master's and doctoral programs in nursing analyze epistemological, philosophical, and methodological aspects of interpretative research, focusing on phenomenology, ethnography, and interactionism. As this analysis has been carried out, it has seen the collaboration of nursing academics and anthropologists, sociologists, and others, to enrich the prevailing understanding of the approach. The phenomenological framework requires analysis of the existential phenomenology of Heidegger and Merleau-Ponty, among others. The ethnographic modality is considered against the backdrop of anthropological tradition, and the approach of symbolic interactionism follows the schema of social psychology laid down by George Herbert Mead and Herbert Blumer. This third approach has been used to investigate the meaning that breast cancer has for women. Phenomenology and ethnography have been used to research topics of adult and family care in cases of Alzheimer's, diabetes, hypertension, cardiovascular illness, gastric cancer, depression, and osteoarticular disease, as well as ethnocultural factors in the Mapuche population, and others.

Future directions

Qualitative nursing research in Chile had a period of slow growth, in both the number of researchers trained in this approach and the number of studies produced. Its inception has been far from straightforward, for various reasons, foremost among which is the mark that has been left by positivism on the health education sphere as a whole (the biomedical paradigm), as well as on individual examples where research funds are secured (CONICYT). Second, there has been uncertainty over how trustworthy its results are, given the number of people involved in its study. A third reason is the lack of training required to carry out such research: we have mentioned above that undergraduate programs do not include qualitative methodology, with few exceptions. A fourth limiting factor for the qualitative approach is the disproportionately strong curative emphasis in undergraduate curricula, at the expense of the humanistic element.

Boemer-Roseira (2001) indicated how important it was that the students "discuss different philosophical trends and scientific traditions." Mariano, in the same volume, identifies certain "essential skills" for learning qualitative research, such as that of "fighting ambiguity," a capacity for "abstraction," and a "humanist bent." On this last skill, the same author stated that "students must have a desire to understand other perspectives and a sense of awareness, in order to see the researcher–subject relationship as a two-way relationship."

The inherent difficulty of qualitative research, which cannot be achieved by following a simple formula with linear and pre-planned stages, requires reflexive thought, in order to discover meanings and explore results with the greatest possible breadth and diversity. These skills do exist in current undergraduate curricula, and the future is therefore promising for qualitative research and the students who will come to move on to postgraduate studies. Chilean nursing "is working hard to produce a body of knowledge that has an impact on the health of the population" (Mendoza-Parra et al., 2009). We as teachers face a great challenge in trying to put incentives into the introductory scientific programs at undergraduate level so that they continue on the path of scientific research, with its various conceptions and worldviews. The teaching practice and academic scientific frontiers should promote further discussion and use of the different modalities of qualitative research. Transforming the low levels of access to available research sources is one of the greatest challenges faced by qualitative nursing research in Chile, in order to promote its empowerment as a social science and to support society, by humanizing nursing care.

Colombia[4]

Historical context

Colombian nurses who have adopted qualitative research as a means of knowledge production have followed various paths which combine to articulate and define four characteristics. The first is that qualitative research has become possible as a result of a network of influences which ultimately derive from local experiences in participatory research (Romero B., 1995), and from the international context, passing then onto universities of standing in Bogotá, Cali and Medellín: the Pontifical Xavieriana University (Pontificia Universidad Javeriana), the National University of Colombia, the University of Valle, the University of Antioquia, and the University of La Sabana. This has branched out into other universities of regional influence in other capital cities, such as the University of Cauca, the Pedagogical and Technological University of Colombia, and the University of Cartagena.

After training on doctoral programs in nursing and social sciences, usually in universities in the United States and Brazil, professors from the most reputable universities have contributed to the design of Master's and doctoral courses, on which other university teachers then began to train to those levels. During their postgraduate training, some teachers learned and adopted qualitative methodologies which they have gradually incorporated into their practice as teachers and researchers. Qualitative research has likewise had a relevant presence in the doctoral programs in nursing offered by the National University of Colombia since 2004, and in those of the University of Antioquia since 2011.

Another network of influences is derived from the theories and methodologies of other disciplines, whether health-related ones, such as critical epidemiology, or from the human and social sciences, such as philosophy, anthropology, and sociology. Of this last group, the influence of certain authors is particularly noteworthy, such as Orlando Fals Borda, Jürgen Habermas, Michel Foucault, Pierre Bourdieu, Susana Guber, Guillermo Hoyos, Humberto Maturana, and Arturo Escobar. In the context of nursing theory, Madeleine Leininger is an author who has had an influence on researchers who work from an ethnographic perspective.

The second characteristic is related to the clear structural inequalities of the country, both social and economic, which, in the field of nursing, are manifest, for example, in the variable levels of access to higher education in nursing (Duque-Páramo & López Maldonado, 2009), and particularly in the dramatically unequal access to knowledge and resources necessary to produce quality research. These two examples are related because, in general, it is the professors from universities of greater standing and wider resources who have had the opportunity to train in other countries, who have greater access to financial and bibliographic resources, as well as research groups, and who then act as teachers on domestic postgraduate programs.

The third characteristic is that the boom in qualitative research in many nursing faculties has gone hand in hand with criticism of the instrumentalization of the practice of nursing, along with an interest in the study of *care* as what defines the profession. This has been related to the interest of certain professors who, skeptical of the power and hegemony of the biomedical perspective over nursing practice, have instead carried out participatory research on the voices and perspectives of the social actors with less power in society: women, children, the disabled, and displaced persons.

The fourth characerestic which has made qualitative research possible is the passion, innovation, and resolve of certain nurses who, recognizing that empirical-analytical approaches are insufficient for the understanding of social reality, especially in contexts that are contrary to their interests and ideologically positivist, ventured to produce research of a participatory or hermeneutic nature. At first, they did this with the bare bones of methodological knowledge behind them, but with the passing of time, the advent of postgraduate students, and the benefits of self-teaching, they have become the points of reference for young professionals and students.

Exemplars and methods

Following a trend in nursing common in the United States until the 1950s and in Latin America until the 1960s (Castrillón Agudelo, 2004), nursing research in Colombia until the 1980s centered on self-knowledge, on looking at oneself as a profession and seeking both to reaffirm the status and to emphasize the role of the nurse in society, and finally on the use of empirical-analytical, quantitative methodologies. In contrast, since the 1990s, qualitative research has contributed to a broadening and diversification of interests, as well as heightening the impact and relevance of Colombian research in nursing.

As researchers have become competent in dealing with a variety of different methodologies, qualitative nursing research has slowly grown and consolidated itself as a practice recognized by other health disciplines, such as medicine, phonoaudiology, and psychology, as well as by some social sciences. This is also reflected in the higher levels of funding available at a national level for research, Master's theses, and doctoral theses which take a qualitative approach. Similarly, there is a growing presence of qualitative research by Colombian nurses at national and international events in nursing, social sciences, and research.

A review of critical literature between 1990 and 2010 reveals 190 relevant studies, on a wide variety of themes and showing an interest in both hospital nursing and public health, as well as including studies of specific groups divided by age, ethnicity, gender, and social class. There is a preponderance of studies on women and expectant mothers, on adults and the elderly; but some studies have been made of children, families, peasants, and students and teachers of nursing.

Among the wide range of studies, we draw attention to three examples which are representative of standard influences, approaches, and methods. The first example is that of participatory research and cultural studies. In this group there are a wide variety of qualitative interviews and pieces of ethnographic research, on the varying cultural practices of different groups, particularly women (Acosta et al., 1997; Argote, Bejarano Beltran, Ruiz de Cárdenas, Muñoz de Rodriguez, & Vásquez, 2004; Castro, Muñoz, Plaza, Rodríguez, & Sepúlveda, 2006), the elderly (Castellanos Soriano & López Díaz, 2010, 2011), indigenous peoples (Alcaraz López & Yagarí Tascón, 2003; Arias Valencia & De la Cuesta-Benjumea, 2004; Duque-Páramo & Salazar, 1994), and marginal and peasant communities (Eslava Albarracín, 1998). Participatory studies have also been carried out with peasants (Romero B., 1995), the elderly (Céspedes Salgado, 2001), and children and young people (Duque-Páramo, 2008). Some researchers have also become interested, on the basis of participatory and Action Research approaches, in analyzing and drawing attention to social inequalities, and in creating forms of empowerment and social inclusion.

The second representative example includes studies of experiences (Canaval, González, Tovar, & Valencia, 2003), of meanings and representations of illness, of carers (Alvarado García, 2007), and of nursing care for people with various health problems such as infectious diseases, chronic illnesses, Alzheimer's, or disabilities (Moreno Fergusson, Rodríguez, Gutiérrez Duque, Ramírez, & Barrera Pardo, 2006), and cancer (Castillo & Chesla, 2003). These studies, a high proportion of which concern adults and the elderly, are largely carried out by means of qualitative interviews, phenomenological studies, and grounded theory.

Carmen de la Cuesta Benjumea, a Spanish nurse who studied nursing in Madrid before taking a Master's in social science and a doctorate in nursing in England, is our third example. When she arrived in Colombia in 1992, and at the University of Antioquia in 1994, she found a place rich with the experience of researchers who had carried out participatory, ethnographic, and phenomenological studies. Until her return to Spain in 2003, Carmen contributed to the development of qualitative research in the country with her own research work, as well as by training other researchers and translating into Spanish four books representing stages of qualitative research that have become reference works for researchers in the country (Coffey & Atkinson, 2003; Morse, 2003; Strauss & Corbin, 2002; Wolcott, 2003). Her influence is also still felt through thematic and methodological publications (De la Cuesta Benjumea, 2003, 2006), as well as being felt in the emphasis on qualitative research now evident in the Nursing Faculty of the University of Antioquia and in the growing use in the academic community of grounded theory as a tool for the analysis of qualitative data.

Contributions

In Colombia, qualitative research has contributed to the criticism of the biological and pathocentric models of biomedicine, as well as to improving nursing practice and humanizing nursing care. It has allowed a widening of nursing's conceptual perspectives towards other disciplines of the social sciences, and contributed to nurses' greater recognition, self-esteem, and vigor; it has had a positive impact on undergraduate and postgraduate courses, and fostered interdisciplinary work in the field of health.

From the point of view of academic development, we are seeing a rise in the number of qualitative research articles in the various journals of Colombian nursing catalogued internationally, of which the outstanding journals are: *Aquichan*; *Investigación y Educación en Enfermería* (*Research and Education in Nursing*); *Investigación en Enfermería* (*Research in Nursing*); *Investigación en Enfermería: Imagen y Desarrollo* (*Nursing Research: Image and Development*); and *Avances en Enfermería* (*Advances in Nursing*).

In contrast to the hierarchical and authoritarian models which are still present in biomedical practice, qualitative research promotes horizontal relationships based on the participation and empowerment of communities, and also has positive emotional effects, such as catharsis, the expression of emotions, and recognizing participants as social actors. It has also contributed to the design of health programs tailored to specific communities, to sensitizing public opinion about childhood in the context of migration, and to the creation of local and regional policy on the issues of violence and sexual and reproductive health.

Limitations, challenges, and future directions

The limitations and challenges are tied up with the social context, the institutions, and the nurses themselves. One problem that is still present, though less so than before, is the ignorance of qualitative studies, or the low value attributed to them, on the part of some researchers, nursing faculties, and financing bodies, in comparison with the greater prestige enjoyed by quantitative studies.

Another set of limitations, this time related to both regional inequalities and those between universities of greater and lesser standing, as well as the varying levels of access to higher education in the country, may be found in the often limited command of English, in the scarcity of resources for bibliographical searches, and in the difficulty itself of qualitative analysis.

We consider the following necessary for the future: greater capacity on the part of researchers and students in the planning, analysis, and rigor of qualitative research; the promotion of regional, national, and international alliances, with the aim of carrying out cross-institutional studies, introducing exchange visits for teachers and students, and fostering a culture of learning and innovating on the basis of experience; and finally, progress towards the construction of theories and models to contribute, from our national reality, to the global development of nursing as a discipline.

The most important challenge is to make our research more applicable and ensure that it has greater impact on the living conditions of the people and communities we work with. In this sense, we consider feedback to be of the highest importance, along with: the submission of reports to those who participate in research; a mixed approach which aims at contributing both quantitative and qualitative evidence to the design of health programs and policies; and the implementation of tools which bring greater participation and joint interpretation with participants, such as methodologies based on games and art.

Mexico

Historical context

Mexico is currently in the midst of an accelerated process leading to the development of an economy based on a knowledge society. Attempts are thus being made to bring about the necessary conditions to reduce the current gaps in education, science, technology transfer and innovation, and social and economic education. The challenge for the country is to consider the various methodological approaches appropriate to social realities, themselves ever more diverse, unfair, and riddled with contradictions. Moreover, there is an intention that knowledge should contribute to social well-being, and to the professions as social practices (Benavides, 2002; Romero & De la Peña, 2007; Verde, Nájera, & Contreras, 2010).

In the discipline of nursing, research was originally associated with gaining a diploma, professional title, or academic qualification, and was marked by North American influence and its positivist perspective. The methods used during the period of 1983–2003 were quantitative in nature and with descriptive designs, where subjects were treated such as the development of human resources, and factors associated with professional practice, with scarcely any attention paid to nursing care (Benavides, 2002).

The great variance in levels of training in the country, which was diverted into questions of the type of nurse required and the need to specify different functions, has been a research priority. This produced studies which were vital in justifying the presence of nursing in universities (Facultad de Enfermería de la UANL, 2011; Verde, Nájera, & Contreras, 2010).

During the late 1980s, research was largely carried out within nursing Master's programs, which began in the Autonomous University of Nuevo León in 1982, and was most strongly driven forward by the First Plan for the Development of Postgraduate Nursing in Mexico, proposed by the Mexican Federation of Nursing Faculties and Schools (Espino, Martínez, Alonso, & Gallegos, 2001). If anything can be criticized in Mexican nursing, it is the late introduction of the research approach of the essence of the discipline, which is *care*.

A change may currently be observed in the interests and approaches of research undertaken. García et al. (2011) report that 77% of this research is still quantitative, with 16% qualitative, and 6% showing a mixture of approaches. In terms of qualitative paradigm, 33.7% of studies carried out between 2005 and 2010 were ethnographic; 32.6% worked with grounded theory; and 33.7% used phenomenology. The subjects studied were largely (60%) on matters of care, and the majority of the researchers had Master's qualifications in nursing, a minority holding doctorates in the subject, coinciding with the introduction of this level of qualification in Mexico in 2002–2003.

The change in nursing research and the use of the qualitative paradigm are a product of recent years, as a result of various factors relating to the introduction of doctoral programs in nursing. The first doctoral training program was developed in the University of Guanajuato (Celaya-Salvatierra Campus) in collaboration with the Riberão Preto School of Nursing of São Paulo University. In 2003, the Autonomous University of Nuevo León began the first doctoral nursing program in a Mexican university. The emphasis of the doctorate is on the study of nursing phenomena, such as integral responses to risk and sickness processes, self-care in health and sickness, integral adaptation to internal and environmental processes, as well as people's behavior in risk processes, contributing thereby to the understanding of national health problems (Facultad de Enfermería, UANL, 2012; Secretaría de Salud, 2007). Another reference point in nursing research is seen in the priorities of the health sector, public health insurance, quality, and patient security (Secretaría de Salud, 2007).

In a context where the positivist perspective and its various approaches are privileged, over three decades had to pass from the early days of research for Mexican nursing to look clearly at the qualitative perspective, and its potential for the understanding of phenomena.

Exemplars and methods

Qualitative research implies the acquisition of a paradigmatic position from which to understand social reality, the product of an historical process of construction viewed through the lens of the logic and subjectivity of the protagonists. In this paradigm, the researcher develops a close relationship with the subject of the research, and with its informants, as well as becoming involved in its social world: the qualitative researcher forms a part of the world which is being investigated, affects it, and is in turn affected by it (De la Cuesta, 2005).

In order to contribute evidence on the development of qualitative research in Mexico, we decided to investigate by means of publications by colleagues in two domestic nursing journals (*Desarrollo Científico de Enfermería* [*Scientific Development in Nursing*] [DCE] and the nursing journal of the Mexican Social Security Institute), and in two international journals in which Mexican nurses publish, one from Colombia (*Aquichan*) and one from Brazil (*Revista Latin Americana de Enfermería* (*Latin American Nursing Journal*) [RLAE]). While searching the domestic journals, we found that one contained 292 research articles published during the five years (2007–2011), of which only 20 featured qualitative research. The other journal, linked to a health institution, ran 129 such articles during the same period, of which only one showed a qualitative approach.

In the Colombian journal in which Mexican nurses publish, two of the 89 published articles were on the basis of qualitative methodology. Finally, in the Brazilian journal, we found 762 articles, of which four were the result of qualitative research done by Mexican nurses.

The phenomena treated by Mexican nurses include the construction of meaning of actions, of lived experience regarding a health problem, and of beliefs about illness, as well as values which have an impact on health practices. The studies emphasize understanding from another's perspective—the dynamics of social relationships established between people who share a life experience such as suffering from a chronic or critical illness, or going through something on a daily basis.

Other studies concern the meaning ascribed to their suffering by people who live with critical diseases such as HIV/AIDS (Calvo, Pérez, Morales, Báez, & Alonso, 2008), and what it means to live with peritoneal dialysis (Medina, García, Martínez, & Alonso, 2009). The starting point for both these studies is symbolic interactionism, and their methodological framework was provided by grounded theory. The authors indicate that people who live through these realities create meanings which are shared through experience of the disease, as well as though interaction with various groups and with their families; these constructions of meaning are therefore derived from their realities.

In the search for professional identity through care, Alonso et al. (2009) investigated how care constructs professional identity and the way that nursing students follow in this construction. Various elements emerged in the study which help to construct this identity, from the voices of teachers as role models, to learning experiences in care, and shared knowledge and norms.

In the article published in the journal of the Mexican Social Security Institute, we see the views of adolescents on the risk of contracting AIDS (Trejo-Franco, Flores-Padilla, & Villaseñor-Farías, 2010). The authors refer in their interpretation to the classical theory of perception and semiotic textual analysis centered on discourse. Their findings derive from the fact that adolescents process what they perceive in an active-constructive way, within an anticipatory schema against which they compare the perceptual stimulus, which is then accepted or rejected according to whether or not it fits with what is proposed by the schema (Neisser & Ato, 1981). Their conclusion is that these adolescents perceive AIDS as a stigmatizing disease of homosexuals or drug addicts, but interpret the risk perception as a matter of bad luck or destiny, exhibiting cognitive dissonance.

In sum, then, three of the four examples presented by the two domestic journals were carried out with the aim of understanding the meaning of living with critical or catastrophic illnesses, of their actions and beliefs, beginning with the social interaction of those who share the same set of problems, and the same territorial, cultural, and historical context.

The article published in *Aquichan* treats the experience of caring for an elderly adult with a chronic illness from a phenomenological perspective (Aldana-González & García-Gómez, 2011). The authors indicate that, by emphasizing the person's subjective experiences, the phenomenological perspective considers their ideas, experiences, and feelings, within the framework of the internal system of reference of the person who experiences them. The results of the carers' discussions speak of the understanding of a concrete existential phenomenon, i.e. caring for the aged (such as elderly relatives), as a filial duty, revealing constant moral contradictions in this role designated by the feminization of care.

Finally, of the articles published by the *Revista Latinoamericana de Enfermería* (*Latin American Nursing Journal*), three were carried out from the perspective of symbolic interactionism and the method of grounded theory, while one was a phenomenological study. In the study of drug consumption as a social practice in gangs (Guzmán, Pedrão, López, Alonso, & Esparza, 2011), the authors indicate that this perspective allowed them to understand how gang members construct the meaning of consuming drugs in their social reality, and in the interaction with their peers. The interpretative paradigm of grounded theory allowed the emergence of certain concepts such as the consumption of drugs as a collective activity, whose origins lie in the influence of gang members and friendship ties. The experience of consumption is shared in a context which facilitates this practice and the distribution of drugs within the same gangs.

Other studies take as their starting point the perspectives and attributions which patients confer on their care of themselves and on the causes of breast cancer and violence. It may also be noted that in Mexico certain groups interested in qualitative research join forces within the nursing faculties which offer postgraduate training at Master's and doctoral level. There is a feeling that during the next few years there will be a systematic and sustained flourishing of qualitative studies, which will broaden and deepen our knowledge of the very phenomena of nursing and health.

Challenges and limitations

Qualitative researchers contribute to the development of the theoretical grounding of care and the delivery of health care services. In the integration of teaching, service, and research, various phenomena of interest for nursing arise, and the integration of these dimensions allows for a more integral analysis. The principal challenge for qualitative research is that it demands a philosophical posture that needs to be developed. Here we may note the low levels of training of research nurses in philosophical and methodological positions, and in qualitative methodologies, which is reflected in the small number of publications during the last five years in the journals treated here.

Linked to the above is the fact that nurses of some institutions are still faced with criticism of the validity and trustworthiness of data obtained by the qualitative method, since the positivist paradigm is still the dominant tradition in most health and education institutions. Equally, the bodies which offer financial support to research projects favor the quantitative method, for its potential to make generalizations which contribute to the health of a greater number of users.

A further challenge is that of managing to get the results of the research into the public eye, in journals which are catalogued in *Journal Citation Reports*. This source does not currently include any of the Mexican nursing journals; one possible option is then to publish in journals that focus on health sciences, but the potential for publishing studies that rely on qualitative methodology is then reduced by the number of quantitative studies presented for publication by other professionals.

Another challenge is presented by language: our first language is Spanish, which causes us to look to Brazilian journals that accept studies written in English, Spanish, and Portuguese, such as the *Revista Latinoamericana de Enfermería* (*Latin American Nursing Journal*). This journal is catalogued on *Journal Citation Reports*, which has brought wider attention to the works published there, but at the same time has led to rising interest in sending work to this prestigious journal to be published, meaning that there is a certain wait involved before publication is possible.

North American journals which publish qualitative work and are catalogued on *Journal Citation Reports* have increased in number considerably more dramatically than those of Brazil or Spain. Nonetheless, there is a language barrier, since the publication process demands a level of proficiency in both languages (Spanish and English), and there are significant costs involved in professional translation. In this light, and granted that qualitative research allows one to understand a phenomenon from the perspective of the person who lives and experiences it, researchers have proposed projects which make use of mixed methods (quantitative and qualitative studies), where both paradigms complement the results of the research and allow a broader conception of the phenomenon. This increases the likelihood of securing funding, but demands a profound knowledge of how both paradigms must be applied.

Future directions

It is undeniable that qualitative nursing research is a recent phenomenon that is linked to postgraduate training. Despite the analysis of publications by Mexican nurses, as well as the increase in nurses with postgraduate qualifications, we can discern a short-term growth in qualitative research. The limitations outlined above on the possibilities for obtaining funding for qualitative studies require nurses to be more creative and competitive when proposing a project, making adjustments to their approaches as required and to participate in different organizations and programs to obtain grants. One possible strategy in this country is for work to be undertaken in groups including both inexperienced research nurses and those of experience and renown, which would drive forward the quality of qualitative research.

Another alternative for the consolidation of this research in Mexico is that of research networks, and there is certainly potential for growth in qualitative methodologies, interdisciplinary work, and the training of postgraduate students.

Conclusion

The positive change during recent decades in the area of knowledge production in nursing in Latin America has been driven by three key factors: first, academic qualifications gained by nursing professionals, and especially postgraduate programs; second, research groups; and third, the availability of funding for research projects.

At the beginning of the 2010s, in terms of qualitative nursing research, the countries studied here present different accomplishments and different levels of development. Brazilian nurses have achieved greater leadership, recognition, and consolidation of this research activity by means of established research centers comprised of undergraduate, Master's, and doctoral students, together with researchers, both in nursing and in other disciplines; moreover, they have also managed to have an impact on professional practice. Colombia has research groups and researchers whose work has an impact on both academic literature and the practice of nursing and public health. Chile is advanced in the focus of development for qualitative research through cross-institutional colloquia and the formation of research groups, while in Mexico some nurses have gradually begun to introduce qualitative studies into research practice.

We close this chapter with some suggestions for the promotion of qualitative research in Latin America, and the establishing of links with other regions:

- to offer greater opportunities for nursing professionals to develop scientific research by consolidating and broadening postgraduate programs, and thus make them more competitive in a globalized world;
- to promote unions, alliances, cross-institutional collaborative projects, and exchanges at a national and international level between researchers and research groups that contribute to the resolution of shared health problems in those countries;
- to achieve a greater social impact through research which draws attention to inequalities of gender, ethnicity, social class, age, and place of origin; furthermore, to incorporate the results of qualitative research on certain ways of caring for people, and to make good quality and more significant contributions to the resolution of health problems faced by the communities we work with;
- to forge a place in the scientific sphere in Latin American nursing, respecting its idiosyncrasies and sharing experiences in the field of research;
- to establish national policies for the creation of coordination mechanisms between the bodies charged with responsibility for science and technology at a national level, to achieve greater

recognition for nursing research and its participation and contribution to the health of those countries' populations;

- to achieve greater cohesion among the various professional and academic levels of development, in order to establish a policy for nursing research, specifying possible lines of approach and research priorities, both at a national level and in a wider, Latin American context;
- to consolidate the position of nursing and health periodicals, by seeking that they be rated in at least two languages, with the aim of making the knowledge produced more widely available;
- to develop reflexive studies of the theoretical-methodological frameworks of qualitative research, seeking approaches to nursing practice.

We agree with Malvárez (2011) that the fostering of research policies, together with continual education and the creation of dialogue spaces between universities and services are the primary strategies that will incentivize change in the services, and produce solutions to health problems and evidence to sustain the policies and practices of nursing care.

Notes

1 This chapter was translated by Richard Rabone, Merton College, Oxford University, UK.
2 The sections were authored as follows:
    - Brazil: Maria Itayra Padilha
    - Chile: Olivia Inés Sanhueza-Alvarado
    - Colombia: María Claudia Duque-Páramo and Fabiola Castellanos Soriano
    - Mexico: María Magdalena Alonso Castillo, Karla Selene López-García, and Yolanda Flores-Peña.
3 We are grateful for the help of Professors María Figueroa F., Magali Roseira Boemer, and Luz Angélica Muñoz, who allowed us to include relevant material to the history of qualitative nursing research in Chile.
4 Research funded by the Pontifical Xavieriana University (Pontificia Universidad Javeriana), with the support of the nurse Diana Carolina Buitrago García. The study includes a review of criticism from 1990 to 2010, and interviews with researchers from Colombian universities with a variety of backgrounds.

References

Acosta, M., Alearia, L., Cajiao, G., Llano, A. M., Valencia, C., & Zuluaga, P. (1997). Creencias populares sobre el autocuidado durante el puerperio en las instituciones de salud Nivel 1 [Popular beliefs regarding self-care during puerperium in level one health institutions]. *Colombia Médica, 28*(1), 42–50.

Agüero, F. (1987). *La reforma en la Universidad de Chile* [Reform in the University of Chile]. Santiago: Eds. Sur.

Ailinger, R. L., Najera, R. M., Castrillón, M. C., & Manfredi, M. (2005). Nursing research in Latin America: 1988–1998. *Revista Latino-Americana de Enfermagem, 13*(6), 925–928.

Alarcón-Muñoz, A. M., & Astudillo-Diaz, P. (2007). La investigación en enfermería en revistas latinoamericanas [Nursing research in Latin American journals]. *Revista Ciencia y Enfermería*, XIII (2).

Alcaraz López, G. M., & Yagarí Tascón, L. (2003). La concepción de la curación Chamánica entre los indígenas Embera de Colombia: un proceso de comunicación socio-cultural y fisiológico [The concept of Shaman healing among the indigenous Embera people of Columbia]. *Investigación y Educación en Enfermería, 21*(2), 60–78.

Aldana-González, G., & García-Gómez, L. (2011). La experiencia de ser cuidadora de un anciano con enfermedad crónica [The experience of being a nurse to the elderly suffering from chronic illness]. *Revista ACUCHIA, 11*(2), 158–172.

Alonso, M. M., López, K. S, Medina, M. R., Esparza, S. E., Alonso, M. T., & Álvarez, M. E. (2009). El cuidado como fundamento de la identidad de Enfermería: Las Voces del Profesorado [Care as the foundation of identity in nursing: The teachers' voice]. *Desarrollo Científico de Enfermería, 17*(9), 386–391.

Alvarado García, A. M. (2007). Adquiriendo habilidad en el cuidado: "De la incertidumbre al nuevo compromiso" [Acquiring skills in care: "From uncertainty to the new agreement"]. *Aquichan*, 7(1), 25–36.

Argote, L. A., Bejarano Beltran, N. L. i., Ruiz de Cárdenas, C. H., Muñoz de Rodriguez, L., & Vásquez, M. L. (2004). Transitando la adolescente por el puerperio [Taking a young woman through puerperium]. *Aquichan* 4(4), 18–29.

Arias Valencia, M. M., & De la Cuesta-Benjumea, C. (2004). El equilibrio inestable. El caso de Los Chamibida de Cristianía en Antioquia, Colombia [The unstable balance: The case of the Chamibida people in Antioquia, Colombia]. *Index de Enfermería*, 13(46), 23–28.

Barreira, I. A., & Baptista, S. S. (2000). La investigación y la documentación en la historia de la enfermería en Brasil [Research and documentation in the history of nursing in Brazil]. *Escola Anna Nery Revista de Enfermagem*, 4(3), 396–403.

Benavides, T. R. A. (2002). La investigación en la enfermería Mexicana [Research in Mexican nursing], *Revista de Enfermería IMSS*, 10(3), 153–158.

Berríos-Cortez, P. (2007). Análisis sobre las profesoras universitarias y desafios para la profesión académica en Chile [Analysis of university professors and challenges facing the academic profession in Chile]. *Calidad en la educación*, 26, 39–53.

Boemer, M. R., & Rocha, S. M. M. (1996). A pesquisa em enfermagem: notas de ordem histórica e metodológica [Nursing research: Historical and methodological notes]. *Saúde e Sociedade*, 5(2), 77–88.

Boemer-Roseira, M. (2001). Paper presented at *Conferência Chile: Investigação Qualitativa em Enfermagem* [Chile conference: Qualitative nursing research]. Departamento de Enfermería, Universidad de Concepción.

Brasil, Ministério da Ciência e Tecnologia. Conselho Nacional de Desenvolvimento Científico e Tecnológico, CNPq [National Council of Scientific and Technological Development]. (2011). *Diretório dos Grupos de Pesquisa*, Séries Históricas [online database]. Retrieved on May 9, 2011 from http://dgp.cnpq.br/censos/series_historicas/index_basicas.htm.

Calvo, M. C., Pérez, E., Morales, M. L., Báez, M. R., & Alonso, M. M. (2008). El significado de vivir con VIH, en la voz de quienes enfrentan esta realidad [The meaning of living with HIV, in the words of those who face this reality]. *Desarrollo Científico de Enfermería*, 16(7), 309–312.

Canaval, G. E., González, M. C., Tovar, M. C., & Valencia, C. (2003). La experiencia de las mujeres gestantes: "Lo invisible" [The experience of pregnant women: "The invisible"]. *Investigación y Educación en Enfermería*, 21(2), 32–46.

Capalbo, C. (1994). Abordando a enfermagem a partir da fenomenologia [Approaching nursing from phenomenology]. *Revista Enfermagem UERJ*, 2(1),70–76.

Cassiani, S. B., Caliri, M. H. L., & Pelá, N. T. R. (1996). A teoria fundamentada nos dados como abordagem da pesquisa interpretativa [Grounded theory as an interpretative research approach]. *Revista Latino-Americana Enfermagem*, 4(3), 75–88.

Castellanos Soriano, F., & López Díaz, A. L. (2010). Mirando pasar la vida desde la ventana: significados de la vejez y la discapacidad de un grupo de ancianos en un contexto de pobreza [Watching life pass by from the window: Meanings of the old age and disability of a group of the elderly in a context of poverty]. *Investigación en Enfermería Imagen y Desarrollo*, 12(2), 37–53.

Castellanos Soriano, F., & López Díaz, A. L. (2011). Tejiendo explicaciones sobre vejez, discapacidad y pobreza en los cerros nororientales de Bogotá, Colombia [Forging explanations for old age, disability, and poverty in the north-eastern hills of Bogotá, Colombia]. *Investigación en Enfermería Imagen y Desarrollo*, 13(2).

Castillo, E., & Chesla, C. A. (2003). Viviendo con el cáncer de un(a) hijo(a) [Living with your child's cancer]. *Colombia Médica*, 34(3), 155–163.

Castrillón Agudelo, M. C. (2004). Trends and priorities in nursing research. *Revista Latino-Americana Enfermagem*, 12(4), 583–588.

Castro, E., Muñoz, S. F., Plaza, G. P., Rodríguez, M., & Sepúlveda, L. J. (2006). Prácticas y creencias tradicionales en torno al puerperio, municipio de Popayán, 2005 [Traditional practices and beliefs concerning puerperium: The town of Popayán, 2005]. *Revista Infancia, adolescencia y familia*, 1(1), 141–152.

Céspedes Salgado, L. M. (2001). Sentido que tiene el anciano, el autocuidado frente a la enfermedad pulmonar obstructiva crónica. Propuesta participativa de autocuidado. [The meaning that an elderly man has: Self-care before chronic obstructive pulmonary disease. A participatory self-care proposal]. *Hacia la Promoción de la Salud*, 6, 87–92.

Coffey, A., & Atkinson, P. (2003). *Encontrar el sentido a los datos cualitativos* [Finding the meaning in qualitative data]. Medellín: Universidad de Antioquia.

De la Cuesta Benjumea, C. (2003). El investigador como instrumento flexible de la indagación [The researcher as a flexible instrument of investigation]. *International Journal of Qualitative Methods, 2*(4), Article 3. Retrieved from http://www.ualberta.ca/~iiqm/backissues/2_4/pdf/delacuesta.pdf.

De la Cuesta Benjumea, C. (2005). La contribución de la Evidencia Cualitativa al campo del cuidado y la salud comunitaria [The contribution of qualitative evidence to the field of care and community health], *Index de Enfermería, 14*(50), 47–52.

De la Cuesta Benjumea, C. (2006). "Aquí cuidamos todos": Asuntos de individualidad versus colectividad en un estudio sobre cuidado en la casa con pacientes de demencia avanzada ["Here we are all carers": Matters of individuality versus collectivity in a study on home care with patients with advanced dementia]. *Forum Qualitative Social Research,* 7(4), 5.

De la Cuesta-Benjumea, C. (2010). La investigación cualitativa y el desarollo del conocimiento en enfermería [Qualitative research and the development of knowledge in nursing]. *Texto Contexto Enferm.* 19(4), 762–726.

Duque-Páramo, M. C. (2008). No me gusta, pero está bien si me porto mal. Voces sobre el castigo de niñas y niños de un barrio de Bogotá [I don't like it, but it's fine if I behave badly. Notes on the punishment of children in a district of Bogotá]. *Investigación en Enfermería Imagen y Desarrollo, 10*(1), 113–134.

Duque-Páramo, M. C., & López Maldonado, M. C. (2009). Nursing in Colombia. In K. L. Breda (Ed.), *Nursing and globalization in the Americas: A critical perspective* (pp. 21–54). Hartford, CT: Baywood Publishers.

Duque-Páramo, M. C., & Salazar, E. (1994). *Cuidado de las personas en los procesos de salud y enfermedad en comunidades indígenas y negras aisladas de Colombia* [Caring for people in health and illness processes in isolated indigenous and Black communities in Columbia]. Bogotá: Javegraf.

Elsen, I., Monticelli, M. (2003). Nas trilhas da etnografia: Reflexões em relação ao saber em enfermagem [On the trail of ethnography: Reflections regarding knowledge in nursing]. *Revista Brasileira de Enfermagem, 56*(2), 193–197.

Eslava Albarracín, D. G. (1998). Los agentes tradicionales de salud: Otra alternativa de salud para las comunidades campesinas el caso de Cundinamarca y Santander [Traditional health agents: Another health alternative for peasant communities. The case of Cundinamarca and Santander]. *Investigación y Educación en Enfermería, 16*(2), 57–70.

Espino, V. M. E., Martínez, M. M. G., Alonso, C. M. M., & Gallegos, C. E. (2001). *Plan de Desarrollo del Posgrado de Enfermería en México* [Development plan for postgraduate nursing programs in Mexico]. Federación Mexicana de Asociaciones de Facultades y Escuelas de Enfermería AC y Universidad de Guanajuato, pp. 1–28.

Facultad de Enfermería, Universidad Autónoma de Nuevo León. (2011). *La Facultad de Enfermería de la UANL: Perspectiva Histórica* [The nursing faculty of the autonomous University of Nuevo León: An historical perspective]. Primera Edición, Monterrey, Nuero León. México: Centro de Documentación y Archivo de la UANL.

Facultad de Enfermería, Universidad Autónoma de Nuevo León. (2012). *Programa de Doctorado en Ciencias de Enfermería, Monterrey, Nuevo León, México* [Doctoral program in nursing sciences: Monterrey, Nuevo León, Mexico]. Monterrey, Nuevo León.

Flores-Montiel, N. (2009). Caracterización, contexto académico y pertinencia al contexto sanitario de las tesis de pregrado de la Escuela de Enfermería de la Universidad Austral de Chile [Characterization, academic context, and relevance to the health context of undergraduate theses in the School of Nursing of the Southern University of Chile]. Thesis for degree in nursing, School of Nursing of the Southern University of Chile in Valdivia. Retrieved from http://cybertesis.uach.cll/tesis/uach/2009/fmf634c/dac/fmf634cpdf.

García, R. M., Gómez, A. M. G., Aguilar P. I., Pérez M. G. P., Velázquez D. L., Soriano S. M., & Landeros, O. E. (2011). Tendencias y características de la investigación en enfermería publicada en México [Tendencies and characteristics of nursing research published in Mexico]. *Revista de Enfermería Universitaria ENEO-UNAM, 8*(1): 7–16.

Gastaldo, D., Mercado-Martinez, F. J., Ramasco-Gutierrez, M., Lizardi-Gomez, A., & Gil-Nebot, M. A. (2002). Qualitative health research in Ibero-America: The current state of the science. *Journal of Transcultural Nursing: Official Journal of the Transcultural Nursing Society/Transcultural Nursing Society, 13*(2), 90–108.

Gelbcke, F.L., Peñà, .Y., & Gallo, E. (2008). Dialéctica y materialismo histórico: su aproximación al estudio del fenómeno salud/enfermedad [Dialectics and historical materialism: Their approximation to the study of the health/illness phenomenon]. In *Investigación cualitativa en Enfermería: contexto y bases conceptuales*

[Qualitative nursing research: Context and conceptual bases]. Washington, DC: Serie Paltex Salud y Sociedad No. 9. Organización Panamericana de La Salud.

Guzmán., F., Pedrão., L., López., K., Alonso., M., & Esparza., S. (2011). El consumo de drogas como una practica cultural dentro de las pandillas [Drug consumption as a cultural practice in gangs]. *Revista Latino-América de Enfermagem, 19*(1), 839–847.

Japiassu, H. (1983). *O mito da neutralidade científica* [The myth of scientific neutrality] (2nd ed.). Rio de Janeiro: Imago.

Jara-Concha, P., Behn-Theune, V., Ortiz-Rebolledo, N., & Valenzuela-Suazo, S. (2009). Nursing in Chile. In K. Breda (Ed.), *Nursing and globalization in the Americas: A critical perspective* (pp. 55–98). Hartford, CT: Baywood Pub. Co.

Malvárez, S. (2011). Editorial. *Texto & Contexto—Enfermagem* [Text and Context—Nursing], *20*, 21–26. Retrieved on June 25, 2012 from http://www.scielo.br/scielo.php?script=sci_arttext&pid=S0104-07072011000500002&lng=en&tlng=en.

Medina, O. M., García, M. A., Martínez, M. G., & Alonso, M. M. (2009). Significado cultural de vivir con diálisis peritoneal ambulatoria continúa [The cultural meaning of living with continuous ambulatory peritoneal dialysis]. *Desarrollo Científico de Enfermería, 17*(8), 342–346.

Mendoza-Parra, S., & Paravic-Klijn, T. (2004). Organización y tendencias del conocimiento de enfermería en Chile [Organization and tendencies of nursing knowledge in Chile]. *Revista Brasileira de Enfermagem, 57*(2): 143–151.

Mendoza-Parra, S., Paravic-Klijn, T., Muñoz Muñoz, A. M., Barriga, O. A., & Jiménez-Contreras, E. (2009). Visibility of Latin American nursing research (1959–2005). *Journal of Nursing Scholarship, 41*(1), 54–63.

Merighi, M. A., Gonçalves, R., & Ferreira, FC. (2007). Bibliometric study on nursing theses and dissertations employing a phenomenological approach: Tendency and perspectives. *Revista Latino-Americana Enfermagem, 15*(4), 645–650.

Moreno Fergusson, M. E., Rodríguez, M. C., Gutiérrez Duque, M., Ramírez, L. Y., & Barrera Pardo, O. (2006). ¿Qué significa la discapacidad? [What does disability mean?] *Aquichan, 6*(1), 78–91.

Morse, J. M. (2003). *Asuntos críticos en los métodos de investigación cualitativa* [Critical issues in the methods of qualitative research]. Medellín: Universidad de Antioquia.

Muñoz, L. A. (1995a). La enfermedad vino para quedarse [Illness has come to stay]. *Revista Ciencia y Enfermería, I* (1), 43–51.

Muñoz, L. A. (1995b). El desafio de investigar en enfermería [The challenge of nursing research]. *Revista Ciencia y Enfermería, I* (1): 17–21.

Muñoz, L. A., & Lorenzini, A. (2008). La fenomenología en la producción de conocimiento en enfermería [Phenomenology in knowledge production in nursing]. In M. L. do Prado, M. Lourdes de Souza, & T. E. Carraro (Eds.), *Investigación Cualitativa en Enfermería: Contexto y Bases Conceptuales* [Qualitative nursing research: Context and conceptual bases], Washington, DC: O.P.S. Serie PALTEX Salud y Sociedad.

Murillo, A. (1899). La mortalidad en Santiago [Mortality in Santiago]. *Revista Chilena de Hijiene, 1899.* Imprenta Cervantes, Chile. Retrieved from http://www.memoriachilena.cl/temas/documento_detalle. asp?id=MC0027488.

Neisser, U., & Ato, M. (1981). *Procesos cognitivos y realidad: Principios e implicaciones de la psicología cognitiva* [Cognitive processes and reality: Origins and implications of cognitive psychology] (trans. M. Ato). Madrid: Marova.

Padilha, M. I. (2011). Translational research: What is its importance to nursing practice? *Texto e Contexto—Enfermagem* [online], *20*(3), 219–224.

Padilha, M. I., Borenstein, M. S., Carvalho, M. A. L., & Ferreira, A. C. (2010). Grupos de pesquisa em história da enfermagem: a realidade Brasileira [Research groups in the history of nursing: The Brazilian reality]. *Revista da Escola de Enfermagem da USP, 46*(1), 192–199 .

Padilha, M. I. C. S., Kletemberg, D. F., Gregório, V. R. P. I., Borges, B., & Borenstein, M. S. (2007). A produção da pesquisa histórica vinculada aos programas de pós-graduação no Brasil, 1972 a 2004 [The production of historical research tied to postgraduate research programs in Brazil, 1972–2004]. *Texto e Contexto—Enfermagem* [online], *16*(4), 671–679 .

Padilha, M. I., & Nelson, S. (2009). Teaching nursing history: The Santa Catarina-Brazil experience. *Nursing Inquiry, 16*(1), 171–180.

Pang, T., et al. (2003). Knowledge for better health: A conceptual framework and foundation for health research systems. *Bulletin of the World Health Organization, 81*(11), 815–820.

Prado, M. L., & Gelbcke, F. L. (2001). Produção do conhecimento em enfermagem no Brasil: As tematicas de investigação [The production of nursing knowledge in Brazil: Research themes]. *Revista Brasileira de Enfermagem 54*(1), 34–42.

Prado, M. L., Souza, M. L., Carraro, T. E., Cisneros, G. R., & Arzuaga, M. A. (2008). Producción del conocimiento en enfermería en América Latina: Un meta-análisis [Knowledge production in nursing in Latin America: A meta-analysis]. In *Investigación cualitativa en Enfermería: Contexto y bases conceptuales* [Qualitative nursing research: Context and conceptual bases]. Washington, DC: Serie Paltex Salud y Sociedad No. 9. Organización Panamericana de La Salud.

Reibnitz, K. S., Prado, M. L., Lima, M. M., & Klock, D. (2012). Estudo bibliométrico das dissertações e teses que utilizaram pesquisa convergente assistencial [Bibliometric study of dissertations and theses using convergent-care research]. *Revista Texto e Contexto Enfermagem*. In press.

Rodrigues, R. M., & Bagnato, M. H. S. (2003). Pesquisa em enfermagem no Brasil: Problematizando a produção de conhecimentos [Nursing research in Brazil: Problematizing knowledge production]. *Revista Brasileira de Enfermagem, 56*(6), 646–650.

Romero, B. M. N. (1995). El saber y las prácticas médicas tradicionales [Knowledge and traditional medical practices]. *Avances en Enfermería, 13*(2), 71–76

Romero, J. C., & De la Peña, J. A. (2007). El CONACYT y la ciencia mexicana de hoy: Logros y retos [CONACYT and current Mexican science: Achievements and challenges]. Retrieved from ABCuniversidades.com.: http:// www.abcuniversidades.com/Articulos/282/el_conacyt_y_la _ciencia_ mexicana_hoy.

Salgado-París, J., & Sanhueza-Alvarado, O. (2010). Enseñanza de la Enfermería y relación docente asistencial en el marco educacional y sanitario chileno [The teaching of nursing and the teacher–carer relationship in the Chilean educational and health context]. *Investigación y Educacióu en Enfermería, 28*(2), 258–266.

Sanhueza-Alvarado, O. (2009). Contribución de la Investigación Cualitativa a Enfermería [The contribution of qualitative research to nursing]. *Ciencia y Enfermería, 15*(3), 15–20.

Sanhueza-Alvarado, O., & Villela-Mamede, M. (2000). Estereotipos de género y cuidado de sí en mujeres mastectomizadas [Gender stereotypes and self-care in mastectomized women]. *Revista Ciencia y Enfermería, 6*(1), 21–31.

Secretaría de Salud. (2007). Programa Sectorial de Salud, 2007–2012: Por un México sano, construyendo alianzas para una mejor salud [Sectorial health program, 2007–2012: For a healthy Mexico: constructing alliances for better health]. México D. F., 1–24. Retrieved from http://portal.salud.gob.mx/ descargas/pdf/plan_sectorial_salud.pdf.

Silva, M. A. (2009). Os contrapontos da produção acadêmica na emergência da pesquisa qualitativa [The counter-arguments of academic production on the emergence of qualitative research]. *Educativa, 12*(1), 163–170.

Strauss, Λ., & Corbin, J. (2002). *Bases de la investigación cualitativa: Técnicas y procedimientos para desarrollar la teoría fundamentada* [The bases of qualitative research: Techniques and procedures to develop grounded theory]. Medellín: Universidad de Antioquia.

Trejo-Franco, J., Flores-Padilla, L., & Villaseñor-Farías, M. (2010). Percepción de riesgo de contraer SIDA en adolescentes de Guadalajara, Jalisco [The perceived risk of contracting AIDS among adolescents in Guadalajara, Jalisco]. *Revista de Enfermería IMSS, 18*(3), 3–8.

Trentini, M., & Paim, L. (2004). Pesquisa convergente assistencial [Convergent-care research]. Florianópolis, Insular: Universidad de Chile. Available at: http://www.memoriachilena.cl/temas/bibliografia.asp?id_ut =launiversidaddechile(1842-2000).

Universidad de Valparaíso, Escuela de Enfermería y Obstetricia Universidad de Valparaíso. (n.d.). *Reseña de la carrera de enfermería Universidad de Valparaíso* [Review of the nursing degree at Valparaíso University]. Retrieved from http://www.uv.cl/enfermeriayobstetricia/docen_enf10.htm.

Velásquez A., Manassero, M., Fernández, M., Picornell, C, Serra, B., & Erice, C. (1999). *Los estereotipos de género en el currículo científico y tecnológico de secundaria: Actitudes y preferencias de alumnado y profesorado* [Gender stereotypes in the secondary science and technology curriculum: The attitudes and preferences of students and teachers]. Madrid: Ministerio de Trabajo y Asuntos Sociales, Instituto de la Mujer de España.

Verde, E., Nájera, N. R. M., & Contreras, G. M. E. (2010). La investigación como generadora de cambios de paradigmas de enfermería [Research as generator of paradigm change in nursing]. *Actualización de Enfermería, 13*(3),16–21.

Wolcott, H. F. (2003). *Mejorar la escritura de la investigación cualitativa* [Writing up qualitative research]. Medellín: Universidad de Antioquia.

37

Qualitative nursing research in Spain

An evolving strategy of resistance

Andreu Bover Bover, Denise Gastaldo,
Margalida Miró, and Concha Zaforteza

Introduction

In the past two decades Spanish nursing research has grown dramatically. The adoption of qualitative research by a large group of Spanish nurses, attested by publications in scientific journals and conference presentations, reveals a rising affinity with critical-social and interpretivist paradigms of knowledge production. In order to understand such growth and the consolidation of Spanish nursing qualitative research, it is important to explore recent Spanish history, scientific policies and research trends, as well as nursing education. Two major phases can be identified in this process: (1) in the 1990s, introductory training and fragmented initiatives, followed by (2) more systematic education in the 2000, which resulted in an increased number of studies and a relative enhancement in quality. In this chapter we describe the movement that led to this increase in research and to the current trends in qualitative research (hereafter QR) in Spanish nursing. In addition, we analyze how QR represented a resistance strategy utilized to produce knowledge about caregiving and nursing, and promote it as an academic discipline. We believe the Spanish case, given both its achievements and the challenges it has faced during this period, can serve as an inspiration for nurses attempting to increase their national or regional research capacity.

Three main sources of information have been used here: (1) the authors' experiences as qualitative researchers and academics over the last 10–15 years; (2) key informant interviews with well-established nursing researchers and leaders of organizations related to QR; and (3) a literature review of 119 qualitative studies into Spanish nursing. The review was conducted for the years 2000 to 2011, using the *EBSCOhost Research Database*, the *Web of Knowledge/Web of Science* and the Spanish database CUIDEN, which together encompass a broad selection of national and international nursing publications (114) and doctoral theses (5).

The making of nursing QR in Spain

For almost 40 years, Spain was under the dictatorship of General Franco (1936–1975). In that period, nursing professionals were unified under the designation of "ATS"—sanitary technical assistants—and their training was delivered in technical schools, not universities (Miró et al., 2011). During this period, women lost significant civil rights, and as members of a female-dominated profession nurses were trained to be subservient and obey physicians' orders (Miró,

2008). If we fast-forward to the twenty-first century, nursing schools have become university institutions, evidence-based practice has become common among practitioners, and teachers in the field are expected to hold PhDs and to undertake research as well as to teach. This dramatic transformation is at the very heart of the development of qualitative research in Spain, and we will now explore some key features of this process.

In the 1990s, nurses were keen to expand their professional horizons and many practitioners were interested in acquiring research skills. Their introduction to qualitative research was mainly through in-service continued education, followed by occasional, small nursing projects related to care issues or through participation in interdisciplinary research projects, predominantly in health promotion (Milagros Ramasco, pers. comm., 2011). In this period, two new journals, *Index de Enfermería* (1992) and *Cultura de los Cuidados* (1997), were created, in both cases along the lines of American journals such as *International Journal of Qualitative Health Research* and *Journal of Transcultural Nursing* (Amezcua & Carricondo, 2000). As these latter authors explain, this was an attempt to mimic successful strategies utilized in North America to consolidate QR, in particular, to create a platform to publish phenomenological studies undertaken by nurse researchers.

Both Milagros Ramasco and Carmen de la Cuesta Benjumea (pers. comm., 2011) describe this period as characterized by awareness raising, brief introduction courses, and informal supervision that resulted in incipient and fragmented projects; however, these in general lacked a clear conceptual framework and had methodological and analytical limitations. Most clinicians, with a technical training, had no background in social sciences or humanities (Carmen de la Cuesta Benjumea, pers. comm., 2011; Mercado et al., 2005) and to undertake short QR projects represented a significant intellectual challenge.

As an illustration of activities developed in the 1990s, one of the co-authors of this chapter (DG) was invited in 1998 by the national nursing research group, Investen, through a partnership with the Université de Montréal, to teach several lectures and intensive QR courses across the country in hospitals, primary health care settings and universities, as well as to present a keynote lecture at the second national nursing research conference. In the 1990s, those involved in capacity building for QR in nursing were mainly professionals from other disciplines, especially social scientists, a few academics from other countries, and Spanish nurses who were trained abroad or had degrees in other disciplines, as is the case with our interviewees de la Cuesta and Ramasco.

Those in administrative positions, such as chief nurses and research coordinators, also played an important role in expanding research opportunities, often having to fight to assure the presence of nurse-researchers in interdisciplinary institutional projects (Milagros Ramasco, pers. comm., 2011). In 1999, the "Laboratorio de Investigación Cualitativa en Salud" was created in Granada, bringing together not only Spanish researchers but also reaching out to Latin American researchers in the field of QR (Manuel Amezcua, pers. comm., 2012; Amezcua, 2000).

Also in this period, under the leadership of Investen, in the Instituto de Salud Carlos III (the educational and research arm of the Ministry of Health), nurses were sent annually to undertake a MSc program at the Université de Montréal (1996–2000), Canada, with a total of 21 Spanish nurses trained in this way, many of whom wrote Master's theses in the area of QR and returned to Spain to be research leaders in clinical settings and practice-oriented research.

The years from 2000 to 2012 were characterized by increasing access to research education, access to funding, and publications. Even though nursing became a university-based diploma in 1977, not until the European Union established the Bologna Agreement could nursing education officially include research content at the undergraduate level (BSc), followed by postgraduate studies (established more recently). The unification of European educational systems led to an intensification and expansion of research education in nursing for many countries. In the Spanish case, the first opportunity for nurses to have a bachelor's degree came from a private university, which trained approximately a hundred nurses in Anthropology (an intensive program). Later, nursing specialization, Master's and a few PhD programs followed, including an interdisciplinary program on qualitative health research, offered for a few years by the Fundación Robert and the Universidad Autónoma de Barcelona (Mercado et al., 2005).

Early in the first decade of the twenty-first century, other activities reflected and supported QR development. For instance, two books collected the contributions of Spanish researchers to qualitative health research, along with Ibero-American scholars (Gastaldo et al., 2002; Mercado et al., 2002), journals received and published more qualitative studies (e.g. *Archivos de la Memoria, Enfermería Clínica, Index de Enfermería*) and conferences on QR were organized, such as the second Ibero-American Qualitative Health Research Conference in Madrid, 2005, and annual meetings at the Reunión Internacional de Investigación Cualitativa, now in their tenth year (Manuel Amezcua, pers. comm., 2012).

Funding was a crucial factor in the development of more robust projects. At first, there was a limited understanding of qualitative research by many reviewers (Carmen de la Cuesta Benjumea, pers. comm., 2011), but gradually more qualitative researchers became reviewers themselves. However, poor evaluation standards or being evaluated according to positivist criteria continued to be problems faced by many qualitative health researchers, both for funding projects or publishing articles (Manuel Amezcua, pers. comm., 2012). Finally, organizations were created to promote qualitative nursing and interdisciplinary research, such as RedICS—Red Española de Investigación Cualitativa en Salud (www.isciii.es/investen)—a virtual space that offers information, opportunity for exchange of ideas and advice on QR.

In this decade, the original emphasis on training and funding for research by health care providers was accompanied by an increase in formal academic training, larger research projects being developed, and some projects being funded at clinical settings and others at faculties of nursing. From the many initiatives that have invigorated QR into nursing, we would like to mention two. At the level of specialization, in the Escuela de Enfermería de la Comunidad de Madrid, mental health and midwifery programs made QR an integral and transversal component of specialists' curricula. This means that for two years nursing residents have to develop a supervised research project and acquire basic research skills. Recent projects (2008–2010) have covered subjects such as gynecological and reproductive issues for lesbian women, home care for severely ill mental health patients, and women as consumers of psychotropic medication (Milagros Ramasco, pers. comm., 2011).

The second example is our own experience of developing nursing QR at the Universitat de les Illes Balears since 2001. After a week-long introduction to QR, taught by Denise Gastaldo, a research project which involved several faculty members received methodological supervision for two years, and resulted in national and international publications. Concomitantly, three authors of the present chapter became Gastaldo's PhD students (AB, MM, CZ) and obtained national funding for their own PhD projects. Funding was decisive in the process of building stronger projects in QR that helped to create programs of research, which in turn generated new projects that were subsequently also funded. All projects have generated national and international publications, several awards, and a number of presentations to different audiences. These authors are now PhD supervisors themselves and members of the doctorate program of their own faculty, whose development was supported by an interuniversity initiative from 2004 to 2011, the INPhD—International Nursing PhD Collaboration, originally composed by the University of Toronto, Canada, the universities of Melbourne and Sydney, Australia, and the Universidad de Nuevo Léon, Mexico. In the last year, they have organized a research group named GICS—Critical Health Research Group—which has local, national and international members, from Latin America and North America.

In summary, the 2000s were characterized by a considerable increase in the number of QR projects and enhancement of the quality of research, especially among studies developed under the supervision of an experienced qualitative researcher (Milagros Ramasco, pers. comm., 2012). Many of the same problems remain, though, such as studies that lack a theoretical orientation or are essentially limited descriptions of a phenomenon, as well as problems already noted regarding funding and publishing. We will now analyze nursing studies published in the last 11 years, exploring themes, methodologies and methods utilized in the twenty-first century in qualitative nursing research in Spain.

Major trends in Spanish nursing qualitative research

As mentioned earlier, with the aim of identifying the main trends in qualitative research into nursing in Spain over the last decade (2000–2011), we have conducted a review of studies published by Spanish nursing practitioners and academics. The search for these included the following descriptors: nursing, qualitative, care, as well as other terms referring to approaches, research methodology and techniques, such as phenomenology, participatory research, discourse analysis, ethnography, interviews, focus groups and life stories.

It should be noted that this form of search has limitations, in that databases do not include all reports of nursing qualitative research, and multidisciplinary or inter-professional publications in which nurses are not the primary author might be missed. The search itself identified 119 studies, and these have been analyzed in terms of the type of article, subject matter, design, and techniques used, as well as the journals in which they were published. This has allowed us to identify topics, methodologies and techniques that are currently dominant and emerging in Spain, and also to better understand the kind of journals in which Spanish nurses typically publish QR. Overall, we have found a high degree of diversity in nursing studies that use qualitative methodologies.

Regarding the types of articles, 65% report on original research. A further 30% are theoretical and methodological studies, 18% being position papers and 12% methodological articles, in which the authors present and describe new methodologies, techniques or methods, or discuss and analyze well-established research techniques. The final 5% of studies are review articles.

In the studies under examination, the authors looked at a wide range of topics, and identified six major categories. In Table 37.1 these are listed, together with example publications for each topic.

The first three categories include articles on perceptions, social factors and relationships established between professionals, users, patients' relatives and caregivers and together are the topics that dominate qualitative studies in Spain over the past 11 years. Studies on perceptions, experiences and needs focus primarily on the following situations: home care, dementia, death and bereavement, palliative care, cancer, surgical procedures, intensive care and hemodialysis. This may be related in part to the fact that since the early 2000s researchers have developed a particular interest in understanding the impact of nursing activities on the perception of members of the public (Amezcua & Carricondo, 2000).

Of the articles that consider the influence of social factors on family caregivers (also known as informal caregivers) and hired caregivers (mainly immigrants) and the impact of these factors on health and well-being, most focus on gender relations and/or caregivers' generational groups as determinants in their perception of caregiving roles and burden, as well as on studies into the accessibility and use of health services by immigrant caregivers. Studies looking at the relationship between nurses and patients' relatives or caregivers are carried out mainly in the areas of primary health care, emergency and intensive care units. The majority of studies on the perceptions and experiences of nursing students focus on the analysis of strategies used by students during

Table 37.1 The main topics of studies, with example publications

Main topics	Examples of publications
The perceptions, experiences and needs of nurses, patients and carers	Vivar, C. G., Orecilla, E., & Gómara, L. (2009). "Es más difícil": experiencias de las enfermeras sobre el cuidado del paciente con recidiva de cáncer. *Enfermería Clínica, 19*(6), 314–321.
	De la Cuesta Benjumea, C. (2010). The legitimacy of rest: Conditions for the relief of burden in advanced dementia caregiving. *Journal of Advanced Nursing, 66*(5), 988–998.
	Palacios, D., Losa, M. E., Salvadores, P., & Fernández, C. (2011). Sudden cardiac death: The perspectives of Spanish survivors. *Nursing & Health Sciences, 13*(2), 149–155.
Social factors and the impact of care on family caregivers and hired (immigrant) caregivers	Bover, A. (2006). El impacto de cuidar en el bienestar percibido por mujeres y varones de mediana edad: Una perspectiva de género. *Enfermería Clínica, 16*(2), 70–77.
	De la Cuesta Benjumea C. (2009). "Estar tranquila." La experiencia del descanso de cuidadoras de pacientes con demencia avanzada. *Enfermería Clínica,19*, 24–30.
	Zabalegui, A., Juandó, C., Sáenz de Ormijana, A., Ramírez, A., Pulpón, A., López, L., Bover, A., Cabrera, E., Corrales, E., Díaz, M., Galart, A., González, M. A., Gual, M. P., & Izquierdo, M. D. (2007). Los cuidadores informales en España: Perfil y cuidados prestados. *Revista Rol de Enfermería, 30*(7–8), 33–38.
Relations between professionals and family members or caregivers and the quality of nursing care offered	López, L., Tolson, D., & Fleming, V. (2001). Exploring Spanish emergency nurses' lived experience of the care provided for suddenly bereaved families. *Journal of Advanced Nursing, 35*(4), 562–570.
	Zaforteza, C., de Pedro, J. E., Gastaldo, D., Lastra, P. M., & Sánchez-Cuenca, P. (2003). ¿Qué perspectiva tienen las enfermeras de unidades de cuidados intensivos de su relación con los familiares del paciente crítico? *Enfermería Intensiva, 14*(3), 109–119.
	Useros, D., Candel, E., Alfaro, A., López, M., & García, C. (2004). Interacción de enfermería y cuidadoras informales de personas dependientes. *Atención Primaria, 33*(4), 193–199.
Perceptions and experiences of student nurses	Pérez, C., Alameda, A., & Albéniz, C. (2002). La formación práctica en enfermería en la Escuela Universitaria de Enfermería de la Comunidad de Madrid. Opinión de los alumnos y de los profesionales asistenciales. *Revista Española de Salud Pública, 76*(5), 517–530.
	Gálvez, A. (2005). Pedagogía de la desmotivación: Soy tonto, me llaman inútil: Dos estrategias de socialización secundaria en el hospital. *Index Enfermería, 14*(48–49), 23–27.
	San Rafael, S., Arreciado, A., Bernaus, E., & Vers, O. (2010). Factores que influyen en la elección de los estudios de enfermería. *Enfermería Clínica, 20*(4), 236–242.

Table 37.1 Continued

Main topics	Examples of publications
Gender, social and professional discourse on nursing	Cánovas, M. A. (2004). Trabajo e ideología de género: Un análisis antropológico de la enfermería en Murcia. *Enfermería Global*, 5 (nov).
	Lillo, M., Casabona, I., Galao, R., & Mora, M. D. (2004). La imagen de la enfermería española en cuidados críticos vista por pacientes europeos—Una aproximación hacia la identidad de los profesionales de los cuidados españoles en el contexto de la UE. *Cultura de los Cuidados,* Año VIII (15), 32–36.
	Miró, M., Gastaldo, D., & Gallego, G. (2008). ¿Porqué somos como somos? Discursos y relaciones de poder en la construcción de la identidad profesional de las enfermeras en España (1956–1976). *Enfermería Clínica*, 18(1), 26–34.
Responsibilities, organization, functions and the efficiency of care given by nurses in primary health care	Corrales, D., Galindo, A., Escobar, M. A., Palomo, L., & Magariño, M. J. (2000). El debate sobre la organización, las funciones y la eficiencia de enfermería en atención primaria: A propósito de un estudio cualitativo. *Atención Primaria, 25*, 34–47.
	Sancho, S., Vidal, C., Cañellas, R., Caldés, M. J., Corcoll, J., & Ramo, M. (2002). Análisis de situación y propuestas de mejora en enfermería de atención primaria de Mallorca: Un estudio con grupos focales. *Revista Española de Salud Pública, 76*, 531–543.
	Raña, C. D., Pita, R., Conceiro, A., Fernández, I., & García, C. M. (2004). Opinión de las enfermeras de atención primaria en el área sanitaria de A Coruña sobre la utilización de los diagnósticos de enfermería. *Enfermería Clínica, 14*(2), 77–82.

socialization, the reasons behind their choice of career, and difficulties faced in the educational process, particularly in their training in clinical settings. With respect to studies on changes and improvements to nursing practice through participatory processes, we note that most are carried out in intensive care units or focus on rehabilitation programs for patients with chronic conditions. Studies into gender, social and the professional discourse on nursing mainly analyze the values and attitudes that characterize the profession, the image that patients have of nursing, and how social and professional discourses, such as gender discourse, have shaped nurses' identity.

The literature also includes articles on methodology. Position papers present a diverse range of issues and controversies, but a dominant concern is that of the usefulness, characteristics and myths of qualitative versus quantitative research in nursing. In such studies the authors discuss the value of qualitative approaches in the study of health and nursing and argue that they are especially important in capturing the most complex and profound meanings of these phenomena, as a means of involving patients and professionals in the improvement of practices as well as to give voice to marginalized or minority groups. QR is described as an alternative to the positivist and biomedical paradigm for the exploration of complex caregiving phenomena (de la Cuesta Benjumea, 2006; Pita & Pértegas, 2002; Zabalegui, 2002). The authors also criticize the lack of consideration given to QR in evidence-based nursing (de la Cuesta Benjumea, 2005; Gálvez, 2003). Besides this central theme (usefulness and characteristics), the majority of other methodological papers focus on the five topics set out in Table 37.2.

Regarding articles on theoretical foundations, techniques and the characteristics and limitations of methods, it should be noted that these deal mainly with grounded theory, phenomenology, ethnography and the group interview (either focus groups or nominal groups). Among the review articles, at first, studies explored the scientific production in QR in Spain broadly (Amezcua & Carricond, 2000; Gálvez, Poyatos, & Estrada, 2000), while more recently they focus on specific topics, such as care of relatives of critically ill patients (Zaforteza et al., 2008).

Table 37.2 Main methodological topics in publications, with examples, 2000–2011

Main topics	Examples of publications
Usefulness and characteristics of QR	De la Cuesta Benjumea, C. (2006). Naturaleza de la investigación cualitativa y su contribución a la práctica de enfermería. *Metas de Enfermeria, 9,* 50–55.
	Amezcua, M., & Gálvez, A. (2002). Los modos de análisis en investigación cualitativa en salud: Perspectiva crítica y reflexiones en voz alta. *Revista Española de Salud Publica, 76,* 423–436.
	Pita, S, Pértegas, S. (2002). Investigación cuantitativa y cualitativa. *Atención Primaria, 9,* 76–78.
Reflexivity as a strategy of rigor in qualitative methodology	De la Cuesta Benjumea, C. (2003). El investigador como instrumento flexible de la indagación. *International Journal of Qualitative Methods, 2*(4) (online).
	De la Cuesta, C. (2004). Formación para la práctica de la investigación cualitativa: Algo más que retocar programas. *Enfermería Clínica, 14,* 111–116.
	Bover, A., Gastaldo, D., Izquierdo, D., Juandó, C., Luengo, R., Robledo, J., Sáenz de Ormijana, A., & Taltavull, J.M. (2006). Rigor metodológico en la investigación cualitativa: La reflexividad como herramienta para grupos de investigación. *Nure Investigación, 27* (online).
Participatory Action Research as an emerging form of health research	Delgado, M. P., Blasco, M., Torrents, R., Mirabete, I., & Solga, A. (2001). Modificación de la práctica enfermera a través de la reflexión: Una investigación–acción participativa. *Enfermería Intensiva, 12*(3), 110–126.
	Abad, E., Delgado, P., & Cabrero, J. (2010). La investigación–acción–participativa. Una forma de investigar en la práctica enfermera. *Investigación y Educación en Enfermería, 28*(3), 464–474.
	Abad, E., Meseguer, C., Martínez, J. T., Zárate, L., Caravaca, A., Paredes, A., Carrillo, A., Delgado, & P., Cabrero, J. (2010). Effectiveness of the implementation of an evidence-based nursing model using participatory action research in oncohematology: Research protocol. *Journal of Advanced Nursing, 66*(8), 1845–1851.

Table 37.2 Continued

Main topics	Examples of publications
Theoretical foundations, characteristics and limitations of methods and techniques	Amezcua, M. (2003). La entrevista en grupo. Características, tipos y utilidades en investigación cualitativa. *Enfermería Clínica, 13*(2), 112–117.
	De la Cuesta, C. (2006). Estrategias cualitativas más usadas en el campo de la salud. *Nure Investigación, 25* (nov–dic).
	Miró, M., & Gastaldo, D. (2010). Teoría fundamentada ¿Es una traducción adecuada para grounded theory? *Enfermería Clínica, 20*(5), 322.
Critical reading in qualitative research	Gálvez, A. (2003). Lectura crítica de un estudio cualitativo interpretativo. *Index de Enfermería, 42*, 39–43.
	Gálvez Toro, A. (2003). Lectura crítica de un estudio cualitativo descriptivo. *Index de Enfermería, 40–41*.

It seems remarkable that of all the articles published in the decade under study here, 24% were found in a diverse range of international journals, as detailed in Table 37.3. Also noteworthy is that the *Journal of Advanced Nursing* had most publications (five papers) and five other international journals have accounted for two articles each, these being *European Journal of Cancer Care, International Journal of Nursing Studies, Journal of Clinical Nursing, Journal of Transcultural Nursing* and *Nursing Science Quarterly*.

Table 37.3 International journals in which Spanish authors have published, 2000–2011

Journal name	Number of publications
BioMed Central Geriatric	1
BioMed Central Health Services Research	1
EDTNA/ERCA Journal	1
European Journal of Cancer Care	2
International Journal of Nursing Knowledge	1
International Journal of Nursing Studies	2
International Journal of Qualitative Methods (online)	1
Journal of Advanced Nursing	5
Journal of Clinical Nursing	2
Journal of Palliative Care	1
Journal of Transcultural Nursing	2
Nurse Researcher	1
Nursing & Health Sciences	1
Nursing Science Quarterly	2
Palliative Medicine	1
Patient Education and Counseling	1
Preventive Medicine	1
Revista Brasileira de Enfermagem	1
Risk Analysis	1
Women's Health (online)	1

Table 37.4 Main Spanish journals for qualitative nursing research publications, 2000–2011

Journal name	Number of publications
Atención Primaria	3
Cultura de los Cuidados	2
Enfermería Clínica	23
Enfermería Global	2
Enfermería Intensiva	9
Index de Enfermería	22
Investigación y Educación en Enfermería	2
Nure Investigación	6
Revista de Calidad Asistencia	2
Revista Española de Salud Pública	5
Revista Rol de Enfermería	2

In terms of Spanish national publications, the majority of studies were found in those journals listed in Table 37.4, with *Enfermería Clínica* (23 papers) and *Index de Enfermería* (22 papers) accounting for the most studies.

Having looked briefly at QR into nursing in Spain since 2000, we can say that it is in a state of rapid growth and consolidation. It can be characterized by its interest in theoretical and methodological debates, with less interest in the transfer, use and impact of research applied to specific problems in clinical and community settings. This is reflected in the number of position papers and of empirical, descriptive studies, as well as the fact that a minority of studies are interpretive and critical in nature. From our point of view, the fact that many authors do not state their theoretical frameworks is a reflection of a transition by researchers from a positivist paradigm, in which the majority of researchers in Spain were trained, to an interpretive or critical one.

However, we must also note that the articles published employ a wide range of methods and techniques, the most prevalent of which is the interview, most often a structured or semi-structured, followed by focus group; we can also see the emergence of ethnographic and evaluative methodologies, document analysis, and case studies. For the moment, though, most studies use techniques of a conversational nature and do not allow for the exploration of what participants actually do in their everyday activities (what could be achieved through observation), implying that the discourses people create about their practices represent their actions. That is consistent with the fact that there is also an emphasis on content analysis, but rarely on discourse analysis.

In numerous studies, a strategy used to ensure methodological rigor is to combine different data collection techniques, in order to obtain a triangulation of sources and methods or to ensure saturation of the data. Finally, we note that only a minority of authors explicitly set out the paradigm, theoretical framework, methodology or design which guides their study. Most simply, they name the methodology as qualitative, and go on to describe only the procedures for data collection and analysis. In the next section, we analyze some of these trends to better understand why they have arisen.

Relevant features of qualitative nursing research in Spain

QR in Spain has not simply been a new methodology to nursing and to the production of knowledge in the area of health care, but rather has represented a political opportunity to re-position nursing as a profession that produces scientific knowledge and engages with research in academic and health care settings, both as a discipline in itself and also in interdisciplinary teams. The emergence of QR as a space for resistance resembles what happened to sociology in the 1960s and early 1970s in Spain, when qualitative research was used to produce alternative discourses to those of the dictatorship, giving voice to marginalized groups in society (Peinado, 2002).

The achievements of the past 20 years have to be understood in the context of nurses' engagement with the national movement of re-democratization and the affirmation of women's rights, of great professional commitment, and significant levels of personal investment (e.g. cost of courses and traveling, studies being conducted in personal/family time), all of which reveals an eagerness for professional growth from a nursing cohort denied access to undergraduate and postgraduate education for many decades.

Within nursing, this meant a challenge to nurses' subordinated position in the health care system, as women and as a professional group, and resulted in a search for strategies towards new ways of thinking, talking, practicing, and producing knowledge in an attempt to overcome the traditional biomedical and positivist approaches in health care. We believe it is fair to say that this resistance and transformation movement tended to relate positivist, quantitative research to traditional values in practice and science, with an alternative to the status quo being the adoption of QR in the study of caregiving. As Pérez (2002) comments, in this context, quantitative and qualitative research confront each other: "the same way health promotion lacks prestige in relation to disease treatment, the work of nurses is in respect to the work of doctors, the same way that qualitative methodology is considered less valuable than quantitative" (p. 377).

As we noted in the literature review, many recent publications have focused on characterizing the differences between qualitative and quantitative research. In most, there is an emphasis on qualitative as the methodological approach of choice for nurses because it allows for overcoming the previous theory–practice gap that characterized the profession, studying complex and holistic caregiving issues, understanding patients' subjectivity to provide quality patient care, to be able to take into account how sociocultural factors shape patients' experiences and thus humanize health care (de la Cuesta Benjumea, 2000, 2010; Ramasco, pers. comm., 2011; Salinas, 2010). Perhaps for this reason there is an emphasis on the study of caregivers, family and professional ones, as a means of giving voice to those who are conceived as marginalized groups, like nurses themselves.

Being more than simply a scientific approach, indeed constituting a political and professional strategy to empower the nursing profession and potentially care users as well, QR has been assumed to offer a positive way of developing and strengthening the nursing discipline. This position, though, is problematic in that it reinforces nurses as a minority group (despite being in a numerical majority in the health care sector) which needs to defend itself in very hierarchical settings. In particular, nurses often claim a research identity as qualitative researchers as a means of differentiating themselves in the field of health care (see Pla, in Mercado et al., 2005). Even in recent studies, a significant trend can be seen towards research which empowers nurses' participation in health care decision-making.

A similar movement can be extrapolated to university settings, where nurses are novices in comparison to those in well-established academic disciplines. Current policies of academic productivity in Spain, such as universal promotion criteria based mainly on publications in high-impact-factor journals (most written in English) and the lack of the positive evaluation of contributions to education and practice, mean that many nurse researchers find themselves at the bottom of the academic enterprise. Again, this reinforces a search for minority survival approaches among these researchers, which interferes with the emergent process of searching for collective strategies to improve the contribution of the discipline to the general health of the population and the care it enjoys.

In summary, rapid growth of the sector over the past 20 years can be attributed to a synergic effect of several factors: (1) educational opportunities, such as in-service, continuing education, and university degrees, in addition to a wave of publications that defined and popularized the field and, more recently, the availability of supervisors for qualitative studies in nursing doctorate programs; (2) the perception that qualitative studies are closely related to nursing and are a tool to address practice settings issues (i.e. a utilitarian view), which led to many descriptive studies; (3) the development of more sophisticated, theory-driven studies, first based on the interpretative/constructivist paradigm (e.g. phenomenology and grounded theory) followed by an increase in studies based on the critical social paradigm (e.g. emancipatory approaches and poststructuralist studies); and (4) in recent years, the incipient organization of research groups.

The historical context and features described so far point to the achievements and limits in the process of developing qualitative nursing research in Spain. In the next section, we discuss current challenges and potential future directions.

Challenges and future directions

In general, qualitative nurse-researchers in Spain face a research glass ceiling and are not seen as scientists by colleagues or by the general public (Carmen de la Cuesta Benjumea, pers. comm., 2011). Nurse-researchers who frequently use qualitative methods in particular face a hidden discrimination in that, whereas the politically correct discourse claims that all methodologies are equally important, these researchers frequently receive less funding and are seen as less rigorous because they address issues related to human subjectivity and do not make positivist claims through the generalization of their findings (Carmen de la Cuesta Benjumea, pers. comm., 2011). Clearly, this context is not unique to Spain, but it intensifies current challenges, such as the need to do the following: (1) strengthen the onto-epistemological and methodological competence of researchers; and (2) move from a nursing-centered research agenda to an ethical-political one to improve the population's health.

Strengthening the onto-epistemological and methodological competence of researchers

Nurses of the younger generation see research as a tool for addressing problems in clinical practice, but often do not know how to connect practice and research and are not technically trained to do so (Amaia Saenz de Ormijana, pers. comm., 2012). Despite their interest, limited research education remains a major barrier (Mercado et al., 2005). However, in general, health care institutions do not seem to accept that research should be an element in nurses' work. Those in academic settings are trying to define levels of research competence to be taught at the undergraduate, Master's and doctorate levels. A problem that remains is that most Master's and PhD students do not have access to scholarships and undertake these courses while working full-time, leading to very extensive periods of training (some leaving the programs after several years of supervision).

Another element to be considered is that, even among those trained as researchers, many are still isolated, working individually, and unable to form research teams because when they attempt to collaborate with other disciplines, the nursing focus tends to disappear, given the dominance of other areas and nurses' less developed research careers. Conversely, teams comprised exclusively of nurse researchers are less likely to be awarded funding (Mercado et al., 2005).

The result of such a scarcity of senior researchers, both in clinical and academic settings, is that those in leading positions have a work overload because they have to act simultaneously as lead researchers, methodological advisors for other studies, and educators of their own co-investigators. Like the nurses of the 1970s, the advancement of nursing research requires a great deal of professional and personal investment from those promoting it.

The current use of Anglo-American texts and applied research to inform the QR curriculum is another problem (Hsiung, 2012). Anglo-American-centered readings may reproduce stereo-typical accounts of the core approaches as superior and the role of the periphery as mere consumers. Qualitative health research articles might in this sense be seen as the product of private, commercial publishing companies with the aim of encouraging others to hold up the research they promote as the standard reference, to the detriment of local publications; this is an additional challenge for training the next generation of Spanish researchers (Mercado et al., 2005).

While in the past a successful strategy was to educate nurses abroad and to invite foreign researchers to teach in Spain, the current European economic crisis poses an additional challenge for such a direction in the future (Bover et al., 2011). In this context, it is important to create stronger alliances between health care research units, nursing chiefs, and university-based researchers to boost educational opportunities. To train students, it is important to link their education to research projects or networks and to bring research findings to the students' everyday classroom experience. Another element that might support training is to develop educational materials, such as textbooks, that incorporate examples from both Spanish research and other studies that could be transferred to this specific teaching context (that is, less expensive ways of conducting QR or examples of studies from other Latin countries).

Finally, there is a need to foster constructive criticism among those in funding agencies and journal review boards to increase awareness about what constitutes quality in QR. The same is true for academic evaluations of qualitative research, which would benefit from a more transparent and stringent mode of evaluation, expecting students to go beyond description to develop rigorous, epistemologically congruent studies.

Moving from a nursing-centered research agenda to an ethical-political one to improve health for all

Some researchers believe "we are dying of success" in nursing QR and that our research agenda is self-centered; that we are spending too much energy justifying qualitative methodologies in a positivist environment, rather than questioning what has been the social impact of QR to date (for example, see Pla, in Mercado et al., 2005). This change in focus assumes that researchers are aware of emerging social trends and that they are flexible in order to be responsive to emerging health needs. For instance, in the current economic crisis faced by many European countries, the gap between the rich and poor has increased noticeably and the health consequences of inequities are a growing problem (Milagros Ramasco, pers. comm., 2011; Bover et al., 2011). In Spain, this year alone universal access to health care was removed (RD 16/2012), excluding several segments of the population who are now only allowed access to emergency services. Only research can document the impact of these measures in the short and medium term and advocate more equitable solutions to the crisis.

However, in the everyday lives of qualitative researchers in Spain, challenges include the logic of research productivity dominated by impact-factor evaluation of scientists' publication records. Adopting an ethical-political agenda for QR could help to promote resistance against such trends and to increase participation and representation of the population in health decision-making (at individual and social levels); also, QR critical approaches may lead nurses into an augmented commitment towards social justice and health equity. They need to address the complexity of such issues by pointing to alternative ways of thinking about and practicing caregiving and health promotion that are simultaneously efficient and critical of the current social modes of production of disease.

Thus, future directions might include addressing the frequent disconnection between research findings and policy or program formulation. Larger research teams, with strategically selected research topics that are responsive to population needs, would be one way of achieving greater outcomes from QR, as would interdisciplinary studies organized as a part of research programs.

Qualitative researchers could also be more inclusive in the formulation of projects, through having users and community or clinical groups as advisors for the development of new projects. In addition, incorporating knowledge translation and exchange strategies to all research, whether they propose a new concept or an intervention, can foster a new mentality of social impact rather than one in which the number of papers published is a gauge of success.

Finally, we believe that the great achievements of the past two decades, as well as the limitations of present QR, mean that Spanish researchers are ideally placed to be partners in a global dialogue of peers on the exchange of experiences about quality improvement and overcoming challenges, as well as embracing a real commitment to equity. Our contribution, we hope, has been to show how QR in nursing is connected to broader social and political contexts and requires a clear vision towards social transformation and resistance strategies in order to become a collective asset with value beyond the nursing profession.

Acknowledgments

The authors are grateful to Dr. Carmen de la Cuesta Benjumea, Manuel Amezcua, Dr. Milagros Ramasco, and Amaia Sáenz de Ormijana, for their in-person or online interviews about the development of qualitative nursing research in Spain. We also want to thank Dr. Teresa Moreno for the information about the Investen group. Finally, we thank Montse Gea for the logistic support during the development of the last version of the chapter.

References

Amezcua, M. (2000). El laboratorio de investigación cualitativa en salud (LIC) un grupo para la humanización de los cuidados [The Qualitative Health Laboratory (LIC): a group for humanizing care]. *Index de Enfermería, 28–29,* 41–44.

Amezcua, M., & Carricondo, A. (2000). Investigación Cualitativa en España: Análisis de la producción bibliográfica en salud [Qualitative research in Spain: Analysis of bibliographic output on health]. *Index de Enfermería, 28–29,* 26–34.

Bover, A., Gastaldo, D., Meyer D. E., Miró, M., Miró R., Moreno, C., Peter, E., & Zaforteza, C. (2011). Economic crisis, austerity discourses and caregiving: How to remain relevant through engagement and social justice. *Nursing Inquiry, 18*(3), 188–190.

de la Cuesta Benjumea, C. (1997). Características de la investigación cualitativa y su relación con la enfermería [Characteristics of qualitative research in relationship to nursing]. *Investigación y Educación en Enfermería, 15*(2), 13–24.

de la Cuesta Benjumea, C. (2000). Investigación cualitativa y enfermería [Qualitative research and nursing]. *Index de Enfermería, 28–29,* 7–8.

de la Cuesta Benjumea, C. (2005). La contribución de la evidencia cualitativa al campo del cuidado y salud comunitaria [The contribution of qualitative evidence to care and community health]. *Index de Enfermería, 14*(50), 47–52.

de la Cuesta Benjumea, C. (2006). Naturaleza de la investigación cualitativa y su contribución a la práctica de enfermería [Nature of qualitative research and its contribution to nursing practice]. *Metas de Enfermería, 9,* 50–55.

de la Cuesta Benjumea, C. (2010). La investigación cualitativa y el desarollo del en enfermería [Qualitative research and the development of knowledge in nursing]. *Texto Contexto Enferm. Florianopolis, 19*(4), 762–766.

Gálvez, A. (2003). Un enfoque crítico para la construcción de una enfermería basada en la evidencia [A critical approach to building evidence-based nursing]. *Investigación y Educación en Enfermería, 21*(1), 50–64.

Gálvez, A., Poyatos, E., & Estrada, J.M. (2000). Evolución de la documentación en enfermería en España: Las bases de datos Cuiden y Bdie [Evolution of nursing documentation in Spain: The Cuiden and Bdie databases]. *El profesional de la información, 9*(12), 13–19.

Gastaldo, D., Mercado, F., Ramasco, M., Lizardi, A., & Gil, M. A. (2002). Qualitative health research in Ibero-America: The current state of the science. *Journal of Transcultural Nursing, 13*(2), 90–108.

Hsiung, P. (2012). The globalization of qualitative research: Challenging Anglo-American domination and local hegemonic discourse. *Forum: Qualitative Social Research, 13*(1), Art. 21.

Mercado, F. J., Bosi, M. L., Robles, L., Wiessenfeld, E., & Pla, M. (2005). La enseñanza de la investigación cualitativa en salud: Voces desde Iberoamérica [Teaching qualitative health research: Voices from Iberoamerica]. *Salud Colectiva, 1*(1), 97–116.

Mercado, F. J., Gastaldo, D., & Calderón, C. (2002.) *Investigación cualitativa en salud en Iberoámerica: Métodos, análisis y ética* [Qualitative health research in Iberoamerica: Methods, analysis and ethics]. Guadalajara: Universidad de Guadalajara.

Miró, M. (2008). ¿Porqué somos como somos? Continuidades y transformaciones de los discursos y las relaciones de poder en la constitución de la identidad profesional de los/as enfermeros/ras en España (1956–1976) [Why are we the way we are? Continuities and transformations in the discourses and power relations in nurses' professional identity in Spain (1956–1976)]. PhD thesis, Palma de Mallorca, Universitat de les Illes Balears.

Miró, M., Gastaldo, D., Nelson, S., & Gallego, G. (2011). Spanish nursing under Franco: Reinvention, modernization and repression (1956–1976). *Nursing Inquiry.* Online. Retrieved on May 28, 2012 from http://onlinelibrary.wiley.com/doi/10.1111/j.1440-1800.2011.00565.x/pdf.

Peinado, A. (2002). La investigación cualitativa en España: De la vida política al maltrato del sentido [Qualitative research in Spain: From political life to maltreatment of senses]. *Revista Española de Salud Pública, 76*, 381–393.

Pérez, C. (2002). Sobre la metodología cualitativa [About qualitative methodology]. *Revista Española de Salud Pública, 76*, 373–380.

Pita, S., & Pértegas, S. (2002). Investigación cuantitativa y cualitativa [Quantitative and qualitative research]. *Atención Primaria, 9*, 76–78.

Salinas, V. (2010). La enfermería y la investigación cualitativa: Un aprendizaje [Nursing and qualitative research: An education]. *Archivos de la Memoria.* Online. Retrieved on May 6, 2012 from http://www.index-f.com/memoria/7/7504.php.

Zabalegui, A. (2002). Más allá del dualismo cualitativo-cuantitativo [Beyond the qualitative-quantitative dualism]. *Enfermería clínica, 12*(2), 74–79.

Zaforteza, C., Sánchez, C., & Lastra, P. (2008). Análisis de la literatura sobre los familiares del paciente crítico: Es necesario desarrollar investigación en cuidados efectivos [Analysis of the literature about the critical patient's relatives: The need to research effective caregiving]. *Enfermería Intensiva, 19*(2), 61–70.

State of the science of qualitative nursing research in Portugal

Marta Lima-Basto

Introduction

The possibility of disseminating some aspects of nursing research in Portugal, mainly qualitative studies, was a challenge accepted with enthusiasm. This chapter starts with a historic background. The main part of the chapter is an analysis of data included in a recent study by the author on doctoral theses in nursing in the three universities offering this qualification, giving special attention to qualitative studies. A personal perspective follows on the impact that some qualitative studies have had, during the past nine years. It must be said that the majority of the research studies have chosen the qualitative paradigm. Some considerations about reasons for a small impact on clinical practice follow. The chapter ends with predictions about future directions of qualitative research in Portugal.

Historic background: nursing education and research, professional, and national context

Landmarks of the development of nursing education and research are pointed out in Table 38.1 as well as the national context that set the scene for the development of nursing research, in order to show what is considered a rapid professional development, mainly at the educational level, but also in direct nursing care and care management in health organizations.

In the 1960s, nursing education remained traditional, though nursing schools were separate from hospitals. Nurse leaders understood the importance of international contacts at a time when the country was closed to the western world and fighting a war in African colonies. There were very few sociologists in the country when sociology was introduced at the post-basic nursing education level.

The 1970s were characterized by the social revolution that started a democratic state and facilitated the move to one level generalist nurse by closing first-level nurse education (two-year program, but with a fewer number of years of secondary education in relation to diploma nurses) and offering an upgrading program. The approval of a national health service introduced health as a right as well as a new organization, increasing the state responsibility.

In the 1980s, nursing education entered higher education, a binary system, university and polytechnic, that remains by law until the present day. Several nursing colleges were meanwhile

Table 38.1 Landmarks in the development of nursing education and research in Portugal

Education and research	Profession	National context
1965 – New nursing care-centered curriculum; admission educ. requirements: 9 years		1965 – Parliament reacts to new curriculum
		Dictatorship continues
1966 – Post-basic programs to prepare leaders; introduction of "nursing research methods" and "sociology"	1969 – Portuguese Nurses Association joins International Council of Nurses	
1973 – Post-basic specialization programs		1974, April 25 – Social revolution. Democratic process starts
	1975 – First level nurse with 2-year education, cancelled.	
1979 – Admission requirements for initial education: preference for 12 years	Upgraded program offered	1979 – National Health Service
1982 – First Portuguese nurse PhD in Public Health (Brazil)	1980 – Portuguese Nurses Association (APE) becomes a member of WENR	
1983 – New curriculum for specialization programs (research, management, education)	1987 – First Nursing Research Conference (APE)	1986 – Portugal becomes a member of European Union
1988 – First degree higher education "bacharelato" (3 years); admission requirements: 12 years of study	1988 – Nursing education integrated into the national educational system at polytechnic level	1988 – Double coordination of nursing education: Ministries of Education and Health
1991 – First Portuguese nurse PhD (Nursing) (São Paulo, Brazil)		1990 – Bologna Declaration (European Union)
1991 – Master's Degree in Nursing Sciences (Catholic University)	1992 – Nurse tutors same career as other higher education tutors	
1993 – Master's Degree in Nursing Science (Porto University)		
1995 – First Portuguese nurse PhD in Portugal (Social Psychology)		
1999 – Bachelor's Degree in Nursing (4 years)	1998 – Nurses' Order (Nurses Regulating Body)	1998 – National Committee on Nursing Research (Ministry of Health)

Table 38.1 Continued

Education & research	Profession	National context
1999 – Study shows "direct care" most frequent object of study in 10 years (Soares & Basto, 1999)		2000 – Bologna Agreement (European Union) (2) adopted by Portuguese legislation
2001 – PhD in Nursing Sciences (University of Porto)	2001 – Nursing Research Units (linked to Nursing Colleges in Lisbon and Coimbra) funded by the Government Research Agency	
2004 – PhD in Nursing (University of Lisbon and Catholic University)		
2009 – Master's Degrees in areas of nursing offered by most nursing colleges	From 2005 – Reorganization of Community Care Services; enlarged nurses intervention	

integrated into polytechnic institutes, others in universities and still others not integrated awaiting the opportunity to enter universities' organizational structure. Several curricular developments took place. The first nursing research conference was launched and has regularly been organized every two years by the Portuguese Nurses Association (APE), at the time representing the country within the International Council of Nurses (ICN). In the beginning, the Workgroup of European Nurse Researchers[1] (WENR) helped, giving credibility to the conferences.

Nursing research developed in the 1990s at the bachelor's and Master's levels. The first two Master's degrees in nursing and the first doctoral program in nursing, as a research degree, the only type of doctoral degree in Portugal, introduced a new era for nursing research in the twenty-first century. Research units, multi-disciplinary but with special emphasis on nursing, were initiated following the government's research funding department orientation. The Bologna Agreement at the European Union level influenced each country member's legislation in all aspects and levels of education, and naturally nursing education and research.[2]

Early efforts in qualitative nursing research

When in 1993 the Master's Degree in Nursing Science (University of Porto) was launched, qualitative methods were introduced, at first as an option but immediately after as a compulsory subject. Emphasis on qualitative methods continued through the three doctoral programs (since 2001). It is also worth mentioning that many nurses completed Master's and doctoral degrees in educational sciences, psychology, sociology, history and communication in health, where most studies used qualitative methods. Most tried to answer research questions related to nursing care or nursing education using qualitative and mixed methods.

An analysis of academic research studies by Portuguese nurses in post-basic programs (clinical specializations, education and management programs, Master's degrees in nursing and other areas) from 1987 to 1996, based on content analysis of 541 abstracts (Soares & Lima-Basto, 1999) showed 435 (27.1%) of the sample were qualitative studies. Later, another study (Lima-Basto & Carvalho, 2003) analyzed research articles published in the eight most read Portuguese nursing journals, from 2000 to 2002. Of the 122 articles, 48 (39%) were qualitative studies. In both studies, the predominant area of study was the clinical setting.

Two Nursing Research Units were created in 2001, both linked to Nursing Colleges in Lisbon and Coimbra and funded by the Government Research Agency. They established lines of research, prioritizing areas and methods of research. The Coimbra Research Unit has three lines of research: education of health professionals and health education; well-being, health and disease; and health systems and organizations. The Lisbon Unit has created new lines of research as the qualifications of the researchers are developed. At present they are: nursing interventions; lived experience; epistemology; history of nursing; emotions in health; health organization climate: quality and management of care; educating and learning in nursing; observatory of human development and professionality. Methods used vary but there has been a preference for qualitative studies in the Lisbon Unit.

Analysis of doctoral theses in nursing

The following data have been drawn from the analysis of 60 doctoral theses in nursing (out of a total of 64) completed until the end of 2011 (Lima-Basto, 2012) in all three universities that offer this qualification. The study shows that 32 (53.3%) opted for the qualitative paradigm, 23 (38.3%) for the quantitative paradigm and 5 (8.3%) opted for the mixed paradigm.

There was no significant correlation between choice of paradigm and specific university, which is not surprising since there are very broad boundaries in each one. None of the universities opted to develop research exclusively in very specific areas, which is usual in some countries. Nevertheless, each of the Portuguese doctoral programs has made an effort to delimit its areas of research in nursing. All use the same resources as theses supervisors, since they are chosen from nurse professors with doctoral degrees and some non-nursing professors.

A possible explanation for the preference for qualitative studies is that the most frequent area of study is "clinical" (Table 38.2) and within it "care process" (Table 38.3). This might mean that there has been greater interest in identifying and understanding nursing phenomena than in testing explanatory hypothesis. There were no studies on the history of nursing at the doctoral level but they are expected in 2012. Studies on nurse education refer to bachelor's degree questions.

The "clinical area" of study refers to direct care and it was categorized as: "care process" referring to the process of nurse–client relationship/clinical decision-making; "needs assessment" of a group of people; "intervention piloting" refers to the impact evaluation of a nursing intervention; "intervention identification" refers to naming and characterizing interventions or confirming known interventions in a different culture; and "intervention implementation" refers to introducing new interventions in the professional practice.

Table 38.2 Frequency of areas of study

Areas of study	Total	
	No.	(%)
Clinical	45	75.0
Lived experience	4	6.7
Care management	5	8.3
Nurse education	5	8.3
Conceptual/theoretical development	1	1.7
Total	60	100.0

Marta Lima-Basto

Table 38.3 Clinical areas of study before and after 2009

Clinical areas	Years		Total	
	2002–2008	2009–2011	No.	(%)
Care process	4	12	16	35.6
Needs assessment	8	4	12	26.7
Intervention piloting	4	7	11	24.4
Intervention identification	1	3	4	8.9
Intervention implementation	1	1	2	4.4
Total	18	27	45	100.0

Table 38.4 Frequency of research designs

Research designs	No.	(%)
Descriptive	20	33.3
Explanatory	19	31.7
Action Research	8	13.3
Quasi-experimental	5	8.3
Experimental	3	5.0
Case study	3	5.0
Mixed methods	2	3.4
Total	60	100.0

Research designs were categorized as: descriptive, explanatory (including relationships among variables/factors), Action Research, quasi-experimental, experimental (including RCT), case study, mixed methods and metasynthesis/meta-analysis (no studies) (Table 38.4).

As expected, there is a great variety of study designs, depending on research questions. An interesting feature is the number of Action Research designs, considered high risk at the doctoral level, even unwelcome in some universities, due to the high degree of participation needed and stability of participants. The eight studies were very successful which may be due to the high involvement of the nurse teams in changing the quality of nursing care.

What do qualitative studies in Portugal study?

Methods used in qualitative studies

The doctoral thesis analysis from which the data were drawn looked at methods used in qualitative studies, based on the typology proposed by the National Centre for Research Methods, in the UK (Beissel-Durant, 2004) as well as Morse (1994). The methods used were grounded theory, interpretative description, phenomenological method, narrative inquiry and discourse analysis (Table 38.5). The preferred software analysis tool was NVivo.

Of the 16 studies using grounded theory, 14 followed Glaser and Strauss (1967) or did not specify, one was according to Strauss (1987), one followed a constructivist framework according to Charmaz (2006) and no one used Glaser (2005) or his follower's orientation. It is possible that

Table 38.5 Frequency of qualitative methods in inductive and mixed studies

Methods	No.	(%)
Grounded theory	16	42.1
Interpretative description	13	34.2
Phenomenological method	6	15.8
Narrative inquiry	2	5.3
Discourse analysis	1	2.6
Total	38	100.0

the authors specified it in the full report though not in the abstract, since Strauss and Corbin (1998) is very popular. Of the six studies that used the phenomenological method, four followed interpretative phenomenology and two descriptive phenomenology. None of the completed theses used ethnography or the historical method, but others using these methods will be completed soon.

The highest frequency of grounded theory in all three doctoral programs might be explained by the influence that Professor Carmen de la Cuesta Benjumea (formerly at the University of Antioquia, Colombia, at present at the University of Alicante, Spain) has had and still has in the whole country.

Central concepts in qualitative studies

In order to understand the object of study of qualitative studies, central concepts were categorized (Table 38.6). The use of the concept "Transition" (Meleis, 2010), is very common. "Transition" refers to transitions, adaptation or preparation for a variety of situations, such as breastfeeding, adolescence, old age, end of life.

"Nurse–client relationship" relates essentially to the nursing care process, ethical decisions, emotional intelligence, use of power. "Nursing intervention" refers to actions or group of actions and includes expressions such as support, being with, referring, venous puncture, Kangaroo technique, humor, patient information, health education, visualization technique, comfort, drug management, and body care. There is a further need to identify nursing interventions clearly for documentation and funding reasons. "Diagnostic evaluation" refers to assessment, such as functionality, suffering, adaptation, pain, confusion, falls, drug abuse, knowledge, attitudes, competencies, anxiety, body image, and coping mechanisms. "Conceptual models" refers to core

Table 38.6 Categorization of central concepts, in decreasing order

- Transition
- Nurse–client relationship
- Nursing intervention
- Conceptual models
- Nursing information systems
- Diagnostic evaluation
- Care intentionality/aims
- Care context
- Nursing/nurse issues

concepts of nursing care, family nursing, informal caregiver as client, as well as well-known nursing conceptual models, such as the Calgary model of family care (Wright & Leahey, 2009) and Roper, Logan, and Tierney's (2000) model based on activities of living, very influential in Europe. "Nursing information systems" refers to documentation, minimum data set, support systems of nursing practice, International Classification of Nursing Practice (International Council of Nurses, 2010). "Care intentionality/aims" refers to care intentions such as quality, change, growing old with quality. "Context of care" refers to expressions such as primary health care, community nursing, home nursing, palliative care, and nurse consultation. "Nursing/Nurse issues" puts together expressions such as nurses' role, competencies, knowledge, and professional behavior.

Studied phenomena in qualitative studies

Analysis of central concepts was not considered enough to clarify what were the qualitative studies' topics of study, probably because abstracts and not the whole theses were analyzed. An analysis of the studied phenomena, defined as aspects of people's lives relevant to nursing practice, expected to being sensitive to nursing care, was done. The analysis was guided by a framework for nursing research represented by a matrix formed by two axis: life transitions and nursing dimensions (priorities related to care of persons or groups, cared for in different contexts and for different levels of prevention) (Lima-Basto, 2009). None of the qualitative studies was categorized as prevention of diseases/incapacities (person, group, community), which was unexpected. The following nursing phenomena were identified in qualitative and mixed studies in the clinical area (interventions and caring process):

- *Lifestyles and environment (physical, social, therapeutic)*, e.g., the therapeutic use of emotions of nurses caring for children, youngsters and families; family interventions; the nurse as mediator and emotional support giver to the family of patients at home; integration of humor in the professional practice of hospitalized patients, partnership between nurse and elderly patient at home.
- *Treatment of acute and chronic conditions*: support groups for parents of children with chronic disease; nature of the relationship between nurses and patients undergoing chemotherapy in a day hospital; support system to clinical decision-making in hospitalized patients; ethical decision in clinical practice; the clinical decision process; protecting the hospitalized elderly's identity.
- *Body function/self-care*, e.g., use of power during hygiene care in a medical unit, strengthening adult patients with progressive disease, caring process of hospitalized persons in the end-of-life stages.

Results of qualitative studies

The following data continue to be drawn from the analysis of study results included in doctoral thesis abstracts (Lima-Basto, 2012). In general, the results of the studies show how important subjective aspects of life, a basis for nursing care, can be identified through qualitative studies. Outcomes of nursing care identified in qualitative studies were categorized as client, client–nurse relationship and management of care outcomes, as follows:

- *Client outcomes* (efficacy of nursing interventions on the client's well-being, the client being a person, a group or a community):

- Felt dignity was preserved; less vulnerable; protected, respected; self-integrity; hope promoted; decreased depression, anxiety and stress.
- Increased knowledge, e.g. about disease prevention; knowledge reinforced, less need for information, favored family adaptation.
- Attitude and behavior change, positive expectations; self-care and care of children; autonomy promoted; increased drug adherence; improvement in disease management; adjustment to somatic symptoms; increased control over life project.
- Facilitated weight gain; increased comfort; less suffering; well-being; environment harmonized, facilitating family and friends presence; satisfying last wishes and spiritual needs.
- *Client–nurse relationship* (expressed in the well-being of the client and the nurse):
  - Understanding caring process as diagnostic evaluation process and therapeutic intervention process; when evaluating experiences lived in the transformed body nurses readjust care; perceiving, identifying, evaluating and intervening therapeutically; evaluates, revises and readjusts care, manage information and feelings; evaluating patient responses and intervening on them.
  - Steps (initial, beginning of a relationship, core of the relationship, end of relationship); welcoming the person and family; synchronized and last encounters.
  - Adequate interventions to each person; personalize discourse; partnership between nurse and client; person-centered care; trust and therapeutic alliance; time is an important dimension.
  - Nurse also suffers; personal and professional development; both grow; contributes to personal development of client and nurse.
  - Clinical decision and structure supporting decision form a methodic and personalized process; use of ethical principles in decision-making; objective improvement in diagnostic quality, better perception of the nature of possible usage of interventions; increased quantity and quality information, definition of models of care in practice, validation of interventions, better risk prevention.
- *Outcomes in the management of care* (strategies to facilitate the clinical decision, such as documentation and language used, guidelines or models of care practice):
  - Positive impact on data production and on describing common aspects of care, starting writing down nursing diagnoses, patient activity, learning, adaptation and "doing for" activities;
  - Better inter-group communication, organizational factors, and work distribution (electronic support documentation support system);
  - Individualized care depends strongly on models in use and on nurses' intention;
  - Few differences between the clinical guideline and performed nurses' interventions.

Examples of qualitative studies that had an impact on nursing research/knowledge development

Among the studies that have clearly influenced qualitative nursing research and practice locally and nationally, five nurse authors, all professors of nursing at graduate and postgraduate levels, were chosen.

Abel Silva was the first Portuguese nurse to qualify with a PhD in nursing sciences (Silva, 2002), with a thesis about nursing information systems and their influence on individualization of care, guided by the constructivist paradigm, using grounded theory. Implementation of the nursing information system in hospitals changed the narrative logic used by nurses into information production—type of data used, common aspects of care, systematic use of nursing diagnosis, with a common language (International Classification of Nursing Practice). The impact on nurses, health administrators, health authorities, the nursing regulating body and tutor colleagues was enormous. Silva has supervised several studies in different parts of the country, dissertations and doctoral theses, following questions regarding clarification of nursing care as "theories in use" (Argyris & Schön, 1974), with emphasis on the concepts "transitions" and "self-care." His contribution to the profession has been extended through the conceptual framework and statements of quality principles disseminated by the regulating body (Ordem dos Enfermeiros, 2003) and by leading an International Council of Nurses-accredited Research Centre for International Classification of Nursing Practice (International Council of Nurses, 2010). Portugal is now one of the leading European countries in the development of the taxonomy.

Maria Antónia Rebelo-Botelho completed her PhD in contemporary philosophy at the New University of Lisbon with a study on the person and health care: ethical understanding and phenomenological "sense" (Rebelo-Botelho, 2003). She is one of a few nurses to influence nursing research using the phenomenological perspective. She has made many nurses recognize the importance of understanding the lived experience of health conditions prior to identifying the nursing care they need. By acquiring this understanding nurses will also tend to personalize care and reflect on their own life experiences. The influence on nursing research and knowledge is mainly through her role as coordinator of a nursing research unit and the doctoral program in nursing of the University of Lisbon, through Master's dissertations and doctoral theses she has supervised in different universities and areas of study, as well as publications (Rebelo-Botelho, 1994, 2006, 2009; Chambers et al., 2010; Pereira & Rebelo-Botelho, 2011).

Margarida Vieira completed her PhD in contemporary philosophy at the New University of Lisbon with a study on vulnerability and respect in the caring of the other (Vieira, 2003). Pursuing her interest in ethical, philosophical and historic questioning, she has been supervising Master's dissertations and doctoral theses and coordinating Master's and doctoral programs at the Portuguese Catholic University, since 2004, where she plays a key role in the development of research and knowledge in nursing. Her influence at the national level was especially relevant when she was president of the jurisdictional council (1999–2003), and has been a member of the committee supporting ethical and deontology reflection (since 2008) of the nursing regulating body.

Maria do Céu Figueiredo completed her PhD in nursing sciences (Figueiredo, 2004) with an Action Research study that showed positive outcomes of a family nursing intervention, based on the Calgary family intervention model on families of children with congenital heart disease. Her continuous contact with international research centers on family nursing and the organization of regular conferences on the subject helped disseminate the principles, strategies and qualitative instrument development to analyze the effects of family-centered nursing. Her study has led nurses to pursue research in this area and she has agreed to supervise several Master's degree dissertations and doctoral theses, becoming a reference in the area. She is a pillar of the doctoral program at the University of Porto, and contributes to the three programs.

Manuel Lopes qualified with a PhD in nursing sciences (Lopes, 2005) with a study using grounded theory according to Strauss and Corbin (1998) to discover the nature and process of the nurse–patient relationship in a day hospital for chemotherapy: the diagnostic evaluation and therapeutic intervention are interwoven, apparently simultaneous and developed through three stages of the relationship. These outcomes were rapidly disseminated through a book, contact with graduate and postgraduate students and the orientation of numerous Master's dissertations and doctoral theses, all over the country. His contribution to multi-professional research teams and efforts to increase collaboration from various research units and universities have clearly influenced knowledge development. Several studies have confirmed the nature and process of nurse–client relationships in various contexts, most of them identifying client's outcomes.

Impact of research on clinical practice

A recent study done in Portugal (Vilelas & Lima-Basto, 2011) confirms the difficulties involved in knowledge transfer. The greatest barriers to the use of research in practice were related to organizational factors: "time at work is insufficient to implement new ideas," congruent with results in other countries. Other barriers were the lack of trust in research studies and type of beliefs related to nursing care.

A very small impact of doctoral research outcomes on practice was expected; nevertheless a focus group[3] was organized in order to listen to practicing nurses' reflections on doctoral thesis results (Lima-Basto, 2012). Their first reaction was surprise at the quantity and quality of the studies. They showed satisfaction at the knowledge organized around interventions, use of power and clinical decision-making. All of them regretted care management issues not being considered a priority. The group considered that the research results did not reflect their clinical practice and acknowledged that practice environments are not always open to new contributions. It must be said that most studies do not aim to describe clinical practice in general, but at uncovering nurses' contribution to the well-being of clients, often coming as a surprise for nurses themselves.

In general, the group identified lack of leadership as a barrier to knowledge transfer. There are barriers related to dissemination of new knowledge and the use of evidence-based guidelines and models of care. Group suggestions for future research and for better use of research outcomes in clinical contexts, many of them common to the suggestions mentioned in the doctoral thesis abstracts, indicate a need for more qualitative studies. They were identified as follows.

Suggestions for future research and for clinical practice

- Multidisciplinary studies on the quality of care and measurement instruments are much valued.
- Need for better conceptualization of care management, issues related to human resources, care organization, clinical governance, nurses' feelings, suffering, self-esteem and leadership.
- More studies about patient information and education, translational knowledge, health gains sensitive to nursing care, nurses' role in health policy, relationship with those in power, cost-effectiveness of nursing care.

Suggestions to increase the use of research results in clinical practice

- Disseminate results in the organizations and not just to the nurses involved, involving participants.
- Sharing study results in clinical meetings (nursing and multidisciplinary) showing nurses' competencies, regular occasions for reflecting clinical practice.
- Better links between colleges and health services, partnerships, care evaluation; introduce evidence-based interventions and evaluate them; better use of research results during educational programs, stimulate nurses teams that are qualified but underutilized; use of measurement instruments.
- Translate knowledge to technology, develop knowledge on patient outcomes sensitive to nursing care, keep the circle going (study–trial–questions–new study–implementation), clarification of models of practice.

Future directions of qualitative nursing research in Portugal

There is already a trend to increase the number of studies that clarify clients' outcomes and it will continue, for professional and management reasons. Because nursing care is by definition subjective and individualized, it might mean that qualitative studies will be the best option to identify clients' outcomes in well-being, sensitive to nursing interventions. Nurses have accumulated experiential knowledge that needs to be uncovered, characterized and named as interventions to persons, groups and communities.

It can be expected that in an era of evidence-based practice, qualitative studies will be needed and accepted in order to understand results of quantitative studies. As Grypdonck (2006) proposed, the concept *evidence-based* should be enlarged to *appropriateness*, when caring possibilities maximize the contribution for the well-being of persons, at a reasonable cost for societies.

These are times for innovation and entrepreneurship and it is possible that new practice development units will take the lead, changing the traditional model of research as essentially academic. An indicator of this possibility in Portugal is the increasing number of practicing nurses qualifying with PhD. Hopefully it will increase knowledge transfer (Pentland et al., 2011; Rolfe, 1998; Woods & Magyary, 2010) in both directions. The type of research to be developed will have to include qualitative methods.

There are various qualitative methods that could be developed further and it is possible that if there were a collaboration agreement between universities, each one could deepen research in specific areas of study, using fully their resources. But this is probably just wishful thinking.

Acknowledgments

The author acknowledges and is grateful to Professor Carmen de la Cuesta Benjumea for her critical review of this chapter.

Notes

1 The Workgroup of European Nurse Researchers (WENR) was created in 1978 when 26 nurses from 18 countries met in Holland, reacting to a need to develop nursing research when it was not well accepted in their own countries.
2 The Bologna Agreement was followed by the Bologna process, a developing process that made educational levels comparable in the European Union by a credit system and a framework of learning principles that guides the regulation of all educational levels in all member states, standardizing competencies acquired in the educational system, continuing education programs, and increasing teacher and student exchanges.
3 Eight nurses were chosen for their interest in quality improvement, experience in direct and management of care, as well as in research, working in various health environments and as probable users of the knowledge developed in doctoral theses.

References

Argyris, C., & Schön, D. (1974). *Theory in practice: Increasing professional effectiveness*. San Francisco, CA: Jossey-Bass Publishers.

Beissel-Durrant, G. (2004). *Typology of research methods within the social sciences*. ESRC National Center for Research Methods Working Paper, UK, Nov 2004. Accessed November 2011.

Chambers, M., Guise, V., Välimäki, M., Botelho, M. A., Scott, A., Staniuliené V., & Zanotti, R. (2010). Nurses' attitudes to mental illness: A comparison of a sample of nurses from five European countries. *International Journal of Nursing Studies, 47*(3), 350–362.

Charmaz, K. (2006). *Constructing grounded theory: A practice guide through qualitative analysis*. Thousand Oaks, CA: Sage Publications.

Figueiredo, M.C. B. (2004). Necessidades em cuidados de enfermagem das famílias de crianças com doença cardíaca congénita [Nursing care needs of families with children with congenital heart disease]. Doctoral thesis in nursing sciences, University of Porto, ICBAS [full text and abstract in English can be accessed online through Repositório aberto, Universidade do Porto, ICBAS, teses de doutoramento].

Glaser, B. G. (2005). *The grounded theory perspective III.* Mill Valley, CA: Sociology Press.

Glaser, B. G., & Strauss, A. (1967). *The discovery of grounded theory.* Chicago: Aldine Publishing.

Grypdonck, M. (2006). Qualitative health research in the era of evidence based practice. *Qualitative Health Research, 16,* 1371–1385.

International Council of Nurses (2010). *International Classification of Nursing Practice.* Version 2. Geneva: International Council of Nurses.

Lima-Basto, M. (2009). Investigação sobre o cuidar de enfermagem e a construção da disciplina: proposta de um percurso [Researching nursing care and constructing the discipline: Proposing a way]. *Pensar Enfermagem, 23*(2), 11–18 [online journal with abstract in English].

Lima-Basto, M. (2012). Qual o objeto de estudo das teses de doutoramento em enfermagem das universidades portuguesas? [What is the focus of study of doctoral theses in nursing in Portuguese universities? An analysis of abstracts]. *Pensar Enfermagem, 16*(1), 1–24 [online, with an English abstract].

Lima-Basto, M., & Carvalho, Z. M. (2003). A produção do conhecimento em enfermagem: o que escrevem os enfermeiros portugueses? [Nursing knowledge production: What do Portuguese nurses write about?] *Pensar Enfermagem, 7*(2), 2nd semestre, 2–14.

Lopes, M. J. (2005). Os utentes e os enfermeiros: construção de uma relação [Clients and nurses: building a relationship]. Doctoral thesis in Nursing Sciences, University of Porto, ICBAS [full text and abstract in English can be accessed online through Repositório aberto, Universidade do Porto, ICBAS, teses de doutoramento].

Meleis, A. (2010). *Transitions theory: Middle range and situation specific theories in nursing research and practice.* New York: Springer.

Morse, J. (1994). *Critical issues in qualitative research methods.* London: Sage.

Ordem dos Enfermeiros. (2003). *Conselho de Enfermagem: Do caminho percorrido e das propostas* [The Nursing Council of the Nurses Order: Accomplishments and proposals]. Lisbon: Ordem dos Enfermeiros.

Pentland, D., Forsyth, K., MacIver, D., Walsh, M., Murray, R., Irvin, L., & Sikora, S. (2011). Key characteristics of knowledge transfer and exchange in health care: Integrative literature review. *Journal of Advanced Nursing, 67*(7), 1408–1425.

Pereira, H. R., & Rebelo-Botelho, M. A. (2011). Sudden informal caregivers: The lived experience of informal caregivers after an unexpected event. *Journal of Clinical Nursing, 20,* 2448–2457.

Rebelo-Botelho, M. A. (1994). A estrutura essencial da interação aluno–doente: Uma análise fenomenológica [The essential structure of student–patient interaction: A phenomenological analysis]. Master's dissertation in Nursing Sciences, Portuguese Catholic University.

Rebelo-Botelho, M. A. (2003). A pessoa e os cuidados de saúde: Compreensão ética e "sentido" fenomenológico [Person and health care: Ethical understanding and phenomenological "meaning"]. Doctoral thesis in Philosophy, New University of Lisbon, FCSH. Available at: repositorio@fct.unl.pt.

Rebelo-Botelho, M. A. (2006). A doença mental em primeira pessoa: uma análise fenomenológica [Mental illness from the person's perspective: A phenomenologic analysis]. In F. Martins & A. Cardoso (Eds.), *A felicidade na fenomenologia da vida* [Happiness in life phenomenology]. Lisbon: Centro de Filosofia da Universidade de Lisboa.

Rebelo-Botelho, M. A. (2009). A questão ética da relação no cuidado [The ethical question of the caring relationship]. In *Razão e liberdade: Homenagem a Manuel José do Carmo Ferreira* [Reason and freedom: Homage to Manuel José Carmo Ferreira]. Lisbon: Centre of Philosophy, University of Lisbon.

Rolfe, G. (1998). The theory–practice gap in nursing: From research-based practice to practitioner-based research. *Journal of Advanced Nursing, 28*(3), 672–679.

Roper, N., Logan, W., & Tierney, A. (2000). *The Roper, Logan & Tierney model of nursing, based on activities of living.* London: Elsevier.

Silva, A. P. (2002). Sistemas de informação em enfermagem: uma teoria explicativa da mudança [Nursing information systems: A theory of change]. Doctoral thesis in nursing sciences, ICBAS, University of Porto [full text and abstract in English can be accessed online through Repositório aberto, Universidade do Porto, ICBAS, teses de doutoramento].

Soares, I., & Lima-Basto, M. (1999). 10 anos de investigação em enfermagem em Portugal [Ten years of nursing research in Portugal]. *Enfermagem, 14*(2), 32–45.

Strauss, A. (1987) *Qualitative analysis for social scientists.* Cambridge: Cambridge University Press.

Strauss, A., & Corbin, J. (1998). *Basics of qualitative research: Techniques and procedures for developing grounded theory* (2nd ed.). London: Sage.

Vieira, M. (2003). Vulnerabilidade e respeito no cuidado do outro [Vulnerability and respect in the care of others]. Doctoral thesis in Philosophy, New University of Lisbon, FCSH. Available at: repositorio@ fct.unl.pt.

Vilelas, J., & Lima-Basto, M.(2011). Validação para a língua Portuguesa da Escala de Funck et al. "Barreiras à utilização da investigação" [Validation for Portuguese of Funck et al.'s scale "Barriers to the use of research"]. *Pensar Enfermagem,15*(1), 1–14 [online journal with abstract in English].

Woods, N., & Magyary, D. (2010). Translational research: Why nursing's interdisciplinary collaboration is essential. *Research and Theory for Nursing Practice: An International Journal, 24*(1), 9–24.

Wright, M. L., & Leahey, M. (2009). *Nurses and families: A guide to family assessment and intervention* (5th ed.). Philadelphia, PA: F.A. Davis Company.

39

Finland and Sweden

Qualitative research from nursing to caring

Terese Bondas

The message of qualitative research in nursing science is of no use unless it is delivered to the patients, their loved ones and their caregivers: DENUNTIATIO SOLUM TRANSLATA VALET.

Introduction

The aim of this chapter is to discuss two decades of qualitative nursing research, and the qualitative methodological developments in nursing science in Finland and Sweden. In Finland, the term for nursing science in Finnish is "hoitotiede" and in Finland-Swedish, which is the second official language, the term is "vårdvetenskap." In Sweden, there is no consensus on the correct vocabulary, as several terms for nursing science are used with different connotations, including "omvårdnad," "omvårdnadsvetenskap" and "vårdvetenskap." To further complicate the disciplinary differences, both "nursing science" and "caring science" are used in English to depict the discipline. There are differing views on the ontological and epistemological foundations, as well as the desirable development of qualitative research, which are intertwined with the disciplinary and educational development. Here, the term "qualitative research" refers to approaches and methods that search for an understanding and illumination of the human experience from a nursing or caring science perspective in all its different variations through description, exploration and interpretation. In research, studies are always rooted in epistemological beliefs, i.e. the view of knowledge, whether explicitly written or possible to read between the lines (Bondas, 2011; Bondas & Hall, 2007b).

Finland and Sweden: neighboring countries

In addition to Denmark, Iceland and Norway, the neighboring countries of Finland and Sweden belong to the Nordic welfare states, with their official health care and education systems paid by taxes. They are situated in Northern Europe, and partly share Northern borders. In Sweden, the official language is Swedish, while in Finland the majority speaks Finnish, with Swedish being the second official language. There is a Finland-Swedish minority group (approximately 6%) in Finland. Finland was part of Sweden from the twelfth to the nineteenth centuries. Statistically, the emigration from Finland to Sweden in recent years shows a population of more than 170,000

Finns living in Sweden. As of 2011, Finland had slightly more than 5.4 million inhabitants (www.stat.fi), whereas Sweden has almost twice as many at 9.4 million (www.scb.se). Finland is a republic and Sweden is a kingdom, while both nations are parliamentary democracies that are governed nationally, regionally and at the European level. According to Eurostat, Sweden changed from an emigration to an immigration country in 2010, with 1.33 million foreign-born residents living in Sweden, comprising 14.3% of the total population. The largest group within that population was actually from Finland (172,218), while over the past 20 years, immigration has increased by more than six times in Finland, with 183,333 (3.4%) foreign nationals living there in 2012 (www.stat.fi). The infant mortality rates in both countries are among the lowest in the world at 3.47% in Finland and 2.75% for Sweden (The World Factbook, 2011).

Qualitative nursing research in Finland and Sweden

Since its inception and the resultant years of steady growth in Finland and Sweden, qualitative research in nursing has come of age in both countries. This chapter looks at the 20-year period from 1991 to 2011, including a short background on the early history of nursing science. Both countries have had different journeys into nursing science and qualitative research, which are explored. Method profiles and university profiles are discussed, and exemplars are provided from studies in both countries. In addition, there is a critical and emancipatory interest (Habermas, 1972) in relation to asking new metaquestions that point to qualitative nursing research and method development.

Method

I have chosen a textual analysis with the help of matrices (Miles & Huberman, 1994). My interest was the aims, approaches and methods of the scientific production over the past two decades, while discussing the originality, rigor and significance of any individual studies to a lesser degree. The conclusions must be viewed from the limitations inherent in a large scientific production and the decisions that were made. Validity is viewed here as something that is supported by convincing and sound evidence. Validation is a process of doing justice to the research and having made an effort that is worthy of thrust and convincingly written (Angen, 2000). It is also about doing something meaningful that furthers our understanding and stimulates us to become more informed, and to be more human in our thoughts and actions. The intention was to maintain an ethically reflective attitude, exhibiting respect for the authors and their choices in relation to the state of development of nursing science, as well as the policies of the journals that also have directed the research (Paterson et al., 2001; Sandelowski & Barroso, 2007).

Criteria for inclusion and exclusion

The primary criteria for inclusion were qualitative nursing research, in addition to qualitative method development in relation to the disciplinary area of Finnish/Swedish nursing and caring science. The publications under review are internationally published, peer-reviewed original research articles in English between 1991 and 2011, with publications on the development of nursing science pertaining to qualitative research in the aforementioned countries completing the primary publications. I chose to omit the qualitative publications in the primary native languages of Finnish and Swedish, which was a conscious choice to enable not only an international audience to retrieve the publications, but also in terms of reading them. Nursing leadership and administration, including occupational health such as the work profiles, nursing documentation and nursing didactics are excluded, not because they are unimportant, but as large areas, they need their own forum. Studies that concern nursing in other disciplines such as public health (among others) are excluded. Mixed studies in which the qualitative is part of a quantitative survey or manifest content analysis applying counting are omitted.

Literature search and analysis

I used recurring database searches with a skilled librarian in combination with the key words "nursing/caring research," "qualitative," "Finland" and "Sweden," in addition to manual searches of various university databases, lists of doctoral dissertations, central journals, author searches and the backtracking of references (cf. Sandelowski & Barroso, 2007). A data extraction table was used to note the data, with the analysis and synthesis processes being connected when the analysis makes room for an overall view; metaphorically speaking, this means seeing the trees but foremost the forest and some of these trees may be pointed out as exemplars and variations. The research process is non-linear, which is similar to any qualitative research endeavor. The analysis was begun by reading the title, the author affiliation, the key words and the abstract, and the entire text was skimmed and the exemplary chosen models were thoroughly read. I proceeded by making notes on the aims and epistemological and methodological characteristics, and also conducting matrix work (Miles & Huberman, 1994). The analysis and grouping processes were ongoing; emerging questions were asked about the data decisions and conclusions were reported, and finally, suggestions for methodological development were made. The research process may be characterized as ambiguous, open-ended and evolving in an enumeration of possibilities in a back and forth movement, asking questions, reflecting and making notes. Moreover, the findings are displayed through argumentative profiles and exemplary models.

From the trembling years to years of steady growth and coming of age

On the basis of the analysis, qualitative nursing research in Finland and Sweden may be classified into three eras:

1 *The Trembling Years*. This is when the first qualitative doctoral theses began to emerge that were written by the second generation of nurse researchers who were supervised by the first generation of professors with a medical, social or educational science education. The use of qualitative methods was heavily criticized by quantitatively oriented nurse researchers, with the method references possibly varying until the middle of the 1990s.
2 *The Years of Steady Growth*. This is when the qualitative theses and publications slowly increased, and researchers who had developed a qualitative research profile emerged in both countries; there were also method references and development from the middle of the 1990s to the first years of the new century.
3 *Coming of Age*. This is when the choice of qualitative methods became a *sine qua non* in nursing science and the use of (some) qualitative methods were criticized within the qualitative research community in itself, while the meta-era led to a new type of development of qualitative methods, even to the point that an anti-method tradition has emerged during recent years.

Courses in different qualitative methods were soon offered at most universities in both countries. In the beginning, priorities for research and nursing science development were discussed by the Nordic professors in a collaborative effort, which also shows how the development of nursing science in one Nordic country most likely influenced developments in another Nordic country. The first meeting took place in 1966 at a Nordic research conference when methodological issues were discussed (Hamrin & Lorensen, 1997). The Nordic Academy of Nursing Science was initiated in 1991 by Nordic professors. The Nordic journals were important in helping to support the publication of the qualitative studies. *Vård i Norden* was not peer-reviewed from the start in the early 1980s. The *Scandinavian Journal of Caring Sciences* (peer-reviewed from its first volume in 1986) is the official journal of the Nordic College of Caring Science, which unites caring science researchers in the Nordic countries (www.nccs.nu). The content of current nursing and caring research in Nordic doctoral dissertations, including Finland and Sweden, a total of 26 in 2003, were investigated by the Swedish researchers Lundgren, Valmari, and Skott (2008). They concluded that the scientific knowledge and the discipline's unique perspective and value system were still evolving. This view is not completely shared, as shown by an evaluation of nursing research by Nordic professors (Larsen & Adamsen, 2009). In their study of international differences in nursing research, Polit and Beck (2009) studied both qualitative and quantitative studies in eight leading English-language research journals in 2005 and 2006. They found that Sweden had quite a bit of qualitative studies in a worldwide comparison, with 92 studies, while Finland had 16 studies in those two years.

Sweden

Swedish nursing and caring science research has developed gradually over the past few decades in combination with the academic education for nurses (Heyman, 1995; Larsen & Adamsen, 2009). Heyman (1995) included a comprehensive bibliography for all 65 theses written by nurses from 1974 to 1991 in Sweden. The deductively developed knowledge was based on scales that were mostly lent from other disciplines, with the majority aligned with medical science and supervised by medical doctors, which resembled their research in quantitative studies. Human values and experiences were not of interest in the early agenda, and the nurses who started the academic development had a quite unindependent start within the medical sciences (Heyman, 1995; Larsen & Adamsen, 2009; Lundgren, Valmari, & Skott, 2008). There are still physicians involved in the doctoral projects, though their role is now that of a co-advisor. The first Professorship in Nursing was established in 1987 in Sweden, and was chaired at Umeå University by Astrid Norberg, who was one of the first nurses in Sweden to take a doctoral degree. Gothenburg, Stockholm, Lund, Uppsala and Örebro soon gained professorships (Hamrin & Lorensen, 1997) and, more recently, Luleå, Karlstad, Sundsvall and Växjö have also joined these other cities. The first qualitative doctoral theses in nursing science were written by the second generation of nurse researchers. It is still a matter of debate as to whether nursing science is an autonomic discipline or a "smorgasbord" of nursing from a cross-disciplinary basis, and thus not important in terms of developing a discipline of its own (Östlinder, Söderberg, & Öhlén, 2007; Larsen & Adamsen, 2009). In 2007, the Swedish National Agency for Higher Education radically denied the examination rights of several universities because its main subject, nursing science, was unclear. In 1998, there were approximately 200 nurses who attained a doctoral degree (Hamrin & Lorensen, 1997). In 2010, the number was 1000, including roughly 60 professors (www. vardforbundet.se). The number of articles and manuscripts in doctoral theses has radically reduced, from seven to eight articles in the early 1990s to as few as three in recent years, with the doctoral students writing with their advisors.

Rahm Hallberg (2006) argued that too many qualitative studies are published. Instead, in her opinion, nurse researchers need to do more multidisciplinary intervention studies and evaluate practice since she thinks that patients want to be approached from a holistic perspective, and are not greatly concerned about the profession. Furthermore, Hallberg takes it for granted that implementing findings from descriptive studies requires a translation into an intervention before the knowledge is of use to practice. Nordic and British researchers answered Hallberg (Galvin et al., 2008) by describing the significance of qualitative research. A successful new journal, the *International Journal of Qualitative Studies in Health and Well-Being*, was initiated by Lillemor Hallberg, a nurse-grounded theorist, and Karin Dahlberg, a nurse phenomenologist in Sweden in 2006. A new critical phase of qualitative nursing research is on its way in Sweden, as seen in the editorials of the leading journals.

Qualitative research profiling in Sweden

The University of Gothenburg, Sahlgrenska Academy is one of the influential Swedish universities in qualitative nursing research, led by Professor Marie Berg, Professor Ingegerd Bergbom, Professor Ella Danielson and Associate Professor Ingela Lundgren, among others. Linda Berg's thesis focuses on the caring relationship and an applied interpretive phenomenology inspired by Benner (Berg, Skott, & Danielson, 2006, 2007) that combines participant observation with field notes and both patients' and nurses' perspectives. Narrative-based methods of interpretation are illuminated by Ekman and Skott (2005) and Frid, Öhlén and Bergbom (2000). Sjöström and Dahlgren (2002) describe phenomenography designed to answer questions about how people make sense of their world. Professor Bergbom has supervised several qualitative studies in intensive care, and recently applied Gadamerian hermeneutics to family visitation (Eriksson, Lindahl, & Bergbom, & 2010), which combines interviews and non-participant observation. Being the relative of a patient diagnosed as brain dead uses Eriksson's theory of suffering for interpretation (Frid, Bergbom, & Haljamäe, 2001) and a follow-up of the primary analysis from 2001 used imagery (Frid, Haljamäe Öhlén, & Bergbom, 2007). The relationship between patients, informal caregivers and health professionals involved in home care (Lindahl, Lidén, & Lindblad, 2011) is illuminated in metasynthesis research. In collaboration with Holmgren, Valmari and Skott (2011), Lundgren used a seldom seen data collection method, that of McDonald's shadowing nurses in their everyday work.

Jönköping, Karlstad, Linköping, Lund, Mid-Sweden, Uppsala and Örebro Universities might not normally be clustered together, but in the case of qualitative methods in nursing, they share some things in common. None of these universities have developed qualitative method profiles in nursing science. At Karlstad University, Lindwall, von Post and Bergbom (2003) followed the hermeneutic tradition from a caring science perspective on the meaning of perioperative nursing care. Linköping University exemplifies pediatric nursing (see Fägerskiöld, 2009). Lund University displays content analysis studies (see Andersson, Hallberg, & Edberg, 2008; Persson, Fridlund, Kvist, & Dykes, 2011) and phenomenographic research (see Sjöström-Strand & Fridlund, 2006, 2007). Uppsala University has had a quantitative psychologically influenced tradition. The early theses in maternal care by Marie Berg and Ingela Lundgren included phenomenological studies (see Lundgren & Dahlberg, 1998, 2002; Berg & Dahlberg, 1998, 2001).

Mid-Sweden University has a qualitative research profile in development that arises through the supervision of Umeå University-educated researchers Kenneth Asplund, Ove Hellzén and Marianne Svedlund. A few examples of this are in Eriksson, Asplund and Svedlund (2010) that concern care for couples after acute myocardial infarction, and Lilja and Hellzén (2008) on psychiatric care when applying narrative picturing.

Örebro University shows a mixed profile when it comes to qualitative approaches and methods. Birgitta Andershed has, in collaboration with researchers from Ersta Sköndal University College, applied different qualitative methods in ethically sensitive end-of-life care and nursing care (see

Dwyer, Andershed, Nordenfelt, & Ternestedt, 2009; Ek, Sahlberg-Blom, Andershed & Ternestedt, 2011; Henriksson, Benzein, Ternestedt, & Andershed, 2011; James, Andershed, & Ternestedt, 2007a, 2007b). An early labor study applied grounded theory (see Carlsson, Hallberg, & Petterson, 2009), and Odencrants, Ehnfors and Grobe (2005, 2007) studied nutritional care by using interviews and case vignettes, while Skovdahl, Kihlgren and Kihlgren (2003) used video recording and stimulated recall interviews in nursing care for patients who suffered from dementia and aggressive behavior. A qualitative methodological study by Carlsson, Paterson, Scott-Findlay, Ehnfors and Ehrenberg (2007) concerned methodological issues (sampling, informed consent, fatigue) in interviews involving people with communication impairments after acquired brain damage.

The Karolinska Institute has produced some exemplary qualitative studies in relation to older people's nursing care that apply phenomenological hermeneutics supervised by Professor Emerita Sirkka-Liisa Ekman (Nilsson, Sarvimäki, & Ekman, 2000; Robinson, Ekman, & Wahlund, 1998), and interpretive phenomenology in the anesthesia care of older patients (Mauleon, Palo-Bengtsson, & Ekman, 2005). The hermeneutic caring science tradition from *Åbo Akademi University* is visible in Associate Professor Maria Arman's postdoctoral research. One example of this is a study (Arman, 2007) that applies Socratic dialogues, while another study (Arman, Hammarqvist, & Rehnsfeldt, 2011) uses face-to-face interviews, telephone follow-up interviews over a period of one year and email interview dialogues with 18 Swedish women and men suffering from burnout.

The Luleå University of Technology has created a profile of qualitative research through the research of Professor Siv Söderberg (see Chapter 6 in this volume), among others. The supervision of Professor Karin Axelsson (currently an Emerita) has furthered content analysis collecting data by using elderly couple interviews supported by scenario vignettes (Harrefors, Sävenstedt, & Axelsson, 2007) and interviews about the care of premature babies (Lindberg, Axelsson, & Öhrling, 2008). In a series of critical care studies, content analysis is applied (see Engström & Söderberg, 2007, 2010).

Finland

Finland was the first Nordic country to establish academic research in nursing science and education at the Master's, licentiate and doctoral levels, starting in Kuopio (currently the University of Eastern Finland) in 1979, which were soon followed by Tampere, Oulu, Turku and the Finland-Swedish Åbo Akademi University in Vasa (see Tuomi, 1997; Leino-Kilpi & Suominen, 1998). From the start, the Finnish doctoral theses in nursing have primarily been supervised by nurse researchers, who unlike their Swedish counterparts, were not influenced by medicine, but instead had graduated from the social (Professor Emerita Sirkka Sinkkonen) or educational sciences (Katie Eriksson, Hertta Kalkas and Sirkka Lauri, all of whom are current Professor Emerita). Survey type research in nursing had started much earlier with the *Finnish Yearbook of Nursing* in 1958. The Nursing Research Institute was established as early as 1966 (see Leino-Kilpi & Suominen, 1998), and some of the first studies were called Action Research, displaying a strong clinical incentive. The Finnish Association of Nursing Science was founded in 1988, creating the peer-reviewed journal *Hoitotiede* (Journal of Nursing Science), which published qualitative studies from its start in 1989. In 1990, the first national conference took place, and has continued as a yearly meeting for Finnish nursing scientists. In Finland, the majority of current professors belong to the second generation, who were educated in qualitative methods and wrote qualitative doctoral theses. In Finland, the academic education does not include a nursing education, which is provided at colleges.

Qualitative research profiling in Finland

The University of Eastern Finland (previously Kuopio University) currently displays an international profile in preventive nursing science, among other research interests. Professor Emerita Sirkka Sinkkonen, whose interest in health care administration in nursing arose from a social science perspective held the first chair and supervised the first doctoral dissertation, Maija Hentinen (currently Professor Emerita) on Action Research in cardiac care. Fridlund et al. (2007) honorably call Hentinen's research the start of cardiovascular nursing. Until 2011, 136 licentiates and doctoral theses, and over 1000 Master's theses in nursing science, have been produced, several qualitatively supervised by full professors such as Pietilä, Turunen and Vehviläinen-Julkunen.

Oulu University is profiled by research in chronic illness and patient education with the leading Professors Isola and Kyngäs. Elo and Kyngäs wrote a method article on content analysis (2008), and Kortesluoma, Hentinen and Nikkonen (2003) wrote one on interviewing children between the ages of 4 and 11 years in their study on pain (Kortesluoma & Nikkonen, 2004). Juntunen, Nikkonen and Janhonen (2000, 2002) include unusual cultural care studies in Tanzanian care, whereas Pesonen, Remes and Isola (2011) describe and reflect on the ethical and methodological issues in dementia care research.

Tampere University has developed an internationally recognized family nursing science led by Professors Åstedt-Kurki and Paavilainen. Programs of research include families' experiences of care received in health care settings, family violence and child maltreatment. Research on the effectiveness of family nursing interventions has put the focus on quantitative methods (Åstedt-Kurki, 2010). Arja Häggman-Laitila's six articles from her doctoral thesis (see 1997, 1999), all of which were published in refereed journals, exemplify the thorough early research in the department, with qualitative methods playing a major role. In a broad study on how Finnish adults understand health, Häggman-Laitila and Åstedt-Kurki (1995) applied a phenomenological research tradition. The large sample was typical for the beginning of the Finnish qualitative research. The researchers were conscientious about explicating the epistemological view of the human being and theoretical starting points indepth, and applied references to nursing science pioneers and not only to philosophy. Maijala's thesis is qualitative, and uses grounded theory in family nursing (see Maijala, Paavilainen, & Åstedt-Kurki, 2003; Maijala, Paavilainen, Väisänen, & Åstedt-Kurki, 2004).

Turku University has its main focus on nursing values and ethics, and has participated in several large-scale EU projects, with a preferred focus on intervention studies. The leading researchers in this regard are Professors Leino-Kilpi, Salanterä, Suhonen and Välimäki, all of whom have supervised qualitative studies.

Unifying geographically spread qualitative nursing paradigms

There are a few traditions in which qualitative epistemology and methods have played a major role in the development of disciplinary knowledge, and they have spread geographically with the doctoral students who have been educated in the tradition, and then continued by advising the next generation.

The hermeneutic caring science tradition

The Finland Swedish *Åbo Akademi University* in Vasa is profiled by hermeneutic caring science research, with a preference for conceptual determination (Sivonen, Kasén, & Eriksson, 2010). No quantitative doctoral theses exist. This tradition was the first to develop outside a medical faculty, and has spread widely under the guidance of its leader, Professor Emerita Katie Eriksson.

The autonomous caring science discipline has an explicit theoretical perspective with an ethos (i.e., the basic values, vision and mission) and ontology that provide a basis for the epistemology (i.e., the view of knowledge), choosing the methodological prerequisites, the choice of methods and the contextual prerequisites (Eriksson, 2002, 2007). The construction of systematic and contextual clinical caring science is combined by the mission of caring as the alleviation of human suffering and the serving of life and health in a spirit of the caritas motive and compassion. The methodological development began with the "Multidimensional Health" project (starting in 1989), and the subsequent "In the Patient's World" (starting in 1995), in which some of the first international qualitative empirical studies arising from the caritative theory were published (see Bondas & Eriksson, 2001; Bondas-Salonen, 1998; Lindholm, 1997). An example of the fruitfulness of the basic hermeneutic research is Kasén's doctoral thesis (2002) on the caring relation as asymmetrical, including touching, connection and story. Fredriksson made a method journey on caring conversations in psychiatric care (see Fredriksson, 1999, among others). The hermeneutic Gadamerian-dominated approach currently prevails, with the research mainly published in doctoral theses (in both Swedish and Norwegian) and postdoctoral. There is a skeptical view towards rigid methods when the philosophical turn combines ontology and epistemology with a striving towards universal models.

The Swedish researcher Maud Söderlund's study is exemplarily hermeneutic, focusing on the relatives of dementia sufferers (2007). The design builds on the American philosopher Charles Sanders Peirce and his idea of abduction, a guiding idea that leads the researcher. The distinction among three types of logical reasoning—deduction, induction and abduction—is the thought that each is correlated to a unique view of valid knowledge, which is irreducible to that of the others. In particular, abductive validity cannot be analyzed in either deductive or inductive terms but when the abductive argumentation is clarified, every phase in the process can be seen in the forms of deduction and induction. The end is a special type of practical inference which, if correct, is deductively valid, while the creative phase is not inferential at all, but instead led by a persistent idea of the researcher. A typical outcome of the hermeneutic research is a theoretical model. Söderlund's model is called "Terra Caritatis," in which suffering is alleviated in an atmosphere of community. When *"seeing the truth"* (Gadamer, 1993) (Söderlund's italicization and reference, 2007, p. 36), it will be possible to alleviate suffering and give the relatives the support needed in order to be able to reach their potential health when reconciled with their suffering.

A methodological article on metaphors in caring science research is written in the hermeneutic tradition by the Swedish researcher Lena Wiklund-Gustin (2010). Understanding is promoted by analyses of narrative content, i.e., what the text talks about that could be revealed by metaphors used by the participants or constructed by the researcher. Metaphors are not only analytic tools, but also the means to communicate findings in their ability to make connections between language and body metaphors. The more complex and abstract a phenomenon, the better suited it is to the use of metaphors because of its ability to reveal something in a new and more tangible way. While at the same time bringing meaning closer by giving it a new gestalt and not trivializing it, oversimplifying it and taking it for granted, the metaphor must be creative, ethical and alive, with metaphors such as "the clown" and "pouring oil over the waves" depicting suffering and caring. The last step is a root metaphor created by the researcher, in this study, "frozen water," and the caregiver is like "an icebreaker" that may be a positive opening, but one that might also ruin the foundations. Wiklund-Gustin (2010) vividly describes how her research was skeptically met by colleagues, including even qualitatively educated persons, as being too speculative.

The phenomenological hermeneutic and content analysis traditions

At *Umeå University*, Professor Emerita Astrid Norberg, was influential in creating a qualitative approach that relied on phenomenological hermeneutics and Ricouer's philosophy. It was developed during the 1990s in several doctoral projects, and geographically spread by many of her doctoral students, who now in turn advise their own students. The new approach was developed in several polygraph theses on the meaning of caring as a narrated, lived and moral experience (see Åström, Jansson, Norberg, & Hallberg, 1993; Åström, Norberg, Hallberg, & Jansson, 1993, among others) and on ethics in intensive care (see Söderberg & Norberg, 1993). The analysis starts with a naïve reading of the data as text to achieve an initial sense of the whole, as well as evoking ideas of how to continue to analyze. The structural analysis is a detailed thematization, meaning unit by meaning unit, to help identify patterns and seek explanations. The comprehensive understanding forms the third part, a critical in-depth understanding, which takes into account the whole and depth, using theory/theories for interpretation.

One of the other early innovative studies was a video-recorded observation of 49 morning sessions of five nursing home patients who suffered from dementia (Kihlgren, Hallgren, Norberg, & Karlsson, 1994). A phenomenological hermeneutic analysis of the interaction of patients and staff was conducted from a theoretical perspective using Erikson's theory and Ricoeur's phenomenological philosophy. Wholeness and common patterns in each person's interactions as a whole, including action, talk, mimics, gesture and the context, were transformed into a text and musical notes (yes, musical notes). Another exemplary research program was published by Pejlert and colleagues. Ten schizophrenic patients were interviewed about their experiences of life in a hospital ward, of their care provider and of the care received (Pejlert, Asplund, & Norberg, 1995). Another study illuminates the meaning of caring for patients on a long-term psychiatric ward as narrated by 17 formal care providers (Pejlert, Asplund, Gilje, & Norberg, 1998), with the results interpreted and discussed in light of a previously published interview study with the patients. In a 1999 study, Pejlert, Asplund and Norberg continued a series of interviews with six clients with a diagnosis of schizophrenia about their lives in a home-like setting, their key care provider and the care received. The next study included nurse interviews one and two years after their patients had moved to a home-like setting in comparison with results from interviews before the move. The final study illuminates the natural caregivers' perspective in relation to being the parent of an adult son or daughter with a severe mental illness receiving professional care (Pejlert, 2001).

Phenomenological hermeneutics is applied in several contexts of care, including palliative care (see Rasmussen, Jansson, & Norberg, 2000; Brännström, Ekman, Boman, & Strandberg, 2007), chronic heart failure (see Ekman, Ehnfors, & Norberg, 2000), care for patients suffering dementia and their relatives (see Kihlgren, Hallgren, Norberg, & Karlsson, 1994), childbearing and care (see Hallgren, Kihlgren, Norberg, & Forslin, 1995), antenatal booking interviews (see Olsson, Jansson, & Norberg, 1998, 2000), patients and nurses in psychiatric care (see Hellzén, Asplund, Sandman, & Norberg, 1999), care for persons who live at home and are dependent on a ventilator (see Lindahl, Sandman, & Rasmussen, 2006), care for parents of a child affected by disability (see Lindblad, Rasmussen, & Sandman, 2007), patients who have suffered a stroke (see Nilsson, Jansson, & Norberg, 1997), old people's care (see Nygren, Norberg, & Lundman, 2007), older people's abuse from the perspective of public health nurses (see Saveman, Hallberg, & Norberg,1993), coercion in psychiatric care (see Olofsson & Jacobsson, 2001), dependency on care (see Strandberg, Norberg, & Jansson, 2000, 2001), patients with communication difficulties (see Sundin, Jansson, & Norberg, 2000, 2002), women's myocardial infarction and their partners (see Svedlund, Danielson, & Norberg, 1999, 2001) and fibromyalgia sufferers (see Chapter 6 by Söderberg).

Content analysis

Content analysis has been developed by Graneheim and Lundman at *Umeå University* in an extensively cited article (2004), while different variations of content analysis using a variety of references have been applied in studies of diabetes care (see Hörnsten, Sandström, & Lundman, 2004), prolonged labor (see Nystedt, Högberg, & Lundman, 2008), old people's bodily experiences (see Santamäki Fischer, Altin, Ragnarsson, & Lundman, 2008), pediatric nursing (Angström-Brännström, Norberg, & Jansson, 2008), and patients who suffer from abdominal aortic aneurysms (see Brännström, Björck, Strandberg, & Wanhainen, 2009). In psychiatric care, a case content analysis with one patient (PAR for 21 months, including journal texts, staff diaries, video tapes and 15 narrative interviews) shows the potential richness of a case study (see Hellzen, Asplund, Gilje, Sandman, & Norberg, 1998).

The phenomenological lifeworld caring science tradition

At *Linnéus University*, the Swedish nurse researcher Karin Dahlberg advocated for a qualitative lifeworld-based research in a caring science tradition. Her doctoral education was based on pedagogy, her thesis is a phenomenographic study from Gothenburg University, and she is connected to Åbo Akademi University in Finland by an adjunct professorship. The striving for lifeworld-led research is developing a continental philosophy regarding health and well-being by exploring developments in care that can enhance individual experiences. In an editorial, Dahlberg (2006a) argues that qualitative studies suffer from being too close to the criteria of a measurable methodology that may confuse many researchers, who end up practicing what she calls a "mixed discourse." Moreover, Dahlberg points to internal paradigmatic problems within qualitative research that pay less attention to the issues of validity, objectivity and generalization that are actually the characteristics of scientific work. The epistemological basis must be sound: we must know what we are doing and how a certain study should be carried out, and why we are doing what we do in research, i.e., a coherent and logical reasoning is pivotal in qualitative research. Dahlberg has written extensively on phenomenology and the reflective lifeworld research method that she has developed (Dahlberg, 2006b, 2007, 2011; Dahlberg, Dahlberg, & Nyström, 2008, among others). Dahlberg continues to supervise doctoral students by applying a reflective lifeworld research. Exemplary studies concern dementia care (Svanström & Dahlberg, 2004), psychiatric care (Carlsson, Dahlberg, Ekebergh, & Dahlberg, 2006), and prehospital care (Wireklint Sundström & Dahlberg, 2011).

Nordic qualitative research network: an exemplary case

BFiN (www.uin.no/bfin) is an acronym for Childbearing in the Nordic Countries, a qualitative research network in the caring sciences initiated in 2002 by Professor Terese Bondas, who at that time was an Associate Professor at Åbo Akademi University, Finland, and Anita Hallgren, from Umeå University in Sweden. The network started with support from Åbo Akademi University, NorFa and a subsequent Nordforsk grant to become a European research network that unites researchers and doctoral students, with more than 80 researchers currently conducting qualitative research from eight countries, with the majority coming from Sweden and Finland. The steering group of researchers from the Nordic countries includes Professor Marie Berg and Associate Professor Ingela Lundgren, at Sahlgrenska Academy at Gothenburg University, who were the first members, together with Professor Emerita Elisabeth Hall at Århus University in Denmark. Researcher mobility, in addition to the collaboration and coordination of research teams in qualitative childbearing research, are priorities. Several qualitative research courses have been organized since 2001 with the participating universities, and it is of importance to contribute to the disciplinary discussion and developments in the field of childbearing and care, as exemplified by an article in which the researchers' steering group advocates for the inclusion of qualitative research findings in evidence-based care (see Berg et al., 2008). The methodological studies on metasynthesis (see Bondas & Hall, 2007a, 2007b) are developed within the research network. Moreover, prominent international guest professors who are well known for their qualitative research and international textbooks, including Cheryl Tatano Beck, Barbara Paterson and Pranee Liamputtong, have been invited to create collaboration.

Discussion

Some critical remarks need to be considered when starting the discussion. The challenge was the large number of publications, as it is not possible to analyze all the details and create an all-inclusive view since there are numerous ways to look at the research area. Peer-reviewed, internationally published research provides a part of the mosaic of qualitative nursing and caring research in Finland and Sweden and the production that is analyzed is not complete. The data, however, are considered to be sufficient enough to provide a picture with examples from qualitative research and method development. The data reflect the work of several distinct investigators in Finland and Sweden, and the Nordic neighboring countries are most definitely at the forefront of qualitative research in nursing and caring science. Choosing refereed international publications while omitting national publications in Finnish or Swedish because of their inaccessibility to an international readership requires national studies. The fields and contexts cover research from birth to the elderly. I have used several examples, although method information was sometimes very difficult to retrieve, particularly in the abstracts from the 1990s, as well as in more recent research. Method slurring is evident, but also creative combinations and applications, when talking about qualitative nursing research coming of age in both Sweden and Finland. The disciplinary orientation of authors was not always easy to discern and the question of discipline still needs some attention, along with the organizational questions of autonomy. The differences in faculty connections, e.g. medical, social science and autonomous faculties (to mention only a few), in conjunction with the advising professors' educational backgrounds, do seem to matter when it comes to qualitative research. The main ideas such as building discipline, contributing to nursing practice, including the trend of evidence-based practice and the views on the contribution of qualitative nursing research, are all differentiated. I suggest that there seem to be three different overarching views of the role of qualitative research in the Finnish and Swedish nursing and caring sciences:

1   *Qualitative nursing and caring research is developed within an autonomous science.* There are several paradigmatic views of an autonomous science in which three traditions are devoted to the development of different qualitative approaches: hermeneutic, phenomenological-hermeneutic and lifeworld research. An underlying assumption seems to be that qualitative studies produce an understanding and provide direction for nursing care and caring as a value in itself. As its main motive, the hermeneutic caring science tradition arising from Åbo Akademi University has had a universal disciplinary development. Theories are developed. There is a body of knowledge with an ontological basis in continuous development and the development of epistemology, methodology and ways to understand and procedures for developing new knowledge are discussed from an epistemological perspective. Philosophical ways of thinking might easily invade qualitative studies, and the interest in substance could turn to an

interpretation of the philosophers' thoughts. Further development of a theory of science may be considered as an urgent need.

2   *Qualitative nursing research is a prelude to intervention studies.* Nursing science is a research area in which intervention studies are the gold standard because of their primary reason for existence: to develop an evidence-based care. The qualitative studies are then seen as a possible pilot in the development of the real study—the intervention or training before the "real" research of doing interventional studies is carried out. There are islands of qualitative research and some skilled researchers.

3   *A"smorgasbord" of qualitative nursing research from a multidisciplinary view.* The characteristics here are that knowledge is developed without an explicit theoretical consciousness or on an ad hoc theoretical basis, in which a scientific identity is difficult to discern. The scientific discussion is often pursued in relation to the research within the area on an ad hoc basis. The disciplinary question may therefore seem irrelevant, even if one adheres to the notion of cumulative knowledge. The interest seems to be an immediate pragmatic good for the nursing profession. Furthermore, there are often cross-disciplinary supervision teams in the doctoral students' projects when they are connected to a diagnosis and a method mix.

Another conclusion is that there seem to be obstacles in the development of qualitative methods in use: (1) equating nursing as a discipline with the nursing profession's entire area of work seems to have led to an emphasis on primary pragmatic interests and non-cumulative knowledge. This is seen even more in Sweden, where nursing education has been part of the academic system from the beginning; (2) postdoctoral research projects primarily focus on educating doctoral students, and international postdoctoral education and a collaboration in qualitative methods need further incentives; (3) an equal cross-disciplinary collaboration is needed when different perspectives within different disciplines may provide a broader and more systematic whole with the concurrent use of theories and knowledge from several disciplines. This seems to be difficult when one's own disciplinary identity is weak and old authorities rule. A double discussion could be possible in relation to the research area and discipline. Scientific borders are useful when the discipline's members maintain an ongoing, healthy constructive discussion, though the opposite occurs when thick walls have been built between the paradigms, thereby inhibiting collaboration and innovation. Research questions might be considered important within the paradigm, but remain uninteresting in the field of nursing and societal development. This situation does not further the development of care and caring for the good of the patients and their families, even if we could create an ethical, esthetical and well-structured body of knowledge. The problematization of perspective and the preunderstanding, both of which are necessary in order to develop a critical scientific attitude, may be difficult. The universities would benefit from collaboration in education, supervision and the integration of doctoral studies in large projects. Cumulative knowledge that benefits the care of patients and their loved ones need not be in conflict with a disciplinary discussion. The research that underpins the writing of this chapter inspired me to reflect on the importance of disciplinary consciousness and cumulative development. My answer is yes, we do need to create and recreate the discipline to inform praxis and to inform health care politics, i.e., to minister to the patients and their loved ones (Bondas, 2003). However, the balance between the clinical nurse researchers and the theory-guided nurse researchers seems to be wide in Finland and Sweden, with both arguing that they are right.

Qualitative approaches and methods are needed to build bridges. The theoretical discussions might need to be informed from the qualitative studies in order to move forward, while the empirical qualitative studies may need to rely on theoretical perspectives to help make their ontological and epistemological starting points more clear to obtain more depth and validity.

Critical synthetic studies are needed to push the renewal of research discourses that may have gone awry in vicious non-fruitful circles, or even come to a dead end like a broken LP (Bondas & Hall, 2007a, 2007b). An heuristic synthesis of several studies in a qualitative research program (Bondas, 2011) might also illuminate a new understanding and help us see what we do not know to start new fruitful studies. My suggestion is to include the study of concepts and language in use and to study findings across contexts in health, suffering, caring, as well as several other phenomena pertinent to nursing. Polit and Beck discuss generalization as an act of reasoning, i.e., "drawing broad conclusions from particular instances—that is making an inference about the unobserved based on the observed" (2010, p. 1451). My suggestion is in accordance with Polit and Beck (2010) when they claim that qualitative research is well suited to reveal higher-level concepts and theories that are not unique to a particular participant or setting, in addition to the rich, highly detailed and potentially insightful findings that make them suitable for extrapolation. Edmund Husserl, the father of phenomenology, called for evidence as insight: seeing the essence (1931/1999). Interventions are not needed in human existential question when the findings convince the reader in either analytic or case-to-case models of the potential transferability of the findings. In turn, this requires thick description according to Geertz's (1973) terms. Polit and Beck (2010) suggest a deliberate replication in a different context: "Knowledge does not come simply by . . . inventing a new construct or the worst scenario, 'giving an inventive label to an old construct'" (p. 1454). Even more confusing is using an old concept in a new context and meaning without discussing the problems that this poses for the research reader. Reflection on the broad research questions and the issues of time, space and relations in the methodological decisions are needed to further the development. When adding to the building of the discipline, the phenomena could be the cornerstones in addition to the concepts in the twofold model of systematic and clinical research (see Eriksson, 2007). Inductive descriptions of experiences might become naïve and endless repetitions, and become lost in superficial structures when there are no cumulative connections to a theoretical perspective or sometimes not even to previous research. The hermeneutical interest might help to open, explore and extract knowledge, but there always lies the threat of circles within circles going bad, not seeing anything new or seeing what one wants to see, obstructed instead of open to the world of the patient, their relatives and the world of care. There are examples of qualitative studies "drowning" in philosophy and not coming up to the surface, with sadly nothing more than the old sayings of the philosophers who may actually have said it better, and the nursing is lost. How could our findings better touch the person reading them?

Implications for the future of qualitative nursing science research

- *Discovery* of new fruitful research questions by listening to the patients, their loved ones and nurses, as well as the media debate and connections between practice and cumulative knowledge.
- *Reading:* not only philosophy, but also our pioneers in nursing and caring science by incorporating history and a history of ideas.
- *Balance* between ontology and theory and the phenomena, and another balance between epistemology and methodology and methods.
- *Time:* looking at the phenomena unfolding over time as well as the connections.
- *Relations:* combine the perspectives of those cared for and care providers in their culture.
- *Renewal* of an in-depth thick description when daring to move from the broad questions to the small questions so relevant for care and the patients and their loved ones.
- *Critical research* endeavors that increase action research, discourse analysis and critical interpretation, thereby enabling changes.

- *Metastudies* that extend across contexts and findings pertinent to nursing, combined with metamethod and metatheory studies to help develop qualitative approaches.
- *International collaborations* in qualitative research, thus enabling cultural nuances and comparisons, and ethical reflections.

Conclusion

Qualitative research has come of age in both Finland and Sweden, and is now entering its fifth decade. The research areas that are pursued in qualitative nursing research in Finland and Sweden concern basic caring science research, pediatric nursing, reproductive care, old people's nursing care, end-of-life care, chronic illness experience and care, health promotion and prevention, transcultural nursing, family nursing, intensive and critical care and cancer care. The most developed methodological contributions are hermeneutics and its conceptual determination, phenomenological hermeneutics, reflective lifeworld research and content analysis, all of which are also applied in the vast majority of research. Research is published in international journals.

This development has started in different ways, and is moving in different directions with the second and third generation of qualitative researchers. The enduring debate of what is nursing science and its philosophical orientations is ongoing. We should also ask: "What are the phenomena that need to be understood in connection to what we know already, and what is our responsibility in research to pursue changes in practice in accordance with this new understanding?" The "how" questions continue, and still take precedence over the "what is" and "what might be" questions. There is some mid-range theory development and some framework theories that are strong, and there is also a trend to decontextualize findings and abstraction, as well as a universal theory development that we have not previously connected to qualitative research. The interest in evidence-based care and health policy remains low, and there is still much work to do in expressing the underlying assumptions, paradigmatic views and research ethics, preferably in an international collaboration in our multicultural world.

References

Andersson, M., Hallberg, I. R., & Edberg, A. K. (2008). Old people receiving municipal care, their experiences of what constitutes a good life in the last phase of life: A qualitative study. *International Journal of Nursing Studies, 45*, 818–828.

Angen, M. J. (2000). Evaluating interpretive inquiry: Reviewing the validity debate and opening the dialogue. *Qualitative Health Research, 10*, 378–395.

Angström-Brännström, C., Norberg, A., & Jansson, L. (2008). Narratives of children with chronic illness about being comforted. *Journal of Pediatric Nursing, 23*, 310–316.

Arman, M. (2007). Bearing witness: An existential position in caring. *Contemporary Nurse, 27*, 84–93.

Arman, M., Hammarqvist, A. S., & Rehnsfeldt, A. (2011). Burnout as an existential deficiency: Lived experiences of burnout sufferers. *Scandinavian Journal of Caring Sciences, 25*, 294–302.

Åstedt-Kurki, P. (2010). Family nursing research for practice: The Finnish perspective. *Journal of Family Nursing, 16*, 256–268.

Åström, G., Jansson, L., Norberg, A., & Hallberg, I. R. (1993). Experienced nurses' narratives of their being in ethically difficult care situations: The problem to act in accordance with one's ethical reasoning and feelings. *Cancer Nursing, 16*, 179–187.

Åström, G., Norberg, A., Hallberg, I. R., & Jansson, L. (1993). Experienced and skilled nurses' narratives of situations where caring action made a difference to the patient. *Journal of Nursing Scholarship, 7*, 183–193; discussion 195–198.

Berg, L., Skott, C., & Danielson, E. (2006). An interpretive phenomenological method for illuminating the meaning of caring relationship. *Scandinavian Journal of Caring Sciences, 20*, 42–50.

Berg, L., Skott, C., & Danielson, E. (2007). Caring relationship in context: Fieldwork in a medical ward. *International Journal of Nursing Practice, 13*, 100–106.

Berg, M., Bondas, T., Hall, E., Lundgren, I. Olafsdottir, O., Støre Brinchmann, B., & Vehviläinen-Julkunen, K. (2008). Evidence based care and childbearing: A critical approach. *International Journal of Qualitative Studies on Health and Wellbeing, 3,* 239–247.

Berg, M., & Dahlberg, K. (1998). A phenomenological study of women's experiences of complicated childbirth. *Midwifery, 14,* 23–29.

Berg, M., & Dahlberg, K. (2001). Swedish midwives' care of women who are at high obstetric risk or who have obstetric complications. *Midwifery, 17,* 259–266.

Bondas, T. (2003). Caritative leadership: Ministering to the patients. *Nursing Administration Quarterly, 27,* 249–255.

Bondas, T. (2011). Husserlian phenomenology reflected in caring science childbearing research. In G. Thomson, S. Downe, & F. Dykes (Eds.), *Qualitative research in midwifery and childbirth: Phenomenological approaches* (pp. 1–18). London: Routledge.

Bondas, T., & Eriksson, K. (2001). Women's lived experiences of pregnancy: A tapestry of health and suffering. *Qualitative Health Research, 11,* 824–840.

Bondas, T., & Hall, E. (2007a). A decade of metasynthesis research: A meta-method study. *International Journal of Qualitative Studies on Health and Wellbeing, 2*(2), 101–113.

Bondas, T., & Hall, E. (2007b). Challenges in the approaches to metasynthesis research. *Qualitative Health Research, 17,* 113–121.

Bondas-Salonen, T. (1998). How women experience the presence of their partners at the birth of their baby. *Qualitative Health Research, 8,* 784–800.

Brännström, M., Björck, M., Strandberg, G. & Wanhainen, A. (2009). Patients' experiences of being informed about having an abdominal aortic aneurysm: A follow-up case study five years after screening. *Journal of Vascular Nursing, 27,* 70–74.

Brännström, M., Ekman, I., Boman, K., & Strandberg, G. (2007). Being a close relative of a person with severe, chronic heart failure in palliative advanced home care: A comfort but also a strain. *Scandinavian Journal of Caring Sciences, 21,* 338–344.

Carlsson, E., Paterson, B. L., Scott-Findlay, S., Ehnfors, M., & Ehrenberg, A. (2007). Methodological issues in interviews involving people with communication impairments after acquired brain damage. *Qualitative Health Research, 17,* 1361–1371.

Carlsson, G., Dahlberg. K., Ekebergh, M., & Dahlberg, H. (2006). Patients longing for authentic personal care: A phenomenological study of violent encounters in psychiatric settings. *Issues in Mental Health Nursing, 27,* 287–305.

Carlsson, I. M., Hallberg, L. R., & Odberg Pettersson, K. (2009). Swedish women's experiences of seeking care and being admitted during the latent phase of labour: A grounded theory study. *Midwifery, 25,* 172–180.

Dahlberg, K. (2006a). Editorial. *International Journal of Qualitative Studies on Health and Well-being, 1,* 130–132.

Dahlberg, K. (2006b). The essence of essences: The search for meaning structures in phenomenological analysis of lifeworld phenomena. *International Journal of Qualitative Studies on Health and Well-being, 1,* 11–19.

Dahlberg, K. (2007). The enigmatic phenomenon of loneliness. *International Journal of Qualitative Studies on Health and Well-being, 2,* 195–207.

Dahlberg, K. (2011). Lifeworld phenomenology for caring and for health care research. In G. Thomson, S. Downe, & F. Dykes (Eds.), *Qualitative research in midwifery and childbirth: Phenomenological approaches* (pp. 19–33). London: Routledge.

Dahlberg, K., Dahlberg, H., & Nyström, M. (2008). *Reflective lifeworld research* (2nd rev. ed.). Lund: Studentlitteratur.

Dwyer, L. L., Andershed, B., Nordenfelt, L., & Ternestedt, B. M. (2009). Dignity as experienced by nursing home staff. *International Journal of Older People Nursing, 4,* 185–193.

Ek, K., Sahlberg-Blom, E., Andershed, B., & Ternestedt, B. M. (2011). Struggling to retain living space: Patients' stories about living with advanced chronic obstructive pulmonary disease. *Journal of Advanced Nursing, 67,* 1480–1490.

Ekman, I., Ehnfors, M., & Norberg, A. (2000). The meaning of living with severe chronic heart failure as narrated by elderly people. *Scandinavian Journal of Caring Sciences, 14,* 130–136.

Ekman, I., & Skott, C. (2005). Developing clinical knowledge through a narrative-based method of interpretation. *European Journal of Cardiovascular Nursing, 4,* 251–256.

Elo, S., & Kyngäs H. (2008). The qualitative content analysis process. *Journal of Advanced Nursing, 62,* 107–115.

Engström, Å., & Söderberg, S. (2007). Close relatives in intensive care from the perspective of critical care nurses. *Journal of Clinical Nursing, 16*, 1651–1659.

Engström, Å., & Söderberg, S. (2010). Critical care nurses' experiences of follow-up visits to an ICU. *Journal of Clinical Nursing, 19*, 2925–2932.

Eriksson, K. (2002). Caring science in a new key. *Nursing Science Quarterly, 15*, 61–65.

Eriksson, K. (2007). Becoming through suffering: The path to health and holiness. *International Journal for Human Caring, 11*, 8–15.

Eriksson, M., Asplund, K., & Svedlund, M. (2010). Couples' thoughts about and expectations of their future life after the patient's hospital discharge following acute myocardial infarction. *Journal of Clinical Nursing, 19*, 3485–3493.

Eriksson, T., Lindahl, B., & Bergbom, I. (2010). Visits in an intensive care unit: An observational hermeneutic study. *Intensive and Critical Care Nursing, 26*, 51–57.

Fägerskiöld, A. (2009.) Support of fathers of infants by the child health nurse. *Scandinavian Journal of Caring Sciences, 23*, 243–250.

Fredriksson, L. (1999). Modes of relating in a caring conversation: A research synthesis on presence, touch and listening. *Journal of Advanced Nursing, 30*, 1167–1176.

Frid, I., Bergbom, I., & Haljamäe, H. (2001). No going back: Narratives by close relatives of the braindead patient. *Intensive and Critical Care Nursing, 17*, 263–278.

Frid, I., Haljamäe, H., Öhlén, J., & Bergbom, I. (2007). Brain death: Close relatives' use of imagery as a descriptor of experience. *Journal of Advanced Nursing, 58*, 63–71.

Frid, I., Öhlén, J., & Bergbom, I. (2000). On the use of narratives in nursing research. *Journal of Advanced Nursing, 32*, 695–703.

Fridlund, B., Hildebrandt, L., Hildingh, C., & Lidell, E. (2007). Status and trends in Swedish dissertations in the area of cardiovascular nursing. *European Journal of Cardiovascular Nursing, 6*, 72–76.

Gadamer, H. G. (1993). *Truth and method.* New York: Continuum,

Galvin, K., Emami, A., Dahlberg, K., Ekebergh, M., Rosser, E., Powell, J., Bach, S., Edlund, B., Bondas, T., & Uhrenfeldt, L. (2008). Challenges for future caring science research: A response to providing evidence for health-care practice. *International Journal of Nursing Studies, 45*, 971–974.

Geertz, C. (1973). *The interpretation of cultures: Selected essays.* New York: Basic Books.

Graneheim, U. H., & Lundman, B. (2004). Qualitative content analysis in nursing research: concepts, procedures and measures to achieve trustworthiness. *Nurse Education Today, 24*, 105–112.

Habermas. J. (1972). *Knowledge and human interests* (trans. J. J. Shapiro). London: Heinemann.

Häggman-Laitila, A. (1997). Health as an individual's way of existence, *Journal of Advanced Nursing, 25*, 45–53.

Häggman-Laitila, A. (1999). The authenticity and ethics of phenomenological research: How to overcome the researcher's own views, *Nursing Ethics, 6*, 12–22.

Häggman-Laitila, A., & Åstedt-Kurki, P. (1995). How Finnish adults understand health. *Western Journal of Nursing Research, 17*, 614–630.

Hallgren, A., Kihlgren, M., Norberg, A., & Forslin, L. (1995). Women's perceptions of childbirth and childbirth education before and after education and birth. *Midwifery, 11*, 130–137.

Hamrin, E., & Lorensen, M. (1997). *Perspectives on priorities in nursing science.* Report 1. Stockholm: Vårdalstiftelsen.

Harrefors, C., Sävenstedt, S. & Axelsson, K. (2007). Elderly people's perceptions of how they want to be cared for: An interview study with healthy elderly couples in Northern Sweden. *Scandinavian Journal of Caring Sciences, 21*, 56–63.

Hellzén, O., Asplund, K., Gilje, F., Sandman, P. O., & Norberg A. (1998). From optimism to pessimism: A case study of a psychiatric patient. *Journal of Clinical Nursing, 7*, 360–370.

Hellzén, O., Asplund, K., Sandman, P. O., & Norberg, A. (1999). The unwillingness to be violated: Carers' experiences of caring for a person acting in a disturbing manner. An interview study. *Journal of Clinical Nursing, 8*, 653–662.

Henriksson, A., Benzein, E., Ternestedt, B. M., & Andershed, B. (2011). Meeting needs of family members of persons with life-threatening illness: A support group program during ongoing palliative care. *Journal of Palliative and Support Care, 9*, 263–271.

Heyman, I. (1995). *Gånge hatt till: omvårdnadsforskningens framväxt i Sverige: sjuksköterskors avhandlingar, 1974–1991* [The emergence of nursing research in Sweden: Doctoral theses written by nurses, 1974–1991]. Gothenburg: Daidalos.

Hörnsten, Å., Sandström, H., & Lundman, B. (2004). Personal understandings of illness among people with type 2 diabetes. *Journal of Advanced Nursing, 47*, 174–182.

Husserl, E. (1999/1931). *Cartesian meditations* (12th ed.) (trans. D. Cairns). Dordrecht: Kluwer.

James, I., Andershed, B., & Ternestedt, B. M. (2007a). A family's beliefs about cancer, dying, and death in the end of life. *Contemporary Nurse, 27*, 61–72.

James, I., Andershed, B., & Ternestedt, B. M. (2007b). The encounter between informal and professional care at the end of life. *Journal of Family Nursing, 13*, 226–252.

Juntunen, A., Nikkonen, M., & Janhonen, S. (2000). Utilising the concept of protection in health maintenance among the Bena in Tanzania. *Journal of Transcultural Nursing, 11*, 174–181.

Juntunen, A., Nikkonen, M., & Janhonen, S. (2002). Respect as the main lay care activity among the Bena in Ilembula village in Tanzania. *International Journal of Nursing Practice, 8*, 210–220.

Kasén, A. (2002). *Den vårdande relationen.* [The caring relationship]. Åbo: Åbo Akademi.

Kihlgren, M., Hallgren, A. Norberg, A., & Karlsson, I. (1994). Integrity promoting care of demented patients: Patterns of interaction during morning care, *International Journal of Aging and Human Development, 39*, 303–319.

Kortesluoma, R-L., Hentinen, M., & Nikkonen, M. (2003). Conducting a qualitative child interview: Methodological considerations, *Journal of Advanced Nursing, 42*, 434–441.

Kortesluoma, R-L., & Nikkonen, M. (2004). "I had this horrible pain": The sources and causes of pain experiences in 4- to 11-year-old hospitalized children. *Journal of Child Health Care, 8*, 210–231.

Larsen, K., & Adamsen, L. (2009). Emergence of Nordic nursing research: No position is an island. *Scandinavian Journal of Caring Sciences, 23*, 757–766.

Leino-Kilpi, H., & Suominen, T. (1998). Nursing research in Finland from 1958 to 1995. *Image: Journal of Nursing Scholarship, 30*, 363–367.

Lilja, L., & Hellzén, O. (2008). Former patients' experience of psychiatric care: A qualitative investigation. *International Journal of Mental Health Nursing, 17*, 279–286.

Lindahl, B., Lidén, E., & Lindblad, B.-M. (2011). A meta-synthesis describing the relationships between patients, informal caregivers and health professionals in home-care settings. *Journal of Clinical Nursing, 20*, 454–463.

Lindahl, B., & Lindblad, B.-M. (2011). Family members' experiences of everyday life when a child is dependent on a ventilator: A metasynthesis study. *Journal of Family Nursing, 17*, 241–269.

Lindahl, B., Sandman, P.-O., & Rasmussen, B. H. (2006). On being dependent on home mechanical ventilation: Depictions of patients' experiences over time. *Qualitative Health Research, 16*, 881–901.

Lindberg, B., Axelsson, K., & Öhrling, K. (2008). Adjusting to being a father to an infant born prematurely: Experiences from Swedish fathers. *Scandinavian Journal of Caring Sciences, 22*, 79–85.

Lindblad, B.-M., Rasmussen, B. H., & Sandman, P.-O. (2007). A life enriching togetherness: Meanings of informal support when being a parent of a child with disability. *Scandinavian Journal of Caring Sciences, 21*, 238–246.

Lindholm, L. (1997). Health motives and life values: A study of young persons' reasons for health. *Scandinavian Journal of Caring Sciences, 11*, 81–89.

Lindwall, L., von Post, I., & Bergbom, I. (2003). Patients' and nurses' experiences of perioperative dialogues. *Journal of Advanced Nursing, 43*, 246–253.

Lundgren, I., & Dahlberg, K. (1998). Women's experience of pain during childbirth. *Midwifery, 14*, 105–110.

Lundgren, I., & Dahlberg, K. (2002). Midwives' experience of the encounter with women and their pain during childbirth. *Midwifery, 18*, 155–164.

Lundgren, S. M., Holmgren, M., Valmari, G., & Skott, C. (2011). Home care encounters in a multicultural context: A diverse space for caring, *International Journal for Human Caring, 15*, 23–30.

Lundgren, S. M., Valmari, G., & Skott, C. (2008). The nature of nursing research: Dissertations in the Nordic countries, *Scandinavian Journal of Caring Sciences, 23*, 402–416.

Maijala, H., Paavilainen, E., & Åstedt-Kurki, P. (2003). The use of grounded theory to study interaction. *Nurse Researcher, 11*, 40–57.

Maijala, H., Paavilainen, E., Väisänen, L., & Åstedt-Kurki, P. (2004). Caregivers' experiences of interaction with families expecting a fetally impaired child. *Journal of Clinical Nursing, 13*, 3, 376–385.

Mauleon, A.-L., Palo-Bengtsson, L., & Ekman S.-L. (2005). Anaesthesia care of older patients as experienced by nurse anaesthetists. *Nursing Ethics, 12*, 263–272.

Miles, M. B., & Huberman, A. M. (1994). *Qualitative data analysis* (2nd ed.). Thousand Oaks, CA: Sage Publications.

Nilsson, I., Jansson, L., & Norberg A. (1997). To meet with a stroke: Patients' experiences and aspects seen through a screen of crises. *Journal of Advanced Nursing, 25*, 953–963.

Nilsson, M., Sarvimäki, A., & Ekman, S.-L. (2000). Feeling old: Being in a phase of transition in later life. *Nursing Inquiry, 7,* 41–49.

Nygren, B., Norberg, A., & Lundman, B. (2007). Inner strength as disclosed in narratives of the oldest old. *Qualitative Health Research, 17,* 1060–1073.

Nystedt, A, Högberg, U., & Lundman, B. (2008). Women's experiences of becoming a mother after prolonged labour. *Journal of Advanced Nursing, 63,* 250–258.

Odencrants, S., Ehnfors, M., & Grobe, S J. (2005). Living with chronic obstructive pulmonary disease: Part I. Struggling with meal-related situations: Experiences among persons with COPD. *Scandinavian Journal of Caring Sciences, 19,* 230–239.

Odencrants, S., Ehnfors, M., & Grobe, S. J. (2007). Living with chronic obstructive pulmonary disease (COPD): Part II. RNs' experience of nursing care for patients with COPD and impaired nutritional status. *Scandinavian Journal of Caring Sciences, 21,* 56–63.

Olofsson, B., & Jacobsson, L. (2001). A plea for respect: Involuntarily hospitalized psychiatric patients' narratives about being subjected to coercion. *Journal of Psychiatric and Mental Health Nursing, 8,* 357–366.

Olsson, P., Jansson, L., & Norberg, A. (1998). Parenthood as talked about in Swedish ante- and postnatal midwifery consultations: A qualitative study of 58 video-recorded consultations. *Scandinavian Journal of Caring Sciences, 12,* 205–214.

Olsson, P., Jansson, L,. & Norberg, A. (2000). A qualitative study of childbirth as spoken about in midwives' ante- and postnatal consultations. *Midwifery, 16,* 123–134.

Östlinder, G., Söderberg, S., & Öhlén, J. (2007). *Omvårdnad som akademiskt ämne* [Nursing as academic subject]. Svensk sjuksköterskeförening SSF report 2007.

Paterson, B., Thorne, S., Canam, C., & Jillings, C. (2001). *Meta-study of qualitative health research.* Thousand Oaks, CA: Sage.

Pejlert, A. (2001). Being a parent of an adult son or daughter with severe mental illness receiving professional care: Parents' narratives. *Health and Social Care in the Community, 9,* 194–204.

Pejlert, A., Asplund, K., Gilje, F., & Norberg, A. (1998). The meaning of caring for patients on a long-term psychiatric ward as narrated by formal care providers. *Journal of Psychiatric and Mental Health Nursing, 5,* 255–264.

Pejlert, A., Asplund, K., & Norberg A. (1995). Stories about living in a hospital ward as narrated by schizophrenic patients. *Journal of Psychiatric and Mental Health Nursing, 2,* 269–277.

Pejlert, A., Asplund, K., & Norberg, A. (1999). Towards recovery: Living in a home-like setting after the move from a hospital ward. *Journal of Clinical Nursing, 8,* 663–673.

Persson, E. K, Fridlund, B., Kvist, L. J., & Dykes, A. K. (2011). Mothers' sense of security in the first postnatal week: Interview study. *Journal of Advanced Nursing, 67,* 105–116.

Pesonen, H.-M., Remes, A. M., & Isola, A. (2011). Ethical aspects of researching subjective experiences in early-stage dementia. *Nursing Ethics, 18,* 651–661.

Polit, D. F., & Beck, C. T. (2009). International differences in nursing research, 2005–2006. *Journal of Nursing Scholarship, 41,* 44–53.

Polit, D. F., & Beck, C. T. (2010). Generalization in quantitative and qualitative research: Myths and strategies. *International Journal of Nursing Studies, 47,* 1451–1458.

Rahm Hallberg, I. (2006). Guest editorial: Challenges for future nursing research: Providing evidence for health-care practice. *International Journal of Nursing Studies, 43,* 923–927.

Rasmussen, B. H, Jansson, L,. & Norberg, A. (2000). Striving for becoming at-home in the midst of dying. *American Journal of Hospice and Palliative Care, 17,* 31–43.

Robinson, P., Ekman, S.-L., & Wahlund, L. O. (1998). Unsettled, uncertain and striving to understand: Toward an understanding of the situation of persons with suspected dementia. *International Journal of Aging and Human Development, 47,* 143–161.

Sandelowski, M., & Barroso, J. (2007). *Handbook for synthesizing qualitative research.* New York: Springer.

Santamäki Fischer, R., Altin, E., Ragnarsson, C., & Lundman, B. (2008). Still going strong: Perceptions of the body among 85-year-old people in Sweden. *International Journal of Older People Nursing, 3,* 14–21.

Saveman, B.-I., Hallberg, I. R., & Norberg, A. (1993). Identifying and defining abuse of elderly people, as seen by witnesses. *Journal of Advanced Nursing, 18,* 1393–1400.

Sivonen, K., Kasén, A., & Eriksson, K. (2010). Semantic analysis according to Peep Koort: A substance-oriented research methodology. *Scandinavian Journal of Caring Sciences, 24*(suppl. 1), 12–20.

Sjöström-Strand, A., & Fridlund, B. (2006). Stress in women's daily life before and after a myocardial infarction: A qualitative analysis. *Canadian Journal of Cardiovascular Nursing, 16,* 5–12.

Sjöström-Strand, A., & Fridlund, B. (2007). Women's descriptions of symptoms and delay reasons in seeking medical care at the time of a first myocardial infarction: A qualitative study. *Scandinavian Journal of Caring Sciences, 21,* 10–17.

Sjöström, B., & Dahlgren, L. O. (2002). Applying phenomenography in nursing research. *Journal of Advanced Nursing, 40,* 339–345.

Skovdahl, K., Kihlgren, A. L., & Kihlgren, M. (2003). Dementia and aggressiveness: Video recorded morning care from different care units. *Journal of Clinical Nursing, 12,* 888–898.

Söderberg, A., & Norberg, A. (1993). Intensive care: Situations of ethical difficulty. *Journal of Advanced Nursing, 18,* 2008–2014,

Söderlund, M. (2007). Terra caritatis: Where suffering is alleviated in an atmosphere of community. *International Journal for Human Caring, 11,* 35–44.

Strandberg, G., Norberg, A., & Jansson, L. (2000). An exemplar of a positive perspective of being dependent on care. *Journal of Nursing Scholarship, 14,* 327–346; discussion 347–353.

Strandberg, G., Norberg, A., & Jansson, L. (2001). Being overwhelmed by the feeling of having a home and family: One aspect of the meaning of being dependent on care: A study of one patient and two of his nurses. *Journal of Advanced Nursing, 35,* 717–727.

Sundin, K., Jansson, L., & Norberg, A. (2000). Communicating with people with stroke and aphasia: Understanding through sensation without words. *Journal of Clinical Nursing, 9,* 481–488.

Sundin, K., Jansson, L., & Norberg, A. (2002). Understanding between care providers and patients with stroke and aphasia: A phenomenological hermeneutic inquiry. *Nursing Inquiry, 9,* 93–103.

Svanström, R., & Dahlberg, K. (2004). Living with dementia yields a heteronomous and lost existence. *Western Journal of Nursing Research, 26,* 671–687.

Svedlund, M., Danielson, E., & Norberg, A. (1999). Nurses' narrations about caring for in patients with acute myocardial infarction. *Intensive & Critical Care Nursing, 15,* 34–43.

Svedlund, M., Danielson, E., & Norberg, A. (2001). Women's narratives during the acute phase of their myocardial infarction. *Journal of Advanced Nursing, 35,* 197–205.

Swedish National Agency for Higher Education (2007). *Utvärdering av grundutbildningar i medicin och vård vid svenska universitet och högskolor* [Evaluation of basic education in medicine and care at Swedish universities and university colleges]. Report 2007:23 R.

Tuomi, J. (1997). *Suomalainen hoitotiedekeskustelu* [The genesis of nursing and caring science in Finland]. English summary, Dissertation, Jyväskylä University.

Wiklund-Gustin, L. (2010). Metaphors: A path to narrative understanding. *International Journal for Human Caring, 14,* 60–68.

Wireklint Sundström, B., & Dahlberg, K. (2011). Caring assessment in the Swedish ambulance services relieves suffering and enables safe decisions. *International Emergency Nursing, 19,* 113–119.

The World Factbook. (2011). www.cia.gov/library/publications/the-world-factbook/.

Electronic resources

www.nccs.nu
www.scb.se
www.stat.fi
www.uin.no/bfin
www.uin.no/niv
www.vardforbundet.se

40

Qualitative nursing research in Norway, Denmark and Iceland

State of the science

Marit Kirkevold

This chapter provides an overview of qualitative research in three of the Nordic countries: Norway, Denmark and Iceland. In all three countries, qualitative research has had an important, or partly, even dominant position. Within the medical profession, some researchers tend, disapprovingly, to equate nursing research with qualitative research. Although this is an overly simplistic picture, it underscores the strong position of qualitative nursing research in these countries. Because of this position, providing a comprehensive review of qualitative research is not possible. Rather, my aim is to illustrate the variety of this research both in terms of philosophical foundation, methodological approach and thematic orientation. As an analytic framework, I will use Kim's (2010) description of the structure of nursing knowledge to illuminate how qualitative research in these three countries has contributed to nursing knowledge.

Brief historical overview of nursing research in Norway, Denmark and Iceland

The history of nursing research in Norway, Denmark and Iceland is relatively short. Iceland started out first by introducing a baccalaureate program in nursing at the University of Iceland in Reykjavik in 1973. From 1986, nursing education has only been offered at the university level (https://english.hi.is/school_of_health_sciences/faculty_of_nursing/about_faculty). In 1987, the University of Akureyri in the northern part of Iceland offered the second program of nursing in Iceland (http://english.unak.is/health-sciences/page/hjukrun_forsida). Initially, graduate nursing education and research training were not available in Iceland and Icelandic nurses traveled abroad for Master's and doctoral education. Icelandic nursing has traditionally had strong ties to the US, but Icelandic nurses have also traveled to Sweden, Norway and other European countries for graduate studies. During the last decades, Master's and doctoral courses have been introduced and nursing research has grown significantly.

In Norway, basic nursing education is the responsibility of colleges of nursing. The first formal university program, dedicated to advanced nursing education, was established at the University of Tromsø in 1977, followed by the University of Bergen in 1979 and the University of Oslo in 1985 (Lerheim, 2000). The first doctoral programs in nursing science were established at the University of Bergen in 1987 and at the University of Oslo in 1993 (Lerheim, 2000). In the past ten years, there has been an exponential growth in doctorally prepared nurses, as the Norwegian government has supported the academic development of nursing particularly through doctoral stipends to the colleges of nursing with the goal of strengthening nursing education. Also in the past ten years, the university hospitals have also encouraged clinical nursing research by supporting increasing numbers of nurses to complete doctoral degrees and continue to do clinical research.

In Denmark, nursing science was not formally established at the university level until 2001, although higher nursing education and research was conducted at the former Danish School of higher education in nursing from the early 1990s. The only university department dedicated to academic training within nursing science in Denmark is located at Aarhus University. In recent years, several hospitals have supported doctoral training of their nurses and have established clinical nursing research positions. Consequently, Denmark has experienced an exponential growth of doctorally prepared nurses during the past ten years. In these three countries then, nursing research is experiencing dramatic growth.

Nursing knowledge needs

Nursing research is closely related to nursing practice. It is nursing practice that generates most of the knowledge needs that nursing research seeks to address. Kim (2010) argues that because of this complexity, nursing encompasses four ontological commitments: the ontologies of human nature, human living, human agency, and practice. Each ontological commitment generates specific cognitive needs with matching knowledge spheres. As the ontologies are fundamentally different, the epistemological foundation of each knowledge sphere is also different. Although this way of structuring nursing knowledge has been questioned and criticized for unnecessarily promoting the knowledge–practice gap (Risjord, 2010), it provides a useful analytic overview of diverse ontologies and epistemologies in nursing. It will be used here to facilitate a systematic presentation of the great variety of qualitative research in nursing. Kim refers to these knowledge spheres as the public knowledge domain of nursing.

The ontology of human nature refers to those general patterns that human beings share as a consequence of being part of nature, e.g., species-specific or group-specific characteristics influenced by innate as well as contextual and experiential forces. According to Kim (2010), knowledge of human nature is inferential and leads to generalized knowledge of common patterns and regularities which individuals and/or groups share. This knowledge makes it possible to understand, explain and predict (theoretically) individual occurrences based on drawing inferences from general theories.

The ontology of human living refers to "understanding of human living as experienced, interpreted, and managed from the totality of the living self, the individual that is conscious, meaning making, historically and contextually embedded, and reflective all at once" (Kim, 2010, p. 49). This generates a referential cognitive need in order to understand the uniqueness, situatedness, meanings and contextuality of human beings. Through situated hermeneutic knowledge, we may gain access to the similarities, differences, commonalities, and uniqueness in human living experiences. This knowledge can give us insights, appreciation, sensibility and in-depth understanding of the experiences of individual persons.

The ontology of human agency is based on the assumption that "humans are agents who are engaged in both independent and coordinated actions in search of certain goals. Human agents are both free and constrained in seeking and moving towards their goals" (Kim, 2010, p. 49). Because human agency is intertwined with "the socially coordinated nature of living" (p. 53), which implies various forms of struggles, constraints, dominations and disharmony, a transformative cognitive need is generated. Through critical hermeneutic knowledge, humans may be emancipated and mutual understanding be achieved.

The ontology of practice is based on the assumption that

> human practice is a human service of one person (the provider or the professional) to another (the patient, the client, the service user) in which the goal is specified for the recipient (the patient), thus requiring ethical, moral, and aesthetic guidelines for practice.
>
> *(Kim, 2010, p. 49)*

This implies both normative and desiderative cognitive needs. The normative cognitive need refers to ethical knowledge about normative values and expectations and ethical principles and standards. This knowledge is required to connect "what is known" with "what must be" (p. 55). The desiderative cognitive need refers to practice as "a form of self-presentation and self-expression" (p. 55). This aspect of nursing practice requires aesthetic knowledge that may foster harmony, beauty and creativity expressed through individualized, unique nursing.

According to Kim (2010), the inferential knowledge need is addressed through empirical and positivist research, usually applying quantitative research methods, which she maintains is still quite dominant in nursing. The other cognitive needs are addressed through research based on other epistemological assumptions (interpretive, constructivist, critical, pragmatic and normative) applying a wide range of qualitative research approaches. In nursing practice, nurses must draw on and synthesize knowledge from all aspects of the public knowledge sphere, as well as from personal knowledge and situation-specific knowledge, in order to deliberate and act in specific situations in nursing practice (Kim, 2010). In the following, I will highlight how qualitative research in Norway, Denmark and Iceland has contributed to the knowledge needs of the nursing discipline within these knowledge spheres.

Qualitative research contributing to normative/ethical knowledge

I will start with highlighting how nurse scholars in Norway, Denmark and Iceland have contributed to the development of normative/ethical knowledge. In my view, nurse researchers from these countries have made significant contributions in this area.

Developing a normative foundation for nursing

It is impossible to describe qualitative research in Norway and Denmark without referring to Norwegian nurse, historian and philosopher Kari Martinsen (Martinsen, 1975, 1984, 1993a, 1996, 2006; Martinsen & Wærness, 1979). From 1975, Martinsen has been a vocal and ardent critic of traditional, positivist research within nursing, arguing for the need for phenomenological knowledge in nursing. Martinsen herself has primarily done theoretical work, analyzing nursing and caring from the perspective of phenomenological and critical philosophy, and historical research, exploring the professional development of the nursing profession at the end of the eighteenth century (Martinsen, 1984). Her work has inspired innumerable nurse researchers in Norway and Denmark to conduct qualitative research. Because of her influential historical and philosophical work, phenomenological and hermeneutic nursing research has gained a strong position in these two countries.

Martinsen's major contribution to nursing practice and research has been her development of a philosophy of caring, inspired by the phenomenological works of Husserl, Merleau-Ponty, Heidegger and Danish philosopher and theologian Knud Løgstrup (Martinsen, 1993, 1996, 2006). Martinsen maintains that the concept of caring essentially is that which maintains and secures life. It is relational, practical and moral. Caring highlights the basic interdependence of human beings and the moral responsibility that human beings have for taking care of one another. Building on Løgstrup and the Danish life philosophy movement (Delmar, 2006; Løgstrup, 1997), Martinsen emphasizes that the moral responsibility of nursing is to respect, promote and protect what Løgstrup called the "sovereign expressions of life," i.e., trust, openness, hope and honesty (Løgstrup, 1997) in their caring relations with patients. Influenced by the phenomenological studies of Merleau-Ponty (2011), Martinsen emphasizes the importance of the senses and bodily knowledge and skills in providing individualized care. Sensitivity is both a bodily and moral skill that nurses must develop through the disciplined reflection on practice (Martinsen, 1993a, 2006).

Martinsen strongly emphasizes the social, cultural and historical context of nursing. Through her critical historical works, which have been influenced by Marx (Marx & Sitton 2010), Weber (2011) and Foucault, Bertani, and Fontana (2004), Martinsen outlines how societal forces and trends impact on the individual nurse as well as the nursing profession. In particular, she has provided fundamental critique of the dominance of positivism on the development of medical science and health care in general and nursing science in particular (Martinsen & Wærness, 1979). She has also provided critique of the economic and individualistic values undergirding the modern health care system and which threaten the integrity of patients and nurses, by neglecting the fundamental responsibility of society and the nursing profession to provide adequate care and support for those in greatest need.

Martinsen's critique has provided the impetus and inspiration for the development of qualitative research in Norway as well as in Denmark. In line with her resistance against the dominant, positivistic ideals of science, Martinsen has systematically refused to play by the scientific rules. She has chosen to publish her work in Norwegian, in books and journals directed primarily towards clinical nurses and educators.

Despite her great influence, surprisingly few research reports published in international research journals refer to her work. One obvious explanation for this is that her students generally have followed her example and published in Norwegian or Danish in the form of monographs (Boge, 2011; Delmar, 1999), books (Alvsvåg & Gjengedal, 2000) and book chapters (Kirkevold et al., 1993; Martinsen, 1993b). This has had the unfortunate consequence that the major ideas of Martinsen have not been recognized internationally until recently (Alvsvåg, 2010; Martinsen 2006).

The students of Martinsen have explored her philosophical/theoretical ideas in a number of phenomenological studies. Danish nurse researcher Delmar (1999, 2006) explored the phenomena of trust and power in hospital units, interviewing patients and nurses. Applying Martinsen's normative theory/philosophy of caring and nursing as moral praxis and the concept of "sovereign expressions of life" from Løgstrup (1997), she highlights the frequently overlooked existential suffering of patients in their encounters with nurses. Gjengedal (2000) explored caring through phenomenological interviews with patients receiving intensive care. Nortvedt (Nortvedt, 1996; Nortvedt et al., 2011) has contributed to the development of phenomenological ethics, focusing on the phenomenon of ethical sensitivity as a necessary foundation for providing good nursing care. Other researchers have focused on body care from the perspective of caring (Boge, 2011; Lomborg et al., 2005).

Sharing the interest for caring as a necessary foundation for good nursing care, but coming from a North American tradition, the Icelandic nursing researcher Haldorsdottir (1996) provided an early phenomenological analysis of caring and uncaring encounters between nurses and patients in a number of different clinical settings, including medical and surgical care, cancer care and maternity care. Based on phenomenological analyses of in-depth dialogues, she proposed a theory of caring and uncaring encounters in nursing and health care. The theory proposed that lack of professional caring leads to disconnection between nurse and patient and subsequent discouragement and decreased sense of well-being and health, whereas professional caring leads to connection between patient and nurse and to empowerment and increased sense of well-being and health. Although Haldorsdottir did not build on the work of Martinsen, her research shares many of Martinsen's basic ideas. Together, the qualitative research carried out by Norwegian, Danish and Icelandic nurse researchers has significantly contributed to comprehensive normative knowledge for nursing practice and stimulated qualitative research into normative questions in nursing practice.

Qualitative research contributing to situated/hermeneutical knowledge

As already mentioned, phenomenological and hermeneutic research has had a strong position in the Nordic countries. This research spans from research into experiences of diverse groups of patients, significant others, informal carers and nurses to historical nursing research. In this section, only a few examples of patient experiences and research into nursing practice are reviewed due to space limitations.

Research focusing on patient experiences

Most of the phenomenological and/or hermeneutical research has focused on patient experiences. The studies have been conducted in a broad range of situations and contexts and span a variety of health problems, health care situations, and patients at different ages and phases of life. Studies focusing on persons with serious, chronic illnesses are predominant.

In Norway, the phenomenological and/or hermeneutical studies have been mostly inspired by the phenomenological descriptive approach of Giorgi (2005), the methodological reflections of Kvale (Kvale & Brinkman, 2009) and the narrative phenomenological–hermeneutic approach of Ricoeur (2004). In Denmark too, Kvale and Ricoeur, as well as van Manen (1997) have been influential. In Iceland, the so-called Vancouver School method has been introduced and applied in a number of studies (Haldorsdottir, 1996). Other Icelandic nurses have drawn on interpretive phenomenology and narrative analysis.

A recent example of a phenomenological study from Iceland is a study of self-identified needs of women in chronic pain (Skuladottir & Haldorsdottir, 2011). Applying the so-called Vancouver School method of phenomenology, they interviewed five women in chronic pain twice, identifying three clusters of needs: the quest to learn to live with the pain, the quest for support, caring and connection and the quest for normalcy. The authors identified the overriding theme to be a quest for well-being: physically, mentally, emotionally and socially. The authors describe the Vancouver School of phenomenology as "a unique blend of description, interpretation, explication and construction" (p. 82) that has been heavily influenced by ideas from constructivism and is "essentially an interpretivist/constructivist school of doing phenomenology" (p. 82). The method is described in 12 steps and data collection and data analysis occur concurrently.

In another Icelandic study of living with cancer, Hjörleifsdóttir and colleagues (2008) interviewed 25 cancer patients with different diagnoses and prognosis about their experiences. Applying manifest and latent content analyses, they identified one core category and three subcategories. Living with cancer was described as an alarming situation and in trying to cope with it, the participants sought to balance life as it was before illness onset against the present situation in order to achieve normality. They underscored that caring encounters promoted well-being whereas factors contributing to inconvenience led to tiredness and irritation.

Ingadóttir and Jonsdottir (2006) explored technological dependency among Icelandic patients using home ventilators and their families. Interviewing six patients, five spouses and one daughter, they applied an interpretive phenomenological and narrative approach. Their participants described the home ventilator as a mixed blessing. Some saw the ventilator as a life-saving "friend" whereas others felt that life had been destroyed and that a ventilator-dependent life was not a "real life." The participants described the sustained work in listening to their body and maintaining the treatment. They underscored the importance of understanding and compassion, but also the tendency of technological thinking in encounters with health care professionals.

In Norway, Giorgi's descriptive phenomenological approach, developed from Husserl's philosophy, has been used by a number of researchers. A recent example of phenomenological research applying this approach is that of Torheim and Gjengedal (2010), exploring the experiences of mask treatment among severely ill patients with chronic obstructive pulmonary disease (COPD). Through in-depth interviews with five patients, the authors uncovered the patients' lived experiences of anxiety, panic and loss of control due to severe breathing difficulties and how they experienced regaining control and trust through the skilled help of nurses when they struggled to deal with the noninvasive positive-pressure ventilation (NPPV) delivered through bi-level positive airway pressure (BPAP).

In Denmark, the hermeneutic-phenomenological method of van Manen has been used in several studies. A recent example is the longitudinal study of Haahr et al. (2010, 2011) of the experiences of living with severe Parkinson's disease and how life is affected following deep brain stimulation (DBS) treatment. Following 11 patients for a year, these studies uncovered how living with advanced Parkinson's disease can be described as leading a life characterized by unpredictability. The participants experienced that the disease gradually took over and they had to struggle with unpredictability on a daily basis. Themes describing the unpredictability were: The body: setting the agenda; Always a struggle to be on time; Living in dependence and compromise: being a burden; and Living with restrained space and changes in social life. The DBS treatment had a major impact on the body. Participants experienced great bodily changes and went through a process of adjustment during the first year that encompassed three phases: Being liberated: a kind of miracle; Changes as a challenge: decline or opportunity; and Reconciliation: redefining life with Parkinson's disease. The authors concluded that patients go through a dramatic process of change affecting their entire lifeworld. Some adjust smoothly to changes while others are affected by loss of control, uncertainty and loss of everyday life as they knew it. The studies highlighted the need to develop a supportive intervention to facilitate the adjustment process.

Research focusing on nursing practice

Hermeneutic and phenomenological research has also explored different aspects of nursing practice. This research has applied in-depth interviews as well as observational approaches, such as ethnographic or fieldwork methods. An example is Danish nurse researcher Buus' (2008, 2009) study of psychiatric nurses' construction of clinical knowledge during "handover" sessions between shifts. Applying an extended fieldwork approach and conversational analysis, Buus highlighted how "the game of constructing clinical knowledge" was a process of negotiating understanding and defining clinical situations and patient problems in which nurses with and without experience and position in the group had different possibilities of participating in the construction of clinical knowledge about the patients.

In a somewhat similar study, the Norwegian nurse researcher Ellefsen and her international colleagues (Ellefsen et al., 2007; Kim et al., 2008) explored clinical decision-making among nurses in acute care hospitals. Using fieldwork and in-depth interviews, they described how nurses interpret and construct clinical situations through their clinical gaze and how clinical deliberations, drawing on diverse types of knowledge, are used to make clinical decisions.

Qualitative research contributing to transformative/critical hermeneutical understanding/knowledge

This section will highlight qualitative research that has been directed to practice development using methods such as Action Research and different critical/deconstructive approaches aimed at increasing insight and critical reflection about nursing practice.

Research focusing on critical aspects of health care ideology

Discourse analysis, inspired by critical theoretical perspectives from the social sciences, has a small, but prominent group of nurse researchers in the Nordic countries of Norway, Denmark and Iceland. As mentioned above, this trend goes back to Martinsen's early work in the 1970s (Martinsen, 1975; Martinsen & Wærness, 1979), in which she critiqued the dominant ideology of the health care system, highlighting its impact on patients and the practice of nurses. This line of work has been further developed by researchers in Iceland, Denmark and Norway.

In a recent study, Gotttfreðsdóttir and Björnsdóttir (2009, 2010) analyzed the consequences for prospective parents of the introduction of prenatal screening for gene abnormalities, inspired by the perspective proposed by Foucault (Foucault, Bertani, & Fontana, 2004). Through in-depth, qualitative interviews with prospective parents (Gotttfreðsdóttir & Björnsdóttir, 2009) as well as a discourse analysis of publications in the public media (newspaper articles and TV shows) (Gottfreðsdóttir & Björnsdóttir 2010), they highlighted how the introduction of routine translucency screening (NT) was a consequence of a dominant discourse that took for granted the obvious benefit of risk reduction that this procedure was assumed to have. Critical public discussion of the ethical and moral aspects of such procedures never took hold in Iceland, although parents of children with disabilities (e.g. with Down's syndrome) tried to raise the issue that gene abnormalities do not automatically lead to poor quality of life for the people involved. Interviewing parents who declined prenatal screening, they found that these parents were "forced" to argue for their choice and that their major line of argument was tied to their personal philosophy of disabilities, the importance of diversity in society as well as the unreliability of the test.

Similarly, Foss and colleagues have conducted several Foucauldian discourse analyses. In one study, she and a colleague (Foss & Kirkevold, 2008) explored how patient participation is portrayed in the media (professional journals and lay health periodicals), focusing on the use of visuals to construct and convey subtle gender attitudes. The authors demonstrate that visuals can be used to unveil how "prevailing dominant discourses of gender silently act upon the subconscious and thereby serve to reinforce existing gendered practices" (p. 306). Such analyses can uncover how nurses both shape and are shaped by discursive practices which they are often unaware of and that such practices may impact on how they come to see and interact with their patients.

In a recent study, Foss (2011) explored user participation as experienced by old people recently discharged from the hospital. Through her Foucauldian discourse analysis, she illuminated how old patients (age 80 or above) constructed patient participation within "an interpretive space" delimited by the theme of hospital professionals as being extremely busy, on the one hand, and themselves as old patients, on the other. These two characteristics, the old, slow patients encountering the extremely high pace of the modern hospital, made patient participation of old people almost impossible. Nevertheless, the participants expressed a wish to participate and described how they applied a number of strategies to make their wishes and opinions known and have a say, at the same time expressing that as old patients they had no choice but to adjust to and trust the power and care of the health professionals.

Knutsen and Foss (2011b) and Knutsen, Terragni, and Foss (2011) used a Foucauldian approach to study the construction of empowerment and identity among participants scheduled to have surgery for morbid obesity. They found that the construction of "empowerment" in a preparatory learning and mastery course aimed at lifestyle changes prior to surgery entailed subtle power transactions and disciplining (including self-disciplining). This was related to the fact that participants could lose the right to surgery both if they were unsuccessful in changing their habits and lose weight and if they were "too successful," losing enough weight so that surgery for obesity was no longer warranted.

Transformative research focusing on nursing practice development

Action Research aimed at transformative change in practice was introduced early in the Nordic countries (Holter & Schwardtz-Barcott, 1993; Wagner, 1992). Inspired by the philosophy of Habermas and the work of Argyris and Schön (Holter, 1988), action-oriented research is aimed at developing better leadership and nursing care. It has been conducted in hospital settings (Fagermoen & Hamilton, 2006), in community care settings (Wagner, 1992) and in cross-institutional studies (Clemensen et al., 2007; Kirkevold, 2008).

In the early 1990s, Wagner (1992) conducted a four-year-long Action Research project in Denmark including the reorganization and coordination of services and facilities for the elderly. The goal was to promote self-care and participation in decision-making. Based on a survey of the social and health service needs and wishes of persons over 67 years of age and comprehensive interdisciplinary training of staff, a 24-hour service was planned, and the former nursing home was converted into a health care center, with sheltered flats, guests flats and a day center, open to all citizens, irrespective of age.

Clemensen et al. (2007) used Participatory Action Research to develop and test a new model of follow-up care of leg ulcers among persons with diabetes living at home in Denmark. This study used information and computer technology to facilitate monitoring, treatment and guidance, where nurses and physicians in a specialized hospital care unit could observe the ulcers and adjust the treatment through close collaboration with patients and home care nurses. Using simple mobile phone technology and a shared electronic ulcer journal, the authors found that the collaboration improved and that both patients and professionals expressed high satisfaction with the new model. It reduced the need for traveling to the hospital among the patients, led to better understanding and collaboration among community care nurses and the specialists and to more equal relations between patients and the staff members involved.

In a comprehensive five-year organizational development study (Kirkevold, 2008), a Norwegian teaching nursing home model was developed, implemented and evaluated, based on Action Research methods, between 1999 and 2003. Inspired by the early teaching nursing home movement in the US in the 1980s, the Norwegian project sought to develop a model in which selected nursing homes, universities and colleges of nursing worked closely together to improve recruitment, reduce turnover, improve the knowledge and skills among the staff and build a culture in the institutions in which continuous quality improvement and critical reflection could take place. The project demonstrated that the new institutions contributed significantly to competence and quality improvement. This project led to the establishment of 20 teaching nursing homes and 20 community care developmental units directed towards home care across Norway.

Despite reports of positive change and substantial enthusiasm among the actors involved (Clemensen, 2007; Kirkevold, 2008), this approach to qualitative research remains limited. This might be due to complexities and time required to conduct Action Research, difficulties getting external funding to conduct this kind of research as well as a discussions about the stringency and validity of Action Research both within and outside the community of qualitative researchers. The evidence-based practice movement, with its emphasis on controlled intervention studies, might also have led to decreased interest in conducting action-oriented, transformative research.

Qualitative research contributing to aesthetic knowledge

Qualitative research aimed at addressing desiderative cognitive needs has been limited in Norway, Denmark and Iceland. However, in an early study, Norwegian nurse researcher Nåden (1998) explored nursing as an art. He described the characteristics of nurses that were considered "artful" in their practice of nursing by their leaders and colleagues.

In recent research, the focus has changed from nurses and nursing to the impact of the surroundings on experiences and well-being among patients. Caspari and colleagues (2011) explored the experienced impact of architecture and art on hospitalized patients' experiences. They found that the qualities of the hospital surroundings impacted significantly on patients and that this aspect of hospital care received limited attention among those responsible for building and maintaining the hospitals.

Other researchers, including Gjengedal and colleagues (Gjengedal et al., 2008) have also explored the phenomenon of room/space and architecture in relation to illness and health care, applying both philosophical and empirical approaches. This research confirms the importance of the surroundings on health and well-being of patients. Although limited, this line of research seems to be on the rise.

Qualitative research contributing to inferential/generalized knowledge

Kim (2010) associates inferential or generalized knowledge with positivist, quantitative research. However, with the introduction of mixed methods research, the espoused gulf between the ontologies and epistemologies of quantitative and qualitative research is increasingly being questioned (Creswell & Plano Clark, 2011). Furthermore, more general patterns also exist in social phenomena and relations, not due to traditional causal relationships, but because of social and individual interactional and transactional processes (Lomborg & Kirkevold, 2003). Consequently, there seems to be increasing boundary blurring between more interpretive and more causal epistemological assumptions. This is also apparent within nursing research. Researchers working primarily within a more traditional, objective tradition increasingly incorporate qualitative approaches into their studies. Within this tradition, qualitative research is primarily used to prepare for or extend quantitative research within a causal paradigm. Traditional qualitative researchers, on the other hand, move towards more generalizing approaches when seeking to apply insights from qualitative research to develop new nursing interventions.

Qualitative research as a foundation for developing nursing interventions

In recent years, a new line of research has emerged within traditional interpretive, qualitative research. Along with the generation of increasing knowledge and understanding of patient experiences and needs through phenomenological and hermeneutic research and grounded theory approaches, researchers have sought to develop nursing interventions to address these needs. In Denmark, Zoffmann and colleagues (Zoffmann et al., 2006, 2007, 2008) have conducted a number of studies, applying a grounded theory approach to develop a guided self-determination intervention to support self-management of difficult diabetes. Similarly, Kirkevold et al. (2012)

introduced a psychosocial nursing intervention developed on the basis of a number of phenomenological and hermeneutic studies of the experiences of living with and adjusting to changes in life following a stroke.

Ruland and colleagues have utilized qualitative research to prepare for quantitative studies. They applied focus group interviews and participatory design to develop web-based support systems aimed at supporting symptom management and patient–provider communication (Ruland, 2008; Ruland et al., 2007). Through qualitative approaches, they interacted with prospective users of the program in order to maximize its relevance and user friendliness. They conclude that the qualitative approaches have been essential in developing interventions that have been found effective in follow-up quantitative studies (Heyn et al., 2012).

Using qualitative research to extend findings from quantitative research

In Denmark, Adamsen et al. (2009) used qualitative research to extend the findings of a controlled trial of a multimodal exercise program for young cancer patients (Adamsen et al., 2006; Andersen et al., 2006). In one study (Midtgaard et al., 2007), they used a phenomenological approach to explore the experienced benefits of participating in the program. In another (Adamsen et al., 2009), they used semi-structured interviews to uncover how the program had impacted on young athletes suffering from cancer. The qualitative studies added insights into the mechanisms by which the program promoted psychological well-being and health among the participants.

In Iceland, Gunnarsdottir and Peden-McAlpine (2010) explored the experienced effect of the complementary treatment of reflexology (foot sole therapy) on pain and other symptoms in persons with fibromyalgia. Applying a multiple case study approach, they offered ten weekly sessions of reflexology to their six women participants. Through in-depth analysis of interviews, observations and diaries both within and across the cases, they uncovered how four of the women first experienced a worsening in their pain, but then around the eighth week experienced significant improvement. Two of the women did not experience any effects from the treatment. The mechanisms explaining the women's experienced benefits of reflexology may be multifactorial and the authors suggest a number of possible explanations. However, the study does not provide a clear answer to this question.

Strengths and weaknesses of qualitative research in Norway, Denmark and Iceland

As illustrated above, qualitative research in Norway, Denmark and Iceland varies widely both in terms of ontological and epistemological foundation, methodological approach and in terms of topics and populations included. A major strength of the research is that Nordic nurse researchers have studied and utilized a wide range of qualitative approaches, giving rise to studies and knowledge within all of the knowledge spheres identified by Kim (2010) as necessary for providing good nursing care. One particular feature of the research is the strong position that normative/ethical knowledge development has had, particularly in Norway and Denmark. This research was initiated by one of the pioneers in nursing research, Kari Martinsen, but has subsequently inspired generations of nurse researchers to conduct qualitative research on a broad range of issues and topics.

Another striking feature of much of the qualitative research reviewed is the strong influence of philosophical theories on the research. In particular, phenomenological and hermeneutic philosophies have inspired nurse researchers in Norway, Denmark and Iceland to conduct descriptive and interpretive research to uncover the lived experiences and meanings of diverse illness and health conditions. Critical theory and deconstructive philosophy have also been influential, leading to a substantial body of transformative knowledge. A recent development is the utilization of knowledge from qualitative studies in developing nursing interventions to support patients in dealing with challenging experiences and situations.

In terms of weaknesses, qualitative research in Norway, Denmark and Iceland has been primarily descriptive. Much of the phenomenological research has provided close-up descriptions of lived experiences of a small number of participants, but without discussing the relevance of the findings for understanding the experiences of larger groups of persons or implications for nursing care. In a majority of the studies, little attention is given to how the sample is selected and to the position and influence of the researcher(s) on the findings. Furthermore, although the context is considered essential in qualitative research, analysis of how the context might have influenced the findings is usually lacking. Another weakness is that theory development is limited. Although grounded theory has been used in a number of studies, most of these studies appear to be single, isolated studies where the theories are not further developed and refined in subsequent research. Attempts to develop theory based on other qualitative approaches are limited and/or lack stringency.

Conclusion

Although nursing science is quite young in Norway, Denmark and Iceland, qualitative research has made significant contributions to nursing knowledge in these countries. Particularly within the knowledge spheres of normative/ethical knowledge, situated-hermeneutic knowledge and transformative knowledge, nurse researchers from these countries have contributed. Further refinement of qualitative methods and combined qualitative and quantitative approaches are underway to strengthen the relevance of this research for nursing practice.

References

Adamsen, L., Andersen, C., Midtgaard, J., Moller, T., Quist, M., & Rorth, M. (2009). Through exercise: Qualitative findings from a supervised group exercise program in cancer patients of mixed gender undergoing chemotherapy. *Scandinavian Journal of Medicine & Science in Sports*, *19*(1): 55–66.

Adamsen, L., Quist, M., Midtgaard, J., Andersen, C., Møller, T., Knutsen, L., Tveterås, A., & Rorth, M. (2006). The effect of a multidimensional exercise intervention on physical capacity, well-being and quality of life in cancer patients undergoing chemotherapy. *Support Care Cancer*, *14*(2):116–127.

Alvsvåg, H. (2010). Kari Martinsen. Philosophy of caring. In M. R. Alligood & A. M. Tomey (Eds.), *Nursing theorists and their work* (pp. 165–189). Maryland Heights, MO: Mosby.

Alvsvåg, H., & Gjengedal, E. (2000). *Omsorgstenkning. En innføring i Kari Martinsens forfatterskap* [Caring perspective. An introduction to the work of Kari Martinsen]. Bergen: Fagbokforlaget.

Andersen, C., Adamsen, L., Moeller, T., Midtgaard, J., Quist, M., Tveteraas, A., & Rorth, M. (2006). The effect of a multidimensional exercise programme on symptoms and side-effects in cancer patients undergoing chemotherapy: the use of semi-structured diaries. *European Journal of Oncology Nursing*, *10*(4): 247–262.

Boge, J. H. (2011). *Kroppsvask i sjukepleie: eit politisk og historisk perspektiv* [Body wash in nursing: A political and historical perspective] Oslo: Akribe.

Buus, N. (2008). Negotiating clinical knowledge: A field study of psychiatric nurses' everyday communication. *Nursing Inquiry*, *15*(3):189–198.

Buus, N. (2009). How writing records reduces clinical knowledge: A field study of psychiatric hospital wards. *Archives of Psychiatric Nursing*, *23*(2): 95–103.

Caspari, S., Eriksson, K., & Nåden, D. (2011). The importance of aesthetic surroundings: A study interviewing experts within different aesthetic fields. *Scandinavian Journal of Caring Sciences*, *25*(1):134–142. doi: 10.1111/j.1471-6712.2010.00803.x.

Clemensen, J., Larsen, S. B., Kyng, M., & Kirkevold, M. (2007). Participatory design in health sciences:

Using cooperative experimental methods in developing health services and computer technology. *Qualitative Health Research*, *17*(1):122–130.

Creswell, J. W., & Plano Clark, V. (2011). *Designing and conducting mixed methods research*. Thousand Oaks, CA: Sage.

Delmar, C. (1999). *Tillid & Magt. En moralsk utfordring* [Trust and power: A moral challenge]. Kopenhagen: Munksgaard.

Delmar, C. (2006). The phenomenology of life phenomena in a nursing context. *Nursing Philosophy*, 7: 235–246.

Ellefsen, B,. Kim, H. S., & Ja Han, K. (2007). Nursing gaze as framework for nursing practice: A study from acute care settings in Korea, Norway and the USA. *Scandinavian Journal of Caring Sciences*, *21*(1): 98–105.

Fagermoen, M. S., & Hamilton, G. (2006). Patient information at discharge: A study of a combined approach. *Patient Education & Counseling*, *63*(1–2): 169–176.

Foss, C. (2011). Elders and patient participation revisited: A discourse analytic approach to older persons' reflections on patient participation. *Journal of Clinical Nursing*, *20*(13–14): 2014–2022.

Foss, C., & Kirkevold, M. (2008). Unfolding the invisible of the visible: Gendered constructions of patient participation. *Nursing Inquiry*, *15*(4): 299–308.

Foucault, M., Bertani, M., & Fontana, A. (2004). *"Society must be defended": Lectures at the Collège de France, 1975–76*. London: Penguin.

Giorgi, A. (2005).The phenomenological movement and research in the human sciences. *Nursing Science Quarterly*, *18*(1): 75–82.

Gjengedal, E. (2000). *Understanding a world of critical illness*. Oslo: Pensumtjeneste.

Gjengedal, E., Schiøtz, A., & Blystad, A. (Eds.). (2008). *Helse i tid og rom* [Health in time and space]. Oslo: Cappelen akademisk forlag.

Gottfreðsdóttir, H., & Björnsdóttir, K. (2009). How do prospective parents who decline prenatal screening account for their decision? A qualitative study. *Social Science and Medicine*, *69*: 274–277.

Gottfreðsdóttir, H., & Björnsdóttir, K. (2010). "Have you had the test?" A discourse analysis of media presentation of prenatal screening in Iceland. *Scandinavian Journal of Caring Sciences*, *24*: 414–421.

Gunnarsdottir, T. J., & Peden-McAlpine, C. (2010). Effect of reflexology on fibromyalgia symptoms: A multiple case study. *Complementary Therapies in Clinical Practice*, *16*: 167–172.

Haahr, A., Kirkevold, M., Hall, E., & Østergaard, K. (2010). From miracle to reconciliation: A hermeneutic phenomenological study exploring the experience of living with Parkinson's disease following Deep Brain Stimulation. *International Journal of Nursing Studies*, *47*(10): 1228–1236.

Haahr, A., Kirkevold, M., Hall, E., & Østergaard, K. (2011). Living with advanced Parkinson's disease: A constant struggle with unpredictability. *Journal of Advanced Nursing*, *67*(2): 408–417. doi: 10.1111/ j.1365-2648.2010.05459.x.

Haldorsdottir, S. (1996). Caring and uncaring encounters in nursing and health care: Developing a theory. Doctoral dissertation, Linköping, Sweden.

Heyn, L., Ruland, C. M., & Finset, A. (2012). Effects of an interactive tailored patient assessment tool on eliciting and responding to cancer patients' cues and concerns in clinical consultations with physicians and nurses. *Patient Education and Counseling*, *86*(2): 158–165.

Hjörleifsdóttir, E., Hallberg, I. R., Gunnarsdóttir, E. D., & Bolmsjö, I. Å. (2008). Living with cancer and perception of care: Icelandic oncology outpatients, a qualitative study. *Support Care Cancer*, *16*: 515–525.

Holter, I. M. (1988). Critical theory: A foundation for the development of nursing theories. *Scholarly Inquiry for Nursing Practice*, *2*(3): 223–236.

Holter, I. M., & Schwartz-Barcott, D. (1993). Action research: what is it? How has it been used and how can it be used in nursing? *Journal of Advanced Nursing*, *18*(2): 298–304.

Ingadóttir, T. S., & Jonsdottir, H. (2006). Technological dependency: The experience of using home ventilators and long-term oxygen therapy: Patients' and families' perspective. *Scandinavian Journal of Caring Science*, *20:* 18–25.

Kim, H. S. (2010). *The nature of theoretical thinking in nursing* (3rd ed.). New York: Springer.

Kim, H. S., Ellefsen, B., Kyung, J. H., & Alves, S. L. (2008). Clinical constructions by nurses in Korea, Norway, and the United States. *Western Journal of Nursing Research*, *30*(1): 54–72.

Kirkevold, M. (2008). The Norwegian teaching home program: Developing a model for systematic practice development in the nursing home sector. *International Journal of Older People Nursing*, *3*(4), 282–286.

Kirkevold, M., Bronken, B. A., Martinsen, R., & Kvigne, K. (2012). Promoting psychosocial well-being following a stroke: Developing a theoretically and empirically sound complex intervention. *International Journal of Nursing Studies*, *49*(4): 386–397.

Kirkevold, M., Nortvedt, F., & Alvsvåg, H. (Eds.) (1993). *Klokskap og kyndighet: Kari Martinsens innflytelse på norsk og dansk sykepleie* [Wisdom and proficiency]. Oslo: Ad notam Gyldendal.

Knutsen, I. R., & Foss, C. (2011a). Caught between conduct and free choice: A field study of an empowering programme in lifestyle change for obese patients. *Scandinavian Journal of Caring Sciences*, 25(1): 126–133. doi: 10.1111/j.1471-6712.2010.00801.x.

Knutsen, I. R., Terragni, L., & Foss, C. (2011b). Morbidly obese patients and lifestyle change: Constructing ethical selves. *Nursing Inquiry*, 4: 348–358. doi: 10.1111/j.1440- 1800.2011.00538.x. Epub 2011 Jul 10.

Kvale, S., & Brinkmann, S. (2009). *Interviews: Learning the craft of qualitative research interviewing*. Los Angeles: Sage.

Lerheim, K. (2000). *Sykepleieforskningen i Norge i fortid og nåtid* [Nursing research in Norway in the past and the future]. Oslo: Forlaget Sykepleien.

Lomborg, K., Bjørn, A., Dahl, R., & Kirkevold, M. (2005). Body care experienced by people hospitalized with severe respiratory disease. *Journal of Advanced Nursing*, 50(3): 262–271.

Lomborg, K., & Kirkevold, M. (2003). Truth and validity in grounded theory: A reconsidered realist interpretation of the criteria: Fit, work, relevance and modifiability. *Nursing Philosophy*, 4(3): 189–200.

Løgstrup, K. E. (1997). *The ethical demand*. Notre Dame, IN: University of Notre Dame Press.

Martinsen, K. (1975). Sykepleie og filosofi. Et marxistisk og fenomenologisk bidrag [Nursing and philosophy: A Marxist and phenomenological contribution]. Thesis, University of Bergen.

Martinsen, K. (1984). *Freidige og uforsagte diakonisser. Et omsorgsyrke vokser frem* 1860–1905 [Courageous and frank deaconesses: A caring profession emerges 1860–1905]. Oslo: Aschehoug/Tanum-Norli.

Martinsen, K. (1993a). *Fra Marx til Løgstrup. Om moral, samfunnskritikk og sanselighet i sykepleien* [From Marx to Løgstrup: On morality, social critique and sensuousness in nursing]. Oslo: Tano.

Martinsen, K. (Ed.). (1993b) *Den omtenksomme sykepleier* [The thoughtful nurse]. Oslo: Tano.

Martinsen, K. (1996). *Fenomenologi og omsorg. Tre dialoger* [Phenomenology and caring: Three dialogues]. Oslo: Tano.

Martinsen, K. (2006). *Care and vulnerability*. Oslo: Akribe.

Martinsen, K., & Wærness K. (1979). *Pleie uten omsorg?* [Care without caring?] Oslo: Pax.

Marx, K., & Sitton, J. F. (2010). *Marx today: Selected works and recent debates*. New York: Palgrave Macmillan.

Merleau-Ponty, M. (2011). *Phenomenology of perception*. London: Routledge.

Midtgaard, J., Stelter, R., Rørth, M., & Adamsen, L. (2007). Regaining a sense of agency and shared self-reliance: The experience of advanced disease cancer patients participating in a multidimensional exercise intervention while undergoing chemotherapy: Analysis of patient diaries. *Scandinavian Journal of Psycholology*, 48(2):181–190.

Nåden, D. (1998). Når sykepleie blir kunstutøvelse [When nursing becomes an art performance]. Doctoral dissertation, Åbo Akademi, Åbo, Finland.

Nordtvedt, P. (1996). *Sensitive judgment: Nursing, moral philosophy and an ethics of care*. Oslo: Tano Aschehoug.

Nortvedt, P., Hem, M. H., & Skirbekk, H. (2011). The ethics of care: Role obligations and moderate partiality in health care. *Nursing Ethics*, 18(2):192–200.

Ricoeur, P. (2004). *The conflict of interpretations: Essays in hermeneutics*. London: Continuum.

Risjord, M. W. (2010). *Nursing knowledge: Science, practice, and philosophy*. Chichester: Wiley-Blackwell.

Ruland, C. M., Jeneson, A., Andersen, T., Andersen, R., Slaughter, L., & Bente-Schjødt, O., & Moore, S. M. (2007). Designing tailored Internet support to assist cancer patients in illness management. *AMIA Annual Symposium Proceedings*, October 11: 635–639.

Ruland, C. M., Starren, J., & Vatne, T. M. (2008). Participatory design with children in the development of a support system for patient-centered care in pediatric oncology. *Journal of Biomedical Information*, 41(4): 624–635.

Skuladottir, H., & Halldorsdottir, S. (2011). The quest for well-being: Self-identified needs of women in chronic pain. *Scandinavian Journal of Caring Sciences*, 25(1): 81–91. doi: 10.1111/j.1471-6712.2010.00793.x.

Torheim, H., & Gjengedal, E. (2010). How to cope with mask treatment in patients with acute chronic obstructive pulmonary disease-exacerbations. *Scandinavian Journal of Caring Sciences*, 24: 499–506.

van Manen, M. (1997). *Researching lived experience: Human science for an action sensitive pedagogy*. London, Ontario: Althouse Press.

Wagner, L. (1992). Non-institutional care for the elderly: A Danish model. *Danish Medical Bulletin*, 39(3): 236–238.

Weber, M. (2011). *The Protestant ethic and the spirit of capitalism*. New York: Oxford University Press.

Zoffmann, V., Harder, I., & Kirkevold, M. (2008). A person-centered communication and reflection model: Sharing decision-making in chronic care. *Qualitative Health Research*, *18*(5): 670–685.

Zoffmann, V., & Kirkevold, M. (2007). Relationships and their potential for change developed in difficult type 1 diabetes. *Qualitative Health Research*, *17*(5): 625–638.

Zoffmann, V., & Lauritzen, T. (2006). Guided self-determination improves life skills with type 1 diabetes and A1C in randomized controlled trial. *Patient Education and Counseling*, *64*(1–3): 78–86.

Resources

https://english.hi.is/school_of_health_sciences/faculty_of_nursing/about_faculty.
http://english.unak.is/health-sciences/page/hjukrun_forsida.

41

Qualitative nursing research in the Netherlands and Flanders

Maria Grypdonck, Marijke C. Kars,
Ann Van Hecke, and Sofie Verhaeghe

In this chapter we will discuss the role and the nature of qualitative research in the field of nursing research in the Netherlands and Flanders, the Dutch-speaking part of Belgium. The Netherlands and Flanders use the same language, Dutch, but have different legislation and a different history of nursing, nursing education and adoption into the academy of nursing. The situation in Flanders is quite different from that in the French-speaking part of Belgium, where nursing research has a different history and qualitative nursing research is less practiced. Before discussing qualitative research in the Netherlands and Flanders, we will provide some background information about nursing, nursing research and nursing education in those countries.

Nursing and nursing research in the Netherlands and Flanders: similarities and differences

The history of nursing education and of nursing research in the Netherlands and Belgium is quite different. Formal nursing education started around the same time, at the end of the nineteenth century, somewhat earlier in the Netherlands than in Belgium, but in a completely different manner. In the Netherlands the emergence of nursing education was linked to the Dutch feminist emancipation movement. Women from very well-to-do families played a major role. They saw nursing as a possible profession for women and as a valuable alternative to waiting at home for the right marital candidate to come along (Bakker-van der Kooij, 1983). They considered a university education the appropriate education for nurses. They did not obtain it, however, due to the objection of physicians, who fully agreed with the need for nursing education, but not at that level. Nurses were forced to be content with an in-service education of which the level was variable: the more candidates that were needed, the lower the entry requirements (Aan de Stegge, 2012). It would take until 1970 for nursing education to become part of the regular education system.

In Belgium, the initiative for formal nursing education came from (anticlerical) physicians who found it difficult to cope with the bossiness of the Catholic sisters who, after the French Revolution, had remained in charge of both the private and the public hospitals (Velle, 1988). Belgium has never known an in-service education for nurses—of course the (anticlerical) doctors did not want their lay nurses to be socialized by the Catholic sisters (Velle, 1988)—and nursing has always been part of the regular educational system. This has been a great advantage for Belgian nursing education, which has been considered advanced compared to other countries in Europe. Indeed, nursing education developed with and within the national educational system. Nurses were admitted to regular university education (in health care management) and given (some) academic credit for their nursing education as early as 1965.

Nursing education and nursing research in a dual system of higher education

Both Belgium and the Netherlands have a dual system of higher education. This organizational model of higher education was in place almost everywhere in Europe, but has been changed in some countries such as Great Britain, Portugal and others.

A dual system of higher education means that there is a separate system of educational institutions for applied subjects (professional education) and for theoretical subjects. The former are referred to as Universities of Applied Sciences (in the Netherlands) or university colleges (in Belgium); the latter are the (old) universities. Sometimes a subject can be studied in both types of institutions: applied economists were educated in the applied institutions for higher education, "pure" economists at the university. Doctors and pharmacists as well as some other professionals have always been educated at the university; nurses are not. Between the applied institutions for higher education and the university there is a difference in level (of difficulty) and in status. The curricula in the applied institutions differ as to degree of difficulty and also in duration. Both in the Netherlands and in Belgium the qualification to practice nursing is obtained in the applied institutions. In Flanders, a bachelor's degree in nursing takes three years; in the Netherlands four. Nurses subsequently can obtain a Master's degree at the university. This can be in nursing science, in health care management, in health education or (sometimes) in another related subject. Since the Bologna Agreement, regulating education in Europe, a Master's degree in Advanced Practice can be obtained in Dutch Universities of Applied Sciences. These programs educate Nurse Practitioners.

Traditionally, research was the province of the university, and university education was characterized by its teachers (professors) being engaged in research. As already mentioned, changes have occurred in the relationship between both types of education, also in those countries where the dual system remains.

The applied institutions now are expected to engage in practice-oriented research, and in the Netherlands lecturers are appointed in specific areas, to undertake such research and to enhance the utilization of research-based knowledge in the teaching of the institution. Nursing is one of the fields that has several such lecturers. PhD education takes place at the university. Thus far, the Dutch and Flemish universities have the system of PhD by dissertation only. This means that formally there are no course requirements above the Master's degree in order to obtain a PhD. The "only" requirement is a substantial piece of research, intensively supervised by the dissertation director, the equivalent of four years' full-time work. In medical faculties, the requirement is to have at least three or four articles published in high-ranking international journals. PhD research is considered to have high status because of the very stringent quality requirements.

The beginnings of nursing research

As the university was the natural habitat for research, and nursing did not move into the university until after 1960 (and 1980 in the Netherlands), little nursing research took place in Belgium and the Netherlands before that time. When in the late 1960s the Center for Hospital Administration and Medical Care Organization was founded at the Katholieke Universiteit (KU) Leuven

(Louvain, Belgium), in order to provide education and do research in hospital management, and nurses were admitted to it, the research agenda also included research about nursing. The first "nursing" research studies pertained to nurse staffing and utilization (Dhaene & Quaethoven, 1988). In 1972, the KU-Leuven started a long-lasting research project, Integrating Nursing (Grypdonck et al., 1979). This study addressed the essence of nursing and how nursing care in the hospital could be organized so as to maximize the benefits of professionalization of nursing for the patients. The study laid the ground for many others, both in the Netherlands and in Flanders (Aukes, Hellema, & Walenkamp, 1992; Berkhout, Boumans, van Breukelen, Abu-Saad, & Nijhuis, 2004; Boumans, Berkhout, & Landeweerd, 2005; Cromphout, 2012; Heeremans, Boumans, Algera, & Landeweerd, 1994; Kitzen & Boumans, 1995; Molleman, 1990; Nissen, Boumans, & Landeweerd, 1997; Swildens & van Keijzerswaard, 1998). In 1975, the KU-Leuven created a Master's program in nursing administration and education and in 1991 in clinical nursing. From then on, Master's theses about nursing proper became the rule rather than the exception. PhD study in nursing, first abroad, later in Belgium, became accessible. The first nurse obtained her degree at the University of Manchester in 1980 (Grypdonck, 1980).

In the Netherlands it would take until 1980 before the first program in nursing science was established. A research program was developed into a multidisciplinary setting. Self-care and Orem's theory were important themes in the beginning of the department (Evers, Isenberg, Philipsen, Senten, & Brouns, 1993; Jaarsma & Dassen, 1994; Schiltmans & Evers, 1988; Senten, 1991; van Achterberg et al., 1991; van der Bruggen, 1991). The first Dutch nurse to obtain a PhD degree in 1985 studied at the University of California, San Francisco. Her PhD thesis dealt with the perception of health in the elderly. It was a qualitative study using a (variant of) grounded theory approach (van Maanen, 1985, 1988). Because after graduation she did not hold an appointment in the Netherlands—she was a professor in Canada and later in Germany—the influence of her work in the Netherlands was not very great.

In 1985, *Verpleegkunde, Nederlands Vlaams wetenschappelijk tijschrift voor verpleegkundigen* (Nursing. Netherlands-Flemish Scientific Journal for Nurses) was founded. It was a collaboration between the Netherlands and Flanders, and its aim was to stimulate publication of nursing research, not in the least by students in the Master's programs in nursing. The journal would make nursing science visible and at the same time accessible for the nurses who held a degree from the Universities of Applied Sciences.

Nursing research in a multidisciplinary context

Both in Belgium and in the Netherlands, nursing research has always been carried out in multi-disciplinary institutes. There are no Faculties of Nursing. In the Netherlands, as the Master's education in nursing science only started in 1980, a considerable number of nurses have obtained a Master's degree in another discipline than nursing and after 1980 several continued to do so. For many of them, their "academic field" is not nursing as in nursing they only have an in-service education. A considerable number of nurses have obtained their PhD with scientists from other disciplines as their dissertation director, and hence in other fields than nursing. In Flanders the situation is different. Flemish universities, as a whole, have much clearer boundaries between disciplines. Almost all nurses who have obtained a PhD did so with a nurse as their dissertation director.

The multidisciplinary embedding of research in nursing makes it difficult to study the characteristics of nursing research. Indeed, what should count as "nursing research" and who should count as a "nurse researcher"? Phenomena of importance to nursing are studied by nurses as well as non-nurses. Some primary investigators have both a nursing background and a background in another discipline. Some nursing topics are studied by nurses under the supervision of persons from other disciplines. Nurses are sometimes hired to carry out studies about nursing as well as about other health topics because as a nurse they know the field. Because of publication pressure in academia many nurses publish their studies in medical journals, which have higher impact factors.

In this chapter we use the following operational definition of nursing research: research that develops knowledge or investigates issues that are directly relevant for the field of nursing reported in scientific journals or books and to which a nurse has made a significant contribution as an author. PhD theses are considered nursing research if the person obtaining the degree is a nurse and the study concerns similar issues. The chapter is based on research published in international journals, in Dutch or Flemish journals or as a book. The latter includes PhD theses which, in the Netherlands, are obligatorily published as a book.

Qualitative nursing research: the first endeavors

Qualitative research in nursing appeared in the Netherlands before it did in Belgium. The first qualitative studies in the Netherlands appeared in the 1980s. They fitted well with the values and assumptions of social science research as it had emerged after the "revolt" of 1968. Indeed, between 1970 and 1980 a large stream of publications emerged on the subject of the method-ological consequences for the social sciences of the new orientation towards the social world. Whether or not the once strong position occupied by phenomenology in psychology and psychiatry in the Netherlands, known as the Utrecht School of Phenomenology (Lynch–Sauer, 2012; van Hezewijk, 2012), encouraged the development of the new, qualitative methodologies is difficult to judge. On the one hand, phenomenological thinking in psychology, education and health was something one was accustomed to, and some of the (older) phenomenologists took part in the debate about the new science (e.g. de Boer, 1980; Strasser, 1963, 1971). On the other hand, the phenomenological orientation not only had been heavily criticized but also had been actively and sometimes vehemently combated. More recent studies, indeed, show that there was no such a thing as *the* phenomenological method or a phenomenological *school* in Utrecht, and that the methods used by the famous phenomenologists were implicit rather than explicit (Dehue, 1995; van Hezewijk, 2012). An oppositional way of thinking had been created, which was reflected in the debate about the legitimacy of qualitative research: one was *pro* or *contra*, and the position was not only based on rational arguments.

When, in 1980 the first Master's program in nursing science was started at the University of Maastricht (NL), the department was part of a modern faculty of Health Sciences, and not of a traditional Faculty of Medicine. With Hans Philipsen, a sociologist and anthropologist as a key player and since 1983 its director, an orientation towards social sciences rather than medical sciences or epidemiology was "natural." This did not mean, however, that in the beginning there was great enthusiasm for qualitative research, and this in spite of the fact that Harry van der Bruggen, the first chairperson of the department, had drawn, and would draw again attention to the value of an existential-phenomenological approach to nursing (van der Bruggen, 1977, 1979, 1987). Qualitative research methodology in the beginning was not part of the curriculum. Later, it became established as a necessary component of a nursing science curriculum.

The first published nursing science study in the Netherlands using a qualitative approach was Corry Bosch's study about interactions between patients, nurses and doctors in a general hospital ward (Bosch, 1984). Bosch did the research for her Master's degree in sociology and her study was published in an accessible version in the series *Verpleegkundige studies* [Nursing Studies]. She used a grounded theory approach. Data were collected through observation and interviews, with an emphasis on the former. *Involvement* appeared as the key concept. Grounded theory was known among social scientists at that time. Already in 1976 *The Discovery of Grounded Theory* had been translated into Dutch (Glaser & Strauss, 1976), three years after the Dutch translation of *Awareness of Dying* was published (Glaser & Strauss, 1973) and had received quite a bit of attention, not so much because of its methodology but because of the clarity with which it brought to light how death was dealt with in hospitals Bosch's study findings, emphasizing the role of human interaction and human relations in the specialized and technical environment that hospitals had become, fitted well with the interests of nursing at that time. As with Glaser and Strauss' study, also in this case the content helped to draw attention to the value of qualitative research for the specific interests of nursing.

In 1988, a study was published by Borgesius, de Lange, and Meurs. The study was commissioned by the National Society of Mental Health (the NcGv) and their assignment was to study psychiatric nurses: not only what they did, but also what the essence of their work was. All three authors were social scientists; de Lange had a nursing background as well. The reasons to choose a qualitative design were the strengths of that type of design given the nature of the study and in pointing them out, de Lange refers to an article by Komter (1983), published in a highly respected Dutch social science methods journal (de Lange, 1990a). The researchers used qualitative methods because the phenomena were studied as processes, often invisible, and of which interactions were a major part. These processes needed to be studied in a broader context, including the historical context, which, of course, would be inaccessible for observation. Moreover, they say they were interested in "differences and nuances" and "as yet not in generalized statements." As did Bosch, Borgesius et al. also used a method "grafted onto the grounded theory approach by Glaser and Strauss" (Glaser & Strauss, 1967), meaning that they followed some but not all of the specific procedures of this methodology, as so many qualitative nursing researchers would do after them. They used both observation and interviews as their method of data collection. De Lange carried out another impressive qualitative study commissioned by the NcGv about persons suffering from dementia in nursing homes (de Lange, 1990b, 1991). In 1990, the Helen Dowling Institute organized a conference to call attention to the value of qualitative research for nursing. According to the organizers, qualitative research did not get the attention in nursing science that it deserved. To make qualitative research better known, the organizers wanted to give qualitative researchers the opportunity to discuss their work with those interested (Francke, 1990). As an institute focusing on holistic health care (de Vries, 1985), qualitative research was, indeed, a logical choice fitting with its mission. Anneke Francke, who organized the conference, would be one of the first nurse researchers in the Netherlands to use qualitative research as part of a doctoral thesis. Francke qualitatively studied nurse pain management in hospital wards and nurses' continuing education needs (Francke et al., 1996). The first Flemish qualitative research study in nursing was published in *Verpleegkunde*, the scientific journal in the Dutch language mentioned above (Vandesande, 1990). The study, based on a Master's dissertation from the KU-Leuven, dealt with the lived experience of patients with lung cancer and their close relatives, and what the manner in which their diagnosis was (not) communicated meant to them. This study was the first one in a long series of studies about the experience of being chronically ill supervised by Maria Grypdonck and mainly carried out at the University of Utrecht (NL) and Ghent University (Belgium).

Nursing and the patient's perspective: the boost for qualitative nursing research

The boost in qualitative research in nursing in the Netherlands and Flanders came when nurse researchers realized the potential of qualitative research for the study of patients' experiences. Already from the start of the KU-Leuven's Integrating Nursing project one of the major tenets was that good nursing care requires the nurse to understand the patient's experiences and to get insight into the meaning the patient gives to his situation, and how he deals with it. Qualitative research proved to be very useful in clarifying this lived experience in such a way that it promoted better nursing care (Grypdonck, 1997). When Maria Grypdonck in 1991 moved from the University of Leuven to Utrecht University, the study of the lived experience of persons with chronic illness was chosen as the core of the research program. In the publication *Lifting Life above Illness* (Grypdonck, 1996), she described, based on a synthesis of the research carried out until then, how persons with a chronic illness tried to reconcile the demands of their illness with those of a good life. This is exactly what the self-management that every person with a chronic illness exercises entails. "Self-management," then, is not an alternative term for "compliance" or "adherence," but refers to the continuous efforts of patients to make decisions that enhance their quality of life. People with a chronic illness should be approached by medical providers in the first place as persons who are trying to live a good life. Nurses and doctors should not make the illness paramount if they want to connect with the way of thinking of the patient. Parsons' description of the sick role may be appropriate for acute illness, but not for persons with a chronic illness (Pool, 1995). *Lifting Life above Illness* was a synthesis of the research Grypdonck had carried out until then; it was also a program for further studies that was carried out in collaboration at Utrecht University and Ghent University. Aart Pool's PhD thesis at the University of Utrecht about autonomy and chronic illness (Pool, 1995) made an important contribution to that program and had a long-lasting influence on Dutch health care for persons with a chronic illness. The approach to persons with a chronic illness these studies showed was well received not only by nurses and other health professionals, but also by persons with a chronic illness, who felt recognized and validated by this approach. In Flanders, the Department of Nursing Science of Ghent University and to a lesser extent and somewhat later, of the KU-Leuven, proceeded along the same lines. In Flanders, however, the nursing science departments were backed up to a much lesser extent than in the Netherlands by a broad societal movement to improve the lot of persons with a chronic illness. Nonetheless, the studies helped to call attention to the way persons with a chronic illness wanted to live their lives and highlighted their vulnerability and their strengths (Grypdonck, 2005; Grypdonck et al., 2000). It also positioned qualitative research as valuable and even indispensable in health care.

The study of the experience of illness and care has proved to be important to understand issues of adherence and to develop adequate interventions (Moser et al., 2008; van der Wal et al., 2010; Van Hecke, 2010; Van Hecke et al., 2011; Vervoort et al., 2009). Van Staa (van Staa, van der Stege, Jedeloo, Moll, & Hilberink, 2011; van Staa, Jedeloo, & van der Stege, 2011) developed a program for adolescents with chronic illness to support them and their parents in the transition from adolescent to adult health care.

Studying the lived experience of persons with a chronic illness revealed the important place of family members of persons with a chronic illness. The studies clearly showed that "a chronic illness you never have alone." Family members also suffer, and often suffer doubly: they suffer with the patient but also suffer their own loss. The PhD study of Sofie Verhaeghe defended at Ghent University (Verhaeghe, 2007; Verhaeghe, Defloor, van Zuuren, Duijnstee, & Grypdonck, 2005; Verhaeghe, van Zuuren, Defloor, Duijnstee, & Grypdonck, 2007a; Verhaeghe, van

Zuuren, Defloor, Duijnstee, & Grypdonck, 2007b; Verhaeghe, van Zuuren, Grypdonck, Duijnstee, & Defloor, 2010a; Verhaeghe, van Zuuren, Grypdonck, Duijnstee, & Defloor, 2010b) and the studies by Marijke Kars of parents of children with serious and with terminal illnesses (Kars, Duijnstee, Pool, van Delden, & Grypdonck, 2008; Kars, Grypdonck, Beishuizen, Meijer-van den Bergh, & van Delden, 2010; Kars et al., 2011) are good examples of this approach. This interest in the lived experience and the suffering of family members was preceded by an interest in the burden of family caregivers in the late 1980s and investigated in the PhD thesis of Duijnstee, a grounded theory study (Duijnstee, 1992) and, later in that of van der Lyke (2000) as well as other studies (van der Smagt-Duijnste, Hamers, & bu-Saad, 2000; van der Smagt-Duijnste, Hamers, bu-Saad, & Zuidhof, 2001; Voorhorst, Grypdonck, & Duijnstee, 2001).

Qualitative research has also been used to understand experiences with illness and care of patients and family members belonging to different cultural groups (de Graaff, Francke, van den Muijsenbergh, & van der Geest, 2010, 2012; Schnepp, 2001; van den Brink, 2003) and thus has contributed to competent culturally sensitive care.

The contribution of qualitative research to understanding patients and family members has greatly contributed to the role qualitative research has acquired not only in nursing, but also more generally in health care. These studies were probably most influential in moving qualitative research from the position of "preliminary research" useful to be carried out in preparation of "true research" (which counts and compares) to research with its own, unique contribution.

Qualitative nursing research: a flourishing tree

The acceptance of qualitative research now seen as a valuable and legitimate research strategy to study the lived experience of patients and their family members was extended to other topics. Its acceptance, however, also requires vigilance. Qualitative research, indeed, is not always used in the best way or to the best effect.

Qualitative research is frequently used to study the perceptions of nurses as well as current practice. Perceptions of practitioners are sometimes deemed an interesting object of study preceding a change process. Such studies can provide understanding of why practices evolve as they do (Anthierens, Grypdonck, De Pauw, & Christiaens, 2009) and can inform the change agents about the ideas that they have to change. However, when the study is limited to organizing a few focus groups and/or the data analysis results in mere description, the results of such studies have limited meaning. Indeed, the findings are highly transient or have only a local significance. Both in the Netherlands and in Flanders there is a temptation to use qualitative research (as well as quantitative research) to document the deplorable state of nursing practice. The studies are said to be necessary to convince those in charge that changes are necessary. One can question, however, whether research, a fine and costly tool, is well used if the findings are limited to mere description and do not provide real insight into the reasons why the situation is as it is.

Qualitative research is also used to bring the processes to light that nurses use in their practice (Koekkoek, van Meijel, Tiemens, Schene, & Hutschemaekers, 2011; Landeweer, Abma, & Widdershoven, 2010; Schoot, Proot, Legius, ter Meulen, & de Witte, 2006; Vervoort et al., 2010). The aim is sometimes to expose what is considered bad practice; sometimes the intent is positive: to understand what is involved in the complex (cognitive) tasks on which nursing is based. It is, however, not always easy to distinguish between good and dubious practices when there is no standard to judge against (Baart & Vosman, 2008).

Empirical ethics has made an important contribution to qualitative research. On the one hand, studies about patients' experiences make clear what the situation is for the patient, which is necessary to decide what is good care (Dierckx de Casterlé, Grypdonck, Cannaerts, & Steeman,

2004). Studying nurses' experience can reveal nurses' ethical intuitions, their reasoning and their behavior (Georges, Grypdonck, & Dierckx de Casterlé, 2002; Smits, 2004; van der Dam, Abma, Kardol, & Widdershoven, 2011) and bring to light ethically taxing situations or ethical dilemmas nurses are confronted with and how nurses deal with them. Especially in the field of euthanasia (De Bal, Dierckx de Casterlé, De Beer, & Gastmans, 2006; Denier, Dierckx de Casterlé, De Bal, & Gastmans, 2009; Denier, Dierckx de Casterlé, De Bal, & Gastmans, 2010a; Denier, Gastmans, De Bal, & Dierckx de Casterlé, 2010b; Dierckx de Casterlé, Verpoort, De Bal, & Gastmans, 2006), qualitative research has made important contributions to the field of nursing ethics. The study of patients' and nurses' interactions has been used to contribute both to principled ethics (Schoot et al., 2006; Verkooijen, 2006) and ethics of care (Timmermann, 2010).

In a few studies qualitative research has been used as a complement to quantitative data analysis in experimental studies (de Lange, 2004; van Meijel, Megens, Koekkoek, Kruitwagen, & Grypdonck, 2009). De Lange (2004) has examined the effect of emotion-oriented care by using a qualitative analysis of observational data comparing the experimental and the control group. She was able to bring to light changes that were not apparent in the RCT. The fine-grained approach seemed very suitable for this task. Although it has long been advised to use mixed methods instead of simple RCTs in order to not only find out whether an intervention works, but also to understand what goes on, it is not really common practice yet.

That the development of interventions should be preceded by an assessment of needs from the patients' perspective and that qualitative research is fit for that purpose, is well accepted nowadays. Studying patients' perspectives has become an integral part of intervention mapping, and, increasingly, qualitative methods are used for this (Koekkoek et al., 2010b; Van Hecke, 2010). However, sometimes the qualitative approach is limited to an inventory of patient needs, rather than attempting to provide understanding of them.

The role of qualitative research in developing interventions has been worked out more fully by van Meijel et al. (2004). These authors emphasize that in complex interventions, interventions consisting of several elements that are delivered as a whole, RCTs provide only partial information. They do not allow the establishment of a causal relation between the elements of the intervention and the outcome. Indeed, it remains completely unclear which parts of the complex intervention contribute to the result, and which do not. Some might even have a negative effect. Van Meijel et al. have developed a strategy, known as the *Utrecht Model of Developing Interventions* to carefully develop and examine interventions before they are included in an RCT (Gamel, 2000; Gamel et al., 2001; Koekkoek et al., 2010a; Van Hecke, 2010; van Meijel et al., 2006; Verhaeghe, 2007; Vervoort, 2010). Qualitative research is used for the assessment of needs from the patients' and sometimes also from the providers' perspective. It can also be used to study existing practices which are considered to give a (partial) answer to the problem under study. In the last phase before the RCT, patients' and providers' experiences with receiving and carrying out the intervention are studied and analyzed. This analysis can give rise to the development of theories to explain the reactions of the beneficiaries of the intervention. Studying the experiences with the intervention in this way allows investigators to judge the contributions of the separate parts of the intervention, and to adapt the intervention before testing it in an RCT. Sometimes testing in an RCT can be considered superfluous because the positive effect of the intervention is clear from the qualitative study. This is more often the case when patients' or family members' experiences or perceptions are the envisaged outcomes of the intervention, such as in supportive interventions. Van Meijel and his co-workers have used (variations of) this approach in several domains of psychiatric nursing to develop an "evidence-based" knowledge base for psychiatric nursing practice (Bakker et al., 2011; Koekkoek, van Meijel, Schene, & Hutschemaekers, 2010a; van Meijel, Kruitwagen, van der Gaag, Kahn, & Grypdonck, 2006; van Omen et al., 2009).

Methodologies

Qualitative nursing researchers in the Netherlands and in Flanders describe their studies most often as (a variation of) a grounded theory approach, and some studies have developed (small-scale) theories. More recently the term "descriptive qualitative research" has become more popular, likely following Sandelowski (Sandelowski, 2000). Most often, as Boeije (2000) has noted experienced qualitative researchers in the Netherlands use a rather pragmatic methodology and do not follow faithfully one of the paradigms or schools of qualitative research (Creswell, 1998; Munhall, 1982; Munhall & Oiler, 1986). Methods are adapted to the needs of the study. As is the case in the international literature, also in the Netherlands and Flanders, a study sometimes is referred to as a grounded theory study without even a very small-scale theory being the outcome (see Sandelowski, 2000). More often qualitative researchers adopt techniques from the grounded theory method rather than the method itself. The small scale of the studies, often Master's dissertations, is certainly at least in part at the basis of this practice. The studies are often worth publishing because they yield insights of value for nursing practice without, in themselves, leading to theory development. "Phenomenological" is often used when a study deals with the experiences of the participants, be it nurses or patients, or when the study tries to reconstruct their perspective. In the latter case "phenomenological" may be considered synonymous with "subjective." Studies using the phenomenological method as explicated by Beekman and Mulderij (1977), in line with the "Utrecht School of Phenomenology," are rather rare. Among the phenomenologists, van Maanen and Giorgi are the ones most often cited, but that does not mean that the methods are really in line with their ideas.

Grypdonck et al. (submitted) developed a variant of grounded theory specially suited to study patients' or family members' experiences with chronic illness or other health-related situations with a high personal impact, such as the threat of the death of a close family member, becoming chronically ill, or having to move to a nursing home. Using grounded theory, they develop small-scale theories explaining the experience and the resulting behavior, but only after they have explored in depth the meaning of the experience for those involved (Dierckx de Casterlé et al., 2011; Kars, Duijnstee, Pool, van Delden, & Grypdonck, 2008; Kars, Grypdonck, Beishuizen, Meijer-van den Bergh, & van Delden, 2010; Kars, Grypdonck, de Korte-Verhoef, Kamps, Meijer-van den Bergh, Verkerk, & van Delden, 2011; Verhaeghe, van Zuuren, Defloor, Duijnstee, & Grypdonck, 2007b; Verhaeghe, van Zuuren, Defloor, Duijnstee, & Grypdonck, 2007a; Vervoort, Grypdonck, De Grauwe, Hoepelman, & Borleffs, 2009). They consider an in-depth study of the lived experience a prerequisite for the validity of the analysis leading to the grounded theory.

Action Research is a strategy not often used in Dutch and Flemish nursing research (Hoogwerf, 2002; Loth et al., 2007; Munten, 2011; Vallenga et al., 2008). It is not easy to explain why. It is also true that in the Netherlands and Flanders the participation of the so-called participants in qualitative studies is often rather limited. The participants have the opportunity to voice their ideas, perceptions, to tell their story, but they are seldom really actively engaged in the analysis. This is so, even though in the Netherlands participation of clients in health care is well advanced.

In contrast to the early days of qualitative research (Borgesius, de Lange, & Meurs, 1988; Bosch, 1984; de Lange, 1990b, 1991; Francke et al., 1996), data collection methods have shifted away from observation. Likely, the time required for observation studies is a major obstacle. Interviews (semi-structured interviews, "semi-structured in depth interviews," loosely structured interviews and narrative interviews) are mentioned most often as the data collection method. As is the case in the international literature, focus groups are increasingly used, not always to the best advantage of the study. It is obvious, but it is also the case in international literature (Vervoort et al., 2007) that focus groups are sometimes used as a cheap alternative to individual interviews and not for the sake of the specific benefits that the interaction in such interviews provides. Regularly, the focus interviews do not result in anything further than the enumeration of opinions disguised as experiences.

Strategies for data analysis particularly useful to novice researchers have been developed by Dierckx de Casterlé et al. (2012) and Boeije's (2005) approach has been used by many inexperienced and experienced qualitative researchers. Grounded theory methods are most often referred to, in particular constant comparative analysis and three levels of coding, sometimes also theoretical saturation. As already pointed out, many studies do not develop theory, and it is not always clear what these methods then entail.

In the Netherlands, and to a lesser extent also in Flanders, consensus methods are in vogue (Grypdonck, 1995). Participants are asked their opinion, and strategies are used to achieve consensus, such as Delphi panels. While such methods certainly have their place, they are improperly used as an alternative to data collection about observable phenomena, while the results are often labeled as "validation" without the "researchers" being aware that the strategy might perpetuate erroneous ideas about what the situation actually is (Grypdonck, 1995). In a similar vein, in some studies professionals are asked about their opinion regarding one or more problems, and a summary of their ideas is given, without proper analysis. It is misleading to present such a study as a true qualitative study instead of as an inventory of opinions. The fact that some handbooks on or inspired by marketing research (such as (Baarda, de Goede, & Theunissen, 1995) are seen as handbooks for academic qualitative research may contribute to the confusion. Especially in the field of management and the study of barriers to implementation of (evidence-based) practices, this approach is used (too often).

Due to the influence of evidence-based practice, there is a "hardening" of qualitative methods, striving for objectivity not in line with the assumptions of qualitative research, as can also be seen in the international literature (Grypdonck, 2006). In order to fit qualitative findings in evidence-based practice, the concept of evidence is stretched and the unavoidable subjective nature of experience and interpretation is overlooked (Cox & Titchen, 2007).

Compared to its beginnings, qualitative research is both recognized and considered to be proper research. This was the case sooner in the Netherlands than in Belgium. The connections and alliances between nursing research and social sciences in the Netherlands certainly contributed to this earlier acceptance as well as the methodological work done in the social sciences in the Netherlands (Maso & Smaling, 1998; Smaling, 1987; Wester, 1987).

Qualitative research has made an indispensable contribution to knowledge and health care practice. In the Netherlands it was mainly the social scientists who carried nurses along in this development; in Flanders, where the interest in qualitative research is from a later date, nursing played a major role in calling attention to this type of research. Qualitative research is now a part of all social science curricula, including nursing.

The future of qualitative nursing research

Qualitative research in the field of nursing is now fully accepted, both in the Netherlands and in Flanders. Qualitative research is judged to meet the high standards applied to PhD theses in the Netherlands and in Flanders. Qualitative research has gained a lot in popularity in the medical field as well. Articles about qualitative research or reporting in trusted medical journals (Mays & Pope, 2000; Pope, Van Royen, & Baker, 2002; Pope, Ziebland, & Mays, 2000; Yamazaki et al., 2009) have contributed, and the exposure to good qualitative studies has probably contributed even more. Doctors find that qualitative studies bring to light what they cannot discover in their quantitative studies and as in medicine, too, interest in the patient's perspective grows, qualitative research becomes more relevant. Where the nursing science department is in the faculty of medicine, this positive attitude of (some) doctors is not unimportant.

In the Netherlands there is a flourishing discussion about methodological issues in qualitative research. There is a Dutch journal on qualitative methodology and there are courses and conferences. Nurses participate, but not proportionate to their share in the field of qualitative research. In university nursing science departments, qualitative researchers are involved as methodological advisors in qualitative studies in other departments of their university and in university colleges.

Based on its present position, qualitative research it is here to stay. The place of the patient and his/her family as relevant actors in the health care field underscores the need for qualitative research, and health care, including medicine, is more inclined than before to lend an ear to it.

However, the popularity of qualitative research has also a drawback. The desire to use qualitative research is sometimes greater than the possibilities for adequate supervision. As has been pointed out in the international literature, the popularity of qualitative research threatens the integrity of its methodology. To some, qualitative research does not seem to require much specialized knowledge or skills, and research project managers often think their researchers can conduct a qualitative investigation without being trained for it (Sandelowski, 2005). Experienced qualitative researchers are often approached by such researchers: they have been given the task to conduct a qualitative study, and after some time they discover it is not that easy. Some students prefer to do a qualitative study to avoid the confrontation with statistics. They too find out soon that it is rather a miscalculation.

The time when nurse researchers were looked at as wearisome and considered poor researchers because they used qualitative methods is gone. Such an attitude now can be pointed out as a problem of such beholders, not of the researchers. The proliferation of qualitative research, however, requires vigilance. Good education and good supervision are essential for qualitative research to play the important role it has in nursing science, in nursing and in health care.

References

Aan de Stegge, C. (2012). *Gekkenwerk. De ontwikkeling van het beroep psychiatrisch verpleegkundige in Nederland 1830–1980* [The development of the occupation of psychiatric nurse in the Netherlands, 1830–1980]. Maastricht: Universitaire Pers Maastricht.

Anthierens, S., Grypdonck, M., De Pauw, L., & Christiaens, T. (2009). Perceptions of nurses in nursing homes on the usage of benzodiazepines. *Journal of Clinical Nursing, 18*(22), 3098–3106.

Aukes, L. C., Hellema, F. G., & Walenkamp, M. J. (1992). *Verpleegkundige zorgvernieuwing. Integrerende verpleegkunde in de praktijk* [Innovation in nursing care. Integrating Nursing in practice]. Groningen: Wolters-Noordhoff.

Baarda, D. B., de Goede, M. P. M., & Theunissen, J. (1995). *Kwalitatief Onderzoek* [Qualitative research]. Stenfert Kroese.

Baart, A., & Vosman, F. (2008). *Aannemelijke zorg: Over het uitzieden en verdringen van praktische wijsheid in de gezondheidszorg* [Plausible care: About boiling down and suppressing practical wisdom in health care]. Amsterdam: Lemma.

Bakker, R., van Meijel, B., Beukers, L., van Omen, J., Meerwijk, E., & van Elburg, A. (2011). Recovery of normal body weight in adolescents with anorexia nervosa: The nurses' perspective on effective interventions. *Journal of Child and Adolescent Psychiatric Nursing, 24*(1), 16–22.

Bakker-van der Kooij, C. (1983). De maatschappelijke positie van verpleegsters in de periode 1880–1940 [The social position of nurses in the period 1880–1940]. *Tijdschrift voor Geschiedenis, 96*, 454–476.

Beekman, T. & Mulderij, K. (1977). *Beleving en ervaring: Werkboek fenomenologie voor de sociale wetenschappen* [Experiencing: Workbook phenomenology for the social sciences]. Meppel: Boom.

Berkhout, A. J., Boumans, N. P., van Breukelen, G. P., Abu-Saad, H. H., & Nijhuis, F. J. (2004). Resident-oriented care in nursing homes: Effects on nurses. *Journal of Advanced Nursing, 45*(6), 621–632.

Boeije, H. (2000). Onderzoek van zorg: benaderingen van kwalitatief verpleegkundig onderzoek [Care research: Approaches in qualitative nursing research]. *Kwalon, 5*(2), 42–45.

Boeije, H. (2005). *Analyseren in kwalitatief onderzoek: Denken en doen* [Analyzing in qualitative research: Thinking and doing]. Amsterdam: Boom.

Borgesius, E., De Lange, J., & Meurs, P. (1988). *Verpleegkundigen zonder uniform; over de pluriformiteit van het beroep van psychiatrisch verpleegkundige* [Nurses without a uniform: About the plurality of the occupation of psychiatric nurse]. Lochem: De Tijdstroom.

Bosch, C. (1984). *Betrokkenheid op de verpleegafdeling* [Commitment in the nursing unit]. Lochem: De Tijdstroom.

Boumans, N., Berkhout, A., & Landeweerd, A. (2005). Effects of resident-oriented care on quality of care, wellbeing and satisfaction with care, *Scandinavian Journal of Caring Sciences, 19*(3), 240–250.

Cox, K., & Titchen, A. (2007). Patiëntenverhalen, een bron van evidence [Patient stories, a source of evidence]. *Nederlands Tijdschrift voor Evidence Based Practice, 5*, 122–124.

Creswell, J. (1998). *Qualitative inquiry and research: Choosing among five traditions*. London: Sage Publications.

Cromphout, L. (2012). Waardebeleving in Integrerende Verpleegkunde. Een eenvoudig arbeidspsychologisch meetinstrument [Values experienced in integrating nursing: A simple instrument from the field of labor psychology]. *Acta Hospitalia, 25*(3), 31–39.

De Bal, N., Dierckx de Casterlé, B., De Beer, T., & Gastmans, C. (2006). Involvement of nurses in caring for patients requesting euthanasia in Flanders (Belgium): A qualitative study. *International Journal of Nursing Studies, 43*(5), 589–599.

de Boer, T. (1980). *Grondslagen van een kritische psychologie* [Foundations of a critical psychology]. Baarn: Ambo.

de Graaff, F. M., Francke, A. L., van den Muijsenbergh, M. E., & van der Geest, S. (2010). "Palliative care": A contradiction in terms? A qualitative study of cancer patients with a Turkish or Moroccan background, their relatives and care providers. *BMC Palliative Care, 9*, 19.

de Graaff, F. M., Francke, A. L., van den Muijsenbergh, M. E., & van der Geest, S. (2012). Understanding and improving communication and decision-making in palliative care for Turkish and Moroccan immigrants: A multiperspective study, *Ethnicity and Health, 17*(4), 363–384.

de Lange, J. (1990a). Verpleegkundigen zonder uniform. Een kwalitatief onderzoek naar de taken van psychiatrische verpleegkundigen [Nurses without a uniform: A qualitative study of the tasks of psychiatric nurses]. In A. L. Francke (Ed.), *Kwalitatief onderzoek in de verpleegkunde*. Amsterdam: Swets & Zeitlinger.

de Lange, J. (1990b). *Vergeten in het verpleeghuis: Dementerende ouderen, hun verzorgenden en familieleden* [Forgetting (and forgotten) in a nursing home. Elderly with dementia, their nursing assistants and family members]. Utrecht: Nationaal centrum voor de Geestelijke volksgezondheid.

de Lange, J. (1991). *Verward in het verzorgingshuis: De zorg voor dementerende en depressieve ouderen* [Disoriented in the nursing home: The care for demented and depressive elderly]. Utrecht: Nationaal centrum voor de Geestelijke volksgezondheid.

de Lange, J. (2004). *Omgaan met dementie; het effect van geïntegreerde belevingsgerichte zorg op adaptatie en coping van mensen met dementie in verpleeghuizen, een kwalitatiefonderzoek binnen een gerandomiseerd experiment* [Caring for persons with dementia: The effect of integrated experience based care on the adaptation and coping of persons with dementia in nursing homes. A qualitative study inside a randomized experiment]. Utrecht: Trimbos-Instutuut.

de Vries, M. (1985). *Het behoud van leven* [The conservation of life]. Utrecht: Bohn-Scheltema en Holkema.

Dehue, T. (1995). *Changing the rules: Psychology in the Netherlands 1900–1985*. Cambridge: Cambridge University Press.

Denier, Y., Dierckx de Casterlé, B., De Bal, N., & Gastmans, C. (2009). Involvement of nurses in the euthanasia care process in Flanders (Belgium): An exploration of two perspectives, *Journal of Palliative Care, 25*(4), 264–274.

Denier, Y., Dierckx de Casterlé, B., De Bal, N., & Gastmans, C. (2010a). "It's intense, you know." Nurses' experiences in caring for patients requesting euthanasia. *Medical Health Care Philosophy, 13*(1), 41–48.

Denier, Y., Gastmans, C., De Bal, N., & Dierckx de Casterlé, B. (2010b). Communication in nursing care for patients requesting euthanasia: A qualitative study. *Journal of Clinical Nursing, 19*(23–24), 3372–3380.

Dhaene, L. & Quaethoven, P. (1988). *Het Centrum voor ziekenhuiswetenschap en 25 jaar vervolmakingscyclus voor beleid van gezondheidsinstellingen 1963–1988* [The Center for Hospital Administration and Medical Care Organization and 25 years of Continuing Education Courses in management of health care organizations, 1963–1988]. Leuven: KU-Leuven, Centrum voor Ziekenhuiswetenschap,

Dierckx de Casterlé, B., Gastmans, C., Bryon, E., & Denier, Y. (2012). QUAGOL: A guide for qualitative data analysis. *International Journal of Nursing Studies, 49*(3), 360–371.

Dierckx de Casterlé, B., Grypdonck, M., Cannaerts, N., & Steeman, E. (2004). Empirical ethics in action: Lessons from two empirical studies in nursing ethics. *Medical Health Care Philosophy,* 7(1), 31–39.

Dierckx de Casterlé, B., Verhaeghe, S. T., Kars, M. C., Coolbrandt, A., Stevens, M., Stubbe, M., et al. (2011). Researching lived experience in health care: Significance for care ethics, *Nursing Ethics, 18*(2), 232–242.

Dierckx de Casterlé, B., Verpoort, C., De Bal, N., & Gastmans, C. (2006). Nurses' views on their involvement in euthanasia: A qualitative study in Flanders (Belgium). *Journal of Medical Ethics, 32*(4), 187–192.

Duijnstee, M. (1992). *De belasting van familieleden van dementerenden* [The burden of members of persons with dementia]. Utrecht: Nederlands Instituut voor Zorg en Welzijn.

Evers, G. C., Isenberg, M. A., Philipsen, H., Senten, M., & Brouns, G. (1993). Validity testing of the Dutch translation of the Appraisal of the Self-care Agency A.S.A.-scale. *International Journal of Nursing Studies, 30*(4), 331–342.

Francke, A. L. (1990). *Kwalitatief onderzoek in de verpleegkunde* [Qualitative research in nursing]. Amsterdam: Swets & Zeitlinger,

Francke, A. L., Garssen, B., Abu-Saad, H. H., & Grypdonck, M. (1996). Qualitative needs assessment prior to a continuing education program. *Journal of Continuing Education in Nursing, 27*(1), 34–41.

Gamel, C. J. (2000). Sexual health care after cancer diagnosis. Doctoral thesis, University of Utrecht.

Gamel, C., Grypdonck, M., Hengeveld, M., & Davis, B. (2001). A method to develop a nursing intervention: The contribution of qualitative studies to the process. *Journal of Advanced Nursing, 33*(6), 806–819.

Georges, J. J., Grypdonck, M., & Dierckx de Casterlé, B. (2002). Being a palliative care nurse in an academic hospital: A qualitative study about nurses' perceptions of palliative care nursing. *Journal of Clinical Nursing,* 11(6), 785–793.

Glaser, B. G., & Strauss, A. (1967). *The discovery of grounded theory.* Chicago: Aldine Atherton.

Glaser, B. G., & Strauss, A. L. (1973). *Besef van de naderende dood* [Awareness of dying]. Alphen aan de Rijn: Samsom.

Glaser, B. G., & Strauss, A. L. (1976). *De ontwikkeling van gefundeerde theorie* [The discovery of grounded theory]. Alphen aan de Rijn: Samsom.

Grypdonck, M. (1980). Theory and research in a practice discipline: The case of nursing. PhD thesis, University of Manchester, Manchester.

Grypdonck, M. (1995), Tien jaar Nederlands-Vlaams Tijdschrift voor Verpleegkundigen: Tien jaar Verplegingswetenschap in Nederland en Vlaanderen [Ten years of the Dutch-Flemish Journal for Nurses: Ten years of nursing science in the Netherlands and Flanders]. *Verpleegkunde. Nederlands-Vlaams wetenschappelijk tijdschrift voor verpleegkundigen, 10*(3/4), 117–125.

Grypdonck, M. (1996). *Het leven boven de ziekte uittillen: De opdracht van de Verpleegkunde en de Verplegingswetenschap voor chronisch zieken* [Lifting life above illness: The mission of nursing and nursing science towards the chronically ill]. Leiden: Spruyt, Van Mantgem & De Does.

Grypdonck, M. (1997). Die Bedeutung qualitativer Forschung für die Pflegekunde und die Pflegewissenschaft [The significance of qualitative research for nursing and nursing science]. *Pflege, 10*(4), 222–228.

Grypdonck, M. (2005). *Tussen verpleegkunde en verplegingswetenschap* [Between nursing and nursing science]. Utrecht: UMC Utrecht.

Grypdonck, M. H. (2006). Qualitative health research in the era of evidence-based practice. *Qualitative Health Research, 16*(10), 1371–1385.

Grypdonck, M., Duijnstee, M., van Linge, R., & Shortridge-Baggett, L. (2000). *10 jaar Verplegingswetenschap in Utrecht: nieuwe accenten in de zorg voor chronisch zieken* [10 years nursing science in Utrecht: New accents in the care for the chronically ill]. Leiden: Spruyt, van Manteghem, de Does.

Grypdonck, M., Koene, G., Rodenbach, M. T., Windey, T., & Blanpain, J. E. (1979). Integrating nursing: A holistic approach to the delivery of nursing care. *International Journal of Nursing Studies,* 16(2), 215–230.

Heeremans, J. G. M., Boumans, N. P. G., Algera, M., & Landeweerd, J. A. (1994). *Integrerende Verpleegkunde in de Praktijk: Resultaten van een experiment in een algemeen ziekenhuis* [Integrating nursing in practice: Results from an experiment in a general hospital]. Maastricht.Universitaire Pers: Maastricht.

Hoogwerf, L. J. R. (2002). Innovation and change in a rehabilitation unit for the elderly: Through action research. PhD thesis, Utrecht University.

Jaarsma, T. & Dassen, P. H. K. M. (1994). Informatiebehoefte en problemen van myocardinfarct- en coronaire-bypass-patiënten; een onderzoek naar informatiebehoefte en problemen vanuit de theorie van Orem [Information needs and problems of patients with a myocardial infarction and of coronary bypass patients: An investigation of information needs and problems using Orem's theory]. *Verpleegkunde. Nederlands-Vlaams wetenschappelijk tijdschrift voor verpleegkundigen, 8*(3), 233–243.

Kars, M. C., Duijnstee, M. S., Pool, A., van Delden, J. J., & Grypdonck, M. H. (2008). Being there: Parenting the child with acute lymphoblastic leukaemia. *Journal of Clinical Nursing, 7*(12), 1553–1562.

Kars, M. C., Grypdonck, M. H., Beishuizen, A., Meijer-van den Bergh, E. M., & van Delden, J. J. (2010). Factors influencing parental readiness to let their child with cancer die. *Pediatric Blood and Cancer, 54*(7), 1000–1008.

Kars, M. C., Grypdonck, M. H., de Korte-Verhoef, M. C., Kamps, W. A., Meijer-van den Bergh, E. M., et al. (2011). Parental experience at the end-of-life in children with cancer: "Preservation" and "letting go" in relation to loss. *Supportive Care Cancer, 19*(1), 27–35.

Kitzen, I. H. J. M. & Boumans, N. P. G. (1995). Integrerende Verpleegkunde en de kwaliteit van zorg. Het effect van de implementatie van Integrerende Verpleegkunde op de kwaliteit van de verpleegkundige zorgverlening en enkele patiëntkenmerken [Integrating Nursing and quality of care: The effect of the implementation of Integrating Nursing on the quality of nursing care and some patient characteristics]. *Verpleegkunde. Nederlands-Vlaams wetenschappelijk tijdschrift voor verpleegkundigen, 10*(2), 73–85.

Koekkoek, B., van Meijel, B., Schene, A., & Hutschemaekers, G. (2010a). Development of an intervention program to increase effective behaviours by patients and clinicians in psychiatric services: Intervention Mapping study. *BMC Health and Services Research, 10,* 293.

Koekkoek, B., van Meijel, B., Tiemens, B., Schene, A., & Hutschemaekers, G. (2011). What makes community psychiatric nurses label non-psychotic chronic patients as "difficult": Patient, professional, treatment and social variables. *Social Psychiatry and Psychiatric Epidemiology, 46*(10), 1045–1053.

Koekkoek, B., van Meijel, B., van Omen, J., Pennings, R., Kaasenbrood, A., Hutschemaekers, G., & Schene, A. (2010b). Ambivalent connections: A qualitative study of the care experiences of non-psychotic chronic patients who are perceived as "difficult" by professionals. *BMC Psychiatry, 10,* 96.

Komter, A. (1983). De onmacht van het getal [The importance of the number]. *Kennis en Methode, 3,* 202–226.

Landeweer, E. G., Abma, T. A., & Widdershoven, G. A. (2010). The essence of psychiatric nursing: Redefining nurses' identity through moral dialogue about reducing the use of coercion and restraint. *Advances in Nursing Science, 33*(4), E31–E42.

Loth, C., Schippers, G. M., Hart, H., & van de Wijngaart, G. (2007). Enhancing the quality of nursing care in methadone substitute clinics using action research: A process valuation. *Journal of Advanced Nursing, 57*(4), 422–431.

Lynch-Sauer, J. (2012). Using a phenomenological research method to study nursing phenomena. In M. M. Leininger (Ed.), *Qualitative research methods in nursing* (pp. 93–107). Orlando, FL: Grune & Stratton.

Maso, I. & Smaling, A. (1998). *Kwalitatief onderzoek: Praktijk en theorie* [Qualitative research: Practice and theory]. Amsterdam: Boom.

Mays, N. & Pope, C. (2000). Qualitative research in health care :Assessing quality in qualitative research. *British Medical Journal, 320*(7226), 50–52.

Molleman, E. (1990). *De organisatie van de verpleegkundige zorg in verandering: Een onderzoek naar de gevolgen van integrerende verpleegkunde* [The organization of nursing care in a process of change: An investigation into the consequences of integrating nursing]. Maastricht: Maastricht Universitaire Pers.

Moser, A., van der, B. H., Widdershoven, G., & Spreeuwenberg, C. (2008). Self-management of type 2 diabetes mellitus: A qualitative investigation from the perspective of participants in a nurse-led, shared-care programme in the Netherlands. *BMC Public Health, 8,* 91.

Munhall, P. L. (1982). Nursing philosophy and nursing research: In apposition or opposition? *Nursing Research, 31*(3), 176–177.

Munhall, P. L. & Oiler, C. J. (1986). *Nursing research: A qualitative perspective.* Norwalk, NJ: Appleton-Century-Crofts.

Munten, G. (2011). Implementeren van EBP in de psychiatrische verpleegkunde door middel van handelingsonderzoek [Implementing EBP in psychiatric nursing by means of action research]. *Nederlands Tijdschrift voor Evidence Based Practice, 8*(3), 16–19.

Nissen, J. M., Boumans, N. P., & Landeweerd, J. A. (1997). Primary nursing and quality of care: A Dutch study. *International Journal of Nursing Studies, 34*(2), 93–102.

Pool, A. (1995). *Autonomie, afhankelijkheid en langdurige zorgverlening* [Autonomy, dependency and long-term care]. Lochem: De Tijdstroom.

Pope, C., Van Royen, P., & Baker, R. (2002). Qualitative methods in research on healthcare quality. *Quality & Safety in Health Care, 11*(2), 148–152.

Pope, C., Ziebland, S., & Mays, N. (2000). Qualitative research in health care: Analysing qualitative data [Reprinted from Qualitative Research in Health Care]. *British Medical Journal, 320* (7227), 114–116.

Sandelowski, M. (2000). Whatever happened to qualitative description? *Research in Nursing and Health, 23*(4), 334–340.

Sandelowski, M. J. (2005). "I speak English, don't I?" *Research in Nursing & Health, 28*(3), 185–186.

Schiltmans, M., & Evers, G. (1988). Zelfzorgvermogen en sociale ondersteuning bij reumapatiënten [Self-care agency, and social support in patients with rheumatoid arthritis]. *Verpleegkunde. Nederlands-Vlaams tijdschrift voor verpleegkundigen, 2,* 195–200.

Schnepp, W. (2001). *Familiale Sorge in der Gruppe der Russlanddeutschen Spätaussiedler* [Family care among Russian-German re-immigrants]. Ghent: Academia Press.

Schoot, T., Proot, I., Legius, M., ter Meulen, R., & de Witte, L. (2006). Client-centered home care: Balancing between competing responsibilities. *Clinical Nursing Research, 15*(4), 231–254.

Senten, M. (1991). *The well-being of patients having CAB-surgery: A test of Orem's self-care nursing theory.* Maastricht: Faculteit der gezondheidszorg.

Smaling, A. (1987). *Methodologische objectiviteit en kwalitatief onderzoek* [Methodological objectivity and qualitative research]. Lisse: Swets & Zeitlinger B.V.

Smits, M. J. (2004). *Zorgen voor een draaglijk bestaan* [Caring for a bearable existence]. Amsterdam: Alsant.

Strasser, S. (1963). *Phenomenology and the human sciences: A contribution to a new scientific ideal.* Pittsburgh, PA: Duquesne University Press.

Strasser, S. (1971). Het probleem van de praktische wetenschap en opvoedkunde. [The problem of the practical science and pedagogics]. *Pedagogische studieën, 48,* 499–512.

Swildens, W., & van Keijzerswaard, A. (1998). Verpleegkunde en rehabilitatie: gaat dat wel samen? [Nursing and rehabilitation, do they fit together?], *Passage,* 3.

Timmermann, M. (2010). *Relationele afstemming: Presentieverrijkte verpleeghuiszorg voor mensen met dementie* [Relational tuning: Presence-enriched nursing home care for persons with dementia]. Utrecht: Lemma.

Vallenga, D., Grypdonck, M. H., Tan, F. I., Lendemeijer, B. H., & Boon, P. A. (2008). Improving decision-making in caring for people with epilepsy and intellectual disability: An action research project. *Journal of Advanced Nursing, 61*(3), 261–272.

van Achterberg, T., Lorensen, M., Isenberg, M. A., Evers, G. C., Levin, E., & Philipsen, H. (1991). The Norwegian, Danish and Dutch version of the Appraisal of Self-care Agency Scale: Comparing reliability aspects. *Scandinavian Journal of Caring Sciences, 5*(2), 101–108.

van den Brink, Y. (2003). Diversity in care values and expressions among Turkish family caregivers and Dutch community nurses in The Netherlands. *Journal of Transcultural Nursing, 14*(2), 146–154.

van der Bruggen, H. (1977). *Leve de zieke* [Long live the ill]. Lochem: De Tijdstroom.

van der Bruggen, H. (1979). *De verpleging in Nederland en het werk van Jan Hendrik van den Berg* [Nursing in the Netherlands and the work of J.H. van den Berg]. Lochem: De Tijdstroom.

van der Bruggen, H. (1987). *Naar een antropologische verpleegkunde* [Towards an anthropological nursing]. Lochem: De Tijdstroom.

van der Bruggen, H. (1991). *Patiënt, privaat en privacy: De stoelgang als gezondheidswetenschappelijk probleem* [Patient, private and privacy: Defecation as a health science problem]. Lochem: De Tijdstroom.

van der Dam, S., Abma, T. A., Kardol, M. J., & Widdershoven, G. A. (2012). "Here's my dilemma": Moral case deliberation as a platform for discussing everyday ethics in elderly care, *Health Care Analysis, 20*(3), 250–267.

van der Lyke, S. (2000). Georganiseerde liefde: Publieke bemoeienis met zorg in de privésfeer [Organized love: Public involvement in the private sphere]. PhD thesis, Maastricht University Van Arkel, Utrecht.

van der Smagt-Duijnste, M. E., Hamers, J. P., & bu-Saad, H. H. (2000). Relatives of stroke patients: Their experiences and needs in hospital. *Scandinavian Journal of Caring Sciences, 14*(1), 44–51.

van der Smagt-Duijnste, M. E., Hamers, J. P. A., bu-Saad, H. H., & Zuidhof, A. (2001). Relatives of hospitalized stroke patients: Their needs for information, counselling and accessibility. *Journal of Advanced Nursing, 33*(3), 307–315.

van der Wal, M. H., Jaarsma, T., Moser, D. K., van Gilst, W. H., & van Veldhuisen, D. J. (2010). Qualitative examination of compliance in heart failure patients in The Netherlands, *Heart and Lung, 39*(2), 121–130.

Van Hecke, A.(2010). Adherence to leg ulcer lifestyle advice: The development of a nursing intervention to enhance adherence in leg ulcer patients. PhD thesis, Ghent University.

Van Hecke, A., Verhaeghe, S., Grypdonck, M., Beele, H., & Defloor, T. (2011). Processes underlying adherence to leg ulcer treatment: A qualitative field study, *International Journal of Nursing Studies*, *48*(2), 145–155.

Van Hezewijk, R. (2012). De geschiedenis van de psychologie [The history of psychology] . Utrecht University, Department of Psychology. Retrieved on February 18, 2012 from http://www.uu.nl/faculty /socialsciences/nl/organisatie/Departementen/Psychologie/Organisatie/Geschiedenis/Documents/Gesc hiedenis_van_de_psychologie.pdf.

Van Maanen, H. M. T. (1985). *Health as perceived by the aged*. San Francisco: University of California.

Van Maanen, H. M. (1988). Being old does not always mean being sick: Perspectives on conditions of health as perceived by British and American elderly. *Journal of Advanced Nursing*, *13*(6), 701–709.

Van Meijel, B., Gamel, C., Swieten-Duijfjes, B., & Grypdonck, M. H. F. (2004). The development of evidence-based nursing interventions: Methodological considerations. *Journal of Advanced Nursing*, *48*(1), 84–92.

Van Meijel, B., Kruitwagen, C., van der Gaag, M., Kahn, R. S., & Grypdonck, M. H. (2006). An intervention study to prevent relapse in patients with schizophrenia. *Journal of Nursing Scholarship*, *38*(1), 42–49.

Van Meijel, B., Megens, Y., Koekkoek, B., de Vogel, W., Kruitwagen, C., & Grypdonck, M. (2009). Effective interaction with patients with schizophrenia: Qualitative evaluation of the interaction skills training programme. *Perspectives in Psychiatric Care*, *45*(4), 254–261.

Van Omen, J., Meerwijk, E. L., Kars, M., van Elburg, A., & van Meijel, B. (2009). Effective nursing care of adolescents diagnosed with anorexia nervosa: The patients' perspective. *Journal of Clinical Nursing*, *18*(20), 2801–2808.

Van Staa, A., Jedeloo, S., & van der Stege, H. (2011). "What we want": Chronically ill adolescents' preferences and priorities for improving health care. *Patient Preference Adherence*, *5*, 291–305.

Van Staa, A., van der Stege, H. A., Jedeloo, S., Moll, H. A., & Hilberink, S. R. (2011). Readiness to transfer to adult care of adolescents with chronic conditions: Exploration of associated factors. *Journal of Adolescent Health*, *48*(3), 295–302.

Vandesande, J. (1990). Posthospitalisatie-onrust: een kwalitatief onderzoek naar de ontslagbeleving van patiënten na ontslag uit een Vlaams ziekenhuis [Post-hospitalization restlessness: A qualitative study of the experience of hospital discharge by patients discharged from a Flemish hospital]. *Verpleegkunde. Nederlands-Vlaams tijdschrift voor verpleegkundigen*, *5*(1), 4–14.

Velle, K. (1988). Kerk, geneeskunde en gezondheidszorg in de 19de en het begin van de 20ste eeuw [Church, medicine and health care in the 19th and the early 20th Century]. In J. Depuydt et al. (Eds.), *Het verbond der Verzorgingsinstellingen 1938–1988* [The Association of Health Care Organizations 1938–1988], Leuven: KADOC, pp. 12–25.

Verhaeghe, S. (2007). *De confrontatie met traumatisch coma: Een onderzoek naar de beleving van familieleden* [The confrontation with traumatic coma: An investigation into the experiences of family members]. PhD thesis, Ghent University.

Verhaeghe, S., Defloor, T., van Zuuren, F., Duijnstee, M., & Grypdonck, M. (2005). The needs and experiences of family members of adult patients in an intensive care unit: A review of the literature. *Journal of Clinical Nursing*, *14*(4), 501–509.

Verhaeghe, S. T., van Zuuren, F. J., Defloor, T., Duijnstee, M. S., & Grypdonck, M. H. (2007a). How does information influence hope in family members of traumatic coma patients in intensive care unit? *Journal of Clinical Nursing*, *16*(8), 1488–1497.

Verhaeghe, S. T., van Zuuren, F. J., Defloor, T., Duijnstee, M. S., & Grypdonck, M. H. (2007b). The process and the meaning of hope for family members of traumatic coma patients in intensive care. *Qualitative Health Research*, *17*(6), 730–743.

Verhaeghe, S. T., van Zuuren, F. J., Grypdonck, M. H., Duijnstee, M. S., & Defloor, T. (2010a). The focus of family members' functioning in the acute phase of traumatic coma: Part one: The initial battle and protecting life. *Journal of Clinical Nursing*, *19*(3–4), 574–582.

Verhaeghe, S. T., van Zuuren, F. J., Grypdonck, M. H., Duijnstee, M. S., & Defloor, T. (2010b). The focus of family members' functioning in the acute phase of traumatic coma: Part two: Protecting from suffering and protecting what remains to rebuild life. *Journal of Clinical Nursing*, *19*(3–4), 583–589.

Verkooijen, H. E. C. (2006). *Ondersteuning, Eigen Regievoering & Vraaggestuurde Zorg* [Support, self-management and demand-based care]. PhD thesis, Universiteit voor Humanistiek Verkooijen & Beima, Jutrijp.

Vervoort, S. C. J. M. (2010). Adherence to HAART. A study of patients' perspectives and HIV nurse consultants' strategies. PhD thesis, Utrecht University.

Vervoort, S. C., Borleffs, J. C., Hoepelman, A. I., & Grypdonck, M. H. (2007). Adherence in antiretroviral therapy: A review of qualitative studies. *AIDS, 21*(3), 271–281.

Vervoort, S. C., Grypdonck, M. H., De Grauwe, A., Hoepelman, A. I., & Borleffs, J. C. (2009). Adherence to HAART: Processes explaining adherence behavior in acceptors and non-acceptors. *AIDS Care, 21*(4), 431–438.

Vervoort, S. C., Grypdonck, M. H., Dijkstra, B. M., Hazelzet, F. E., Fledderus, B., Borleffs, J. C., & Hoepelman, A. I. (2010). Strategies to promote adherence to antiretroviral therapy applied by Dutch HIV nurse consultants: A descriptive qualitative study. *Journal of the Association of Nurses in AIDS Care, 21*(6), 489–502.

Voorhorst, W. M. J., Grypdonck, M., & Duijnstee, M. H. S. (2001). Mantelzorgers van chronische zieken in zicht? De opvattingen van wijkverpleegkundigen over hun rol ten aanzien van de ondersteuning van primaire verzorgers [Family carers of chronically ill in sight? Views of home care nurses on their role in supporting primary family carers]. *Verpleegkunde. Nederlands-Vlaams wetenschappelijk tijdschrift voor verpleegkundigen, 15*(3), 155–165.

Wester, F. (1987). *Strategieën voor kwalitatief onderzoek* [Strategies for qualitative research]. Muiderberg: Countinho.

Yamazaki, H., Slingsby, B. T., Takahashi, M., Hayashi, Y., Sugimori, H., & Nakayama, T. (2009). Characteristics of qualitative studies in influential journals of general medicine: A critical review. *Bioscience Trends, 3*(6), 202–209.

42

Qualitative nursing research in Korea

Kyung Rim Shin, Miyoung Kim, and Seung Eun Chung

Since the early 1990s, qualitative research methods have been actively adopted in nursing research. Qualitative nursing research in Korea not only has significantly increased in number, but also a wide range of methodological approaches have been developed. This research method has contributed greatly in terms of nursing research as well as nursing theory, nursing practice and nursing education. It is worthwhile analyzing and examining the research papers that have been previously conducted in order to determine their usefulness or value. Thus, this chapter briefly examines the historical background of qualitative nursing research in Korea for the last 20 years, and analyzes the trends. This will enable us to identify the degree to which qualitative research has contributed to nursing in Korea, and to suggest new qualitative research directions so as to develop a knowledge system of nursing science.

Historical background

Since 1970s, nursing scholars had begun to become interested in qualitative nursing research as they pointed out the overall problems of quantitative research methods applied to natural sciences. In the 1980s, a wider approach to studying various nursing phenomena was accepted. From the mid-1980s, several nursing schools in Korea started a new educational course on qualitative research for Master's and doctoral degree-seeking students. At the time, quantitative nursing research was dominant, so the graduate students who took the course were surprised by this new approach and it encouraged them to actually conduct qualitative research. Graduate students took other relevant courses including cultural anthropology, philosophy and sociology, to acquire philosophical and methodological knowledge of research in these disciplines. The educational materials and references used for the course were mainly books and theses published by foreign qualitative researchers.

Since 1990, the nursing professors teaching qualitative research have written Korean textbooks for students to promote their understanding of this approach. Some of the books released at the time included *Nursing and Korean Culture* (Choi, 1992) and *Qualitative Nursing Research* (Choi, 1993). Along with this effort, several professors published translated versions of books overseas. The nursing professors, researchers and graduate students who were interested in qualitative research published a few qualitative nursing research papers. Most of the initial qualitative research adopted an ethnographic approach targeting mostly seniors and women and were theses on nursing in Korea, investigations on health and diseases and various responses by patients on diseases (Cho, 1992; Chung, 1990; Kim, 1987; Kim, 1993; Lee, 1990; Lee, 1993). Since 2000, qualitative nurse researchers in Korea have been publishing qualitative research at domestic and/or overseas symposia and in renowned academic journals. Graduate students are adopting qualitative research methods in their Master's or doctoral dissertations.

Meanwhile, professors, researchers and graduate students from various fields who became interested in qualitative research wanted to organize support groups to study, discuss and share information. To do so, Professor Kyung Rim Shin from the Division of Health Science, Ewha Womans University, took the main role. She formed a small yet important group called the "Korea Qualitative Research Group" in the Division of Health Science, Ewha Womans University, in February 1998. After two years after its establishment in 2000, this group was officially authorized as the "Korea Center for Qualitative Methodology (KCQM)," a representative website in Asia, which is linked to the "International Institute for Qualitative Methodology (IIQM)" in the University of Alberta, Canada. KCQM is firmly established as a qualitative research group that incorporates various academic fields including pedagogy, psychology, sociology and social welfare. KCQM officially conducts a "qualitative research colloquium," a small group of professors, researchers and graduate students interested in qualitative research who freely attend it to listen to lectures on qualitative research and share research experiences with one another. This is held on the second Friday of every month.

In addition, KCQM invites eminent qualitative researchers from all over the world every year and holds a large-scale workshop. Many Korean qualitative researchers are given opportunities to directly experience the group work by absorbing theoretical background and practical approaches regarding qualitative research. Some of the scholars invited to Korea and their workshop topics were as follows: Janice Morse (1998, 2005) for ethnography and mixed methods design; Max van Manen (1999) for phenomenology; Juliet Corbin (2000, 2004, 2007) for grounded theory and qualitative analysis; Steiner Kvale (2001) for interview methods; Arthur Frank (2001) for narrative inquiry; Phyllis Noerager Stern (2002) for grounded theory; Marilyn Mardiros (2002) for participatory action research; Amedeo Peter Giorgi (2003, 2004) for descriptive phenomenological method; Carol Jillings (2006) for meta-study of qualitative research; Martha Ann Carey (2008) for focus group research; Maria Mayan (2009) for introduction to the essential of qualitative inquiry; and Julianne Cheek (2010) for current issues in qualitative research. Furthermore, KCQM held the 7th and 13th Qualitative Health Research Conferences in 2001, 2007, and the 1st Global Congress for Qualitative Health Research in 2011, standing proudly as an international academic group, and plays a key role in exchanging qualitative research for qualitative researchers including nursing scholars in Korea and abroad.

Qualitative research methods

For the years from 1991 to 2010, two major academic journals in Korea were chosen to extract qualitative research papers in order to analyze the qualitative nursing research that had been published. The first journal is the *Journal of Korean Academy of Nursing* (hereinafter referred to as *JKAN*), an official academic journal of the Korean Society of Nursing Science, which is an academic research group composed of Korean nursing scholars. *JKAN* is an academic journal that publishes creative research on nursing theory, practice and education, issued bi-monthly for six times a year since 1970. The qualitative research studies included since 1991 were the target for this analysis. The second journal is the *Journal of Qualitative Research* (hereinafter referred to as *JQR*), an official academic journal of the Academy of Qualitative Research and the KCQM. *JQR* is an academic journal that publishes multidisciplinary qualitative studies on theory, practice and education of nursing, medicine, health science, social welfare and pedagogy, which has been published twice a year since 2000.

We selected 124 research papers from *JKAN* that informed major nursing research in Korea and 117 papers from *JQR* that focused on multidisciplinary approaches to qualitative research, 241 papers in total. We analyzed the qualitative nursing research studies to identify the trends and to suggest future research directions. The objective framework applied for analyses included annual number of research studies, type of research, number of keywords and classification, data analysis by methodology and author, research participants and research evaluation.

Number of qualitative research publications by year

Since the characteristics of each academic journal (*JKAN* and *JQR*) differ, the respective number of issues per year was examined. *JKAN* was published 3 times in 1991, 4 times in 1992–1998, 6 times in 1999, 7 times 2000–2002, 8 times in 2003–2006, 7 times in 2007 and 6 times in 2008–2010. For the past 20 years, 1,832 articles in total were published, approximately 28–150 articles per year, and 124 studies out of the total articles were on qualitative research, which accounted for only 6.78%, a fairly small percentage when compared to that of quantitative research. Shin, Sung, Jeong, and Kim (2008) analyzed the doctoral dissertations from six nursing schools in Korea from 2000 to 2006, and discovered that qualitative research among all theses accounted for 18%. It is very encouraging that the number of qualitative research studies in nursing for doctoral dissertations has increased since 2000. However, it is difficult to publish qualitative doctoral dissertations in academic journals because in general the number of pages is limited to 20 pages for it to be included in such journals. Thus, it is believed that only a few dissertations are included in journals as it is insufficient to describe the procedures and results of qualitative research in depth.

JQR has been published 2 times per year since 2000, and for the past 20 years about 12~20 articles were published annually. In total 149 articles were published and 117 papers out of the total articles were on nursing research which accounted for 78.5%. This journal only publishes qualitative research, so it reflects the interest of Korean nursing scholars in qualitative research. In examining these two different journals (Figure 42.1), qualitative nursing research has definitely increased since 2000 when compared to quantitative research. It is expected to steadily increase in the future.

Type of research

As shown in Figure 42.2, research studies were classified into general theses, dissertations and funded theses. There are 169 general theses which accounted for 70.1% of the total, 6 Master's dissertations and 20 doctoral dissertations which accounted for 10.8% of the total, and 46 theses that were funded by universities and academic research foundations which accounted for 19.1%. When we supervise dissertations written by graduate students, there is pressure that the qualitative dissertations must be carried out within the limited period. There are often cases in which the graduate students complain that it is difficult to choose the right qualitative methodology depending on the research topic and they become overwhelmed. It is important to encourage students to complete lectures on various approaches to qualitative research during their Master's/doctoral degree courses and actively participate in domestic/international symposiums, seminars or workshops to be trained as qualitative researchers. The number of funded quantitative research studies accounted for 35% of the total (Choi et al., 2000), which is much more than that of qualitative research.

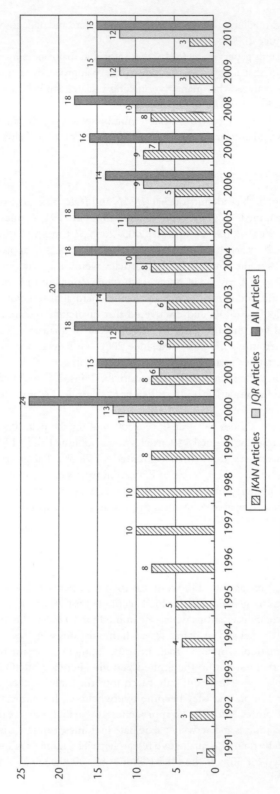

Figure 42.1 Qualitative research published in *JKAN* and *JQR*

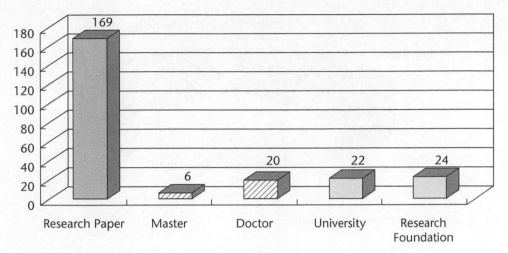

Figure 42.2 Type of research undertaken

When looking into the researchers involved in the theses and dissertations, 106 papers were conducted individually (44%) and 135 papers (56%) were with joint researchers composed of 2–17 researchers.

Number of keywords and classification

In total, 684 keywords were included in 241 articles, and 2.8 keywords on average per thesis. Academic journals specify the number of research-relevant keywords that can be used, which is 5, and this is more than that which appeared in the articles. Keywords should be registered in MeSH for all nursing research studies, yet since 2000 there are many researchers who include keywords driven from the concepts suggested in the research titles. Since keywords imply significant meanings for researchers in searching for previously conducted studies, it is desirable to suggest up to five keywords registered in MeSH from now on.

Keywords were classified into human, health, nursing and environment, which are the meta-paradigm of the science of nursing, and as a result of this analysis, 212 keywords (31.0%) were related to health/diseases followed by 170 human-related keywords (24.9%). This analysis revealed 93 nursing-related keywords (13.6%) and 23 environment-related keywords (3.4%) (Figure 42.3).

Keywords that appeared most often were health/diseases-related words that suggested physical, psychological, social and spiritual health and various disease-related experiences. In particular, keywords on physical aspects mainly dealt with menopause, aging, physical changes and crises which are the potential health problems generated during the life stages. Also, it is anticipated that qualitative research on specific diseases experienced by patients is to be actively conducted.

Human-related keywords included research participants, such as infants, teenagers, adults and seniors categorized by human growth and development cycle, and also included patients' family and nurses. This indicated that research on patients' experiences is inadequate when compared to research on experiences of people in general or nurses.

Nursing-related keywords included not only nursing practice but also nursing intervention, administration and education-related terms. Some of the nursing research studies took into account interpersonal relations, conflicts, identity, nursing expertise and clinical training issues rather than the nursing practice itself.

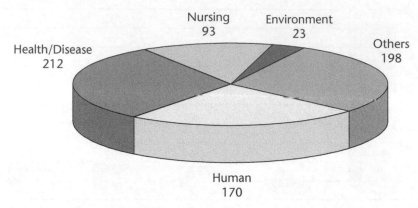

Figure 42.3 Keywords found in research

Environment-related keywords were used the least frequently and included hospital, nursing facility; intensive care unit, neonate room; doctor-less farm villages, forest; mainstream society for women, culture; and Internet. There are very few nursing environment-related keywords when compared to health/disease, human, and nursing keywords. Therefore, it is expected that nurse researchers focus on the patient's environment.

Finally, the research-related keywords excluded from the meta-paradigm of the science of nursing accounted for the majority of keywords, and some of those keywords included qualitative research, approaches (phenomenology, grounded theory, ethnography, etc.) and experience, 198 keywords (28.9%) in total.

Data analysis by methodology and author

One hundred and thirteen studies (46.9%) using the phenomenological method out of 241 research articles in total accounted for the majority of studies, followed by 56 grounded theory research studies (23.2%), 47 descriptive qualitative research (19.5%) and 15 ethnographies (6.2%). Other research included focus groups, narrative, behavioral study and conversation analysis (Table 42.1). Unlike the *Qualitative Health Research*, an international academic journal that carries qualitative research articles that do not propose specific research methods, specific research methods such as phenomenology, grounded theory and ethnography are suggested for qualitative researchers in Korea (Shin, Kim, & Chung, 2009).

Regarding phenomenological research methods, studies conducted using Colaizzi's method were the most frequent, followed by van Manen, Giorgi, and van Kaam. As described in the historical background, *KCQM* invited well-known scholars for systematic learning based on qualitative research so that qualitative researchers are given the opportunity to listen to lectures and to apply this knowledge for practical use. Especially, van Manen and Giorgi visited Korea to discuss phenomenological research methods at workshops and international symposia. They organized lectures on practical, concrete research and analysis methods for professors, graduate students and researchers who were greatly interested in phenomenology and provided opportunities for group work as well. One of the representative scholars in the field of grounded theory, Corbin has also conducted a workshop in Korea. In addition to the scholars mentioned above, many others have visited Korea for lectures and workshops targeting qualitative research. Although there have been learning opportunities on various research methods and strategies organized by these prominent scholars, research using ethnography, focus groups and narratives are less frequently used than those using phenomenology or grounded theory.

Table 42.1 Methods of data analysis

Methods		Number of articles (%)
Phenomenology	van Kaam	6 (2.5)
	van Manen	28 (11.6)
	Colaizzi	47 (19.5)
	Giorgi	19 (7.9)
	Others	13 (5.4)
Grounded theory	Strauss and Corbin	55 (22.8)
	Glaser and Strauss	1 (0.4)
Ethnography	Spradley	15 (6.2)
Focus group		4 (1.7)
Narrative analysis		4 (1.7)
Action research		1 (0.4)
Conversation analysis		1 (0.4)
Qualitative research		47 (19.5)

There was only one qualitative research study conducted with a computer program (NUDIST 4.0) for the purpose of data analysis. It is still unfamiliar for Korean qualitative researchers to use computer programs to analyze qualitative research data. Most of the existing programs are developed in English, so if the raw data in Korean were collected targeting Koreans, it may be very difficult to input such data into the program.

Research participants

Excluding the review articles from the total research reviewed, 228 research studies targeted 78 healthy people (34.2%), which account for the most, followed by 48 patients (21.0%), 42 nurses (18.4%), 31 family members (13.6%), 20 nursing students (8.8%) and 9 others (essays, research papers and etc) (3.9%) (Figure 42.4). The sum of healthy people and patients accounted for the majority of participants, and there were more healthy people than patients as subjects of the research because at the initial stage of qualitative research, the researchers were more easily able to access healthy individuals.

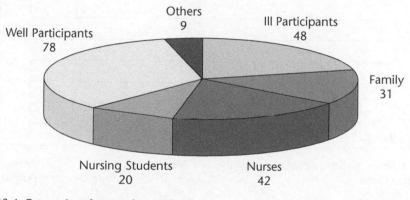

Others
9

Ill Participants
48

Well Participants
78

Family
31

Nursing Students
20

Nurses
42

Figure 42.4 Categories of research participants

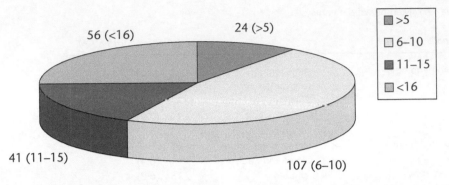

Figure 42.5 Number of research participants

In the qualitative studies reviewed, 6–10 research participants per thesis accounted for 46.2%, representing the highest percentage (Figure 42.5). The number of qualitative research participants is not predetermined but instead the number is determined by appropriateness and sufficiency during data collection process (Morse & Field, 1995).

Research evaluation

Reliability and validity checks are extremely important for qualitative research evaluation. The evaluation criteria suggested by Lincoln and Guba were applied to most research studies (Figure 42.6). Some of the other criteria suggested by Sandelowski, Giorgi, Morse, and others were also used in the research studies. Many research studies did not suggest clear evaluation criteria, yet they did imply that an overall evaluation process had been conducted between researchers, or experts and participants when describing the research procedure. Checking the reliability and validity is the basis for systematic research and is essential for the development of nursing knowledge (Hinshaw, 1989).

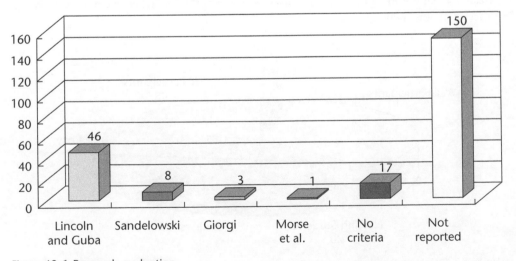

Figure 42.6 Research evaluation

Specific contributions

Qualitative research is a means to understand and study the human issues as individuals or in groups. The qualitative nurse researchers in Korea have studied nursing phenomena for the past 20 years and steadily published qualitative research papers. We would like to examine the contribution of published qualitative research to the field of nursing science, and its implications.

QHR is a global journal, publishing research papers on a wide range of fields using qualitative research methods. QHR publishes research on diseases, analysis, health and health pursuing behaviors, nurses' experiences, socio-cultural organization on health management and policy as well as conceptual, theoretical, methodological and ethical issues in terms of qualitative research. Shin, Kim, and Chung (2009) compared and analyzed the qualitative research published in QHR and JQR in terms of data analysis types and processes based on the research methodology and scholars. When it comes to the data analysis type per research methodology and scholar, 29% of the research studies included in the QHR were descriptive qualitative research which accounted for the most studies, followed by grounded theory (23%), phenomenology (14%) and ethnography (8%). Some of the other types included in order: narrative inquiry, content analysis, focus group, meta-synthesis, case study, participatory research, mixed methods, behavioral research, constructive approach, and anthropological study.

The research included in JQR was mostly studies using a phenomenological approach, followed by grounded theory, descriptive qualitative research, ethnography, focus group, narrative, behavioral research and conversation analysis. The research articles published in QHR are mostly descriptive qualitative researches that did not use specific methods, while specific research methodology were used in those studies published in JQR. Furthermore, there were no meta-syntheses, mixed methods, constructive or anthropological approaches published in JQR. In other words, unlike the research methodologies used in qualitative research studies in QHR, there were less varied approaches used in Korea. Thus, it is desirable to conduct research projects using various qualitative research methods depending on the research topic(s).

As part of this process, we would like to conduct nursing research based on a mixed methods design. It is desirable to use two types of methods rather than one in order to understand complicated phenomena on human experiences and behavioral responses. In particular, research using mixed methods is very useful in fields related to nursing, health service, health promotion, education, policy and evaluation. Also, mixed methods are suitable for measuring changes such as aging or for building mutual interaction among individuals, communication and nursing theory. Researchers should be flexible in selecting methodologies to conduct research based on mixed methods designs. That is, researchers should have abundant experiences and knowledge with both qualitative and quantitative research. The researchers should be fully aware of the project's theoretical drive or conceptual direction. The qualitative or quantitative drive shall be determined by the research questions. In other words, when you are to study and describe a certain phenomenon, an inductive research should be the project's core component, whereas a deductive research should be the core component when you are focusing on theoretical verification. Moreover, researchers should perform another research strategy which is either qualitative or quantitative as a supplemental component to acquire supplementary information. The core component and the supplemental component can be conducted simultaneously/ concurrently or sequentially. In accordance with a wide range of combinations, there are eight types of mixed method designs (Morse & Niehaus, 2009). Nursing research using mixed methods in Korea is in its initial stage, so it is necessary to examine and study the published research papers using these various approaches. If mixed methods studies are carried out with interesting research topics regarding diverse yet complicated nursing phenomena, there may be more funding opportunities, contributing to expanding nursing knowledge.

Since the early 1990s, qualitative research has been actively accepted. It is becoming more and more popular. Considering the usefulness of accumulated qualitative data, this is now the time to look into secondary analysis. The secondary analysis of qualitative data generates concepts that were not dealt within the primary analysis, having an advantage of building nursing knowledge. In other words, secondary analysis is intended to draw out scientific results from existing data to solve new questions, develop theories through advanced analysis and expand concepts. Furthermore, secondary analysis can be carried out without spending too much time, effort and cost for data collection, utilizing the existing qualitative data as much as possible. It provides an opportunity to analyze and interpret the data without being restricted to primary data yet following new intuition. However, for the secondary analysis to be fully scientific and valid, the following matters should be considered: whether it corresponds to the primary research question(s); whether there are enough data; whether any inquiry on primary data can be clearly answered by primary researchers; and whether ethical issues can be resolved without consent from research participants for secondary analysis (Lee, 2004; Thorne, 1998; Yi, 2003). Thus, by conducting qualitative research using secondary analysis based on the qualitative data accumulated for the past 20 years, the nursing knowledge system of Korea can be built.

Future directions

Based on the analysis results, we would like to propose some future research directions by limiting it to research evaluation and qualitative research funding. First of all, research evaluation is a fundamental aspect of research quality and development. As a result of analyzing two journals the qualitative studies that did not suggest clear evaluation criteria accounted for 66%, exceeding the majority. This trend is similar to the context that major aspects of research designs have not been reported from the systematic investigation of qualitative research (Mills, Jadad, Ross, & Wilson, 2005). However, qualitative research explores complicated phenomena that cannot be explained using a quantitative design. Thus, insufficient design and inappropriate reports may lead to unsuitable application of qualitative research including decision-making, health care, health policy and future research (Tong, Sainsbury, & Craig, 2007). Recently, criteria or checklists on qualitative research have been suggested as a guideline for qualitative research to assist researchers, so that they will not miss any critical aspects. Yet this requires attention as the reflexivity of researchers may be overlooked when conforming to this criteria.

Next is the necessity of various strategies to obtain funding for qualitative researches. It is still a challenge for many researchers to achieve funding for qualitative research, yet it is also true that evaluators of many organizations actually granting research funds are now admitting the potential value of qualitative research. Therefore, it is necessary for researchers to first identify which qualitative research has been funded up to now. It has been pointed out that qualitative researchers have not comprehensively dealt with literature reviews in their qualitative research proposals. It is important for qualitative researchers to explore a wide range of literature since advance knowledge to check the research topics, methods and participants are required for funding. Moreover, although originality and creativity of a research topic are critical for qualitative research, the research question that guides such topic should also be clear. Who is conducting the research, and how and why such research is conducted should be clearly described. It is recommended to conduct a case study, if necessary, to suggest a concrete, clear research question. It is also important to acknowledge the academic contribution of research results and limitations, and clearly identify them.

References

Carey, M. A. (2008). Basic and beyond for focus group. Workshop conducted at qualitative research workshop of the Korea Center for Qualitative Methodology, Seoul, Korea.

Cheek, J. (2010). Current issues in qualitative research: Challenging the idea of the deceptive simplicity of qualitative research. Workshop conducted at qualitative research workshop of the Korea Center for Qualitative Methodology, Seoul, Korea.

Cho, M. O. (1992). An ethnographic study of caring for the elderly in a traditional community. Unpublished doctoral dissertation, Ewha Womans University, Seoul.

Choi, K. S., Song, M. S., Hwant, A. R., Kim, K. H., Chung, M. S., Shin, S. R., & Kim, N. C. (2000). The trends of nursing research in the *Journal of the Korean Academy of Nursing*. *Journal of Korean Academy of Nursing*, *30*(5), 1270–1218.

Choi, Y. H. (1992). *Nursing and Korean culture*. Seoul: Soo Moon Sa.

Choi, Y. H. (1993). *Qualitative nursing research*. Seoul: Soo Moon Sa.

Corbin, J. (2000). Grounded theory. Workshop conducted at qualitative research workshop of the Korea Center for Qualitative Methodology, Seoul, Korea.

Corbin, J. (2004). Grounded theory: Qualitative analysis. Workshop conducted at qualitative research workshop of the Korea Center for Qualitative Methodology, Seoul, Korea.

Corbin, J. (2007). Advanced workshop in qualitative analysis: How to go from description to theorizing. Workshop conducted at qualitative research workshop of the Korea Center for Qualitative Methodology, Seoul, Korea.

Chung, S. E. (1990). Experience of powerlessness among patients with spinal cord injury: A phenomenological study. Unpublished Master's dissertation, Ewha Womans University, Seoul.

Frank, A. (2001). Narrative inquiry. Workshop conducted at qualitative research workshop of the Korea Center for Qualitative Methodology, Seoul, Korea.

Giorgi, A. (1997). The theory, practice, and evaluation of the phenomenology method as a qualitative research. *Journal of Phenomenological Psychology*, *28*(2), 235–261.

Giorgi, A. P. (2003). Descriptive phenomenological method. Workshop conducted at qualitative research workshop of the Korea Center for Qualitative Methodology, Seoul, Korea.

Giorgi, A. P. (2004). Advanced workshop on descriptive phenomenological method. Workshop conducted at qualitative research workshop of the Korea Center for Qualitative Methodology, Seoul, Korea.

Hinshaw, A. S. (1989). *Nursing science: The challenge to develop knowledge*. Philadelphia, PA: Williams and Wilkins Publishing Co.

Jillings, C. (2006). Meta-study of qualitative research: Meta-analysis and meta-synthesis. Workshop conducted at qualitative research workshop of the Korea Center for Qualitative Methodology, Seoul, Korea.

Kim, N. S. (1987). The concepts of illness of rural Korean people. Unpublished Master's dissertation, Ewha Womans University, Seoul.

Kim, N. S. (1993). A study of woman's caring as a phenomenon of gender. Unpublished doctoral dissertation, Ewha Womans University, Seoul.

Kvale, S. (2001). Data collection for qualitative research: Interview method. Workshop conducted at qualitative research workshop of the Korea Center for Qualitative Methodology, Seoul, Korea.

Lee, M. S. (1990). Phenomenological nursing study on the critical ill patients' feeling of hopelessness. Unpublished Master's dissertation, Ewha Womans University, Seoul.

Lee, M. S. (2004). Secondary analysis: focusing on qualitative research. *Journal of Korean Academy of Nursing*, *34*(1), 35–44.

Lee, Y. H. (1993). Health lifestyle of Korean elders. Unpublished doctoral dissertation, Ewha Womans University, Seoul.

Lincoln, Y. S., & Guba, E. G. (1985). *Naturalistic inquiry*. Newbury Park, CA: Sage Publications.

Mardiros, M. (2002). Qualitative research workshop: Participatory action research. Workshop conducted at qualitative research workshop of the Korea Center for Qualitative Methodology, Seoul, Korea.

Mayan, M. (2009). Introduction to the essentials of qualitative inquiry. Workshop conducted at qualitative research workshop of the Korea Center for Qualitative Methodology, Seoul, Korea.

Mills, E., Jadad, A. R., Ross, C., & Wilson, K. (2005). Systematic review of qualitative studies exploring parental beliefs and attitudes toward childhood vaccination identified common barriers to vaccination. *Journal of Clinical Epidemiology*, *58*, 1081–1088.

Morse, J. M. (1998). Qualitative research methodology. Workshop conducted at qualitative research workshop of the Korea Center for Qualitative Methodology, Seoul, Korea.

Morse, J. M. (2005). Ethnography and issues in design. Workshop conducted at qualitative research workshop of the Korea Center for Qualitative Methodology, Seoul, Korea.

Morse, J. M., & Field, P. A. (1995). *Qualitative research methods for health professionals* (2nd ed.). London: Chapman & Hall.

Morse, J. M., Hutchinson, S., & Penrod, J. (1998). From theory to practice: The development of assessment guides from qualitatively derived theory. *Qualitative Health Research, 8*, 329–340.

Morse, J. M., & Niehaus, L. (2009). *Mixed method design: Principles and procedures*. CA: Left Coast Press.

Shin, H., Sung, K. M., Jeong, S. H., & Kim D. R. (2008). Trends of doctoral dissertations in nursing science: focused on studies submitted since 2000. *Journal of Korean Academy of Nursing, 38*(1), 74–82.

Shin, K. R., Kim, M. Y., & Chung, S. E. (2009). Methods and strategies utilized in published qualitative research. *Qualitative Health Research, 19*(6), 850–858.

Stern, P. N. (2002). Grounded theory. Workshop conducted at qualitative research workshop of the Korea Center for Qualitative Methodology, Seoul, Korea.

Thorne, S. (1998). Ethical and representational issues in qualitative secondary analysis. *Qualitative Health Research, 8*(4), 547–555.

Tong, A., Sainsbury, P., & Craig, J. (2007). Consolidated criteria for reporting qualitative research (COREQ): A 32-item checklist for interviews and focus groups. *International Journal for Quality in Health Care, 19*(6), 349–357.

Van Manen, M. (1999). Interpretative phenomenology. Workshop conducted at qualitative research workshop of the Korea Center for Qualitative Methodology, Seoul, Korea.

Yi. M. (2003). Secondary analysis of qualitative data: Methodological issues and implications. *Nursing Inquiry, 12*(1), 82–96.

Appendix: journal articles

Journal of Korean Academy of Nursing

Ahn, Y. H., Kim, D. R., Seo, B. N., Lee, K. E., Lee, E. H., & Yim, E. S. (2002). Clinical nurses' lived experience of interpersonal relations in the ward setting of the hospital. *Journal of Korean Academy of Nursing, 32*(3), 295–304.

Bai, J. L. (1996). The experience of the postpartum depression: A grounded theory approach. *Journal of Korean Academy of Nursing, 26*(1), 10–126.

Byeon, Y. S., & Kim, M. (2008). Re-employment experience of nurses who have left the profession. *Journal of Korean Academy of Nursing, 38*(5), 768–778.

Cha, J., & Kim, S. (2009). Healing effects of the forest experience on alcoholics. *Journal of Korean Academy of Nursing, 39*(3), 338–348.

Cho, Y. S. (1994). A phenomenological study on the stresses and the experiences of pregnant women and postpartum mothers who had immigrated to the United States. *Journal of Korean Academy of Nursing, 24*(3), 432–447.

Cho, Y. S., Kim, S., & Martinson, I. (1992). The experience of parents whose child is dying with cancer. *Journal of Korean Academy of Nursing, 22*(4), 491–505.

Choi, K., & Eun, Y. (2000). A theory construction on the care experience for spouses of patients with chronic illness. *Journal of Korean Academy of Nursing, 30*(1), 122–136.

Choi, M. H. (1998). Caring experience of mothers with IDDM children. *Journal of Korean Academy of Nursing, 28*(1), 81–92.

Choi, N. (2005). Narrative analysis on survivor's experience of Daegu subway fire disaster: The hypothetical suggestions for disaster nursing practice. *Journal of Korean Academy of Nursing, 35*(2), 407–418.

Chung, H. K. (2001). A phenomenological approach to high school students' smoking experiencing. *Journal of Korean Academy of Nursing, 31*(4), 610–618.

Chung, H. S. (1996). Menstrual experience of adolescent girls. *Journal of Korean Academy of Nursing, 26*(2), 257–270.

Gong, S. J. (2004). Health as expanding consciousness: Based on the experiences of victims of sexual violence. *Journal of Korean Academy of Nursing, 34*(6), 913–923.

Han, K. J. (1991). A phenomenological study on mother–infant interacting behavior patterns related to newborn infant feeding in Korea. *Journal of Korean Academy of Nursing, 21*(1), 89–116.

Han, K. J., Choe, M. A., Kang, H. J., Park, S. H., Kim, Y. M., Kim, S. G., Kwon, W. K., & Ahn, H. Y. (1996). Content analysis of the nursing interventions and telephone calls to the pediatric nursing unit. *Journal of Korean Academy of Nursing, 26*(3), 515–530.

Han, K. S., & Cho, J. Y. (1999). A study on the experience of fundamental nursing practice. *Journal of Korean Academy of Nursing, 29*(2), 293–303.

Han, Y. R., & Kim, Y. H. (2004). Grounded theory approach to health care of older adults at a doctorless farm village. *Journal of Korean Academy of Nursing, 34*(5), 771–780.

Hong, S. W., & Son, H. M. (2007). Family caregivers' experiences utilizing a nursing home for their elderly family members. *Journal of Korean Academy of Nursing, 37*(5), 724–735.

Hong, Y. H., Cho, M. O., & Tae, Y. S. (2005). An ethnographic study on eating styles of adult diabetics in Korea. *Journal of Korean Academy of Nursing, 35*(2), 313–322.

Hur, H. K. (1997). An exploration of the life experiences of patients with chronic pain: Women with rheumatoid arthritis. *Journal of Korean Academy of Nursing, 27*(1), 13–25.

Hur, H. K., Choi, S. S., Ahn, Y. H., Lim, Y. M., Shin, Y. H., Park, S. M., Kim, G. Y., Song, H. Y., & Kim, K. K. (2004). Content analysis of the experience of preceptors in clinical education for senior student nurses. *Journal of Korean Academy of Nursing, 34*(5), 859–868.

Hwang, H. Y. (2000). Caring related to health in Korea: Ethnography-centered Wichon-ri, Kangwon-do . *Journal of Korean Academy of Nursing, 30*(1), 194–201.

Hwang, S. Y., & Jang, K. S. (2005). Perception about problem-based learning in reflective journals among undergraduate nursing students. *Journal of Korean Academy of Nursing, 35*(1), 65–76.

Im, E. O. (1999). Neglecting and ignoring menopause within a gendered multiple transitional context: Low income Korean immigrant women. *Journal of Korean Academy of Nursing, 29*(6), 1336–1354.

Jo, K. H., & Han, H. J. (2001). Nurses' painful experiences through terminal patient. *Journal of Korean Academy of Nursing, 31*(6), 1055–1066.

Jo, K. H., & Kim, Y. K. (2008). A phenomenological study on the restoration experience for suicide ideation of Korean elders. *Journal of Korean Academy of Nursing, 38*(2), 258–269.

Jo, K. H., Sung, K. W., & Kim, Y. K. (2008). A phenomenological study on the experience of hurt and forgiveness of clinical nurses in Korea after loss of employment. *Journal of Korean Academy of Nursing, 38*(4), 561–572.

Jung, M. S., Choi, H. W., & Li, D. M. (2010). Analysis of nursing-related content portrayed in middle and high school textbooks under the national common basic curriculum in Korea. *Journal of Korean Academy of Nursing, 40*(1), 33–42.

Kang, H. S., Cho, K. J., Choe, N. H., & Kim, W. O. (2002). Reconstruction of professional identity in clinical nurses. *Journal of Korean Academy of Nursing, 32*(4), 470–481.

Kang, H. S., Koh, J. E., & Suh, Y. O. (2000). Model construction of sexual adjustment of patients with spinal cord injury. *Journal of Korean Academy of Nursing, 30*(4), 1018–1034.

Kang, S. R. (2007). The experiences of job stress on head nurses in general hospitals. *Journal of Korean Academy of Nursing, 37*(4), 501–509.

Kang, S. Y. (2008). The lived experience of struggling against illness for patients with amyotrophic lateral sclerosis. *Journal of Korean Academy of Nursing, 38*(6), 802-812.

Kim, A. K. (1998). The study of the process of smoking cessation in adults. *Journal of Korean Academy of Nursing, 28*(2), 319–328.

Kim, A. K. (2003). Experience in nausea and vomiting of pregnancy (NVP) in women: Grounded theory approach. *Journal of Korean Academy of Nursing, 33*(7), 94–953.

Kim, B. H., Kim, K. J., Park, I. S., Lee, K. J., Kim, J. K., Hong, J. J., Lee, M. W., Kim, Y. H., Yoo, I. Y., & Lee, H. Y. (1999). A comparison of phenomenological research methodology: Focused on Giorgi, Colaizzi, Van Kaam methods. *Journal of Korean Academy of Nursing, 29*(6), 1208–1220.

Kim, B. S., Ryu, E. J., Kim, K. H., Chung, H. K., Song, M. S., & Choi, K. S. (1999). A study on the experience of nurses' socialization process in the hospital setting. *Journal of Korean Academy of Nursing, 29*(2), 393–404.

Kim, J. H., Yoo, I. S., & Kim, M. H. (1995). The phenomenological study of kidney donors' experiences. *Journal of Korean Academy of Nursing, 25*(2), 222–243.

Kim, J. S. (2006). Experiences of being tied with drugs in the elderly women in the community. *Journal of Korean Academy of Nursing, 36*(7), 1215–1223.

Kim, K. B., & Lee, K. H. (1998). Ethnography of caring experience for the senile dementia. *Journal of Korean Academy of Nursing, 28*(4), 1047–1059.

Kim, K. B., & Lee, K. H. (2000). The adolescents' experience in drug abuse. *Journal of Korean Academy of Nursing, 30*(4), 917–931.

Kim, K. B., Yoo, J. H., & Lee, E. J. (2002). The experiences of the middle-aged women's crisis. *Journal of Korean Academy of Nursing, 32*(3), 305–316.

Kim, K. H. (1998). A study on the adolescent's experiences in domestic violence. *Journal of Korean Academy of Nursing*, *28*(1), 70–80.

Kim, K. H., Kim, K. S., Kang, K. S., Kang, H. S., Kim, W. O., Paik, H. J., Won, J. S., Lim, N. Y., Jeong, I. S., & Kwon, H. J. (2000). A grounded theory approach to the comfort experience of hospitalized patients. *Journal of Korean Academy of Nursing*, *30*(3), 750–763.

Kim, M. (2007). A study of the caregiving burden on grandmothers who raise their grandchildren: A phenomenological research. *Journal of Korean Academy of Nursing*, *37*(6), 914–923.

Kim, M. H. (2000). A study on subjective experience of drug abuse adolescents. *Journal of Korean Academy of Nursing*, *30*(1), 7–17.

Kim, M. S., & Kim, A. K. (1997). The study of smoking behavior in college women: A grounded theory approach. *Journal of Korean Academy of Nursing*, *27*(2), 315–328.

Kim, M. S., & Shin, Y. H. (1992). Patients' perceptions of health professionals' unkind behavior. *Journal of Korean Academy of Nursing*, *22*(4), 421–443.

Kim, M. Y., Choi, S. J., & Yang, S. A. (1999). A study of women's menopausal experiences. *Journal of Korean Academy of Nursing*, *29*(6), 1263–1272.

Kim, S. (1997). An action research study on measures to mobilize inactive nurses. *Journal of Korean Academy of Nursing*, *27*(4), 880–891.

Kim, S. J., & Yang, S. J. (1997). A study of primiparous women's breastfeeding experience. *Journal of Korean Academy of Nursing*, *27*(3), 477–488.

Kim, S. Y. (1995). Phenomenological approach of self-regulation related to health of patients with adult disease. *Journal of Korean Academy of Nursing*, *25*(3), 562–580.

Kim, W. O., Kang, H. S., & Yi, M. S. (2004). Adjustment patterns of illness process of people with hemophilia in Korea. *Journal of Korean Academy of Nursing*, *34*(1), 5–14.

Kim, Y. H., Chang, K. O., Koo, M. J., Kim, S. H., Kim, Y. M., & Lee, N. Y. (2007). The experiences of mental health hospital workers. *Journal of Korean Academy of Nursing*, *37*(3), 381–390.

Kim, Y. H., Koo, M. J., Kim, S. H., Kim, Y. M., Lee, N. Y., & Chang, K. O. (2007). The experiences of patients in intensive care units (ICU). *Journal of Korean Academy of Nursing*, *37*(6), 924–931.

Kim, Y. H., Park, K. Y., Kim, M. Y., & Kim, M. O. (2004). The experiences of perioperative patients with cancer. *Journal of Korean Academy of Nursing*, *34*(6), 945–953.

Koh, M. H. (2005). Experiences of hope in clients with chronic schizophrenia. *Journal of Korean Academy of Nursing*, *35*(3), 555–564.

Koh, M. S. (1997). The observational experience of labor and delivery by student nurses in the clinical setting. *Journal of Korean Academy of Nursing*, *27*(4), 892–900.

Kweon, Y. R., & Lee, C. S. (2009). Health experience of depressive adolescents: Reflected from Newman's praxis methodology. *Journal of Korean Academy of Nursing*, *39*(2), 217–228.

Kwon, B. S., & Park, H. K. (1997). A producing process for Korean nursing knowledge and discourse on analytic prospects. *Journal of Korean Academy of Nursing*, 27(1),13–25.

Kwon, S. B., Chi, S. A., Back, K. S., Yu, S. O., Ju, S. N., Kim, B. J., Lee, H. S., & Ann, O. H. (2001). Content analysis of quality nursing care perceived by nurses. *Journal of Korean Academy of Nursing*, *31*(3), 380–390.

Lee, B. S., Kang, S. R., & Kim, H. O. (2007). Experience of job satisfaction in clinical nurses: Application of focus group methodology. *Journal of Korean Academy of Nursing*, *37*(1), 114–124.

Lee, G. E. (2002). A grounded theory approach to the adjustment process of the institutionalized elderly: The control of reluctance. *Journal of Korean Academy of Nursing*, *32*(5), 624–632.

Lee, H. J. (2006). A paradigm analysis related to spiritual experiences focused on Christianity of patients with terminal cancer. *Journal of Korean Academy of Nursing*, *36*(2), 299–309.

Lee, J. H., & Chi, S. A. (1993). Patients' experiences about their nurses' healing relations. *Journal of Korean Academy of Nursing*, *23*(3), 356–368.

Lee, J. S., & Kim, S. S. (1994). The experience of the family whose child has died of cancer. *Journal of Korean Academy of Nursing*, *24*(3), 413–431.

Lee, J. S., Oh, S. Y., Han, H. S., & Yi, Y. J. (2001). The coping experience in hypertensive clients. *Journal of Korean Academy of Nursing*, *31*(5), 759–769.

Lee, J. S., Ro, S. O., Shin, D. S., Kim, M. H., & Jung, Y. M. (2000). The experience of life in with diabetics. *Journal of Korean Academy of Nursing*, *30*(5), 1219–1229.

Lee, K. H., & Koh, M. S. (1994). Women's experience of abortion: Phenomenological perspectives. *Journal of Korean Academy of Nursing*, *24*(2), 157–174.

Lee, K. S. (1997). A study on the experience of the life of caregivers with mentally ill children. *Journal of Korean Academy of Nursing*, *27*(4), 953–960.

Lee, K. Y., & Kim, S. Y. (1999). A study on the patterns of alternative therapy experienced by the aged. *Journal of Korean Academy of Nursing, 29*(2), 336–345.

Lee, M. L., & Cho, J. Y. (1996). Women's view on pregnancy. *Journal of Korean Academy of Nursing, 26*(1), 5–14.

Lee, M. S. (1998). Experience of mothers of mentally handicapped children having menarche. *Journal of Korean Academy of Nursing, 28*(1), 7–16.

Lee, M. S. (1999). The lived experience of mothers mentally handicapped daughters having menarche at puberty. *Journal of Korean Academy of Nursing, 29*(3), 494–506.

Lee, O. J. (1995). Lived experience of patients with terminal cancer: Parse's human becoming methodology. *Journal of Korean Academy of Nursing, 25*(3), 510–537.

Lee, Y. J., & Kim, K. B. (2008). Experiences of nurse turnover. *Journal of Korean Academy of Nursing, 38*(2), 248–257.

Lee, Y. S. (2000). A phenomenological study on orphans' lived experience of their parents. *Journal of Korean Academy of Nursing, 30*(2), 452–462.

Min, S. Y. (2005). The daily experiences of people with chronic schizophrenia. *Journal of Korean Academy of Nursing, 35*(6), 1125–1134.

Nam, S. Y. (1998). A study of CVA patients' experience of the illness. *Journal of Korean Academy of Nursing, 28*(2), 479–489.

Oh, J. J. (2000). The experience of nursing staff on the dementia patients' aggressive behavior. *Journal of Korean Academy of Nursing, 30*(2), 293–306.

Oh, P. J. (1998). The meaning of quality of life for bone marrow transplant survivors. *Journal of Korean Academy of Nursing, 28*(3), 760–772.

Oh, P. J., & Kang, K. A. (2001). The experience of spirituality. *Journal of Korean Academy of Nursing, 31*(6), 967–977.

Oh, W. O., & Park, E. S. (2007). Parenting experiences of parents of children with ADHD: Approaching the normal. *Journal of Korean Academy of Nursing, 37*(1), 91–104.

Park, E. J., & Kim, C. (2008). Case management process identified from experience of nurse case managers. *Journal of Korean Academy of Nursing, 38*(6), 789–801.

Park, N. H., Cho, Y. R., Choi, W. H., Moon, N. J., An, H. G., & Shin, J. S. (2004). Immersion experience of the cyber world of adolescents. *Journal of Korean Academy of Nursing, 34*(1), 15–24.

Shin, J. S., An, H. G., Kim, H. M., Yoo, Y. J., Kim, K. H., Chong, I. K., & Lee, Y. M. (2001). Pain of elderly women with osteoarthritis. *Journal of Korean Academy of Nursing, 31*(2), 180–193.

Shin, K. R. (1995). A phenomenological perspective and discovery of meaning in middle-aged women's experience of mastectomy. *Journal of Korean Academy of Nursing, 25*(2), 295–315.

Shin, K. R. (1996). Criteria for critique of qualitative nursing research. *Journal of Korean Academy of Nursing, 26*(2), 497–506.

Shin, K. R. (1998). The lived changing body experience of postmenopausal women. *Journal of Korean Academy of Nursing, 28*(2), 414–430.

Shin, K. R., Cha, E. J., & Kim, Y. H. (2003). The lived experience of a student transferring into the nursing program. *Journal of Korean Academy of Nursing, 33*(6), 722–730.

Shin, K. R., Kong, E. S., Kim, G. B., Kim, N. C., Kim, C. H., Kim, C. K., Kim, H. K., Ro, Y. J., Song, M. S., Ahn, S. Y., Lee, K. J., Lee, Y. W., Chang, S. O., Chon, S. J., Cho, N. O., Cho, M. O., & Choi, K. S. (2002). Lived experience with aging in middle-aged women. *Journal of Korean Academy of Nursing, 32*(6), 878–887.

Shin, M. J. (1996). An analysis of health problems experienced by the clients receiving hemodialysis. *Journal of Korean Academy of Nursing, 26*(4), 903–916.

Shin, M. J. (1997). A study of the lived experiences of clients receiving long-term hemodialysis. *Journal of Korean Academy of Nursing, 27*(2), 444–453.

Son, H. M. (2010). Evaluation of nurses' competency in nurse–patient communication about medications: Conversational analysis approach. *Journal of Korean Academy of Nursing, 40*(1), 1–13.

Son, H. M., Kim, J. H., & Kim, J. H. (2005). The experiences of recovery from disease in patients doing meditation. *Journal of Korean Academy of Nursing, 35*(6), 1025-1035.

Son, H. M., Koh, M. H., Kim, C. M., & Moon, J. H. (2001). The clinical experiences of adaptation as a new nursing staff. *Journal of Korean Academy of Nursing, 31*(6), 988–997.

Son, H. M., Koh, M. H., Kim, C. M., & Yi, M. S. (2006). The experiences of transplantation coordinators' practice. *Journal of Korean Academy of Nursing, 36*(6), 1012–1022.

Son, H. M., Koh, M. H., Kim, C. M., Moon, J. H., & Yi, M. S. (2003). The male nurses' experiences of adaptation in clinical setting. *Journal of Korean Academy of Nursing, 33*(1), 17–25.

Song, M. R., Lee, Y. M., & Cheon, S. H. (2010). An analysis of the meaning of respite for family caregivers of elderly with dementia. *Journal of Korean Academy of Nursing, 40*(4), 482–449.

Song, M. S., & Lee, M. L. (1992). The meaning of vaginal delivery to primiparous mothers. *Journal of Korean Academy of Nursing, 22*(4), 444–453.

Suh, M. J., Yun, S. N., Yoo, J. S., Song, J. H., & Choi, K. S. (1996). A content analysis of the test of the national examination for registration nurses in Korea over 3 years. *Journal of Korean Academy of Nursing, 26*(1), 73–93.

Sung, M. H. (1997). The loss experience in women with hysterectomy. *Journal of Korean Academy of Nursing, 27*(1), 128–140.

Tae, Y. S., Cho, M. O., & Hong, Y. H. (2003). The illness experience of women in advanced uterine cancer. *Journal of Korean Academy of Nursing, 33*(7), 917–927.

Yang, J. H. (2002). A study on health behavior experience of middle-aged women in rural areas. *Journal of Korean Academy of Nursing, 32*(5), 694–705.

Yang, J. H. (2005). The experience of life experiences among patients with chronic low back and extremity pain. *Journal of Korean Academy of Nursing, 35*(5), 955–966.

Yang, J. H. (2008). The actual experiences of the living world among cancer patients. *Journal of Korean Academy of Nursing, 38*(1), 140–151.

Yeo, J. H. (2003). College women's meaning of women: Phenomenological method. *Journal of Korean Academy of Nursing, 33*(1), 34–41.

Yi, M. (2003). Nurses' experience of caring for dying patients in hospitals. *Journal of Korean Academy of Nursing, 33*(5), 553–561.

Yi, M. (2007). Conversation analysis for improving nursing communication. *Journal of Korean Academy of Nursing, 37*(5), 772–780.

Yi, M. S. (1994). A phenomenological study on psychosocial nursing care in Korea. *Journal of Korean Academy of Nursing, 24*(2), 226–240.

Yi, M. S. (1996). Overcoming language barrier by Korean nurses in US hospital settings. *Journal of Korean Academy of Nursing, 26*(2), 483–496.

Yi, M. S. (1997). Lived experience of the family members of gastric cancer patients. *Journal of Korean Academy of Nursing, 27*(2), 275–288.

Yi, M. S. (1998). A comparison of hospital nursing practice in Korea and the US as experienced by Korean nurses. *Journal of Korean Academy of Nursing, 28*(1), 60–69.

Yi, M. S. (1998). Psychosocial adjustment after kidney transplantation. *Journal of Korean Academy of Nursing, 28*(2), 291–302.

Yi, M. S. (1999). Psychosocial adjustment in families with kidney donor or recipient. *Journal of Korean Academy of Nursing, 29*(4), 790–801.

Yi, M. S. (2000). The pattern of decision-making to donate a living kidney. *Journal of Korean Academy of Nursing, 30*(1), 47–59.

Yi, M. S. (2004). Secondary analysis: Focusing on qualitative research. *Journal of Korean Academy of Nursing, 34*(1), 35–44.

Yi, M. S., Lee, E. O., Choi, M. A., Kim, K. S., Ko, M. H., Kim, M. J., Kim, H. S., Son, J. T., Eom, M. R., Oh, S. E., Lee, K. S., Jang, E. H., Cho, G. J., & Choe, J. S. (2000). Expertise in ICU nursing: A qualitative approach. *Journal of Korean Academy of Nursing, 30*(5), 1230–1242.

Yi, M. S., Lee, S. W., Choe, M. A., Kim, K. S., & Kim, Y. M. (2001). Experience of mothers with babies by in vitro fertilization. *Journal of Korean Academy of Nursing, 31*(1), 55–67.

Yi, M., & Yih, B. S. (2006). A conversation analysis of communication between patients with dementia and their professional nurses. *Journal of Korean Academy of Nursing, 36*(7), 1253–1264.

Yi, M., Choe, M. A., Hah, Y. S., Kim, K. S., Yih, B. S., & Kim, J. (2006). Mothers' experience of caregiving for their children with schizophrenia. *Journal of Korean Academy of Nursing, 36*(1), 45–54.

Yi, M., Choi, E. O., Paik, S. W., Kim, K. S., Kwak, S., & Lee, H. J. (2007). Illness experience of people with chronic hepatitis B in Korea. *Journal of Korean Academy of Nursing, 37*(5), 665–675.

Yi, M., Oh, S. E., Choi, E. O., Kwon, I. G., Kwon, S., Cho, K. M., Kang, Y., & Ok, J. (2008). Hospital nurses' experience of do-not-resuscitate in Korea. *Journal of Korean Academy of Nursing, 38*(2), 298–309.

Yih, B. S., & Yi, M. (2009). The life stories of elderly Korean women with urinary incontinence: A narrative study approach. *Journal of Korean Academy of Nursing, 39*(2), 237–248.

Yih, B. S., Kim, C. M., & Yi, M. (2004). Women caregivers' experiences in caring at home for a family member with dementia: A feminist approach. *Journal of Korean Academy of Nursing, 34*(5), 881–890.

Yoo, E. H. (1995). An ethnographic study of sanhubyung experienced by women in Korean postpartal culture. *Journal of Korean Academy of Nursing, 25*(4), 825–836.

Journal of Qualitative Research

Bae, K. E., & Park, C. H. (2007). Experiences of infertile women in artificial insemination. *Journal of Qualitative Research*, 8(2), 23–35.

Baek, K. S. (2006). Experiences of newborn nursery care practice among the male nursing students. *Journal of Qualitative Research*, 7(1), 25–37.

Baek, K. S., & Choi, K. S. (2000). Understanding about mothers' parenting experience in their child of cerebral palsy. *Journal of Qualitative Research*, 1(2), 50–59.

Baek, K. S., & Lee, S. Y. (2010). A study on the breastfeeding experience of mothers. *Journal of Qualitative Research*, 11(2), 69–79.

Byeon, Y. S., & Kim, M. (2009). Interpersonal conflict experiences of nurses. *Journal of Qualitative Research*, 10(2), 142–151.

Byeon, Y. S., & Lee, K. H. (2006). The life change events of patients with AIDS in Korea. *Journal of Qualitative Research*, 7(2), 1–11.

Chang, M. K., Jo, H. K., & Lee, S. K. (2007). A phenomenological study on housewives' experience in two-working-parent family. *Journal of Qualitative Research*, 8(1), 39–54.

Cho, B. S. (2000). A phenomenological perspective and discovery of meaning in mid-aged men's experience of the change of body. *Journal of Qualitative Research*, 1(1), 79–98.

Cho, M. O. (2000). An ethnography of succession of folk caring behaviors for the elderly. *Journal of Qualitative Research*, 1(1), 12–28.

Cho, M. O. (2002). The world views on the after-world and human spirits in Korean folk tales. *Journal of Qualitative Research*, 3(2), 28–39.

Cho, M. O. (2004). Nursing students' learning experience of disabilities. *Journal of Qualitative Research*, 5(1), 61–74.

Cho, M. O. (2005). Quality insurance in qualitative nursing research in the process of preparing research. *Journal of Qualitative Research*, 6(2), 79–92.

Cho, M. O. (2005). The experience of crisis in everyday life among the women with chronic health problem. *Journal of Qualitative Research*, 6(1), 33–45.

Cho, M. O. (2009). A review on micro-ethnography as a nursing research methods. *Journal of Qualitative Research*, 10(2), 130–141.

Cho, M. O. (2010). Decision on treatment modality among the middle-aged in the weight control program. *Journal of Qualitative Research*, 11(1), 1–12.

Cho, M. O. (2010). Experiences of ICU nurses on temporality and spatiality in caring for dying patients. *Journal of Qualitative Research*, 11(2), 80–93.

Cho, M. O., & Kim, H. O. (2006). Meaning of death reflected in nursing students' essay. *Journal of Qualitative Research*, 7(2), 73–83.

Cho, M. O., Kim, Y. K., Kim, Y. H., Kim, Y. S., Yang, J. H., Yoo, Y. G., & Tae, Y. S. (2004). Cosmetic surgery and the nursing students' experiences of body. *Journal of Qualitative Research*, 5(2), 90–103.

Choi, K. S. & Eun, Y. (2000). A companionship of the spouses of patients with arthritis. *Journal of Qualitative Research*, 1(1), 59–74.

Choi, K. S., Youn, M. S., & Choi, J. Y. (2003). Decision that follow antenatal diagnosis of congenital heart disease. *Journal of Qualitative Research*, 4(1), 103–114.

Choi, S. H., Lee, K. S., Jun, I. S., & Kim, Y. S. (2002). Early hemodialysis experience of patients undergoing maintenance hemodialysis. *Journal of Qualitative Research*, 3(2), 47–57.

Choi, S. J. (2003). Male students' lived experience in the female-dominant nursing college. *Journal of Qualitative Research*, 4(1), 52–63.

Chu, M. S. (2000). Discovering island women's experience of urinary incontinence. *Journal of Qualitative Research*, 1(2), 134–142.

Chu, M. S., & Kim, H. Y. (2003). The caregiver's experience for the chronic illness patient. *Journal of Qualitative Research*, 4(1), 41–51.

Chung, S. E. (2005). Health behaviors among elderly Korean immigrants in Canada. *Journal of Qualitative Research*, 6(1), 1–13.

Chung, S. E., Choi, C. H. (2005). The noise exposure experience of concrete manufacturing workers. *Journal of Qualitative Research*, 6(2), 65–78.

Chung, S. E., & Choi, C. H. (2008). University students' experience of noise exposure by personal audio system. *Journal of Qualitative Research*, 9(2), 87–98.

Chung, S. E., & Lee, S. H. (2010). Nursing students' experience of education using simulation. *Journal of Qualitative Research*, 11(1), 50–59.

Gong, B. H. (2007). Phenomenological approach and clinical ethics. *Journal of Qualitative Research*, 8(1), 11–19.

Han, J. S. (2003). A phenomenological study on pregnancy experience of unmarried teenage mothers. *Journal of Qualitative Research, 4*(2), 44–60.

Han, K. S., & Jung, Y. K. (2000). The study on the sexual experience of spinal cord injury patient's spouse. *Journal of Qualitative Research, 1*(2), 109–124.

Hong, Y. H., Oh, H. K., & Han, Y. I. (2007). The lived socialization experience of the diploma nursing students. *Journal of Qualitative Research, 8*(2), 37–50.

Hwang, L. J., Kim, Y H., Eo, Y. S., Kim, H. H., Song, M. G., & Cho, G. Y. (2002). The lived experience of the women suffering from rheumatoid arthritis. *Journal of Qualitative Research, 3*(1), 1–14.

Hwangbo, S. J., & Yang, J. H. (2004). A study on the experience process of health behavior among Korean elderly women. *Journal of Qualitative Research, 5*(1), 50–61.

Jang, W. S. (2002). Ethnography on the daily life of ICU nursing. *Journal of Qualitative Research, 3*(1), 77–93.

Jeon, H. O. (2008). Grounded theory approach on the women's adaptation experience with their retired husbands. *Journal of Qualitative Research, 9*(2), 120–128.

Jeong, J. I. (2003). Head nurse's experience connected with clinical practice education. *Journal of Qualitative Research, 4*(1), 88–102.

Kang, H. L., Lee, S. Y., & Sung, M. S. (2009). A study on the recovery process of stroke in middle-aged men patients. *Journal of Qualitative Research, 10*(2), 152–165.

Kang, M. J., Kim, Y. H., Kim, K. R., Kim, S. G., Kim, Y. S., Lee, S. R., & Cho, Y. S. (2003). A phenomenological study on the experience of female doctoral candidates in nursing. *Journal of Qualitative Research, 4*(1), 27–40.

Kang, S., & Kim, J. S. (2010). Experiences of insomnia of the elderly women in community. *Journal of Qualitative Research, 11*(1), 13–25.

Kim, B. H., & Choi, P. S. (2000). Life experience on the middle-aged man spouse of terminal cancer. *Journal of Qualitative Research, 1*(2), 60–73.

Kim, E. H. (2008). Experience of maternity as divorced women. *Journal of Qualitative Research, 9*(1), 57–70.

Kim, G. (2000). A phenomenological perspective and meaning of joint pains experience of women on an island. *Journal of Qualitative Research, 1*(1), 150–164.

Kim, H. O., & Cho, M. O. (2006). Experiences of conflicts on job identity among the nurses of medium-sized hospitals. *Journal of Qualitative Research, 7*(2), 13–25.

Kim, H. O., & Shin, S. C. (2004). Nurses' work experience in an individual medium-sized hospital. *Journal of Qualitative Research, 5*(2), 15–32.

Kim, H. S. (2008). The lived experience of Ho-Sang of elderly women. *Journal of Qualitative Research, 9*(1), 11–29.

Kim, H., & Hong, C. (2009). A grounded approach on continuous weight control process of women in normal body weight. *Journal of Qualitative Research, 10*(1), 28–38.

Kim, J. S. (2002). The lived experience of male mid-life in men. *Journal of Qualitative Research, 3*(2), 55–67.

Kim, J. S. (2006). The patterns of drug use in the elderly women with chronic disease in community. *Journal of Qualitative Research, 7*(1), 67–76.

Kim, J. S. (2008). A study on health promotion experience of elderly women in community health center. *Journal of Qualitative Research, 9*(1), 71–85.

Kim, J. S., Gong, S. J., Kim, H. S., Rho, Y. H., Kim, O. H., Park, K. S., & Sun, J. J. (2006). A phenomenological study on the elderly's life of bliss. *Journal of Qualitative Research, 7*(1), 39–55.

Kim, J. S., Seo, I. S., & Yang, S. A. (2002). The lived experience of hormone therapy in menopausal women. *Journal of Qualitative Research, 3*(1), 41–55.

Kim, J. S., Sun, J. J., & Kim, H. S. (2009). Clinical practice experiences of nursing students. *Journal of Qualitative Research, 10*(1), 63–76.

Kim, K. H., Yang, S. A., & Shin, S. J. (2006). A phenomenological study on the clinical experience in a rehabilitation center. *Journal of Qualitative Research, 7*(1), 57–65.

Kim, M. H. (2002). A study on the recovery experience of drug abuse adolescent. *Journal of Qualitative Research, 3*(2), 40–54.

Kim, M. H. (2003). Case study on adult children who have been living with a disabled parent. *Journal of Qualitative Research, 4*(1), 76–87.

Kim, M. H. (2006). The lived experience of adult children living with disabled parent. *Journal of Qualitative Research, 7*(1), 15–24.

Kim, M. J., Yang, I. S., & Kim, B. Y. (2010). The experiences of horticulture therapy among the elderly patients with stroke. *Journal of Qualitative Research, 11*(1), 36–49.

Kim, M. S., Lee, S. H., & Kim, S. Y. (2002). The meaning of nursing in the freshmen of nursing school. *Journal of Qualitative Research, 3*(2), 1–9.

Kim, M. Y. (2001). The nurses' experience process caring for the demented elderly. *Journal of Qualitative Research*, 2(1), 65–76.

Kim, N. S. (2000). Gender and illness through the analysis of patriarchal discourse. *Journal of Qualitative Research*, 1(1), 29–57.

Kim, O., Hwang, J. W., Kim, K. R., & Kang, J. S. (2008). The experiences of daily life among elderly women with cataracts. *Journal of Qualitative Research*, 9(2), 129–141.

Kim, S. Y., Kim, S. M., & Yang, S. H. (2001). Nursing students' lived experience of demented elderly. *Journal of Qualitative Research*, 2(1), 55–69.

Kim, Y. H. (2003). Exploring the health behavior of elderly women. *Journal of Qualitative Research*, 4(1), 64–75.

Kim, Y. H., Byunk, E. K., Jeon, Y. S., & Kim, Y. H. (2004). Experiences of parents who take care of schizophrenic children. *Journal of Qualitative Research*, 5(2), 75–89.

Kim, Y. J., & Kim, B. H. (2007). Meaning of experienced life in middle-aged men. *Journal of Qualitative Research*, 8(2), 51–63.

Kim, Y. J., & Kim, I. O. (2003). A phenomenological perspective and discovery of meaning in primipara's spouse's experience of the participation during labor. *Journal of Qualitative Research*, 4(2), 61–73.

Kim, Y. K., & Lee, J. W. (2005). Meaning of fatigue experienced by nursing students. *Journal of Qualitative Research*, 6(2), 15–33.

Kim, Y. K., Cho, M. O., & Yang, J. H. (2005). The experiences of identity developing among enrolled nursing students. *Journal of Qualitative Research*, 6(1), 15–31.

Kim, Y. K., Yang, J. H., Yoo, Y. J., Cho, M. O., & Tae, Y. S. (2004). A phenomenological study on Korean drug addicts' experiences. *Journal of Qualitative Research*, 5(1), 20–29.

Kim, Y., Kim, Y., Yang, J., Yoo, Y., & Tae, Y. (2004). A phenomenological study of the abuse experience among Korean elderly women. *Journal of Qualitative Research*, 5(1), 1–9.

Kong, B. H. (2001). On aesthetical research method on philosophy. *Journal of Qualitative Research*, 2(1), 7–18.

Kong, B. H., & Park, S. A. (2009). Philosophical background of the qualitative research interview. *Journal of Qualitative Research*, 10(2), 77–85.

Kwon, B. S. (2000). A study of discourse on Lao-Chuang's health promotion. *Journal of Qualitative Research*, 1(1), 121–130.

Lee, E. K., Jung, C. H., & Jeon, H. J. (2010). Experiences of nurses in medication errors. *Journal of Qualitative Research*, 11(2), 94–105.

Lee, J. H., Lee, K. H., Um, H., Nobuko, H., & Yuko, O. H. (2005). Gender-based stress of Korean and Japanese married nurses. *Journal of Qualitative Research*, 6(2), 1–14.

Lee, K. S. (2003). Experience of the women who succeeded natural birth after cesarean section: Based on the deliveries at the midwifes clinic. *Journal of Qualitative Research*, 4(2), 20–30.

Lee, K. Y., & Park, I. S. (2007). The experience of the family members with mentally retarded children. *Journal of Qualitative Research*, 8(1), 21–37.

Lee, M. H. (2002). Independence of institutionalized elderly women: Ethnomethodological approach. *Journal of Qualitative Research*, 3(1), 27–40.

Lee, M. H. (2008). A phenomenological study on the enduring experiences in a life-pattern of the institutionalized elderly women. *Journal of Qualitative Research*, 9(2), 142–154.

Lee, O. J., & Choi, Y. S. (2006). Family's conquest experience of person with chronic mental disorder. *Journal of Qualitative Research*, 7(2), 55–71.

Lee, S. A., Lee, Y. S., Cho, S. J., Shin, Y. S., Lee, S. Y., Kim, I. S., Park, Y. S., & Kim, H. K. (2004). The lived experience of adolescent smoking. *Journal of Qualitative Research*, 5(1), 39–49.

Lee, S. H., Chung, S. E. (2007). The experience of verbal violence between nurses. *Journal of Qualitative Research*, 8(1), 79–89.

Lee, S. H., Shin, J. Y., & Lee, Y. J. (2002). A study on middle-aged obese women's weight control experiences. *Journal of Qualitative Research*, 3(1), 65–76.

Lee, S. K. (2010). The value of nurses' professionalism: From the perspective of the health care consumer. *Journal of Qualitative Research*, 11(2), 119–133.

Lee, S. W., Kim, M. J., Yun, E. S., & Park, J. D. (2009). Re-employment adaptation experience of nurses. *Journal of Qualitative Research*, 10(1), 39–50.

Lee, Y. H. (2008). The experience of the consumption behavior of health supplement in the elderly. *Journal of Qualitative Research*, 9(1), 45–56.

Lee, Y. J., & Shin, J. Y. (2001). The experiences of the family caregivers of bone marrow transplantation patients. *Journal of Qualitative Research*, 2(1), 77–89.

Lee, Y. S. (2000). A phenomenological study on orphans' experience of their parents. *Journal of Qualitative Research*, 1(1), 108–120.

Lim, E. J., Jung, S. Y., Choi, M. S., Jo, S. H., & Hur, J. (2009). Approach of grounded theory on regimen experience process through diet among elderly women. *Journal of Qualitative Research*, 10(2), 117–129.

Lim, T. Y. (2000). A phenomenological perspective and discovery of meaning in middle-aged women's experience of the change of body. *Journal of Qualitative Research*, 1(2), 125–133.

Noh, J. H., Eom, J. Y., Yang, K. S., & Park, H. S. (2009). New nurses' experiences on care of dying patients. *Journal of Qualitative Research*, 10(1), 51–62.

Noh, Y. H. (2003). Breast cancer survivor's conquest experience. *Journal of Qualitative Research*, 4(1), 7–26.

Park, H. S., Park, N. H., & Eo, Y. S. (2004). Notes on types and characteristics of literature reviews. *Journal of Qualitative Research*, 5(2), 50–62.

Park, J. A., Park, K. J., & Jin, L. H. (2010). The meaning of cardiopulmonary resuscitation experienced by nurses. *Journal of Qualitative Research*, 11(2), 134–145.

Park, J. H., & Chun, I. S. (2008). The lived experience of newly employed nurses: Phenomenological study. *Journal of Qualitative Research*, 9(2), 99–110.

Park, K. J. (2001). A phenomenological perspective and discovery of meaning in nursing clients' experience of the coronary angiography. *Journal of Qualitative Research*, 2(1), 70–88.

Park, S. I., & Seo, E. H. (2010). Experience of male students majoring in nursing. *Journal of Qualitative Research*, 11(1), 60–68.

Park, S. Y. (2005). Participatory action research for the healthcare of menopausal women. *Journal of Qualitative Research*, 6(1), 91–102.

Park, Y. S., & Choi, K. S. (2002). The experience of patient role in adults with diabetes. *Journal of Qualitative Research*, 3(1), 15–26.

Seo, I. S. (2003). The experiences of daughters-in-law taking care of their demented mothers-in-law: Narrative inquiry. *Journal of Qualitative Research*, 4(2), 74–86.

Shin, K. R. (2000). Writing a proposal using qualitative research method. *Journal of Qualitative Research*, 1(1), 165–171.

Shin, K. R., Kang, Y., Jung, D., Park, H. J., Eom, J. Y., Yun, E. S., & Kim, M. J. (2010). Experiences among older adults who have fallen. *Journal of Qualitative Research*, 11(1), 26–35.

Song, M. R., Kim, I. K., & Kim, Y. K. (2010). Experience of clinical practice faculty and nurses on clinical nursing practicum for nursing students. *Journal of Qualitative Research*, 11(2), 106–118.

Sung, M. S. (2010). The experience of friendship in the Korean aged female. *Journal of Qualitative Research*, 5(2), 63–74.

Woo, M. K., Kim, H. S., & Ji, E. J. (2009). The experience process of obese women in workplace. *Journal of Qualitative Research*, 10(2), 86–102.

Yang, B. S. (2002). A study of experiences for the middle-aged widow. *Journal of Qualitative Research*, 3(1), 56–64.

Yang, J. H. (2001). Yangsaeng experience through dietary practice among Korean women. *Journal of Qualitative Research*, 2(1), 51–63.

Yang, J. H. (2005). A review on culturalism and ethnoscience nursing research. *Journal of Qualitative Research*, 6(1), 65–75.

Yang, J. H. (2005). The experience of fundamental nursing practice among nursing students. *Journal of Qualitative Research*, 6(2), 51–64.

Yang, J. H. (2008). The lived experiences of illness among people living with HIV. *Journal of Qualitative Research*, 9(2), 111–119.

Yang, J. H., Kim, Y. K., Kim, Y. H., Cho, M. O., Yoo, Y. J., & Tae, Y. S. (2003). The lived experience of health behavior in Korean elderly women. *Journal of Qualitative Research*, 4(2), 31–43.

Yang, J. H., Shin, K. R. (2003). An analysis on phenomenological research in the *Journal of the Korean Academy of Nursing* (1998–2002) and desirable writing. *Journal of Qualitative Research*, 4(2), 87–99.

Yang, N. Y. (2001). The phenomenological perspective and meaning of comfort experience of cancer patients in chemotherapy. *Journal of Qualitative Research*, 2(2), 38–54.

Yee, O. H., Ha, J. Y., Lee, J. R., & Whang, E. H. (2009). Lived experiences of grandmothers caring for grandchildren whose parents are working together. *Journal of Qualitative Research*, 10(1), 1–13.

Yi, M. (2000). Qualitative data analysis using computers. *Journal of Qualitative Research*, 1(1), 52–68.

Yoo, Y. J., Kim, Y. K., Kim, Y. H., Kim, Y. S., Cho, M. O., Yang, J. H., & Tae, Y. S. (2005). The meaning of well-aging in elderly women: Approach with a phenomenological study. *Journal of Qualitative Research*, 6(1), 77–89.

Yoon, J. H., & Kim, Y. K. (2009). Elderly spouses' experience in caring for their veteran husband. *Journal of Qualitative Research*, 10(2), 103–116.

43

Qualitative nursing research in Japan

A state of the science and indications for future directions

Shigeko Saiki-Craighill

Introduction

This chapter will briefly review the history of qualitative research and its relationship to nursing academics in Japan, analyze a survey of qualitative research conducted in the field of health care, and focus on a critique of how one representative method was applied. Based on this survey and analysis, some implications will be inferred as to what developments should be made as we move forward.

Historical context

In Japan, the development of qualitative research techniques happened almost precisely concurrently with the development of nursing as an academic discipline. Qualitative research began to be acknowledged within the social sciences as an independent approach in the late 1980s. It expanded and subdivided in the mid-1990s, and was established as an important approach in the 2000s (Oda, 2011). A symbolic event in this development was the establishment of the Nihon Shitsuteki Shinri Gakkai (Japanese Association of Qualitative Psychology) in 2004, a significant turning point in the history of Japanese qualitative research.

At the same time, nursing as an academic subject was also developing rapidly. Although four-year university programs in nursing were first established in 1952, there have not been many schools of nursing in such universities until very recently. In specific terms, there were only 11 such programs in 1991, but by 2010 there were 188 university-level undergraduate programs, 127 Master's courses and 61 PhD programs.[1]

With this dramatic increase in nursing academia, there was a growing recognition that many nursing phenomena could not be adequately addressed by only quantitative methods. This led many in the field to look to qualitative methods for research tools. Therefore, when considering the development of qualitative research within nursing sciences in Japan, a key point to keep in mind is that nursing science as an academic discipline and qualitative research as an investigative approach were undergoing rapid development at precisely the same time. Figure 43.1 illustrates the parallel growth of university nursing programs with the rapid increase in the number of qualitative research articles published each year in the health sciences.

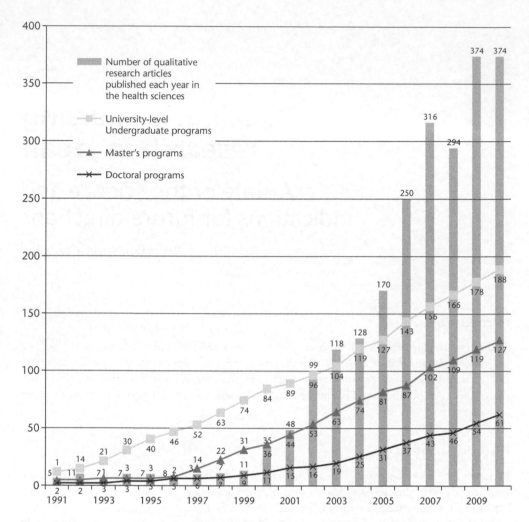

Figure 43.1 A comparison of the growth in university nursing programs with the number of qualitative research articles in the health sciences

Sources: Japana Centra Revuo Medicina: Ichushi database; Japanese Ministry of Education, Culture, Sports, Science and Technology (2003); and Japanese Ministry of Education, Culture, Sports, Science and Technology (2011).

The aim of this chapter is to provide an overview of both the quantity and quality of the qualitative research done by nursing researchers in Japan in the two decades since it was recognized as an independent approach. By coincidence, this is also the two decades that saw nursing science rapidly emerge and become established as an independent academic field. As this chapter will demonstrate, this rapid concurrent development has led to some problems in the implementation of proper research procedures. This will be analyzed in two steps. First, the issue of quantity will be addressed by looking at the number of original articles in medical journals and their growth in number over time. Then the quality issues will be reviewed by taking a close look at the use of grounded theory approach as an example of qualitative research methods.

The range of research in the past two decades

The first objective of this investigation was to find the qualitative research articles written by nursing researchers. For this purpose, the Ichushi (Japan Medical Abstracts Society) website, the largest medical bibliography database in Japan, was used.[2] However, it was impossible to isolate articles written by nursing researchers, since they were usually not identified as such. Nevertheless, within the medical community, nursing researchers are by far the most inclined to use qualitative methods. Therefore, for the purpose of this chapter, the analysis was broadened to all qualitative research done in the health sciences, as this body of research can be taken to be at least roughly equivalent to the qualitative research conducted by nursing researchers.

The growth of original articles using qualitative research

Since there were a very limited number of articles that used qualitative methods before 1990, the search covered original articles published from 1990 to 2010. Because the database did not yield a significant number of articles when the search term "qualitative research" was used,[3] a further search was conducted using the 11 qualitative research methods that are the most used in Japan.[4]

To get a sense of the rate of growth in qualitative research, note that from 1990 to 1999, a total of 35 articles that were based on qualitative research were published, using only six of the 11 methodologies in the search. Then, in the year 2000 alone, another 35 such articles were published. By 2003, nine of the 11 methodologies were represented and the number of articles exceeded 100. By 2006, the number of articles using qualitative research reached 250 and, in 2007, the number exceeded 300. When comparing the years 2000 and 2010, the difference is remarkable—more than a ten fold increase in the number of qualitative research articles published within the year.

If articles that describe the use of other qualitative research methods and articles that do not describe the use of any method are included, the total number of articles is much greater. Nevertheless, if this number is compared with all original articles in the health care sciences,[5] the proportion of those describing qualitative research is still less than 1%.

The methodologies used and their relative popularity

Table 43.1 shows the total number of original articles and the number that used each qualitative research method. The KJ method was the most used (27.6%), followed by, in order of popularity, grounded theory approach (GTA; 19.3%), content analysis (17.4%), narrative (15.0%), and life story/life history (10.0%). In other words, 90% of the articles used one of these five methods. Then, phenomenology (3.3%), action research (2.6%), fieldwork (2.3%), ethnography (1.4%), ethno-methodology and communication analysis (0.7%), and discourse analysis (0.4%) account for the remainder of the articles.

The KJ method deserves a special note, since it is both the most popular method in the survey and also one that is unique to Japan. It was developed by the anthropologist Jiro Kawakita, and the name of the technique derives from his initials. In this method, data are summarized in one phrase and written on separate cards, then similar cards are merged into groups, then each group is labeled and connected to each other in a diagram (Kawakita, 1970, 1995).

This method became popular because of its strength in developing new ideas and sorting them out. It was adopted for use not only in academia, but also in many areas including marketing and business development. An institution was established in Kawakita's name to try to gain strict

Table 43.1 Number of articles by qualitative method

Year of publication	Original articles	KJ method[1]	Grounded theory approach[2]	Content analysis	Narrative	Life story/ life history	Phenom- enology	Action research	Field- work	Ethnog- raphy	Ethnometh- ology and communication analysis	Discourse analysis	Total
1990	106314	0	0	0	0	0	0	0	1	0	0	0	1
1991	102249	0	0	0	0	0	0	0	1	0	0	0	1
1992	103736	0	0	0	0	0	0	0	2	0	1	0	3
1993	101601	0	0	0	0	0	0	0	1	0	0	0	1
1994	102284	0	0	0	0	1	1	0	1	0	0	0	3
1995	71462	0	0	0	0	0	1	0	1	1	0	0	3
1996	52057	0	0	0	0	0	0	0	2	0	0	0	2
1997	51405	1	0	0	0	1	1	0	0	0	0	0	3
1998	52355	2	0	0	0	1	2	0	1	0	1	0	7
1999	50854	0	1	0	0	7	2	0	2	0	0	0	11
2000	51925	8	7	4	0	13	8	1	0	0	0	0	35
2001	49288	15	7	7	0	8	7	2	0	1	0	1	48
2002	49528	31	16	19	0	20	8	1	2	2	0	0	99
2003	48493	40	15	27	0	20	6	2	5	1	0	2	118
2004	48994	39	20	40	1	14	8	1	1	2	1	1	128
2005	50025	65	37	30	3	19	4	6	2	1	3	0	170
2006	48076	85	42	55	21	21	2	7	12	2	3	0	250
2007	49194	103	59	31	68	22	7	12	3	7	3	1	316
2008	48842	72	59	40	70	24	2	16	4	4	1	2	294
2009	48815	88	86	63	78	26	10	7	6	5	3	2	374
2010	48716	69	90	74	96	26	6	3	4	5	1	0	374
Total	1336213	618	432	390	337	223	75	58	51	31	17	9	2241
%		27.6	19.3	17.4	15.0	10.0	3.3	2.6	2.3	1.4	0.7	0.4	100.0

Notes
1 Method developed by Jiro Kawakita.
2 Including modified grounded theory approach.

control of its usage, but this resulted in decreasing its development in academic circles and an increase in its misuse. As an illustration, currently there are nine books on the KJ method available for sale. However, Kawakita himself wrote five of these nine books. This demonstrates how this method has not been very open to input and modification by others—unusual for a method that is as prominent as the KJ method is in Japan.

Nevertheless, it has largely maintained its popularity in nursing research. Some examples of the research topics this method was applied to include emotional experience and anticipatory grief of caregivers of a parent or spouse; home-visit care provided by public health nurses and their skills, and nursing care of elderly care based on common ethics.

Since all procedures in the KJ method depend mainly on the investigators' assessment, there is an illusion that KJ method is easy to use. However, this also means that if the investigator is not skilled, problems can easily develop at any step of the process. Many studies which used this method share similar problems, such as using inappropriate names when the data are summarized, putting data in the same group when they had different meanings, applying labels with inappropriate abstracted names, and/or making connections in a diagram based on chronological order. As a result, only obvious connections could be demonstrated. This may happen with other methods such as GTA, but since there are not enough rules to avoid these pitfalls in the KJ method, studies tended not to show unique results.

Usually, the popularity of a method tends to be related to the number of publications that are available in Japanese. Once a method becomes popular, publishers became interested in publishing books on it, so they make a strong effort to translate existing work and develop original books in Japanese. To investigate the availability of books on each research method and the monographs that were developed using each method, Oda's website, *Nihongo de Yomeru Shitsuteki Kenkyu no Bunken* (Qualitative Research Documents Available in Japanese), was used.[6] A brief overview of the books available on the primary methods will indicate the nature of their relative popularity.

According to this site, there are 13 books regarding the methodology of GTA currently available. Four of them are translations, such as *Discovery of Grounded Theory: Strategies for Qualitative Research* by Glaser and Strauss, *Basics of Qualitative Research: Grounded Theory Procedures and Techniques* and *Basics of Qualitative Research: Techniques and Procedures for Developing Grounded Theory* by Strauss and Corbin, and *Constructing Grounded Theory: A Practical Guide through Qualitative Analysis* by Charmaz. Since several Japanese nursing researchers graduated from the University of California at San Francisco where Strauss taught, the Strauss (and/or Strauss and Corbin) version has been more influential than Glaser's. It is interesting to note that there are nine books on methodology and background that were written by Japanese authors.

There are four monographs available that used GTA, with three of them being translations. Therefore, by comparison, there are over three times more GTA methodology books than GTA-based monographs. This can be taken as an indicator of a strong interest in learning and applying the method.

Narrative became popular as a method in the late 1990s and early 2000s after *The Illness Narratives: Suffering, Healing, and the Human Condition* by Kleinman was translated in 1996 and *Narrative Based Medicine: Dialogue and Discourse in Clinical Practice* by Greenhalgh and Hurwitz was translated in 2001. There are eight books concerning the background of the method and Japanese authors wrote three of them. Seven monographs were also published and five of them were original works by Japanese authors.

Twenty-seven books concerning life history and/or life story were published. There were 11 books regarding methodology and its background and 16 monographs. It is notable that a higher proportion of these are original works by Japanese authors than in any other method (19 out of 27 books).

A special note should be made about the extreme lack of books concerning content analysis, given its ranking as the third most popular method (17.4%) used in the publication of qualitative research articles in the health sciences. Essentially, a translation of *Content Analysis: An Introduction to its Methodology* by Krippendorff, which was published in 1989, is the only one cited. Although a second edition of this book was published in 2004, it has not been translated. Besides this, there is only one book written by a Japanese author on content analysis. However, this book has not been very well regarded, so the translation of the Krippendorff book is almost exclusively the only one referred to. It is hard to imagine methodological rigor being applied well when there are such limited resources.

In contrast, although it is much less represented in the health sciences in terms of original articles published, the number of books on ethnography far exceeds the other methods, although most of these are monographs. A total of 168 books were published, but only seven of these were on methodology, and the rest were monographs. It is also interesting to note that a large portion of these monographs (113) were original studies conducted by Japanese.

A review of the implementation of methodology

For the purposes of this chapter, an in-depth analysis will be performed on how one particular representative method has been used. Although the KJ method has been the most popular method within Japan, it was felt that it was not appropriate to select it for this analysis. The main reason is that it would be unfamiliar to anyone outside of Japan, and so there would be no reference as to the validity of such an analysis. Instead, the second most popular method in Japan, grounded theory approach (GTA), a method that is well established worldwide, will be reviewed. In this chapter, the version of GTA that is referred to is that which is developed in Strauss (1987), Strauss and Corbin (1998), Corbin and Strauss (2008), and Saiki-Craighill (2006, 2008).

In this section, a critique of the original articles that used GTA will be provided. Many problems were found with how GTA was used. These issues will be briefly reviewed.

Confusion between methods

The first problem arose when it came to identifying the articles that use GTA. Table 43.1 indicates that 432 original articles that used GTA were published from 2000 to 2010. However, in Table 43.2, it can be seen that only 213 of these articles (49.3%) actually used GTA. Another 213 articles used a method referred to as modified grounded theory approach (M-GTA). Nevertheless, since their names are similar, 179 (84.0%) articles that used or mentioned the use of M-GTA were grouped with GTA in the Ichushi database. The problem was that 34 (16.0%) articles whose authors seemed to be unaware that they were using M-GTA instead of GTA. This demonstrates the significant confusion between GTA and M-GTA in Japan.

M-GTA can be clearly distinguished from GTA in the following ways: First, it does not involve the analysis of words, phrases, or sentences. Second, it does not use the concepts of property, dimension, and labels. Third, it skips axial coding. Fourth, it does not alternate the collection and analysis of data within the same time frame. The stated objective in omitting these steps is to shorten the time required for analysis (Kinoshita, 2003). If readers are not sufficiently familiar with GTA, they may misunderstand that M-GTA is an improvement that replaces GTA.

M-GTA appeared at an opportune time in 1999. By then, GTA was well known, but there were few resources for GTA available in Japanese. There were only two translated GTA books

Table 43.2 Breakdown of articles attributed to grounded theory approach in the Ichushi database[1]

Research method used	Number of articles	(%)	Number of articles	(%)
Grounded theory approach			213	49.3
Modified grounded theory Approach			213	49.3
self-identified as using GTA[2]	34	16.0		
self-identified as using M-GTA[3]	179	84.0		
Sub-total	213	100.0		
Quantitative research[4]			6	1.4
Total			432	100.0

Notes:

GTA = grounded theory approach

M-GTA = modified grounded theory approach

[1] Searched by using "grounded theory approach" as a search term in the Ichushi database.

[2] Articles which identified themselves as using GTA, although they used M-GTA.

[3] Articles which identified themselves as using M-GTA, but the database identified them as using GTA..

[4] These articles were attributed because they used word of GTA in their abstract, although they were quantitative research projects.

at this time: *Discovery of Grounded Theory: Strategies for Qualitative Research* (translated in 1996) by Glaser and Strauss and *From Practice to Grounded Theory: Qualitative Research in Nursing* (translated in 1992) by Chenitz and Swanson. Neither book covered research procedures in detail.

In 1999, *Grounded Theory Approach: Shitsu-teki Jisho Kenkyu No Saisei* (Regenerating Empirical Qualitative Research) was published by Yasuhito Kinoshita, a Japanese sociologist. The book introduced a Modified Strauss-Glaser version of grounded theory approach, which became the prototype of "Modified Grounded Theory Approach (M-GTA)." This was the first GTA book written in Japanese. In the literature review, it was found that whether a source was available in Japanese strongly determined whether it was cited or not. Therefore, this book was often cited as a resource.

In subsequent years, the same author published two books using GTA in the title in 2003 and 2005,[7] compounding the confusion. Even though a translation of Strauss and Corbin's *Basics of Qualitative Research: Grounded Theory Procedures and Techniques* was published in the same year that M-GTA appeared (1999), a translation of the second version of the same book was published in 2004, and books written by Japanese authors covering grounded theory in detail were published later, the confusion between GTA and M-GTA continued.

Therefore, for the purposes of this critique, the 213 articles that used M-GTA were culled from the 432 articles which the online search produced. In addition, 53 other articles were omitted from this group since they were not presented in the format of original research and two were literature reviews. As a result, 160 articles were used in the following critique.

Lack of attention to how the research method was chosen

Each research method has its own philosophy and background. When a method is chosen, it should be appropriate for the purpose of the study. However, 65.0% of the articles did not mention any reason why GTA was selected for the study and 8.1% gave explanations that indicated the authors did not understand GTA very well (Table 43.3). For example, GTA, when properly applied, highlights the process of change and its variations. However, some studies only used the participant's perceptions at one point in time. In other studies, there were no exploration of the variations in the processes, and only one uniform response was shown.

Table 43.3 Articles that used grounded theory approach sorted by year and appropriateness of methodological rationale

Year	Number of published articles	Rationale for method		
		Appropriate	*Not appropriate*	*Not mentioned*
2001	2	0	0	2
2002	7	3	0	4
2003	7	1	0	6
2004	11	1	0	10
2005	11	5	0	6
2006	18	2	4	12
2007	21	1	3	17
2008	16	6	0	10
2009	30	12	5	13
2010	37	12	1	24
Total (%)	160 (100)	43 (26.9)	13 (8.1)	104 (65.0)

Note: n = 160.

Also, 30.6% of the articles did not cite any books regarding methodology and half of them did not explain the steps used in collecting and analyzing data (Table 43.4). Therefore, there is no way to evaluate and confirm the findings. These findings indicate that the research method was not chosen or used carefully.

Lack of attention to methods of collecting data

The type of data collected depends on how it is to be analyzed, so they are paired in research methods. The importance of explaining how and why study participants were selected for developing theory was described by Strauss and Corbin (1990). It is also important for data to maintain credibility, dependability, and authenticity (Beck, 2009). If there is no explanation about data collection, its adequacy cannot be evaluated.

In GTA, since data are analyzed very closely, collecting in-depth, detailed data and transcribing it correctly are very important. However, many of the articles did not explain how data were collected. It was noted that some researchers did not record their interviews and used transcriptions that were developed from the researcher's memory. This led to results that did not go beyond the summary level, so appropriate concepts did not appear.

Table 43.4. Adequacy of citation

Articles citing any source on methodology		111 (69.4)
Articles not citing any source on methodology		49 (30.6)
with appropriate explanation of process	26 (53.1)	
without appropriate explanation of process	23 (46.9)	
Total	49 (100%)	
Total		160 (100%)

Notes:
n = 160.
Original articles that used GTA which were published from 2001 to 2010.

Two articles did not mention the number and character of subjects. Also, one-third did not use an appropriate number of participants—often less than ten—even when participants seemed to be readily available. However, some of these articles stated that theoretical saturation had been reached. Theoretical saturation is "the point in analysis when all categories are well developed in terms of properties, dimensions, and variations" (Corbin & Strauss, 2008). Of course, the actual number of subjects is not the condition of theoretical saturation. It depends on the richness of data and topic. Nevertheless, it is difficult to imagine studies that used less than ten subjects would have reached this point. The results from these studies did not demonstrate this level of analysis.

In addition, grasping the interaction between the main participant and others, as well as the environment, culture, etc., is important in GTA and collecting data from all of these sources is recommended. At minimum, data should be collected not only from the main participant, but also from those surrounding the participant, that are related to the phenomena. In addition, observational data are also important. Nevertheless, not many studies included these kinds of data.

It should be noted, however, that the collection of data was done in rigorous compliance with established standards for research on human subjects. All of the research studies described in these articles were granted permission from human research committees and the study procedures to protect the rights of the participants were provided.

Problems in explaining and using methods in analysis

Although the analytical steps in GTA are not discrete but are interwoven, in this section the following six points of data analysis procedure are critiqued one by one: line-by-line coding, concept development, concept linkage, comparisons, theoretical sampling, and theoretical saturation.

Explanations and usage of these six points were evaluated. Concerning the explanations, each article was evaluated according to whether procedures were appropriately explained, not appropriately explained, or not mentioned. Usage was evaluated as appropriately used as described in the article, not appropriately used, or not mentioned (Table 43.5).

1 **Line-by-line coding:** In GTA, since analysis is done closely for the development of concepts, line-by-line coding (or phrase by phrase, depending on the richness of the data) is used. Whether it was appropriately used or not was evaluated according to the data described in the articles. It was found that about one-third (37.5%) of the articles explained line-by-line coding appropriately and also one-third (35.6%) used it correctly.

2 **Concept development:** More than half of the articles (58.1%) correctly explained the step of raising the level of abstraction of concepts from label to category. However, 80.0% of the articles used inappropriate names for labels and/or categories, such as using names for labels and categories that did not fit the data and/or referred to only one part of the data. These articles lost sight of the dictum that "coding is more than paraphrasing" (Corbin & Strauss, 2008, p. 66).

3 **Concept linkage:** Concept linkage was the most problematic step. An evaluation of the diagrams in the articles revealed that 40.6% of the articles explained it correctly. However, 61.3% of them demonstrated inappropriate usage such as categories that were connected according to the author's ideas and not according to the appropriate use of property and dimensions. Furthermore, another 36.9% did not even explain how concept linkage was implemented. Therefore, it was found that correct usage could only be confirmed in only 1.9% of the articles (three out of 160 articles).

Table 43.5 Explanation and usage of steps of analysis

	Line-by-line coding (%)		Concept development (%)		Concept linkage (%)		Comparisons (%)		Theoretical sampling (%)		Theoretical saturation (%)	
Explanation												
Appropriate	60	37.5	93	58.1	65	40.6	88	55.0	38	23.8	36	22.5
Not appropriate	17	10.6	48	30.0	30	18.8	1	0.6	1	0.6	4	2.5
Not mentioned	83	51.9	19	11.9	65	40.6	71	44.4	121	75.6	120	75.0
Usage												
Appropriate[1,4,5]	57	35.6	29	18.1	3	1.9	33	20.6	19	11.9	9	5.6
Not appropriate[2]	42	26.3	128	80.0	98	61.3	10	6.3	14	8.8	6	3.8
No way to evaluate[3]	61	38.1	3	1.9	59	36.9	117	73.1	127	79.4	145	90.6
	160		160		160		160		160		160	

Note: Steps in the analytical process are not discrete but are interwoven.
1   Evaluated as appropriately used in the description in article.
2   Evaluated as not appropriately used in the description in article.
3   These articles could not be evaluated because there was no explanation of how the usage was implemented.
4   If there was a reason for not doing an appropriate theoretical sampling it was evaluated as "appropriate".
5   If there was a reason for not doing an appropriate theoretical saturation, it was evaluated as "appropriate".

4 **Comparisons:** Both the making of constant comparisons and the making of theoretical comparisons are important in GTA (Corbin & Strauss, 2008). More than half of the articles explained this point appropriately. However, almost three-quarters of the articles (73.1%) did not describe how such comparisons were developed in their study. Another 6.3% explained their use of comparisons, but in a way that demonstrated inappropriate usage. Therefore, it could be determined that only 20.6% used it correctly.

5 **Theoretical sampling:** Theoretical sampling is one of the unique features of GTA. The purpose is to collect data for developing concepts and identifying relationships among them (Corbin & Strauss, 2008). However, only 23.8% of articles explained its use correctly. When evaluating the usage of theoretical sampling, if there was an explanation for why it was not done appropriately, it was evaluated as "appropriate." Nevertheless, only 11.9% of the articles could be evaluated as demonstrating an appropriate use of theoretical sampling. Almost four-fifths (79.4%) made no mention of how they conducted theoretical sampling. Of those that did, another 8.8% revealed inappropriate usage.

6 **Theoretical saturation:** As explained before, theoretical saturation is the point when all categories are well developed. It is a very important goal, but not easy to reach; 22.5% explained this correctly. When evaluating its usage, if there was an explanation for not reaching theoretical saturation, it was evaluated as an "appropriate usage." Nevertheless, only nine articles (5.6%) could be determined as doing so. Some 90.6% did not mention an attempt at theoretical saturation in their study, and of those that did, six of the 15 (3.8%) failed to apply the concept correctly.

Lack of new findings

Basically, qualitative research should be used to study topics where basic concepts need to be defined through the findings. However, very few of the articles (20.0%) showed new findings.

Many articles stated that their results were similar to those of previous studies or concepts. Then the question arises as to why they had to conduct the qualitative research study.

Future directions

This review of how one of the most popular methods in qualitative research is being used indicates the challenges faced by the rapid development of nursing academia. Although it only covers one of the 11 methods found in the survey, the same dynamics that generated these problems can be inferred to be occurring across the discipline. As new four-year programs and graduate-level programs were being rapidly developed, there has been an intense need for nurses with advanced degrees. However, the infrastructure and human resources needed to insure the quality of the graduate-level training are still struggling to catch up. This has been especially exacerbated in the training of qualitative research methods. Although qualitative research can seem to be deceptively easy to accomplish, as anyone who has made a serious attempt to truly master one of the methods knows, establishing rigor, verifiability, and significant results through the appropriate use of qualitative methods is an extreme challenge requiring extensive training.

This is an area where graduate level nursing academics is in great need of improvement. There were 136 Master's and 62 PhD programs in Japan in 2011(Japanese Ministry of Education, Culture, Sports, Science and Technology, 2011). In a survey of how research methods were taught in 12 doctoral courses in Japan, 58.3% of the courses provided lectures in qualitative research methods and the average time in these lectures was 27.6 hours. Only 33.3% had laboratories in qualitative research methods such as how to collect data through interview and participant observation. Of those that did, the average time spent in these laboratories was only five hours (Takagi, 2009).

This demonstrates that although qualitative research lectures were included in more than half of the courses, only a small amount included laboratory hours, and when they did, these hours were minimal.[8] This is woefully inadequate training for advanced-level research.

Given the importance of the qualitative approach for truly understanding and improving nursing, it is of utmost importance for nursing programs throughout the country, especially the advanced degree programs, to focus on the development of curricula that emphasize a rigorous approach to the proper training of qualitative research techniques. This must also extend to higher standards of peer review for publications, and a renewed effort among researchers to properly understand and implement qualitative research techniques.

Conclusion

This chapter has aimed to put the development of qualitative nursing research in the context of the concurrent rapid growth of both qualitative research and nursing academics. By focusing on how one particular method has been used, it has highlighted several weaknesses in how qualitative research techniques have been used in the health sciences in Japan, although the amount of such work has grown exponentially.

Specifically, within the body of published GTA articles, research methods were not clearly distinguished and there was confusion between different methods. Second, it often seemed that the research methods had not been chosen carefully. Third, there was a distinct lack of attention paid to data collection methods. Fourth, the explanations and use of analytical methods were problematic. For the majority of articles reviewed, procedures were not appropriately explained. As far as usage, the situation was more serious. If concept development and concept linkage are not adequate, theory development is not possible. Consequently, the results only reflected the author's perceptions and were not grounded in the data. Since the goal of GTA is to develop theory, this is problematic.

Although this conclusion is based on a critique of original articles that used GTA, articles that used other methods can be inferred to have similar problems. When this is put in the context of rapid growth of nursing academics in the country, and the dearth of well-developed curricula for training in qualitative techniques, the challenges facing the field become clear.

Acknowledgments

Some parts of this chapter were also used in the following articles: Saiki-Craighill, S., Mito, Y., & Seki, M. *Nihon no Iryou Bunya ni okeru Shituteki Kenkyu no Kentou: Parts 1–3* [Investigation of Qualitative Research in Health Sciences, Parts 1–3]. *Kango Kenkyu* (Vol. 45: pp. 481–489, 578–586, 694–703; 2012).

Notes

1   Japanese Ministry of Education, Culture, Sports, Science and Technology (2011). *Daigaku ni okeru kango-kei jinzai yousei no arikata ni kansuru kentou kai-Saishu houkoku* [Report of the investigative meeting on the development of nursing at the university level: Final report], March 2011.
2   Japana Centra Revuo Medicina (website): Ichushi database of the Japan Medical Abstracts Society [July 2011 ver.]. Available at: http://www.jamas.or.jp.
3   In the hierarchical structure of the Ichushi database, "qualitative research" is a lower level search term than the specific methods, so that a search with this term will not include the specific methods that constitute the various types of qualitative research. Therefore, a search with "qualitative research" as the term actually resulted in somewhat fewer articles than the combined search of the 11 methods mentioned.
4   Nine of the eleven were selected based on Oda's website, which lists books on qualitative research, including GTA, narrative, life story/life history, phenomenology, action research, fieldwork, ethnography, ethno-methodology and communication analysis, and discourse analysis. The articles using KJ method and content analysis were then added based on an investigation of the number of original articles published by Sekijima and others (2005).
5   Because the Ichushi database changed its rules on how articles were counted in 1995, the number of original articles prior to 1995 was greater than the number of articles after 1995.
6   Oda periodically revises his list. The data here are based on the information on the web site as of February 25, 2012.
7   *Grounded Theory Approach No Jissen: Shitsu-teki Kenkyu Eno Izanai* [Practice of Grounded Theory Approach: Invitation to Qualitative Research], 2003, Tokyo: Kobundo. *Bunya Betsu Jissen Hen Grounded Theory Approach* [Compiled by Field Grounded Theory Approach], 2005, Tokyo: Kobundo.
8   This survey was of 110 selected graduate schools in Japan in 2008. Although the rate of response was very low (31.8%) and only 12 out of 35 schools which answered the survey had a PhD program, this is the only resource available to understand how research methods are being taught. The same article indicated that 50% of the programs taught quantitative research methods and the average time in these lectures was 31.6 hours. The results from a survey of 35 Master's courses were also described. All courses provided lectures of quantitative research methods and the average number of lecture hours was 18.6 hours. 76.5% provided laboratory time and the average was 10.2 hours. However, 97% of Master's courses provided lectures on qualitative research techniques and an average of 11 hours was spent on these lectures.

References

Beck, C. T. (2009). Critiquing qualitative research. *AORN Journal, 90*, 543–554.
Charmaz, K. (2006).*Constructing grounded theory approach: A practical guide through qualitative analysis.* Thousand Oaks, CA: SAGE/(translation) Kakai, N., & Sueda, K. (2008). Kyoto: Nakanishiya Shuppan.
Chenitz, W. C. & Swanson, J. M. (1986). *From practice to grounded theory: Qualitative research in nursing.*

Reading, MA: Addison-Wesley Publishing/(translation) Higuchi, Y. & Inaoka, F. (1992). Tokyo: Igakushoin.

Corbin, J. M., & Strauss, A. L. (2008). *Basics of qualitative research: Techniques and procedures for developing grounded theory* (3rd ed.). Thousand Oaks, CA: Sage Publications.

Glaser, B. G., & Strauss, A. L. (1967). *Discovery of grounded theory: Strategies for qualitative research.* New York: Aldine De Gruyter/(translation) Goto, T., Ode, H., & Mizuno, S. (1996). Tokyo: Shinyosha.

Greenhalgh, T., & Hurwitz, B. (1998). *Narrative based medicine: Dialogue and discourse in clinical practice.* London; BMJ Books/(translation) Saito, S., Kishimoto, H., & Yamamoto, K. (2001). Tokyo: Kongo Syuppan.

Japana Centra Revuo Medicina. (website). Ichushi database of the Japan Medical Abstracts Society [July 2011 ver.]. Available at: http://www.jamas.or.jp.

Japanese Ministry of Education, Culture, Sports, Science and Technology. (2003). *Kango-gaku kyoiku no arikatani kansuru kentoukai: Dai 1-kai gijiroku* [Minutes of the investigative meeting on the education of nursing at the university level, First meeting]. July 2003.

Japanese Ministry of Education, Culture, Sports, Science and Technology. (2011). *Daigaku ni okeru kango-kei jinzai yousei no arikata ni kansuru kentou kai-Saishu houkoku* [Report of the investigative meeting on the development of nursing at the university level: Final report]. March 2011.

Kawakita, J. (1970). *Zoku Hasso-ho* [Method of generating ideas again]. Tokyo: Chuo-kouronsha.

Kawakita, J. (1995). *Hassoho no Kagaku* [Science of generating ideas]. Tokyo: Chuo-kouronsha.

Kinoshita, Y. (1999). *Grounded theory approach: Shitsu-teki Jisho Kenkyu No Saisei* [Regenerating empirical qualitative research]. Tokyo: Kobundo.

Kinoshita, Y. (2003). *Grounded theory approach No Jissen: Shitsu Teki Kenkyu Eno Izanai* [Practice of grounded theory approach: Invitation to qualitative research]. Tokyo: Kobundo.

Kinoshita, Y. (2005). *Bunya betsu jissen hen grounded theory approach* [Grounded theory approach: Compiled by field]. Tokyo: Kobundo.

Kleinman, A. (1989). *The illness narratives: Suffering, healing, and the human condition.* New York: Basic Books /(translation) Eguchi, S., Ueno, T., & Gokita, S. (1996). Tokyo: Seishin-Shobo.

Krippendorff, K. (1981). *Content analysis: An introduction to its methodology* (1st ed.) Thousand Oaks, CA: Sage/(translation) Mikami, S., Hashimoto, Y., & Shina, N. (1989). Tokyo: Keiso-shobo.

Oda, H. (2011). Appendix to translation (pp. 608–615) of Flick, U. (2007), *Qualitative Sozialforschung.* Reinbeck bei Hamburg: Rowohlt Verlag GmbH., Tokyo: Syunjyusha,

Oda, H. (web site). *Nihongo de Yomeru Shitsuteki Kenkyu no Bunken* [Qualitative research documents available in Japanese]. [February 25, 2012 ver.]. Available at: http://www13.ocn.ne.jp/~hoda/literature.html.

Saiki-Craighill, S. (2006). *Grounded theory approach: Riron wo Umidasu made* [Grounded theory approach: Toward the development of theory]. Tokyo: Shinyosha.

Saiki-Craighill, S. (2008). *Jissen Grounded theory approach: Gensho wo toraeru* [The practice of grounded theory approach: Grasping the phenomena]. Tokyo: Shinyosha.

Sekijima, K., Kagawa, F., Takagi, H., et al. (2005). *Igaku Chuo Zashi ni miru kango kenkyu ni okeru shitsu-teki kenkyu no doukou* [Qualitative research trend in the nursing research in the Igaku Chuo Zassi]. Departmental Bulletin Paper of Niigata University: School of Health Sciences, Faculty of Medicine, 8(1), 63–68.

Strauss, A. L. (1987). *Qualitative analysis for social scientists.* New York: Cambridge University Press.

Strauss, A. L., & Corbin, J. M. (1990). *Basics of qualitative research: Grounded theory procedures and techniques.* Thousand Oaks: Sage Publications/(translation) Minami, H., & Misao, H. (Eds.) (1999). Tokyo: Igakushoin.

Strauss, A. L., & Corbin, J. M. (1998). *Basics of qualitative research: Techniques and procedures for developing grounded theory* (2nd ed.). Thousand Oaks, CA: Sage Publications/(translation) Misao, H. & Morioka, T. (Eds.) (2004). Tokyo: Igakushoin.

Takagi, H. (2009). *Kangokei daigakuin ni okeru kango kenkyu-hou no kyouiku jittai* [Educational situation of nursing research methods in graduate schools of nursing]. INR 32(2), 6–10.

44

Qualitative nursing research in South-East Asia, China and Taiwan

David Arthur

Towards a research continuum

As I started writing this chapter, a debate between my understanding of quantitative and qualitative research as two ends of one continuum began to simmer in the recesses of my mind. How did a dichotomy ever occur? How could a qualitative "school" emerge in research? Lumping research methods such as phenomenology, ethnography or grounded theory under an umbrella term really does little justice to each of the methods. Yet this has developed, as has its own jargon that engenders automatic responses to the semantics. For example, the common saying: "quality not quantity"; "follow your head not your heart," "be scientific," or "a logical argument is sounder than an emotional argument," are all loaded statements, which imply that traditional scientific problem solving is sounder than examinations of people's experiences. Of course, this doesn't necessarily apply to research but using the terms qualitative and quantitative does trigger preconceived responses. We all want quality but not necessarily quantity in many aspects of our lives, but how does life quality equate with research quality? Are randomized controlled trials not of quality? Is there quantity in ethnographic studies? Indeed, can such a difference exist?

Then, in parallel, there is the right brain–left brain proposition. The popular, and more recently refereed literature would have us believe that one side of the brain has a stronger influence on emotion than logic, and vice versa. Is it really the right brain that which has more influence on our emotional intelligence, our ability to engage in emotional interactions, to be aware of our own emotions, to judge others emotions, to influence others emotions (Mayer, Salovey & Caruso, 2004a, 2004b)? The idea of intelligent quotient (IQ) and emotional intelligence (EI) as existing to different degrees in individuals has become popular. Is it, as Mayer, Salovey, and Caruso (2004a) propose in their four-branch model of EI, that the person with higher EI is better equipped to move along the continuum of emotional abilities from being able to perceive emotions in oneself accurately, to use emotions to facilitate thinking, understanding emotions, emotional language, and the signals conveyed by emotions, through to managing emotions so as to attain specific goals? Can this be applied to research? Is there a continuum of research from the "intelligent to the emotional"? Is the person with higher EI better able to manage qualitative research, and vice versa? Food for thought!

Deep in the crevices of the left hemisphere of my brain came a groan:

"Aarrrhhh . . . come on, get back to writing this chapter on qualitative research in Asia. Stop asking questions, which have no answers. We are supposed to write a piece on qualitative research in Asia. Now let's look at it logically. How can one possibly, adequately sample this vast geographical area and articulate the state of the science of qualitative research? There are at least 13 countries in Asia with some qualitative nursing research activity, many more languages, and an unknown number of publications at the refereed, non-refereed, and gray literature levels. Not to mention conferences and seminars. China alone has at least two million nurses, hundreds of Chinese language publications, and several conferences each year where thousands of nurses from around the country gather to present their research to each other, in Chinese. Most never make it to print, beyond an abstract, in any language, let alone one the international community can share. So forget about trying to generalize this state of the art, the research tools alone would need a huge toolbox, a small fortune to fund it, and that commodity all researchers crave, productive time!"

"Hear, hear . . . go Lefty!" came an echo from the recesses of the right brain. "You're right At last, it's time to be creative, time to come up with something attractive to the readers."

I could almost see the barely suppressed smirk, and feel the ripple of neuronal activity from the cubby-hole nestled in the crevasses of my right brain.

"So why don't you do what you always tell your students to do? Follow your research questions and be loyal to your method," quipped Right One.

"Ahhh, yes, always so emotionally clever, aren't you?" Lefty acquiesced cynically, but countered: "We haven't got the time to interview a reasonable number of experts from 13 countries in 13 languages, and certainly not enough resources to find 13 different samples through snowballing then aim for saturation of the interview data. Case studies, theory development, phenomenology, ethnography, focus groups! Aaahhhh! What a dilemma! Can't we just search CINAHL and come up with some numbers?"

"There you go again. Lefty, . . . now simmer down . . . take a deep breath, relax."

"I say, let's ask an expert," countered the one from the right side, rubbing hands together at the delight of the task ahead.

"Just sit back and listen and let me explain to you what we are going to do," followed Right One.

"What? Relax, sit back . . . are you kidding? . . . we've got a deadline . . . dates . . . reputation to uphold," moaned Lefty sensing the quantitative arsenal was looking sadly underequipped. "It's alright for you sitting back there making bullets and expecting me to fire them, you are supposed to be the creative one but you never stick your neck out!"

"Come on!" coaxed Right One. "Let's do this together, be true to the method, let's conduct an in-depth interview with an expert. Us! We are two parts of a brain supposedly connected, even joined on a continuum, we now find out. We have been slaving away here for nearly 60 years; let's get the body moving, the hands typing, he will do as we say. I will ask the questions and he can answer. Let his thoughts and feelings flow freely. Then we, more me than you, can examine the themes as they emerge, compare and contrast them with the literature and see what develops. Let the subjective nature of the material come straight from our rich center you guard and dilute with your figures, numbers and concrete arguments."

"OK. Go ahead, oh, wise one, you're always right!" quipped Lefty, feeling not quite as uncomfortable as Right One thought. For over the years quite a cosy relationship had developed, and while each side argued passionately for "their" beliefs and methods of best understanding the world, a core of comfort, of mutual respect and understanding, had grown.

"Okey dokey. Let's go. I would like to interview us about qualitative research in Asia. I am interested in our experiences, thoughts and feelings on the issue. Please feel free to talk openly and honestly and be reassured that we will not be able to be identified in any way through the data. With your permission we will record the data, then transcribe it and then show us a copy so that we can verify that it is what we meant. We can stop any time and withdraw if we wish with no penalty. Is that OK?"

"OK."

Tell me about your experience with qualitative research in the Asian region.
Wow, that's a big task, where shall I start?

That's up to you . . . go on . . .
OK, I will start with my experience in Australia, which is these days considered part of the Asia-Pacific region. I started nursing in 1973 when we were still in apprentice-type training in hospitals. Research itself, let alone qualitative research, was never mentioned in our training. By the time we had moved into college and university nursing education in Australia, in the mid-1980s, we were all still pretty green in research matters. Many of us were bachelor-prepared yet were working as academics in universities with high expectations of research as well as teaching and service. So there was a lot of pressure to research and it was quite a scramble really, the blind leading the blind, almost.

In the late 1980s, there was a strong push toward qualitative research. Professor Allan Pearson (Pearson, Durant, & Punton, 1989) then recently from the UK, was working in a university in the south of Australia and several quite senior nurses were studying their higher degrees with him. Apparently he was advocating a "new" form of research. There was a lot of excitement, as a catchy language seemed to be emerging, with philosophical terms like "phenomenology," "ethnography," "etic," "emic," etc., terms which were new to me. I was after all groomed for basic science before I rebelled and became more humanistic in my approach to life and work. Alan Pearson's work was brave, eclectic and innovative. His publication record in the 1980s and 1990s was outstanding and reflected the importance of using whatever research method is necessary to answer the question and provide evidence for practice, and for nurse-led practice (Baker & Pearson, 1991). Yet 25 years on, nursing is still laboring under medical dominance in many countries and the adoption and use of clinical nursing units, nurse-led clinics and the like are still not widespread enough.

I studied research in my bachelor program and conducted quantitative research in my Master's degree but qualitative research was not discussed, that I can remember. I was on one university ethics committee in 1989 and one of the studies involved interviews and the traditional empirical scientists took the view that this was not research, rather an "audit" and didn't need consideration by the committee! Things began to snowball, and for me having studied nursing in a hospital-based program where research of any form was never mentioned, the learning curve was steep.

Although having studied education, the idea of listening to and utilizing people's experiences to bolster teaching and learning was not new. I guess the language was different or I wasn't paying attention. In the early 1990s I had a student from Korea who wanted to do a phenomenological study (Jeon, 1995). She came across the method through her contacts in the education faculty, which was at the time providing an avenue for us to complete higher degrees. The expert supervisor was in education and I was the supervisor ensuring the clinical and academic quality of the nursing material. Several of our faculty in the nursing school were becoming strong advocates of qualitative research, strong almost to the point of denigrating more conventional forms of research.

Tell us about the development of publication of qualitative research in refereed literature in the Asian Pacific region.

You will have to check, but I would say the early 1990s is pretty close. Remember that the language was relatively new and people were doing interviews and data analysis, which would qualify for qualitative research, but the use of the jargon was not established. Not having mentors of our own, we were learning from the disciplines of education sociology and psychology, as we were simply novices in research. Jeon (1995) was the first Master's student I supervised. We collected the data in interviews with patients living in the community and her thesis was published in 1995 and her first paper in the English literature in 1994. She also produced some papers in Korean but where or if they were ever referenced I can't be sure. She is now a senior academic in the University of Sydney and is a prolific qualitative researcher, who also participates in projects using different methods.

Also keep in mind that the nursing qualification available around Asia was at the sub-degree level. They still had hospital training in Hong Kong; Singapore admitted students from year ten to a diploma; China was still struggling with the backlash of the scholarly cringe that resulted in universities ceasing most programs around 1945. Nurses were trained on the job. These countries were the more developed in the region so you can imagine what the state of nursing education was like in other developing countries such as Indonesia, Vietnam and Malaysia. So little nursing research was conducted, and even less published prior to the 1990s.

It was in the mid-1990s that Australian nursing schools began reaching out to our colleagues in Asia and the government encouraged us to feel and be part of the Asia Pacific Region. Australian degrees were conducted offshore and many Asian nurses studied bachelor, Master's and PhDs in Australia. With this came the emergence of research and its dissemination.

On reflection, even then we were using interviews of individuals in multi-method studies, which were certainly qualitative, we didn't use the jargon, and unfortunately we were slow to publish.

Horses for courses

Unfortunately, during that period, research methods became a bit political. By that, I mean people took sides. It seemed that you were either a qualitative researcher or a quantitative researcher and the whole issue became tangled up in gender politics. Sort of like the men were the hard-nosed empirical types and the women more into exploratory, in-depth, methods of unearthing rich data. I never felt strongly one way or the other. I had studied math and physics and statistics at school then in my bachelor degree and I was at home with "quantitative methods" and could and still do see the importance of the subjective, phenomenological experience in nursing.

I really think a lot of it had to do with the fact that many of my colleagues had not completed math or science subjects at school and therefore were intimidated by "numbers" or "sums" as some of my nursing colleagues used to call the physics subject at university. So for many, heading the qualitative route was more comfortable especially if your "science" background was weak and, as many of our colleagues seem to be, stronger in emotional intelligence.

I remember another landmark study (Lawler, 1990), which was played like a ball in a tennis match between the qualitative research side and the quantitative research side. The study used participant and non-participant observation and interviews with 35 nurses and was an early contribution to qualitative research. Unfortunately it was not published in the refereed literature, but it really did stir up some strong responses from both camps.

Things these days have become a lot more sensible, more a case of choosing a method that suits your research questions, or to put in horse-racing parlance, choosing "horses for courses."

613

On a wet track choose a horse that does well in that milieu, and if it's a hot, dry track, choose a horse that has a record of performing well in those conditions. In other words let the task at hand and the questions you ask drive your choice of method.

OK, thanks. Then tell me more your experiences with qualitative research.

Sure, well, if you look at the picture now the amount of qualitative research (mainly phenomenological but also ethnographic, grounded theory but rarely case study) produced in this region is quite impressive. In the universities with which I am most familiar in China, Hong Kong, Philippines, Thailand and Singapore, the nursing degrees are of four years duration, except the latter which is three. In the students' final year they are required to conduct a research study. Some universities allow group work, others insist on individual studies. In the three Philippine universities where I work, until recently the total number of graduates was around 700 per year and I would venture to say that 70% of these, that is around 500 qualitative studies are conducted each year. In July 2010 nearly 90,000 nurses at the board exam! Imagine how many pieces of research were conducted. What a resource this would be if they were published or electronically accessible, but unfortunately they rarely see the light of day, rather the dust of libraries, and certainly are not entered into dissertation indices.

The Philippines

A search of the titles of studies that were conducted by fourth year nursing students, at Angeles University Foundation, the Philippines, for 2009, 2010 and 2011, revealed 160 completed group research projects of which 13 (23%), 12 (21%) and 25 (52%) respectively were qualitative in nature. Over the three years this totaled 50 (31%) which included either "the lived experience" or "phenomenological" in the title. No clear theme emerged in terms of subjects; rather the studies all looked at difficult nursing issues such as obesity, death and dying, stroke, renal disorder, abortion, transsexuals, overseas workers, diabetes, stillborn babies, various issues in mother-hood, and specific disorders such as Asperger's syndrome, Alzheimer's disease, hemophilia, schizophrenia, homunculi, Tourette syndrome and Moebius syndrome.

These students and their supervisors do impressive work involving much effort which, although being a valuable exercise and part of the students' degree, is probably only read by a few students and to the best of my knowledge none of it has been published. However, four of the studies were presented at the First International Conference on Qualitative Research in Nursing and Health in Thailand in 2010, which incidentally was held again in the Philippines in 2012.

What a waste of good material. If it were shared internationally and expanded upon, it would give nursing and health care in the Philippines a boost. It's ironic really, when you think that the Philippines is the largest exporter of nurses in the world and as such strongly influences health care internationally! Students choose subjects that represent an area of interest and most seem very important local nursing issues. Why they are not published is not really clear except to say that the students lack the confidence and experience and are more than ready to move on once they finish their final year. And their supervisors have neither research track records, nor the confidence nor experience in publication. This is really a hard cycle to break.

My experience in the Philippines has led me to be able to make a couple of cautious generalizations. First, the main aim of gaining a nursing degree in the Philippines is to be able to use it to move and work overseas so the family can have a reasonable income and break the poverty cycle. Families frequently devote everything to getting their kids a degree for that purpose. So the brain drain is endless. The better nurses, and doctors who become nurses, and other degree holders who become nurses, leave and the health care system suffers. As soon as possible, they borrow money, barely gain enough clinical experience, and then apply overseas. Obviously research is low on the agenda if your main professional aim is to get a job anywhere but at home, so you can feed the family. Second, for those that are left behind the news is gloomy. There is little work. The health care system is in a mess. Hugely overcrowded public hospitals have poor facilities and equipment and can barely afford to employ a skeleton nursing staff. Nurses volunteer to work in hospitals so they can gain clinical experience! University nursing students and faculty in communities provide outstanding nursing care, and caring communities manage to look after themselves. Yet serious surgical and medical disorders spell doom for families who simply can't afford procedures, equipment or medicine. Either the family goes into debt or they are left to fend for themselves.

Hong Kong

When I reached Hong Kong in 1995, they were in the process of moving from hospital schools of nursing to universities and in the case of the Hong Kong Polytechnic to university status. I was really pleased when I arrived about the supportive attitude toward research. There didn't seem to be factions, none of the nursing faculty was yet PhD qualified, but they held research in high esteem and seemed quite *au fait* with quantitative methods. I somehow had the reputation of being a qualitative researcher. Certainly I had been doing qualitative research but wasn't familiar with the literature, apart from focus groups and in-depth interviews with interview guidelines and I searched for themes manually using my own sorting method (Arthur, 1999). But as the Master's and bachelor honors students were interested in qualitative methods, again mainly phenomenological, as in most of my career, I learned alongside my students, just managing to keep one step ahead (Leung & Arthur, 2004; Wong & Arthur, 2000). Interestingly, and worth considering, was that both these studies utilized individual interviews and phenomenology, and focus groups and phenomenology respectively, yet both slip under the radar if one is looking for qualitative or phenomenological research. So here's a tip: if you want people who are searching the titles in the literature to recognize your research method, choose the words in the paper titles carefully.

By 2006, just ten years after I arrived, the majority of the faculty had obtained PhDs, many in quantitative methods and some were then publishing their work (Wong & Lee, 2000) and gaining their own reputations as qualitative researchers.

In this ten-year period, from 1995 to 2006 there was a huge growth in scholarship in the region. Thailand, Taiwan, Hong Kong, Philippines and China were conducting nursing bachelor programs and developing Master's and PhDs. And there were some healthy collaborations developed utilizing the spectrum of research methods, mixed methods and of course qualitative research. This had a knock-on effect in China where we, in Hong Kong were taking a lead role in helping certain universities develop their research degrees and research agendas. This is nearly impossible to quantify but in 1996 the first four-year bachelor degree in nursing commenced at Peking Union Medical College. Research output was negligible and the first home-grown PhD, via the Hong Kong Polytechnic graduated in 1999 (Li, 1999).

The evidence: Hong Kong, China, and Taiwan

A search of the CINAHL data base from 1986 to 2012 using the search terms (qualitative OR phenomenolog* or ethnograph* OR grounded theory OR lived experience OR action research OR focus group) and (Hong Kong OR China OR Philippines OR Taiwan OR Singapore), revealed 69 papers published in English which reported qualitative research conducted in the above countries or addressed issues related to qualitative research in those countries.

It is difficult to be exhaustive because this was a title search and some studies have not used the above research terms that indicate a qualitative study.

Papers from the People's Republic of China totaled 24, followed by Taiwan (15), Hong Kong (14), Thailand (15), Singapore (3), and the Philippines (3). There were no outstanding themes in terms of topic with the exception of 6 out of 24 papers from Taiwan addressing mental health issues featuring the author Huang et al. (2008, 2009). Interestingly most of these were published between 2010 and 2012.

Interestingly one of the phenomenological papers featuring the lived experiences of academics working in primary health care curriculum in a rural nursing school was used in a recent research text (Arthur et al., 2006) where the authors demonstrated how to critique a piece of qualitative research using various criteria. This study (Arthur et al., 2006) was critiqued as an example of phenomenological research.

China

I'm very fortunate to have been regularly visiting Peking Union Medical College (PUMC) for many years and have observed, like most things it seems in China, a boom in research not only qualitative but also quantitative. From a nursing culture in the mid-1990s where conservatism and caution ruled, there is now an adventurous spirit among nurse researchers in the better universities and many outstanding researchers are examining issues which are in need of change.

It is important to remember that while the overall medicine and nursing in China are very active, the most active and developed is very often confined to more urban areas, so the quality of health care and nursing in one region or city may differ greatly to that of a more remote, lesser-developed area.

Unfortunately, unless you are a Chinese speaker and/or reader, it's very difficult to find out exactly what is happening or, in other words to quantify the output of Chinese nursing scholars. There are many nursing journals, mainly published in Chinese and not that many Chinese nurses are competent at publishing in English without editing help.

It's quite easy to search CINAHL and see how much has been published in English about issues in China, but I don't know how much has been published in the local refereed literature. I do know that I have attended many conferences, probably around 50 in the last ten years. In the early days it was mainly overseas nurses presenting in English, locals in Chinese. But in the last, say, five years, I have seen hundreds of abstracts of qualitative research studies, most of which I doubt have been published. If I had the time I would do a study looking at the uptake of research by refereed journals, from papers presented at conferences. This would be really valuable evidence for publication bias, and ammunition for senior scholars who really need to help junior colleagues, and their universities move on with their publication output.

The evidence: Chinese language publications

Professsor Li Zheng, the first "home-grown" (she studied in Hong Kong) PhD graduate in China conducted a search of the Chinese nursing literature databases, from 1985 to 2012, using the same parameters (translated into Chinese) as that for the CINAHL search noted above, revealed a total of 508 qualitative nursing research studies of which: 311 were "phenomenology and nursing," 12 for "grounded theory and nursing," 17 "action research and nursing," and 168 "qualitative research and nursing."

There were at least 23 journals accessed. As expected for a profession which is rediscovering itself there were many papers published on professional and educational issues, numbering 118. These were on characteristics of nurses, their backgrounds, educational issues and their responses to certain situations. There were several on men in nursing, several on burnout, stress, night shift and satisfaction. Others explored specific educational issues such as communication, empathy and simulated learning.

The remaining 390 were specifically related to clinical issues. For example, there were 40 studies addressing clinical cancer issues, many of which were breast cancer.

Interestingly the increase over the years is worth mentioning: from one paper in 2002, 156 were published in 2011.

Tell me more about quantity and quality of qualitative research in Asia.

That has a ring to it! Two things stand out in Asia. First, the desire of students and faculty to do qualitative research and, second, the usefulness of such research.

In BN programs in Hong Kong, Thailand and the Philippines there is a strong emphasis on getting students starting research in the fourth year of their program. I think it makes sense to do a qualitative study at the bachelor level, just as much as it does to do an instrument reliability and/or validity test. But for some reason I think many students, novices and experienced nurses alike think the former type of study is easier. So quality will always suffer if there are insufficient, inexperienced or, worse, negligent supervisors. Honestly I think some of our earlier attempts were "loose" in terms of rigor and this has no doubt improved as qualitative research has improved its "status" as a reputable research method, and some leaders have emerged to promote the method.

The use of more structured techniques of organizing data such as that of Colaizzi (1978) have improved reliability by providing data trails and the like, as has metasynthesis.

I have supervised at least 20 honors and Master's qualitative theses and managed to publish several and have presented at conferences and have had a good hit rate. Probably due to the fact that much of the research we do in Asia is new, in this context. There are so many research opportunities in health care and nursing. Often, because of the poor standard of health care there is an absence of good nursing and medicine, let alone research, and a study examining the reasons for this or trying to do a cultural validation of an overseas study is interesting, challenging and good reading.

From a pragmatic point of view as a senior researcher, to have a student helping a larger multi-method study by examining an issue in depth in order to culturally validate, or see if a complex concept is replicable, is of great value: the students get a good supervisor, a good topic and the outcome is relatively quick and should be publishable.

So you asked about quality. In the above scenario, in my experience it has been a boon having bachelor and Master's students working on these projects. The drawback is twofold. First, too many students, very junior and naïve in research, come to the table with ideas that don't fit with the department's research agendas, or the supervisors' agenda. This needs to be very carefully managed. Students should be encouraged to take part in larger team studies and discouraged from doing it alone. This creates alienation of the students and a risk to quality.

Over the years, I have noticed the tendency for students to want to study something of professional interest, which has emerged from their own personal experiences. It used to be stress. "I want to study stress in ICU nurses" or "stress in nurses doing shift work." Now it seems to be "quality of life of nursing students, or students in university." I use the question "So what?" to try to tease out the usefulness or otherwise of these ideas. There is no need to do a literature review to find out that nurses in high-pressure situations experience stress and that stress is not always a positive experience. We know that so why study it again? Do something about it! There are far too many measures of stress and anxiety and quality of life as it is. And, there is far too little replication. Add to this the students who in their *naïveté* desire to develop their own instruments, there is a further possibility of clouding the picture. Really, there should be much tighter direction given to students in terms of methods and topics and replication should be strongly encouraged. I use the idea that at the undergraduate level and to a degree in course work Master's research, the student is doing an apprenticeship in research and works with the "master" to learn the techniques and work on small parts of a larger project. The student can also learn a method by replicating previous work.

The future

It's time to implement and test well-designed interventions, those have been developed over the decades and are very qualitative in nature, and at the same time very measurable quantitatively. What about a lifestyle program for groups of stressed nurses, that: presents cognitive behavioral strategies to examine mood and behavioral responses; conducts problem solving, creative thinking, and lateral thinking exercises; expands emotional intelligence, provides training for systematic relaxation, yoga and mindfulness meditation; as well as diet exercise and alternatives to managing the unhealthy responses to stress? Now, there's a large study to get your teeth into! Get your students to take a segment of that and tie it all together into something of use, of value to the individual within the profession. Take it into another culture and you can double the amount of publications with translation, validation, reliability testing, and cultural interpretation

Asia is a perfect setting for using qualitative studies when trying to interpret/translate material used overseas into complex languages and cultures such as China, and Thai. I find this type of research really fascinating and satisfying.

Tell me more about that.

Learning from experience

Well, expressed emotion is a good example. This idea that there is an emotional climate in the family, which can affect the recovery and relapse rate of patients with schizophrenia was researched from the 1960s in the UK. The Camberwell Family Interview (Vaughn & Leff, 1976) expressed emotion instrument was carefully developed from multiple interviews and the experiences of some very clever researchers and clinicians who were able to synthesize the qualitative findings into an instrument for assessing expressed emotion which in turn helped develop strategies for family therapy which in turn has helped improve the re-hospitalization and relapse rates of patients, and further helped a lot of families cope better with a truly debilitating disorder. It all started with a clever fellow by the name of Brown (Brown & Rutter, 1966), who in the 1960s noticed that patients who were discharged to the family home fared worse than those discharged to a hostel or more distant relative.

So think about how the concept and tool were developed. It grew from samples of patients and families and their Anglo-Saxon/Celtic carers. The social environment was one of increasing tolerance and acceptance of patients with mental disorder and the treatment facilities were moving into the communities. Tolerance, humane treatment and government support where abundant. The concepts used were very clearly verbal patterns of expressed emotion captured as homogeneous commonalities in this sample of patients and their families. On reflection, it would seem impossible to take this to another country and culture. The Camberwell Family Interview instrument itself took around an hour to administer.

True to form and in their inimitable style, the Americans were able to take the concepts and the tools and produce a 10-minute interview for family expressed emotion and demonstrated this abbreviated version's reliability and validity.

We were really excited by this because even in the mid-1990s little had been done in Hong Kong relating to improving family communication to help the patient discharged home. While there were attempts to improve community-based mental health care in HK, in mainland China the institutions were still huge and community care negligible.

Now, imagine the context in Beijing. From around 1946 or so onwards to around 1980 the country was ruled by fear and terror. Talking about the wrong topic to the wrong person could mean incarceration of a person and even the family. Creative thought and debate were off the agenda. There were no such things as friends; there were classmates, workmates, children, and wives and husbands. Wives and husbands were very careful about what they said to each other. Trust was non-existent. A generation of people was forced into emotionless, routine servants of the regime, ever fearful of the violent and swift recriminations of deviating from the norm. As an aside, I was intrigued when I first went to Beijing to Peking Union Medical College in 1996, and met their first graduate of the new degree and the last graduate of the last degree, made extinct by the revolution. They were something like 50 years' difference in age.

So imagine, along comes the foreigner with all these great ideas, seeded from the USA, about communication, assertiveness, talking openly, trust, and empathy. They must have thought we were nuts when we started to help with the first bachelor programs in Beijing in 1996. Encouraging group meetings, open, honest interaction . . . wow, we were naïve.

Anyway, we persevered over the years, developed a bit of our own insight and understanding of culture and were not surprised when families were suspicious of filling out forms, especially having to do them twice (in the case of pre-post-test studies). Coming into their homes was a clear threat to their safety, and having the man of the family identified by other community members as mentally ill was a disaster, one which would have meant indefinite incarceration only some 10 or 20 years earlier.

So expressed emotion (EE) was a very difficult concept to translate not only in language but also across a culture steeped in ancient history, recently stagnated by oppression and terror. It sounds grim, but since our first research in the mid-1990s things have really improved and some excellent research is developing both within institutions and out in the community, and I'm proud to say there is a healthy balance of both qualitative and quantitative research methods being used in Hong Kong and China.

Methodological issues and exemplars

Culture and context play a major role in the application of qualitative research. Jeon (1995), for example, when exploring the experiences of parents of patients with serious mental illness in Australia, was readily invited into home in the community. Li and Arthur (2005b) on the other hand struggled to get follow-up interviews with patients discharged to the family home in Beijing. The families, she explains, were ashamed because of the stigma of mental illness particularly for males and the reluctance to trust questionnaires and reluctance to have interviews conducted outside the hospital. Li and Arthur's (2005a) study on the effects of a family intervention program on the outcomes of patients with schizophrenia in China, is an exemplar of how qualitative research can be used to set a solid foundation for developing a later trial. Li was the first home-grown PhD in China, graduating from Hong Kong, and the second after her colleague who graduated from a US university.

Li and Arthur's qualitative studies involved interviews and analysis of data from patients, and nurses in Beijing mental health settings, exploring the concept of EE both in HK and Beijing (2005b) and translation of several outcome measures and their testing with samples of experts for their validity and reliability. She was rewarded with publication of the qualitative data (Li & Arthur, 2005b) and the quantitative data in the prestigious *British Journal of Psychiatry* (Li & Arthur, 2005a).

Another clinical issue of importance, and understudied in Chinese samples is that of perinatal depression. As is often the case, the concepts were first defined and extrapolated from patients in English-speaking countries in largely European cultures. Leung et al. (2005) noticed a trend in mothers in the postnatal period and began to examine the experience of Hong Kong mothers with depression. She conducted a phenomenological examination of a large sample of women in clinics and at home and drew some interesting conclusions: (1) that the incidence of PND in HK is at least as high as other countries, and (2) that there are certain cultural practices which impact on some mothers and their development and management of depression. A clash between the modern "Western" way of life, and the traditional way of "doing the month" after birth with the mother-in-law. Leung's work (2005) has developed steadily and is moving toward a trial of an intervention for susceptible mothers.

Since its first exploration in the mid-1990s in Hong Kong, it has been picked up in Singapore, where again, because of the three main cultural groups, Indian, Chinese and Malay, a deeper understanding through phenomenology was necessary to first provide the foundation for later clinical intervention studies (Nasear et al., 2012). This is an area of study which lends itself to phenomenology, grounded theory or ethnography.

OK, this has been really interesting. In the last few minutes, would you comment on the future of qualitative research in Asia?

OK. Let me take the gloves off here for a minute. It's early days for Singapore, and their scholarly development is hampered by their polytechnic diploma education, lack of innovative research leadership, and heavily medically dominated health care and an overly bureaucratic nursing education system. Despite progressive government thinking in terms of lifestyle-related disorders and interventions, little seems to filter into the scope of nursing practice. They are a long way from making an impression on the refereed literature.

Hong Kong has the resources and the talent, but is losing the bountiful research opportunities in greater China as locals take over. It also has a troubled health care system, plagued with overcrowding and well-reported nursing bungles. They need to practice some mindful approaches to leadership in nursing and health care and replace the paternalistic, medically dominated system, with one which is more flexible, creative and better prepared for the further growth of the aging population and lifestyle-related disorders. Turning their research agenda on themselves would give nurses a golden opportunity for qualitative research. For example, complaints about nursing shortages are ongoing and clearly the current education and/or recruitment system is inadequate. Importing nurses from the Philippines should be high on the agenda. Filipino nurses are well educated, flexible, can speak English and would integrate and perform well in Hong Kong where there are already hundreds of thousands working in various service industries. The problem is that the registration board requires competence in Cantonese, which is an antiquated requirement given that the method of tuition for nurses is in English and virtually everyone in the health care system can speak English. Besides, a three-month immersion course would provide new nurses with sufficient Cantonese to work in the hospitals and community. The whole issue is, however, clouded with political and legal mist but nevertheless would provide plenty of opportunities for qualitative research.

Unfortunately Taiwan is not a major player in the international qualitative research field despite their excellent nursing programs, scholars and leaders. They are hampered by language, or maybe we are hampered by language—at any rate it is hard for us to share their research due to language barriers.

Thailand has a healthy research and nursing university culture and shares productive collaborations with many universities around the globe. Their research is innovative and focused on the needs of the people. Unfortunately again, much of their dissemination is in the gray literature and in conferences and seminars, and language is a barrier. A search of CINAHL does not do them justice.

In harmony with the global economic and political shift toward China, there will be a huge expansion of nursing knowledge and literature in the Asian region. The issues high on their agenda already, apart from HIV/AIDS research, which is already underway, are lifestyle-related disorders: cancer, heart disease, cardiovascular disease, obesity, diabetes, alcohol-related disorders, and mental health. Nurses will examine the use of innovative interventions, many of which will be in harmony with traditional Chinese medicine (TCM), using herbal, plant remedies and adjunctive acupuncture and acupressure. Congruently there are several cross-cultural interpretive studies which should be well suited to qualitative research designs including the concept of empathy, reflective listening, humanistic counseling and interactive student-driven education strategies—all issues which are foreign to conventional Asian communication and education values.

The Philippines is another sleeping research giant. One of the few countries in the world still experiencing population growth, it is conceivable that they will become a valuable, worldwide source of professionals in the future. As developed countries experience epidemics of aging and lifestyle-related disorders, Filipinos will be needed to provide the nursing care. Their education is of a high standard, their English language skills are good and they are mobile people. Their services will not always be as cheap as they are now and this will fuel local development of the profession and contribute in no small part to the country's economic recovery.

Well, thanks for sharing your experiences and ideas with us.
You are very welcome. I enjoyed it, it was almost cathartic.

"There you are, Lefty, how was that?" asked Right One.

"I must say, it was well done. And we have been a part of all that? It's impressive how much we have been party to over the years. You cosy in your corner and me in mine. We even sneaked some figures in there, I liked that!" responded Lefty.

"Everybody has the capacity to use their right and left parts of their brain. Call it IQ or EQ, the smart researcher chooses from a creative arsenal of research strategies. People become smart researchers by keeping an open mind, by learning from experts and wide reading." said Right One.

"Just as solving a life problem can be done by either of the hemispheres of the brain, or by both, depending on the problem, be it logical sequential or in need of abstract inspiration, so too qualitative research has its place either with or next to quantitative research in solving research problems, some more mathematically sequential, others more abstract and in need of deeper creative work. The smart researcher is like the human benefiting from input from both."

"Well, thank you, wise Right One, and thank you, Sir, in the middle, it was fun. Do you think we answered all the questions he started with, if I may be pedantic? But I suppose you on the right side would say, they were rhetorical questions producing seedling ideas which need to be left to sit and germinate, until the reader, one day can see the wood for the trees. How's that for a right hook from the left camp?"

Well, that was the easiest chapter I have ever written. All I needed to do was let the creative and logical parts of my brain work together in harmony. There is a lesson there!

References

Arthur, D. (1999). Assessing nursing students' basic communication skills: The development and testing of a rating scale. *Journal of Advanced Nursing*, *29*(3), 658–665.

Arthur, D., Drury, J., Sy-Sinda, M.T., Nakao, R., Lopez, A., Gloria, G., Turtal, R., & Luna, E. (2006). The lived experience of primary health care nurses in a school of nursing in the Philippines: A phenomenological study. *International Journal of Nursing Studies*, *43*(1), 107–112.

Baker, H., & Pearson, A. (1991). The experience of patients in a professorial nursing unit. *Australian Journal of Advanced Nursing*, *9*(1), 15–19.

Brown, G. W., & Rutter, M. L. (1966). The measurement of family activities and relationships. *Human Relationships*, *19*, 241.

Colaizzi, P. (1978). Psychological research as the phenomenologist views it. In R. Valle & M. King (Eds.), *Existential-phenomenological alternatives for psychology* (pp. 48–71). New York: Oxford University Press.

Huang, X., Lin M., Yang, T., & Sun, F. (2009). Hospital-based home care for people with severe mental illness in Taiwan: A substantive grounded theory. *Journal of Clinical Nursing*, *18*(21), 2956–2968.

Huang, X., Yen, W., Liu, S., & Lin, C. (2008). The role of community mental health nurses caring for people with schizophrenia in Taiwan: A substantive grounded theory. *Journal of Clinical Nursing*, *17*(5), 654–666.

Jeon, Y. H. (1994). Respite care for people with a chronic mental disorder and their caregivers: A critical review. *Australian Journal of Mental Health Nursing*, *3*(1), 10–15.

Jeon, Y. H. (1995). The lived experience of caring for a family member with chronic mental illness: A phenomenological study. Master of Nursing thesis, University of Newcastle, Newcastle, NSW.

Lawler, J. (1990). A social construction of the body: Nurses' experiences. PhD thesis, University of New South Wales, Australia.

Leung, J., & Arthur, D. (2004) Clients and facilitators' experiences of participating in HK self-help group for people recovering from mental illness. *International Journal of Mental Health Nursing*, *13*(4), 232–242.

Leung, S., Martinson, I., & Arthur, D. (2005). Postpartum depression and related psychosocial variables in Hong Kong Chinese women: Findings from a prospective study. *Research in Nursing and Health*, *28*, 27–38.

Li, Z. (1999). The effect of an education programme on family members and patients with schizophrenia in Beijing. Unpublished doctoral thesis, The Hong Kong Polytechnic University, Hong Kong.

Li, Z., & Arthur, D. (2005a). A controlled trial of family education for people with schizophrenia in Beijing, China. *British Journal of Psychiatry*, *187*, 339–345.

Li, Z. & Arthur, D. (2005b). A study of three measures of expressed emotion in a sample of Chinese families of people with schizophrenia. *Journal of Psychiatric and Mental Health Nursing*, *12*, 431–438.

Mayer, J. D., Salovey, P., & Caruso, D. R. (2004a). Emotional intelligence: Theory, findings and implications. *Psychological Inquiry*, *15*(3), 197–215.

Mayer, J. D., Salovey, P., & Caruso, D. R. (2004b). A further consideration of the issues of emotional intelligence. *Psychological Inquiry*, *15*(3) 249–255.

Nasear, E., Makay, S. & Arthur, D., et al. (2012). An exploratory study of traditional birthing practices of Chinese, Malay and Indian women in Singapore. *Midwifery*, *28*, e865–e871.

Pearson. A., Durant, I., & Punton, S. (1989). Determining quality in a unit where nursing is the primary intervention. *Journal of Advanced Nursing*, *14*(4), 269–273.

Vaughn, C., & Leff, J. (1976). The measurement of expressed emotion in the families of psychiatric patients. *British Journal of Social Clinical Psychology*, *15*, 157.

Wong, F. K. Y., & Lee, W. M. (2000). A phenomenological study of early nursing experiences in Hong Kong. *Journal of Advanced Nursing*, *6*, 1509–1517.

Wong, Y. K., & Arthur, D. G. (2000). Hong Kong patients' experiences of intensive care after surgery: Nurses' and patient's views. *Intensive and Critical Care Nursing*, *16*, 290–303.

45

Future directions in international qualitative nursing research

Cheryl Tatano Beck

In this final chapter of the *Routledge International Handbook of Qualitative Nursing Research* attention is focused on future directions for nursing research. As evidenced by the international qualitative research addressed in this handbook, we in nursing have reason to celebrate how far we have come in regards to qualitative research. We cannot, however, rest on our laurels. Qualitative methods are continuing to evolve, be modified, and become essential to knowledge development. Funding for qualitative research must be increased for this movement to be sustained and grow. This chapter is a compilation of the directions for future qualitative research around the globe that the nursing contributors of this handbook identified that merit our consideration in order to advance qualitative research in nursing.

Qualitative nurse researchers in the future need to focus on elevating qualitative research into the forefront of evidenced based practice. In Chapter 2, Morse calls for increased utilization of methods of synthesis and also use of mixed methods to facilitate this process. Morse contends that qualitative nurse scholars also need to use "harder" data such as microanalytic analysis of video data and not just focus on inferential methods. Qualitative contributions for assessing evidence have great potential for nursing practice.

In order for researchers and clinicians to be able to access the valuable qualitative findings from nursing studies conducting throughout the world, Beck in Chapter 10 calls for breaking down the language barriers so that the powerful research conducted by qualitative nurse researchers in non-English-speaking countries can also be published in English journals. Munhall in Chapter 11 points out that in nursing research there is worldwide interest in understanding what it means to be human. Meaning in turn creates worldviews. She tells us that interpretive phenomenology is not only a research method but also a nursing worldview which allows possibilities and different meanings to be understood.

Debates among grounded theorists in nursing will continue regarding whether to stay with the classic Glaserian method, as Stern in Chapter 12 is a proponent of, or explore ways of modifying and enhancing this original method. Corbin (Chapter 13) contents that grounded theory is most useful for studying and explaining the contextual factors or conditions that facilitate or hinder individuals' ability by evolving action/interaction to enable control over personal and professional problems. Future grounded theorists can discover concepts that can be used for discourse about pertinent professional phenomena and concepts that will be the foundation for practice and research in our profession.

Schreiber and Martin in Chapter 14 explore new directions in the future regarding the use of grounded theory. They note some challenges that face nursing grounded theorists in the future. The complexity of grounded theory requires novice researchers to go back to the original references for grounded theory and to examine its roots in order to have a thorough comprehension of the method. It is no longer adequate to just indicate you are using grounded theory. Nurse researchers must identify their own philosophy regarding the method they choose (i.e. Glaserian vs. Straussian), describe what grounded theory means, and provide a rationale for its use in a specific study. It is not acceptable to just state that you are using grounded theory approaches or that your study is informed by grounded theory.

Regarding traditional ethnography in nursing, Brink in Chapter 15 warns U.S. nurse researchers that this method is fading from American nursing research literature but appears to be thriving outside the United States. Leininger's ethnonursing method is maintaining its popularity. In Chapter 16, Ray and colleagues describe the new meta-ethnonursing research method that was developed from analyzing and synthesizing 23 dissertations that used the theory of Culture Care Diversity and Universality and the ethnonursing method. This new meta-ethnonursing method will enhance the conceptual development of the culture care method. In the future ethnonursing method will continue to enhance the understanding of the commonalities and diversities of cultures around the globe and help provide opportunities for humanized health care.

In Chapter 17, Breda reports that critical ethnographic research is increasing in popularity in nursing, especially in Canada and Australia. In the future this method will help nursing to address more health and social issues for unequal and vulnerable populations. We as a nursing profession across the globe have an ethic of care. Critical ethnography will promote nurse researchers to help change social conditions for disenfranchised groups.

Institutional ethnography studies are beginning to appear in nursing literature. In Chapter 18, Rankin tells us that institutional ethnography is challenging and absorbing; however, there is not a step-by-step recipe for conducting this type of ethnography. As nurse researchers use the method in the future, Rankin advises us to stay grounded in people and their actions, not theoretical categories or phenomenological interpretation. Our analytical gaze should be on the broad institutional practices to help build knowledge to illuminate how current health care practices create difficulties for not only the caregivers but also patients. Institutional ethnography will provide a refreshingly new understanding to entrenched problems.

In Chapter 19, Lewenson warns us that if our profession is to value what nursing history has to offer, we need to teach future generations of nurses to value our historical evidence and continue to conduct historical research. The path nurse historians have taken over time has led them from mainly recording chronological happenings and describing our nursing leaders' lives to critiquing our past which requires reflecting and critical thinking.

Over the past 20 years narrative inquiry has become a popular method in nursing research. Bailey, Montgomery and Mossey in Chapter 20 alert us that this growth has not been matched by the nurse researchers specifying the underlying methodological rigor of their narrative inquiry studies. In the future, everyday storytelling needs to be differentiated from stories as units of analysis within narrative inquiry. Nurse researchers who are going to use this qualitative method need to explicitly describe credible methodological processes.

Traynor in Chapter 21 presents discourse analysis as an exciting but complex and challenging approach for nurse researchers who want to focus on language and subjectivity. He warns that discourse analysis is far from settled as far as the method is concerned. Differences of opinions among qualitative researchers characterize this method.

Thorne's interpretive description (Chapter 22) is one of the newer qualitative methods that nurse researchers now have as an option. She believes that interpretive description is well positioned to be part of a new era in our discipline where we grapple as qualitative researchers with ideas such as social justice, vulnerability, human frailty, to name a few.

Use of focus groups is prevalent in nursing literature. Côté-Arsenault (Chapter 23) stresses that in future nurse researchers need to be careful to use focus groups in their studies that are congruent with their use. Meticulous planning and rigorous analysis of group data are necessary.

Young in Chapter 24 offers some suggestions for future directions of Participatory Action Research which focuses on inequities and injustices. Clarification and refining of this innovative research approach are needed to allow theory and nursing practice to interact in new ways. Young alerts nurse researchers undertaking PAR to develop strategies to address the challenges facing them. Use of mixed methods research designs in PAR holds exciting promise but Young cautions there are challenges to research when combining qualitative and quantitative methods in one PAR study since these methods are based in contrasting scientific paradigms.

In Chapter 25, Paterson addresses the fact that metasynthesis has not yet reached a state of clarity. However, the values of metasyntheses are many, such as generating insights that nurses can apply in clinical practice, theory development, and policy revisions. In future research metasyntheses can be used to evaluate the outcomes of processes of particular interventions to help increase the efficacy of these interventions. Paterson highlights several areas regarding metasyntheses that are in need of future discussion and study by nurse researchers, such as the use of a research team vs. an individual researcher in conducting a metasynthesis. Metasyntheses have primarily been published in English. Paterson questions the inclusion of translated articles written in languages other than English in a metasynthesis since a metasynthesis is already an interpretation of interpretations. Translated data can add another layer of interpretation. Use of translation in metasynthesis is an area for further study. Definitive guidelines also need to be developed to help nurse researchers decide which metasynthesis approach fits their research goals.

The mixed research synthesis field is a dynamic one in the future of nursing research. In Chapter 26, Sandelowski and colleagues alert nurse researchers to the need for methodological craftsmanship and flexibility in order to produce findings from mixed research syntheses that are credible and usable for clinical practice. Nurse researchers who attempt mixed research syntheses in the future must be cognizant of the implications of adhering to or transcending the qualitative/quantitative divide.

When considering ethical issues in qualitative nursing research as we move forward Austin (Chapter 27) identifies two pressing needs: (1) for nurse researchers to act with humility and vigilance regarding how they are with their research participants, colleagues, and communities, and (2) for research environments to be sites where nurse researchers feel safe to raise difficult ethical issues and where dialogue is welcomed and accepted.

Johnson in Chapter 28 alerts qualitative nurse researchers to how extremely challenging it will be to overcome the power dynamics involved in the research process. A key component in the politics of qualitative nursing research is negotiation and maintaining strong partnerships. Johnson reminds us of the need to understand that qualitative nursing research is a political endeavor and to carefully position our research as we seek funding and to understand the nuances of the peer review process.

In Im and Chee's Chapter 29 on Internet qualitative research, they suggest that nurse researchers continue to experiment with multiple qualitative methods as advances in new computer and Internet technologies continue to be developed. Use of Internet research with individuals with stigmatized conditions is a great match for qualitative nurse researchers in the future. Nurse researchers need to develop creative strategies to overcome low response rates, selection bias, and feasibility issues. In the future, nurse researchers also need to increase theoretical saturation by means of multiple qualitative methods.

Thorne in Chapter 30 points out that even though qualitative secondary analysis is becoming quite popular; we are still in need of developing a shared theoretical and methodological framework to evaluate the quality of these studies.

Bowers contends in Chapter 31 that complete engagement in the development of an evidence base requires qualitative nurse researchers to understand the intellectual bases informing their methodologies, to match their research questions with the most appropriate methodologies, and to actively engage in debates about generalizability and possible dangers of co-opting qualitative researchers into a narrow view of evidence.

In Chapter 32, Freshwater and Cahill purport that most critical for the future of qualitative research in England, Scotland, and Wales in taking its rightful place in the hierarchy of evidence is developing and refining a discourse of qualitative research. They contend that discourses of evidence have perpetuated the evidence-based practice paradigm where in qualitative research has played a secondary role. Another area that needs to be considered in the future of qualitative research is the paradigm of mixed methods research. Freshwater and Cahill refer back to the four components of learning to be part of the discourse: reading, writing, academic development, and critical ability. It is the current reading and writing practices of mixed methods that they warn will stymie the discourse and lead to ossification of advances in academia.

Tobin in Chapter 33 cautions that the future growth of qualitative nursing research in Ireland is contingent on sustaining the investment that has been made in nursing research in academia. The trend toward funding quantitative nursing research in Ireland needs to be balanced to ensure that Irish nurse researchers continue to value the contribution of qualitative research.

Anderson addresses the future of qualitative research in Canada (Chapter 34) which includes a shift in nursing research discourse that includes ontologies and epistemologies based on the voices of Indigenous peoples, persons from the Global South, and the subaltern within Canadian society. Anderson contends that this inclusion is critical as we focus on issues of equity and social justice in nursing not only as discourse but also as praxis and clinical practice.

Regarding recommendations for future qualitative nursing research in Australia and New Zealand, Barr (Chapter 35) provides some general suggestions that nurse researchers can explore, such as the impact of change, new ways of practice, rich detail to help develop conceptual/theoretical frameworks and define variables to measure effectiveness of change strategies in quantitative research. Specific areas of qualitative research for Australasia that Barr recommends include an increased understanding of health care needs of persons with refugee status and a focus on increasing concerns of infections.

In promoting the future of qualitative nursing research in Latin America Duque-Páramo and colleagues (Chapter 36) offer some of the following suggestions: (1) combining and expanding postgraduate programs to make them more competitive globally; (2) promoting cross-institutional collaborative research projects and promoting exchanges at national and international levels between researchers; (3) conducting research on inequalities of gender, ethnicity, social class, etc.; (4) establishing a policy for nursing research including research priorities; (5) achieving greater recognition for nursing research and its contribution to the health of the people of Latin America; and (6) making research findings more widely available by encouraging nurse researchers to know at least two languages.

Bover Bover and colleagues in Chapter 37 identify two challenges in the future that will face qualitative nurse researchers in Spain. First is strengthening the ontological-epistemological and methodological competence of nurse researchers. Limited research education for nurses is a major barrier along with the use of Anglo-American texts to inform the qualitative research curricula. There needs to be an increased awareness among funding agencies and journal reviewers regarding what constitutes quality in qualitative research. Second is moving from a nursing-centered research agenda to an ethical-political one to improve the health for all. Qualitative nursing research in Spain and globally is connected to larger social and political contexts and needs a direct vision towards social transformation.

Regarding future directions of qualitative nursing research in Portugal, Lima-Basto (Chapter 38) suggests: (1) continuing qualitative studies to identify patients' outcomes in well-being sensitive to nursing interventions; and (2) developing further a variety of qualitative methods by collaboration among universities where each university could focus on research in specific areas of study.

In Chapter 39, Bondas contends that for the future of qualitative nursing research in Sweden and Finland the following areas need to be considered. Nurse researchers can: (1) study phenomena that unfold over time; (2) combine perspectives of patients' care for themselves and their care providers; (3) conduct more action research, discourse analysis and metastudies; and (4) collaborate with international qualitative researchers.

In the countries of Norway, Denmark, and Iceland (Chapter 40) Kirkevold calls for the further refining of qualitative methods and combining qualitative and quantitative approaches in future research in order to enhance the relevance of research findings for nursing practice.

When looking at the future of qualitative nursing research in the Netherlands and Flanders, Grypdonck and colleagues (Chapter 41) note that the popularity that qualitative research has gained also threatens the integrity of its methodology. Vigilance is required to ensure rigorous qualitative research. Education and supervision provided by experienced qualitative researchers are essential for qualitative research to play a vital role in developing nursing scholarship in Norway, Denmark, and Iceland.

Shin and colleagues focus their proposed future research directions in Korea to research evaluation and qualitative research funding (Chapter 42). Korean qualitative nurse researchers need to address clear evaluation criteria in their studies they publish. Various strategies to help obtain funding for qualitative research also need to be focused on in the future.

In Japan, Saiki-Craighill (Chapter 43) calls for nursing advanced degree programs in her country to enhance their curricula to focus on rigorous approaches to qualitative research. Higher standards of peer review of qualitative publications are also needed in the future.

Arthur in Chapter 44 focuses on concentrating efforts in the future for qualitative nurse researches in the Asian region to become major players in the international qualitative research field by overcoming language barriers. To date, much of their qualitative research is disseminated in the gray literature and in conference abstracts.

In his suggestions for future directions for qualitative nursing research, Arthur offers, for example, conducting cross-cultural interpretive studies of empathy, reflective listening, humanistic counseling, and interactive student-driven education strategies.

Conclusion

A groundbreaking first step has been taken by qualitative nurse researchers from around the world in collaborating in this handbook. Further advancement of qualitative nursing research will be enhanced by continuing to promote this international collaboration. We can learn much from each other through the research we are conducting in the different countries across the globe. In reviewing the directions for future research that the contributors of the chapters offered, a few repetitive patterns seemed to emerge: (1) conducting qualitative research that focuses on issues of equity and social justice; (2) making certain of the methodological rigor of the different qualitative methods; and (3) promoting exchanges at the international level among qualitative nurse researchers.

Index

Aamodt, A. M. 206
abductive reasoning 185
Aboriginal people 247, 323–4, 328n3; *see also* indigenous people
abuse: domestic 4, 32–46; sexual 26–7, 48–9, 53
Acculturation Health Care Assessment Enabler 223
Action Research (AR) 6, 319–20, 325, 328n2, 364, 539; Australasia 474, 475; Australia 470; Brazil 479, 482; Finland 533; Ireland 443; Japan 599–600; Korea 583; Netherlands and Flanders 568; Norway, Denmark, and Iceland 553–4; Portugal 518, 522; South-East Asia 616; United Kingdom 423, 425–6; *see also* Participatory Action Research
active learning 270
Adams, Henry 371
Adams, Trevor 290
Adamsen, L. 555
adaptive capacity 69–71, 195
Adaptive Capacity Index 25, 69, 72
Addington-Hall, J. 422, 425
Adler, C. L. 384, 389
admission forms 250–1
adolescence 314–15
advocacy 38, 43, 55
African Americans 55, 57, 139, 178, 317
Agar, M. 204
agency 193, 237, 296, 305, 547
aggregation, research synthesis by 350–1, 353
Aistars, J. 67
Alarcón-Muñoz, A. M. 484
alcohol use 47–8, 56
Aléx, L. 177
Allbutt, H. 206
Allen, M. N. 339
Allen, Moyra 453, 454
Allen, S. 237
Alonso, M. M. 492
Althusser, Louis 286
Alvesson, Mats 284, 287, 290, 409, 411
Alzheimer's disease 398

Amar, A. F. 317
American Association for the History of Nursing (AAHN) 263–4, 266n3
Amman, N. 237
amplified sampling 399
analytic chunks 253
analytic expansion 397
An Bord Altranais 438, 448
Andershed, Birgitta 531–2
Anderson, B. 456–7
Anderson, Joan M. 8, 451–67, 626
Anderson, R. A. 197
Angus, J. 246, 458
Annells, M. 474
anthropology 14, 16, 163, 283, 307, 406; applied 207; ethical and legal issues 396; ethnography 203–6, 210, 231, 232–3, 234–5; human science paradigm 214; Korea 585; lack of generalizability 413; Leininger 214–16; paradigm shift 232; Spain 501–2
anxiety disorders 122–3
Argyris, C. 553
Arman, Maria 532
armchair induction 398
Arsalani, N. 178
Arthur, David 9, 139, 610–22, 627
Artinian, B. M. 164–5
Asplund, Kenneth 531, 535
assessment 72, 223
Åstedt-Kurki, P. 533
Astudillo-Díaz, P. 484
attachment theory 247
audio recordings 313
Austin, Wendy 7, 359–70, 625
Australia 8, 468–77, 612, 613, 619, 626; critical ethnography 237, 239; descriptive phenomenology 135, 139, 140; Internet research 389; methodologies 408; postpartum depression 127; qualitative research methods books 17, 20; situational analysis 191
Australian Nursing and Midwifery Council (ANMC) 469–70
authenticity 156, 381

auto–ethnography 422, 424
Avis, M. 432
Axelsson, Karin 532

Bacon, Francis 326
Baer, Hans 240n3
Bailey, Patricia Hill 6, 268–81, 624
Baker, C. 459
Bakitas, Marie 303
Bargiela-Chiappini, F. 288
Barlett, F. 67
Barr, Jennieffer 8, 468–77, 626
Barr, R. G. 108
Barroso, J. 21, 26
Barthes, Roland 284, 291
Bartley, S. 67
Barton, S. 178
Barwick, D. 457
basic social psychological processes (BSP) 33, 88, 194
bathing 94–5
Baumbusch, J. 238, 457
Bayesian synthesis 334, 338
Baylis, F. 374
Beard, G. 66
Beck, Cheryl Tatano 1–10, 133–44, 151, 152, 365, 384, 442, 530, 537, 539, 623–7
Beck Depression Inventory-II (BDI-II) 125
bedsores 257
Beekman, T. 568
Begley, C. M. 444–6
behavioral research 585
Belgium 560–76
beliefs: cultural 222; ethnoscience 68; interpretive description 297; Latino childhood obesity 104, 112, 114, 115
Bellevue and Mills School of Nursing 263
Benedict, Ruth 14
Benjamin, Kathleen 246, 249–50
Benjumea, Carmen de la Cuesta 489, 501, 519
Benner, M. 374
Benner, Patricia 148, 459, 531
Benoliel, Jeanne Quint 3, 27, 183, 191
Benson, A. 423, 426
Berg, Linda 531
Berg, Marie 531, 536
Bergbom, Ingegerd 531
Bergum, V. 360
Berman, H. 238, 459
Bernstein, Richard 455
Bertani, M. 549
Bess, R. 317
Bhabha, Homi 458
Bhujoharry, C. 474
bias 76, 231, 238–9, 263; selection 389
biographical frameworks 261–2
Björnsdóttir, K. 552

Black feminism 458
Bland, B. 474
Bland, Marian 237
Blumer, Herbert 162–3, 170, 184, 486
Bochner, A. P. 271
body-mass-index (BMI) 103, 110
Boehmke, M. 397
Boeije, H. 568, 569
Boemer, Magali 486
Boemer-Roseira, M. 486
Bohannan, Laura (Eleanor Bowen) 16, 204
Bohr, N. 217
Boisjoly, C. 108
Bokovoy, J. 208
Bol, N. 458
Bolding, G. 387
Bolin, R. 165
Bondas, Terese 9, 527–45, 627
Bonner, A. 191
Borbasi,S. 470
Borda, Orlando Fals 479, 487
Borgesius, E. 564
Bosch, Corry 563–4
Boschma, G. 263, 457
bottle feeding 111
Bottorff, J. L. 397, 452, 456, 457
Bouchard, L. 140
boundary issues 361
Bourdieu, Pierre 457, 487
Bournemouth Centre for Qualitative Research 427–8
Bousfield, L. 270
Bover Bover, Andreu 8, 500–13, 626
Bowen, Eleanor 16, 204
Bowers, Barbara 7, 165, 405–16, 626
Boyle, J. S. 206, 208
bracketing 14, 134, 151, 187
Brah, A. 458
Bray, J. 208–9
Brazil 8, 17, 18, 19, 478–83, 491, 494
breast cancer 176, 397
breastfeeding 53, 111, 115, 331, 475
Breda, Karen Lucas 6, 230–41, 624
bricoleur 399
Briggs Report (1972) 420
Brink, Pamela 5, 16, 203–12, 456, 624
Brown, Gillian 284, 618
Brown, J. 422, 425
Brown, L. M. 272
Browne, A. 321–3, 324, 327
Browne, A. J. 459
Broyles, Lauren 95
Bruner, J. S. 269
Buck, Joy 259–60, 261
Buckley, J. 387
Bungay, V. 462
Buus, Niels 289, 290, 551

Byerly, E. L. 206

Caelli, K. 149
Cahill, Jane 8, 419–36, 626
Camberwell Family Interview 618
Cameron, C. 67, 177
Campbell, Marie L. 242, 245–6, 254n1
Campbell, R. 341
Canada 8, 451–67, 626; Aboriginal people 178,
    247, 323–4, 328n3; condom campaign 190;
    critical ethnography 237–8, 239; descriptive
    phenomenology 135, 139, 140; fatigue 71;
    grounded theory 167, 178, 183; interpretive
    phenomenology 146; nurse practitioner role
    195; politics 371, 373; postpartum depression
    127; qualitative research methods books 17, 18,
    19, 20; SARS 195; Women's Health Effects
    Study 34, 39
Canadian Institutes of Health Research (CIHR)
    360, 364, 365, 375, 377, 378, 452
Canadian Triage and Acuity Scale (CTAS) 249
cancer 54, 56–7, 550, 555; breast cancer 176, 397;
    descriptive phenomenology 140; interpretive
    description 297; Ireland 446; patient fatigue
    64–6, 67, 68, 71; side effects 374
Capitulo, K. L. 384, 387
Capra, F. 192, 193
care, concept of 208, 209, 215, 216–17, 218,
    221
care process 517, 518, 521
caregivers 177, 503, 504, 509, 520
Carey, Mary Anne 307, 578
caring 23–4, 42, 150–1, 215, 216–17, 533–4,
    548–50
Carlsson, I. M. 532
Carpenter, D. Rinaldi 245
Carspecken, Phil 235, 237, 238–9
Carter, B. 422, 425
Caruso, D. R. 610
case studies 52, 300, 323–4, 423, 426, 508, 585
Casey, D. 186
Casey, M. A. 315
Cashin, A. 209
Caspari, S. 554
Castellani, B. 192, 196, 197
Castellani, J. 196
Castillo, María Magdalena Alonso 8, 478–99
categories 164, 172–3
causality 51–3
Cayne, J. 154
Centre for Health Information, Research and
    Evaluation (CHIRAL) 428
Chaffee, M. W. 195
Chaiyawat, W. 177
Champion. J. D. 126
Chang, E. 474
Chapman, Y. 191, 237

Charlebois, S. 140
Charmaz, K. 165, 184, 185, 187, 198, 518, 601
Chee, Wonshik 7, 380–92, 625
Cheek, Julianne 578
chemotherapy 56–7, 140, 297, 303, 397
child sexual abuse (CSA) 26–7, 48–9, 53
Childbearing in the Nordic Countries (BFiN)
    536–7
childbirth experiences 139–41
childhood maltreatment (CM) 48–9, 50, 52, 54
children: Colombia 488, 489; ethical issues 365;
    Finland 533; grounded theory 177; informed
    consent 363; Ireland 442, 444; obesity 4,
    103–18; United Kingdom 422, 425
Chile 8, 126, 478–9, 483–7, 494
China 9, 176, 611, 613–17, 619–21; descriptive
    phenomenology 135, 139, 140; historical
    research 265; qualitative research methods
    books 18, 20
Ching, S. S. Y. 176
Chou, C. C. 139
Chrisman, Noel 16
chronic fatigue syndrome (CFS) 67, 68
chronic pain syndrome 4, 75–85
Chubin, D. E. 375
Chung, Seung Eun 9, 577–96
Chung-Park, M. 177
Chute, E. 67
Cilliers, P. 192
citation 402
Clair, J. M. 188
Clark, A. M. 177
Clark, Lauren 4, 103–18
Clarke, A. E. 165, 187–90, 191, 193, 426
Clarke, C. 423, 474
Clarke, J. M. 368
class: Colombia 488; historical research 261, 263;
    ideological practices 243; inequalities 494;
    intersectionality 458; oppression 234
Cleary, M. 474
Clemensen, J. 553
Clifford, J. 232–3
Cloherty, M. 422, 424
Clune, L. 246
Cochrane Qualitative Research Methods group
    410
coding of data 36, 109–10, 164, 171–2, 297, 424;
    costs 54; focus groups 315; line-by-line 605;
    thematic content analysis 82
co-evolution 194, 196
Cohen, D. J. 376
Colaizzi, P. 119, 122, 133, 135–8, 140, 142, 297,
    388, 582, 583, 617
Collins, Patricia Hill 458
Colombia 8, 177, 478–9, 484, 487–90, 491,
    494
commonality 48, 296

communication: communication analysis 599–600; interpretive phenomenology 153–4; ventilator-dependent patients 96–8, 99; voicelessness 89–90
community clinics 115
compathy 25
complex adaptive systems (CAS) 192–7
complexity science 217
concept mapping 197
concepts 15, 171, 172, 174, 180, 519–20, 605–6, 607
conclusions, logical 302–3
concurrent analysis 187
Conditional/Consequential Matrix 175
condoms 190
Cone, P. H. 164–5
confidentiality 364, 366, 367, 396
configuration, research synthesis by 351, 352, 353
confirmability 223, 315, 399
Congo, Democratic Republic of 127
Connolly, Cindy 259, 260, 266n1
consensus methods 569
consent 220, 362–4, 366, 367, 395–6
constant comparison 34, 36–9, 44, 164, 191, 198, 606; focus groups 309; postpartum depression 119–20; secondary data analysis 400
constructionism 242, 288
constructivism 52, 184–7, 188, 191, 304, 347, 421; agency 193; Australia 470; Canada 459; Korea 585; Portugal 521; secondary data analysis 400; Spain 510
content analysis 19, 75, 301, 508; Finland and Sweden 529, 531, 532, 533, 536; focus groups 315; Internet research 365, 387, 389; Japan 599–600, 602; Korea 585; Portugal 516; secondary data analysis 394; thematic 77, 82; ventilator-dependent patients 96–7
context 170–1, 173–4, 175, 180, 187, 258, 549
converging assistance research 482
Conversation Analysis (CA) 284–5, 551, 583, 585
conversations 75
Cook, A. 426
Cooke, B. 321
Coombs, M. 209
Corbin, Juliet 5, 162, 165, 169–82, 578, 623; coding technique 297; context 187; data collection 604; Japan 601, 602, 603; Korea 582, 583; Portugal 519, 522; power issues in research 361; translation of books 20
core categories 173
co-researchers 137, 138
Côté-Arsenault, Denise 6, 307–18, 625
Coulson, N. S. 385
Council of Nursing and Anthropology (CONAA) 3, 16
counternarratives 55, 57

Cowles, E. 66–7
Cowles, K. V. 367
Cowley, S. 457
Cox, H. 474
Coyne, A. B. 3
Crabtree, B. F. 376
Crandell, Jamie 7, 347–56
Crawford, M. 456
credibility 223, 295, 396; focus groups 315; interpretive description 303; mixed research 354; narrative inquiry 271–2, 275, 277; participatory approaches 327; secondary data analysis 401
Creswell, J. W. 433
Critchley, Simon 292n1
Critical Discourse Analysis (CDA) 285–6, 289, 290, 406
critical ethnography 6, 47–8, 53, 230–41, 408, 457, 460, 624
critical interpretive synthesis 334, 338
Critical Medical Anthropology (CMA) 240n3
Critical Participatory Research 323–4
critical race theory 55, 233, 234
critical realism 52, 236, 337
critical theory 232, 239n2, 462, 510, 539, 556
cross-validation 398
Crouch, M. 348
Cuba 484
Cuellar, Pavon 291–2
culture: anthropology 406; Australasia 472–3; Colombia 488; ethnography 231, 233, 406; ethnonursing 213, 214–16, 218, 220–3, 227; historical research 261; postpartum depression 128, 620
Culture Care Theory (CCT) 213, 216, 218–19, 220–2, 226–7, 624
Cumulative Index of Nursing and Allied Health Literature (CINAHL) 68, 134, 439, 615–16; constructivism 186; discourse analysis 289; focus groups 316; grounded theory 187; Internet research 383; situational analysis 190

Dahlberg, Karin 531, 536
Dahlgren, L. O. 531
Daly, B. J. 90
Dangdomyouth, P. 166–7
Danielson, Ella 531
D'Antonio, P. 257, 258–9, 260, 261
Darbyshire, P. 360
data analysis: Data Analysis Enabler 223; descriptive phenomenology 137–8; ethnonursing 223, 226; focus groups 314–15, 317; grounded theory 166, 171, 172, 174–5, 179; institutional ethnography 252–3; Internet research 387, 389; interpretive description 301–2; Latino childhood obesity 109–10; phenomenology 297; researcher distress 367;

traditional ethnography 206; United Kingdom 421; *see also* secondary data analysis
data collection 43, 403, 411; anthropological field work 203–4; ethnography 205–6; ethnonursing 220, 223; focus groups 308–9, 314, 315, 316; grounded theory 164, 604–5, 607; Internet research 382–3, 384–6, 389, 390; interpretive description 299, 300; Latino childhood obesity 105–9; mixed research 349; Netherlands and Flanders 568–9; postpartum depression 119, 122; Spain 508; United Kingdom 421; ventilator-dependent patients 87–8, 90, 91–2, 96, 98; *see also* methods
data protection issues 363–4
Davidson, P. M. 472
Davies, Celia 261, 266n2
Davies, J. 423, 425
Davis, M. 385, 387
De la Cuesta, C. 177
De Lange, J. 564, 567
De Santis, J. 177
De Witte, L. 178
death 27, 56–7, 564
de-centering 153, 154, 155, 158
decision making: patient involvement 93
decolonization 458, 460–1, 463
deconstruction 287, 296, 556
Deitrick, L. 208
Delmar, C. 549
dementia 177, 398, 423, 426; Australasia 474; Canada 457–8, 459; discourse analysis 290; Finland and Sweden 534, 535, 536; Netherlands 564; Sweden 532
Denmark 9, 140, 264–5, 546–59, 627
Denzin, N. 399
depression: abused women 39; narrative inquiry 275; patient fatigue 67, 68, 69; postpartum 5, 119–29, 152, 471, 620
Derrida, Jacques 287
Descartes, René 326
descriptive phenomenology 133–44, 156, 157, 550, 551; interpretive phenomenology distinction 151–2; literature search 134–9; Norway, Denmark, and Iceland 555–6; postpartum depression 122; topics studied 139–40
descriptive research designs 443, 518, 568, 582, 585
DeVault, M. 251
Developmental Model of Health and Nursing 37
Dewey, John 170
Dexheimer-Pharris, M. 218
Dey, P. 376
diabetes 104, 177, 317, 399, 536, 554
diagrams 176
dialectics 481
dialogue 153, 456

Diamond, T. 250
Dickerson, S. 397
Dierckx de Casterlé, B. 569
Diers, D. 455
DiGiacomo, M. 473
dignity 79, 83, 359, 521
disciplinary logic 302
discourse analysis 6, 57, 282–94, 539, 624; definition of 283; Ireland 443; Japan 599–600; Norway, Denmark, and Iceland 552; Portugal 518–19; United Kingdom 423, 426–7
discourse development 430–2
diversity 48, 159, 219
Doane, G. H. 324–5
Docherty, S. 332
documentation 256, 257, 520
Domain of Inquiry (DOI) Enabler 222
dominant narratives 269
Dougherty, M. 207
Dreher, Melanie 16
Drew, N. 83
Dreyfus, H. 150
Ducharme, F. 177
Duggleby, W. 341–2, 459
Duijnstee, M. S. 566
Duque-Páramo, María Claudia 8, 478–99, 626
Dussault, R. 328n3
Dyjur, Louise 253

Earle, V. 157
Eason, M. 209
ecological restoration 195
Edinburgh Postnatal Depression Scale (EPDS) 124, 125
education: Australasia 468–70, 473; Brazil 479, 480; Canada 454–6; Chile 483, 484, 485–7; Colombia 487–8; Denmark 547; fatigue 72; Finland 532; historical research 258, 262, 263; Iceland 546; Ireland 438–9, 442, 448; Japan 597–8, 607; Korea 577; Mexico 490–1; Netherlands and Flanders 560–1, 562; Norway 546–7; Portugal 514–17; South-East Asia 613, 614, 617, 621; Spain 500–2, 509–11; Sweden 530, 538; United Kingdom 420, 421; ventilator-dependent patients 99
Edwards, N. 195
Ehnfors, M. 532
Ehrenberg, A. 532
Eisner, E. W. 1
Ekman, I. 531
Ekman, Sirkka-Liisa 532
elderly care 177, 474, 489, 552, 553
Elena, L. 246
Elford, J. 387
Ellefsen, B. 551
Elliott, J. 238
Elo, S. 533

emails 382–3, 384, 386, 390
Emami, A. 186
Emblen, J. D. 178
Emden, C. 332
emergence 194, 196
emergent fit 36, 37, 44
emotional intelligence (EI) 610, 618
emotions 25–6, 170
empathy 15, 23, 153, 361, 425
enablers 220–3
Engels, Friedrich 243
England 8, 146, 419–36, 626; *see also* United Kingdom
epistemology 150, 187–8, 304, 321, 405, 430, 527; Canada 462, 463; Finland and Sweden 534, 537, 539; indigenous 461; *see also* knowledge
equity 451, 452, 463, 511, 627
Erasmus, G. 328n3
Erikson, A. 191
Eriksson, Katie 531, 532, 533–4
errors 22
Ersser, S. J. 209
Escadón, S. 177
Escobar, Arturo 487
Estabrooks, C. 35
ethic of care 159
ethics 7, 359–70, 461, 625; benefits to participants 365; Canada 452, 456, 459; consent 362–4; Finland and Sweden 535; international historical research 265; interpretive phenomenology 151; Netherlands and Flanders 566–7; Participatory Action Research 324–5; patient involvement in decision making 93; Portugal 522; privacy and confidentiality 364, 366, 367; research team relationships 362; researcher competence 360; researcher-participant relationships 360–1; risks 365–7; secondary data analysis 395–6
Ethics Review Boards 206
Ethiopia 127
ethnicity 263, 381, 488, 494; *see also* race
ethnography 5–6, 14, 54, 183, 203–12, 406, 408, 459, 624; Australia 470; books on 18; Brazil 481; Canada 457, 460; Chile 484, 485, 486; Colombia 488; combined with phenomenology 50; controversial uses of 207; critical 6, 47–8, 53, 230–41, 408, 457, 460, 624; ethnonursing 219; focus groups 314, 316, 317; future directions 209–10; institutional 6, 242–55, 458, 624; Internet research 387; interpretive description 297; Ireland 443; Japan 599–600, 602; Korea 577–8, 582, 583, 585; Latino childhood obesity 105–16; Leininger 216; literature review 208–9; meta-ethnography 332, 333, 335, 338, 339, 351, 352; Mexico 491; social environment 53;

South-East Asia 620; Spain 506, 508; United Kingdom 422, 424; ventilator-dependent patients 91–6
ethnomethodology 289, 290, 599–600
ethnonursing 6, 21, 213–29, 624
ethnoscience 68, 71, 216
European Nursing History Group (ENHG) 264
Evans-Pritchard, E. E. 14
event analysis 91
everyday experiences 250
evidence 52, 412, 414, 430; assessment of 22; interpretive description 304; policy-making 377; politics of 371–3
evidence-based practice 7, 52, 226, 303, 405–16, 524; Australasia 470; critique of 461; as dominant discourse 327; ethnonursing 227; fatigue 72; Leininger 218, 219; mixed research 347; Netherlands and Flanders 569; psychiatric nursing 567; United Kingdom 421, 430–2
exhaustion 69
expanded genre stories 269
experimental research designs 518
explanatory research 518
expressed emotion (EE) 618–19, 620

Fairclough, Norman 285–6
Fairman, Julie 257, 258
Fallahi-Khoshknab, M. 178
family members 520, 565–6; bedside visitation 93–4; Camberwell Family Interview 618; care giving by 177; focus groups 311; Portugal 522; women and men with fibromyalgia 82–3
Farrelly, M. 442
Fatemeh, D. 178
Fatemeh, O. S. 178
fatigue 4, 25, 64–74; abused women 39; Revised Edmonton Fatigue Framework 69–70, 72; women with fibromyalgia 79, 81
feminism 33, 36, 49, 53–4, 55; Black 458; Canada 458, 459, 462; critical 233, 234; Feminist Participatory Research 320; grounded theory 183–4; institutional ethnography 243; Internet research 388; Lacanian thought 291; Netherlands 560; reciprocity 185; *see also* gender; women
Feminist Participatory Action Research (FPAR) 321–3
Feng, J-Y. 178
Fenwick, S. 422, 424
Ferguson, L. M. 119
Fetterman, D. M. 106
fibromyalgia (FM) 76–83, 555; *see also* chronic pain syndrome
Field, P. A. 3, 20
fieldnotes 106, 109, 185, 313, 315, 531
fieldwork 14, 106, 203–6, 208, 231, 250, 551, 599–600

Figueiredo, Maria do Céu 522
Figueroa, María 484
Finfgeld, D.L. 333, 339, 340, 342
Finland 9, 135, 139, 527–30, 532–40, 627
Finlay, L. 423, 425
Finlayson, M. P. 474
Finn, R. 288–9
First Nations 247, 459
fit 36, 37, 40, 42, 44, 400
Fitzpatrick, Louise 262–3
Fitzpatrick, N. 423, 425
Flanders 9, 560–76, 627
Flores-Montiel, N. 485
Flores-Peña, Yolanda 8, 478–99
focus groups 6, 207, 307–18, 411, 625;
    advantages and disadvantages 309; Australasia
    470, 472; Canada 457; controversies 316; data
    analysis 314–15, 317; data protection issues
    364; ground rules 312; group and sample size
    311; Internet research 383; interpretive
    description 299; Ireland 447; Korea 582, 583,
    585; Latino childhood obesity 106, 107, 109,
    110, 114; moderators 308, 311–12;
    Netherlands and Flanders 568–9; research
    design 313–14; research team 311, 313;
    sample characteristic considerations 310–11;
    South-East Asia 615; Spain 506, 508;
    trustworthiness 315
Fontana, A. 549
Ford-Gilboe, Marilyn 4, 32–46
Forsyth, D. 398
Foss, C. 552, 553
Foucault, Michel 188, 286–7, 289, 290, 427, 471,
    479, 487, 549, 552
framework analysis 334–5, 339
frameworks, in historical research 259–62
Francis, K. 191, 237
Francke, Anneke 564
Frank, A. 578
Fraser, Nancy 291
Fredriksson, L. 534
freelisting 109, 110, 113–14
Freeman, D. 394
Freire, Paulo 320, 378, 479
French, S. 454
Freshwater, Dawn 8, 419–36, 626
Fretheim, A. 377
Freud, Sigmund 291
Frid, I. 531
Fridlund, B. 533
Friedemann, M. 388
Fudge, N. 422, 424
funding 14, 16, 54–5, 58, 209, 623; AAHN 264;
    anthropology 204; Australasia 468; Canada
    452; Internet research 384–6, 388, 390;
    Ireland 438–9, 440–2; Korea 586; Mexico
    494; politics of 373–5; Spain 502, 510; tenure

issues 380; United Kingdom 420, 421;
    ventilator-dependent patients 98
Fyles, G. 457

Gadamer, H. G. 150, 471
Gaddis, J. L. 257, 258
Gagnon, M. 190
Galavan, E. 444–6
Gallop, R. 246
Galvani, L. 66
Gandhi, M. K. 458
García, R. M. 491
Gardner, A. 186
Garfinkel, H. 285
Gass, J. 421, 422
Gastaldo, Denise 8, 20, 457, 500–13
Gazaway, R. 207
Gee, J. P. 268–9
Geertz, Clifford 185, 232, 352, 539
gender: Brazil 480; Canada 458; Chile 484;
    Colombia 488; historical research 259, 261,
    263; ideological practices 243; inequalities 494;
    Internet research 381; interpretive
    phenomenology 456; intersectionality 49, 458;
    Latino childhood obesity 112–13; oppression
    234; Spain 505; see also feminism; women
general adaptation syndrome (GAS) 67
General Nursing Council (GNC) 428
generalizability 33, 50, 51, 179, 413–14; case
    studies 426; Internet research 382;
    metasynthesis 338; politics of evidence 372;
    secondary data analysis 401
Germain, C. 206, 207
Germany 18, 20
Ghezeljeh, T. M. 186
Gibb, C. 423, 426
Giddens, Anthony 237, 455
Giorgi, A. 133, 135–7, 142, 550–1, 568, 578, 582,
    583, 584
Giron, E. R. I. 459
Giske, T. 164–5
Given, L. 410
Gjengedal, E. 549, 551, 554
Glaser, Barney 3, 15–16, 27, 166, 170, 184, 444;
    bracketing 187; Canada 455; constant
    comparison 119; core concepts 194; Glaserian
    grounded theory 162–8; grab 35; Japan 601,
    603; Korea 583; metasynthesis 332;
    modifiability of theory 39, 126–7; Netherlands
    564; Portugal 518; quantitative and qualitative
    data 34; secondary data analysis 394; theoretical
    codes 164
Glaus, A. 67
Glittenberg, J. 207
Goldstein, J. A. 194
Gonzales-Guarda, R. M. 177
Gooden, A. 457

Gotttfredsdóttir , H. 552
Gottlieb, Laurie 453
Goulet, J-G. 178
Gournay, K. 432
grab 32, 34, 35, 43, 44
Grace, W. 427
Graffigna, G. 71
Graham, J. 361
Grandjean, E. 67
Graneheim, U. H. 536
Grealish, A. 186
Great Britain: critical ethnography 237;
    ethnography 210; qualitative research
    methods books 17, 18, 20; see also United
    Kingdom
Green, L. W. 319, 327
Greenhalgh, T. 601
Greenwood, D. J. 327
Gregor, F. 254n1
Gregory, D. 246
Griffiths, P. 206, 432
Grigg, E. 190
Grinspun, D. 195
Grobe, S. J. 532
grounded theory 4, 5, 15, 54, 183–202, 405–6,
    409, 411, 459; abused women 32–46;
    Australia 470; books on 18, 20; Brazil 481;
    Canada 455, 457, 459; Colombia 489;
    complex adaptive systems 192–7;
    constructivism 184–7; criticisms of 178–80;
    fatigue 65, 68, 69; Finland 533; focus groups
    308–9, 316, 317; future directions 623–4;
    Glaserian 162–8, 187; Internet research 387;
    interpretive complexity 348; interpretive
    description 297; Ireland 443–4; Japan
    599–600, 601, 602–6, 607; Korea 582, 583,
    585; literature review 176–8; metasynthesis
    332, 334, 339, 340; Mexico 491, 492; mixed
    research 197, 351, 352; modification of
    126–8; Netherlands and Flanders 563–4,
    566, 568, 569; Norway, Denmark, and
    Iceland 554, 556; origins of 162–3; Portugal
    518–19, 521, 522; postpartum depression
    119–22, 126–8; predominance of 408;
    situational analysis 187–92; South-East
    Asia 616, 620; Spain 506, 510; Straussian
    169–82, 187; Sweden 532; United
    Kingdom 421–4; ventilator-dependent
    patients 86–91
Grypdonck, Maria 9, 411, 524, 560–76, 627
Grypma, S. 262, 263, 265
Guba, E. G. 584
Guber, Susana 487
Gunderson, L. H. 195
Gunnarsdottir, T. J. 555
Guruge, S. 457
Gustavsen, B. 325, 326, 328n2

Haahr, A. 551
Habermas, J. 378, 487, 553
Hackett, E. J. 375
Hafferty, F. 192
Häggman-Laitila, A. 533
Haldorsdottir, S. 549–50
Hall, Elisabeth 536
Hall, Joanne 4, 26–7, 47–63
Hall, W. 40, 238–9
Hallberg, Lillemor 531
Hallberg, Rahm 530–1
Hallgren, Anita 536
Halpin, M. 462
Halpin, P. 462
Hamilton, P. 246, 250
Hammarström, A. 177
Hammersley, M. 402
Hankin, S. 178
Hantikainen, V. 139
Happ, Mary Beth 4, 86–102
Harding, S. 411
Hare, R. D. 124, 332, 333
Harmer, Bertha 15, 256, 257, 265–6
Harrington, A. 432
Harrowing, J. N. 238
Hart, G. 387
Hayder, D. 176
healing 178
health care services 115, 253–4
health promotion 33–6, 39, 40, 116, 319
health science 295, 407
Heaton, J. 394, 402
Hegel, Friedrich 291
Heidegger, Martin 14, 134, 145, 149, 150, 151,
    154–5, 471, 486, 548
Hellzén, Ove 531
Henderson, Virginia 15
Hentinen, Maija 533
hermeneutics 183, 184, 233, 539; Australasia 470,
    471; Canada 456–7, 459; Colombia 488;
    Finland and Sweden 533–4, 535, 537, 540;
    focus groups 317; interpretive phenomenology
    146, 147, 149, 151–2; Ireland 446; Norway,
    Denmark, and Iceland 550, 551, 554–5;
    Participatory Action Research 324; Sweden
    531, 532; women with fibromyalgia 78, 79,
    81, 82
Herrmann, Eleanor K. 265
Heyman, I. 530
Hiestand, Wanda 262
Higgins, A. 442
Higgins, P. A. 90, 317
Hilliard, C. 139
Hilton, B. A. 459
historical materialism 481
historical research 6, 256–67, 481–2, 624
HIV/AIDS 188–90, 339; Canada 459; Hispanics

177; institutional ethnography 248; Internet research 385; metasynthesis 26; Mexico 492; South-East Asia 621

Hjörleifsdóttir, E. 550
Hodges, H. F. 178
Holland, J. H. 194
Holling, C. S. 195
Holloway, I. 422, 432
Holmes, C. 238
Holmes, D. 457, 461
Holmes, S. 140, 190
Holmgren, M. 531
Holtslander, L. F. 186
Homer, Sean 291
Hong Kong 613, 614, 615–16, 617, 619–20
hope 341–2, 444–6
Hossein, K. M. 178
Houghton, C. E. 363
Howard, J. A. 242
Hoyos, Guillermo 487
Hsieh, H.-F. 398
Hsu, T-W. 178
Huang, X-Y. 139, 176–7, 178
Hui, A. 423, 427
human science paradigm 214, 217, 218
Hung, B. J. 139
Hunter, A. 186
Hunter, L. M. 178
Hunter College Department of Nursing 263
Hurwitz, B. 601
Husserl, Edmund 14, 133–4, 135, 138, 149, 151, 152, 471, 539, 548
Hutchinson, S. A. 3
Hyde, A. 440, 441, 447–8
hygiene care 94–5
Hyman, I. 457

Iceland 9, 135, 546–59, 627
identity 261, 289, 290, 492, 505
ideology 243, 286, 287
Iedema, Rick 287–8
illness, living with 75, 76, 176–7, 565
Im, Eun-Ok 7, 380–92, 625
implementation science 218, 226, 227
inclusion 463
indigenous people 204; Australasia 472–3; Canada 452, 456, 458, 461, 463; Colombia 488; see also Aboriginal people
Indonesia 127
induction 398
inequities: Canada 452, 456, 458, 460, 462; Colombia 487–8, 489, 490; Latin America 494; Spain 511
infections 475
information systems 519, 520, 521–2
informed consent 220, 363, 395–6
Ingadóttir, T. S. 550–1

Ingstrup, Andrea 247
in vivo codes 172
"insiders" 1, 2, 76, 233
Institute of Health Promotion Research (IHPR) 319
institutional ethnography (IE) 6, 242–55, 458, 624
integrated knowledge translation (iKT) 378
integrated research design 353–4, 432–3
integrity 401, 402, 410
intensive care unit (ICU) patients 4, 86–102, 177
interactionism 484, 485, 486
interconnections 193
International Congress for Qualitative Inquiry (ICQI) 16
International Council of Nursing (ICN) 264, 469
international historical research 264–5
International Institute for Qualitative Methodology (IIQM) 16
Internet research 7, 140, 365, 366, 380–92, 625
interpretive description 6, 18, 21, 295–306, 457, 518–19, 624–5
interpretive phenomenology 5, 145–61, 623; books on 19; Canada 456; descriptive phenomenology distinction 151–2; exemplars of method 157–9; international studies 146–7; meaning of human understanding 147–8; meaning of the interpretive project 150–1; as method 148–50; Norway, Denmark, and Iceland 550–1, 555–6; researcher as "unknower" 154–5; Sweden 532
"interpretive repertoires" 285, 288
interpretivism 184–5, 421, 471, 510; see also interpretive phenomenology
intersectionality 49, 58, 458, 461
intersubjectivity 145, 146, 154, 155
Intervention for Health Enhancement After Leaving (iHEAL) 33, 35–44
interventions 26–7, 43, 409; fatigue 72; Finland and Sweden 538; grounded theory 44; Norway, Denmark, and Iceland 554–5; Portugal 517, 518, 519, 521; Sweden 530–1; Utrecht model of developing 567; ventilator-dependent patients 96–8
interviews 49, 153, 307, 411; Australasia 472; chronic pain syndrome 77; Colombia 489; conversations distinction 75; ethical issues 364; fatigue 72; institutional ethnography 250, 251–2; Internet research 386, 387; interpretive description 299, 300; Latino childhood obesity 105, 106, 109, 110; mixed research 349; narrative inquiry 272, 275; Netherlands and Flanders 568; over-reliance on 300; postpartum depression 119; researcher-participant relationships 361; Spain 506, 508; ventilator-dependent patients 87–8, 90, 91–2, 96–7; see also focus groups

intrusion 33–4, 35, 39, 42, 44
Ip, H. 457
Iran 178
Ireland 8, 135, 139, 140, 437–50, 626
Irish Nursing Research Interest Group (INRIG) 437–8
Isola, A. 533

Jacelon, C. S. 177
Jacob, J. D. 190
Jakubec, S. 457–8
James, Janet Wilson 261
Jantzen, D. 194
Japan 9, 135, 597–609, 627
Jensen, L. A. 339
Jeon, Y. H. 613, 619
Jeong, S. H. 579
Jezewski, M. A. 177, 178
Jiang, R. S. 139
Jillings, Carol 578
Johnson, B. 368
Johnson, Joy 7, 371–9, 457, 625
Johnson, Susan 4, 103–18
Johnston, B. 139
Johnstone, P. L. 432–3
Jones, D. 218
Jones, K. 423, 428
Jonsdottir, H. 550–1
Josephson, M. 178
journals 3, 4, 16, 163, 198, 263, 327, 410–11; Canada 453, 456, 459; China 616; discourse analysis 289–90; ethnography 209, 210; Finland and Sweden 528–9, 530, 531, 532; Ireland 439–40; Korea 578–82, 585, 586; language barriers 142, 623; Latin America 484, 485, 489, 491–2, 493, 495; Netherlands and Flanders 562, 563, 564; Participatory Action Research 328; peer review 376; politics of evidence 372; secondary data analysis 401; Spain 501, 502, 507–8
Juuso, P. 79

Kalaw, C. 457
Kalkas, Hertta 532
Kapp, S. 474
Kappeli, S. 139
Karreman, Dan 284, 287, 290
Kars, Marijke 9, 560–76
Kasén, A. 534
Katri, V. J. 178
Kauffman, S. 192
Kavanaugh, K. 398
Kawakita, Jiro 599–601
Kay, Margareta 16
Kayser-Jones, J. 21, 207, 406
Keady, J. 186
Kean, S. 311

Kearney, M. H. 191, 332, 333
Keddy, B. 183–4
Keeley, A. C. 178
Keeling, A. W. 265
Keen, E. 138
Keen, S. 423
Keller, H. 366
Kelly, M. T. 457
Kenny, A. J. 385, 389, 472
Kevern, J. 316
Khanlou, N. 320
Kidd, J. D. 474
Kidd, T. 472
Kihlgren, A. L. 532
Kihlgren, M. 532
Kilbride, C. 423, 425–6
Killion, C. 317
Kim, H. S. 546, 547–8, 554, 555
Kim, Miyoung 9, 577–96
Kim, S. S. 177, 237–8
Kinch, J. L. 457–8
Kindy, D. 139
King, I. M. 195
Kinoshita, Yasuhito 603
Kipp, W. 238
Kirkevold, Marit 9, 177, 546–59, 627
Kitzinger, Jenny 307, 308
KJ method 599–601, 602
Kleffel, D. 195
Kleinman, A. 601
Knafl, Kathy 22
"knowing" 154
knowledge 22–4; Canada 461–2; critical ethnography 230, 236; cultural 109, 110, 115; emic and etic 216; ethnonursing 213; Foucauldian discourse analysis 286; historical research 257, 265; inferential/generalized 554; integrated knowledge translation 378; interpretive description 295–6, 301, 304–5; as interpretive framework 454; narrative inquiry 271, 277; nontraditional types of 58; nursing knowledge needs 547–8; Participatory Action Research 320, 324–5, 328; phenomenology 152; politics of evidence 371–2, 373; psychological 448; research outcomes 521; texts 244; transfer of 523, 524; transformative 556; triage 249; see also epistemology
Knutsen, I. R. 553
Koch, J. 385–6
Koch, T. 432
Komter, A. 564
Kondora, Lori 49
Korea 9, 577–96, 627; descriptive phenomenology 135, 139; qualitative research methods books 18, 19, 20
Kortesluoma, R-L. 533
Kothari, U. 321

Kozinets, R. V. 383
Kramer, M. S. 106, 108
Krippendorff, K. 602
Kris, A. 21
Kristeva, Julia 283, 291
Krueger, Richard A. 307, 315
Kuhn, Thomas 49, 232, 235, 429
Kulig, J. 238
Kushner, K. E. 183
Kushner, Rose 374
Kuyper, M. B. 83
Kuzel, A. J. 1
Kvale, K. 140
Kvale, S. 75, 550, 578
Kyngäs, H. 533

Labov, W. 272
Labun, E. 178
Lacan, Jacques 283, 291
Lagemann, Ellen Condliffe 260–1
Lagerström, M. 178
Lalor, J. 444–6
Lambert, S. D. 314
Lane, A. 246
language 56–7, 217–18, 234, 623; Conversation
    Analysis 284–5; deconstruction 287;
    discourse analysis 282, 283–4, 285, 286, 287,
    288–9, 291–2; English journals 142;
    institutional ethnography 252; international
    historical research 265; interpretive
    phenomenology 149, 150; Latin America
    493, 495; Latino childhood obesity 114;
    metaphorical 80; metasynthesis 342, 625;
    policies 427; psychological knowledge 448;
    Taiwan 621
Larsson, M. 140
Lasiuk, G. C. 119
Lassetter, Jane 4, 103–18
Latin America 8, 237, 478–99, 626
Latinos 4, 103–18
Lauri, Sirkka 532
Lauterbach, Sarah 152
Lauzon, C. L. M. 208
Lavis, J. N. 377
Lazarfield, Paul 163
learning 270
Leduc, D. G. 108
Lee, R. 365–6
Lee, S. 366
Leeman, Jennifer 7, 347–56
legal issues 395–6
Legault, A. 177
legitimacy 271, 275, 371–2
Legius, M. 178
Lehane, E. 438
Leininger, Madeleine 6, 16, 21, 195, 206, 213–27,
    375, 455, 487, 624

Leino-Kilpi, H. 533
Leone, Lucile Petry 260
lesbians 47–8, 54–5, 56, 457, 459
Leung, S. 620
Levin, M. 327
Lévi-Strauss, C. 399
Lewenson, Sandra B. 6, 256 67, 624
Lewin, Kurt 320
Lewin, S. 377
Lewis, J. 361
Lewis, L. M. 178
Li, H-F. 178
Li, H-J. 177
Li Zheng 616, 619–20
Liamputtong, Pranee 537
life stage issues 177
life story approach 599–600
lifeworld-based research 536, 537, 540
Light, S. S. 195
Lilja, L. 531
Lima-Basto, Marta 9, 514–26, 627
limited genre stories 269–70, 272–3
Limoges, J. 246
Lin, M. J. 139, 176–7
Lincoln, Y. 399, 584
Lindseth, A. 78
Lindwall, L. 531
Listening to Mothers II survey 126
lived experience 149, 408, 409, 522, 535, 555–6;
    Netherlands and Flanders 565–6, 568; Portugal
    517; South-East Asia 614
Locke, John 326
Loewenthal, D. 154
Logan, Elizabeth 453–4
Logan, J. 178
Logan, W. 441, 520
logic model 296, 297
logical conclusions 302–3
logics of research synthesis 350–2
Løgstrup, Knud 548–9
Loiselle, C. G. 314
longitudinal case analysis 87, 90, 91, 95
Lopes, Manuel 522
Lopez, K. A. 149
Lopez, R. P. 177
López-Garcia, Karla Selene 8, 478–99
Lorenzini, A. 485
loss of control 119–20, 122, 123, 276
Lovato, C. Y. 457
Lovato, L. C. 51
Love, K. L. 139
Luce, A. 423, 426
Lundgren, Ingela 531, 536
Lundgren, S. M. 530
Lundman, B. 78, 177, 536
Lynam, J. 457
Lyndon, A. 191

Lyons, W. L. 21

Ma, W-F. 178
Mac Neela, P. M. 447–8
MacDonald, M. A. 183, 184
MacDonnell, J. A. 457
Macgregor, F. C. 206
MacKinnon, K. 246
Madison, S. 236
Maguire, P. 320
Maijala, H. 533
Malinowski, B. 14, 203
Malinsky, L. 246
Malone, R. E. 459
Malvárez, S. 495
managerialism 287
Manias, E. 238, 432
Manicom, A. 242
Mantzoukas, S. 421
Maoris 473
maps 188–90, 191, 197
Marcellus, L. 186
Marck, P. 195
Marcus, G. 232–3
Mardiros, Marilyn 578
marginalized groups 4, 47–9, 54–8, 320; Colombia
    488–9; Feminist Participatory Action Research
    321–3; Participatory Action Research 327;
    Spain 509
Mariano, - 486
Marroquin, A. P. 459
Martin, B. 374
Martin, C. R. 186
Martin, W. L. 457
Martin, Wanda 5, 183–202, 624
Martinsen, Kari 548–50, 552, 555
Martinson, I. 176
Marx, Karl 243, 549
Marxism 286, 291
Mason, R. 457
Massaquoi, N. 457
Masters, H. 206
materiality 242, 243
Mathew, S. 386
Mattingly, C. 269
Maturana, Humberto 479, 487
May, K. 40
Mayan, Maria 578
Mayer, J. D. 610
McCarthy, G. 438
McClowry, S. 177
McCoy, L. 251
McCurdy, D. W. 204
McDonald, C. 456–7, 459
McDonald, Heather 453, 460–2
McFarland, Marilyn 6, 213–29
McGeorge, S. J. 187

McGibbon, E. 246
McHoul, A. 427
McIntyre, M. 456–7
McKellar, L. 475
McKenzie, H. 348
McNeill, M. M. 195
McVeigh, C. 177
Mead, George Herbert 162–3, 170, 486
Mead, Margaret 14, 394
mealtimes 249–50
meaning: culture 215; deconstruction 287;
    discourse analysis 282, 284, 287; grounded
    theory 170, 174–5, 198; historical research
    256; human science paradigm 214; interpretive
    phenomenology 145–6, 147–8, 150, 152–3,
    154, 156–7, 158–9; meaning-in-context 223;
    stories 273, 274, 275
Mechan-Andrews, T. 472
medication 54, 253
Melchior, F. 263
Meleis, A. J. 77
Melon, Karen 246, 249
memos 176, 179, 198
men: chronic pain syndrome 80–1, 82–3; fathers
    140
Mendoza-Parra, S. 484, 487
mental health: community mental health nurses
    178; Ireland 441, 442–3, 444, 447–8; narrative
    inquiry 275–7; Netherlands 564; United
    Kingdom 422, 423, 424, 426–7;
    ventilator-dependent patients 95
Merighi, J. R. 459
Merleau-Ponty, Maurice 14, 150, 155, 486, 548,
    549
Merritt-Gray, Marilyn 4, 32–46, 183
Merryfeather, L. 457
Merton, Robert K. 163, 307
meta-aggregation 335
meta-analysis 351, 353
meta-ethnography 332, 333, 335, 338, 339, 351,
    352
meta-ethnonursing method 227
metaphors 80, 534
meta-study 332–3, 335, 338, 339, 540
metasummary 336, 351, 353
metasynthesis 7, 22, 23, 26, 331–46, 625; best
    practices 341; challenges 339–41; Finland and
    Sweden 537; future directions 341–3; historical
    overview 332–3; Korea 585; methods 333–9,
    341, 342–3; mixed research 353; postpartum
    depression 124; South-East Asia 617;
    ventilator-dependent patients 98
methodologies 405–13, 626
methods 4, 5–7, 13; Australasia 470–2; Brazil
    480–2; Chile 484–6; Colombia 488–9;
    confusion with methodologies 411; critical
    ethnography 238; descriptive phenomenology

133, 135–9, 142, 151; development of 14–15, 16–19; ethnonursing 219–20; global dissemination of 20; grounded theory 171; Internet research 383; interpretive description 299–300; interpretive phenomenology 148–50, 157–9; Japan 599–607; Latino childhood obesity 106–9; metasynthesis 333–9, 341, 342–3; Mexico 491–3; Netherlands and Flanders 568–9, 570; nurses' contribution to 20–1; Portugal 518–19; secondary data analysis 394; Spain 505–8; ventilator-dependent patients 87, 91–2; *see also* data collection

Meurs, P. 564

Mexico 8, 478–9, 490–4

Miaskowski, C. A. 21

microanalysis 22

midwifery 437, 438, 439, 442–3, 444, 448, 468–9, 475

Mikandawire-Valhmu, L. 237

Mill, J. 238

Mills, C. W. 411

Mills, J. 186, 191

Miranda, J. 459

Miró, Margalida 8, 500–13

misconduct 368

mixed methods research 7, 55, 347–56, 409, 554, 623, 625; books on 19; Canada 459; fatigue 65–6; focus groups 314, 317; grounded theory 197; Internet research 387, 390; Ireland 443; Korea 585; Mexico 493; Netherlands and Flanders 567; nurses' contribution to 21; Participatory Action Research 327; Portugal 517, 518; qualitative metasummary 336; United Kingdom 426, 428, 432–3; ventilator-dependent patients 86

mode of research synthesis 350

moderators of focus groups 308, 311–12

modification of theory 39, 44, 126–8

modified grounded theory approach (M-GTA) 602–3

Montag, Mildred 262–3

Montgomery, Phyllis 6, 268–81, 624

Moore-Dempsey, L. 459

Morgan, David L. 307, 316

Morris, Edith 6, 213–29

Morrow, R. 183

Morse, Janice, M. 1–2, 3, 162, 165, 186, 419, 456, 578, 623; anthropology 163; development of qualitative nursing research 4, 13–31; evidence 412; multi-method design 69; power issues in research 361; pragmatic utility approach 68; purposive sampling 75–6; research evaluation 584; risks to research participants 365, 367

Mortimer, Barbara 261

Mossey, Sharolyn 6, 268–81, 624

motherhood 26, 275–7; *see also* postpartum depression

mother-infant interactions 122

Moustakas, C. 135, 138

Mozambique 188–90

Mulderij, K. 568

multidisciplinarity 16, 237, 283, 341; Australasia 473–4; Finland and Sweden 538; Ireland 447, 448; Netherlands and Flanders 562–3; Portugal 523; Spain 503; Sweden 530–1

multi-method design 69

Muncey, T. 422, 424

Munhall, Patricia L. 3, 5, 16–17, 145–61, 206, 623

Muñoz, L.A. 484, 485

Murphy, K. 186, 441

Murrock, C. J. 317

Mykhalovskiy, E. 248

Nåden, D. 554

Nahm, E. S. 386, 389

narrative analysis 406, 408

narrative inquiry/research 6, 27, 52, 54, 268–81, 400, 624; Australia 470; Canada 457; Japan 599–600, 601; Korea 582, 583, 585; Portugal 518–19; Sweden 531; United Kingdom 422, 425; women with fibromyalgia 79, 81

narrative synthesis 336

National Council for the Professional Development of Nursing and Midwifery (NCPDNM), Ireland 438, 439, 448

National Health Service (NHS) 420, 421

National Institute for Nursing Research (NINR) 50, 58

National Institute of Health (NIH) 373, 380, 388

naturalistic data 52, 395

naturalistic inquiry 459

Nelson, Sioban 261, 262

Nentwich, J. 376

neo-Marxism 234

Netherlands 9, 135, 560–76, 627

netnography 383

network sampling 324

Neville, S. 474

New Zealand 8, 127, 468–77, 626; critical ethnography 237; descriptive phenomenology 135, 139, 140; indigenous scholars 458

Newell, C. 422, 424

Newman, C. 209

Newman, M. A. 218, 326–7

Nicolaas, G. 361

Niehaus, L. 21

Nietzsche, Friedrich 291

Nightingale, Florence 15, 205, 216–17, 239, 420, 483

Nikkonen, M. 533

Noblit, G. W. 124, 332, 333

non-linearity 194–5, 196

non-naturalistic data 395

Norberg, Astrid 78, 80, 82, 177, 530, 535

Nordic Academy of Nursing Science 530
Nortvedt, P. 549
Norway 9, 19, 135, 140, 546–59, 627
nurse-patient relationships 23, 196, 519, 521, 522
Nursing Council of New Zealand (NCNZ) 470
nursing gestalt 166
nursing homes 237, 553

obesity 4, 103–18, 553
objectivity 233, 263, 326, 347, 411, 569
observational research 21, 87, 90, 91, 96–7, 250;
    see also participant observation
Observation-Participation-Reflection (O-P-R)
    Enabler 222, 223
O'Connell, B. 178
O'Connor, M. 237
O'Connor, Mary E. 4, 103–18, 398
Odencrants, S. 532
O'Discoll, C. 209
Ogden Burke, S. 455
Ogedegbe, G. 178
Öhlén, J. 531
Oiler, C. 3, 206
Oliffe, J. L. 457
Olson, Karin 4, 25, 64–74
Olsson, M. 79
Omery, A. 206
oncology 140, 178, 325, 387, 442, 443
O'Neill, M. 139
ontology 150, 321, 405, 463, 534, 539; Finland
    and Sweden 537; grounded theory 184–5, 187;
    ontological commitments 547–8
oppression 234, 284, 286, 319, 448
oral histories 262–3, 265
Orem, Dorothea 15, 562
Ortega, J. 177
Osborne, M. 246
the Other 291
Oudshoorn, A. 458
oversight 368
Oxman, A. 377

Paavilainen, E. 533
Padilha, Maria Itayra 8, 478–99
Paim, Lygia 482
pain 25, 39, 550; neuropathic 331; UK studies
    422, 425, 429; vulnerability of research
    participants 365; see also chronic pain syndrome
Paley, J. 23–4
palliative care 27, 139, 423, 426; Australasia 474;
    Canada 459; Finland and Sweden 535; Ireland
    442, 443; ventilator-dependent patients 95
Pan American Health Organization (PAHO) 478
panarchy 195
Pang, S. M. 139
panic disorder 122–3
Panik, A. 208

Papleau, Hildegard 15
paradigms 49, 429–30, 455
paraphrasing 172
Paravic-Klijn, T. 484
parenting programs 247
Parker, Ian 291
Parkhurst, D. 139
Parkinson's disease 551
Parse, Rosemarie Rizzo 3, 484
participant observation 203–6, 207, 231; focus
    groups 316; interpretive description 299;
    Latino childhood obesity 106; postpartum
    depression 119; researcher competence 360;
    Sweden 531; see also observational research
Participatory Action Research (PAR) 6, 55,
    319–30, 378, 625; Australasia 470; Brazil 479;
    Canada 457, 460; Colombia 489; Critical
    Participatory Research 323–4; defining
    319–21; Denmark 553; ethics 324–5; feminist
    320, 321–3; focus groups 314, 316; Spain 506
partnership 377–8, 463, 476, 482, 523
Paterson, Barbara L. 7, 246, 331–46, 367, 456,
    532, 537, 625
patterns 194, 223
Patton, M. Q. 119
Paulson, M. 80, 82, 333
Pauly, B. 324–5
Pavlish, C. P. 327
payback model 373
Pearson, Allan 612
Pêcheau, Michel 286
Peden-McAlpine, C. 555
Pederson, A. 321–3, 324, 327
peer review 375–6, 607
peer support 317
Peirce, Charles Sanders 534
Pejlert, A. 535
Pereira, A. T. 126
Pérez, C. 509
Performative Social Science 423, 428
Perron, A. 457, 461
Perry, J.-A. 398
Pesonen, H-M. 533
Peter, E. 246
Peters, E. 398
Petersen, S. 139
Pharris, M. D. 327
phenomenography 470, 531
phenomenology 5, 54, 122, 183, 406, 411, 459;
    Australasia 470, 471; books on 19, 20; Brazil
    480, 481; Canada 455, 456–7, 460; Chile 485,
    486; Colombia 489; combined with
    ethnography 50; Finland and Sweden 531,
    532, 533, 535, 536, 537, 540; focus groups
    316, 317; Internet research 387, 388;
    interpretive complexity 348; interpretive
    description 297; Ireland 443–4, 446; Japan

599–600; Korea 582, 583, 585; metasynthesis
340; Mexico 491, 492; Netherlands and
Flanders 563, 568; Norway, Denmark, and
Iceland 549, 550, 551, 554–6; philosophy of
14, 133–4, 149–50, 151, 152; Portugal 518–19;
postpartum depression 119–23; predominance
of 408; South East Asia 614, 615, 616, 620;
Spain 506, 510; United Kingdom 422–3, 425;
women with fibromyalgia 78, 79, 81, 82; *see
also* descriptive phenomenology; interpretive
phenomenology
Philippines 139, 614–15, 616, 617, 620, 621
Philipsen, Hans 563
philosophy 291, 406, 539; Anglo-Saxon/
Continental split 292; grounded theory 170;
human science paradigm 214; phenomenology
14, 133–4, 149–50, 151, 152
Phoenix, A. 458
Piaget, Jean 14
Pless, I. B. 108
policy frameworks 259–60
policy-making 376–7
Polit, D. F. 442, 530, 539
politics 7, 371–9, 625; Critical Discourse Analysis
285–6; of funding 373–5; of partnership
377–8; peer review 375–6; policy-making
376–7
Pool, Aart 565
Porr, Caroline 164, 165, 167
Porter, E. J. 135, 138–9
Porter, Sam 236, 237
Portugal 9, 126, 514–26, 627
positional maps 189–90, 197
positivism 271, 347, 372, 419, 462; Australia 470;
Canada 454, 455; Chile 484, 486; criticism of
479, 549; Mexico 493; Spain 509, 510; *see also*
quantitative research
postcolonialism 55, 233, 234, 320, 323, 458,
462
postmodernism 51–2, 184, 188, 191, 296;
Australasia 471; complexity science 192; critical
ethnography 233, 234; interpretive description
304; mixed methods 432; Participatory Action
Research 326
postpartum depression 5, 119–29, 152, 471, 620
Postpartum Depression Screening Scale (PDSS) 5,
124–6, 128
post-positivism 49, 51–2, 304, 461
post-structuralism 283, 296; Australasia 471;
Canada 457; critical ethnography 233, 234,
238; discourse analysis 285, 287, 291; Spain
510
posttraumatic stress disorder (PTSD) 39, 123, 140
power relations 185, 371, 625; critical
ethnography 230, 231, 234, 236–7, 238–9;
discourse analysis 286–7, 427; focus groups
310; historical research 259; institutional

ethnography 243; Latino childhood obesity
115; researcher-participant relationships 361
pragmatic utility approach 68
pragmatism 170, 184, 187–8, 233, 253
praxis 55, 378
praxis theory of suffering 26
prediction 51
prenatal screening 552
Prigogine, I. 193
primary research 257, 339–40, 341, 399, 400,
401–2
privacy 364, 366, 367
private duty nurses 259
probability sampling 348–9, 413
problematics 248–9, 251
process 174
professional identity 261, 492, 505
professionalization of nursing 260, 562
project maps 190
Proot, I. 178
Pryor, J. 178
psychoanalysis 291, 292
psychology 283, 291, 292, 405, 406, 563
PUBMED 68, 134, 289, 383
purposive sampling 75–6, 87, 348–9
Pyles, Sue 166

Qualitative Health Research Unit (QUARU)
428–9
qualitative nursing research 1–2; definition of 14,
419; development of 13–31; emergence of
3–4; future directions 623–7; methods and
methodologies 4, 5–7, 13, 405–13
qualitative research centres 427–9
quality 340, 372, 376, 511, 610
Quance, M. 246
quantitative research 408, 409, 462, 610;
Australasia 468, 470; Brazil 480, 482–3;
building on 412–13; Canada 454, 455, 459;
causality 52; Chile 484, 485–6; Colombia 488,
490; focus groups 307; generalizability 413–14;
Internet research 380, 382, 387, 389; Japan
603; metasynthesis 333, 338; Mexico 490, 491;
mixed methods research 21, 55, 347–54;
Norway, Denmark, and Iceland 555;
Participatory Action Research 327; politics of
evidence 372; Portugal 517; postpartum
depression 128; South-East Asia 613, 615;
Spain 505, 509; ventilator-dependent patients
96; Women's Health Effects Study 34; *see also*
positivism
quasi-experimental research designs 518
queer theory 55
Quelopana, A. M. 126
questionnaires 153, 349
questions, asking 175
Quiney, L. 457

Quint, Jean 163

race: Black feminism 458; historical research 261, 263; ideological practices 243; Internet research 381; intersectionality 49, 458; oppression 234; *see also* ethnicity
Racine, L. 458
racism 57, 459
Radwin, L. 178
Rafferty, A. 420
Ramasco, Milagros 501
Ramsden, I. 458
randomized controlled trials (RCTs) 51, 52, 342, 409, 411, 412, 421, 567
Rankin, Janet 6, 242–55, 458, 624
Ray, Marilyn A. 6, 195–6, 213–29, 624
realist review 337, 339
realist synthesis 351, 352
Reason, P. 321
Rebelo-Botelho, Maria António 522
reciprocity 185
recurrent patterning 223, 226
reduction 133–4, 135–7
reductionism 192
Reeves, Christopher 257
reflexivity 231, 232, 236, 238, 239, 506, 586
Reimer-Kirkham, Sheryl 453, 460–2
Reiter, Frances 262
relational ethics 7, 360
relationships 218
relativism 184–5
reliability 206, 271, 584
religion 461–2
Remes, A. M. 533
Renzetti, C. 365–6
representation 396–7
research centres 427–9
research ethics boards (REBs) 359, 361, 363, 364
research evaluation 584, 586
research question, articulation of 298
research team relationships 362
researcher competence 360
researcher-participant relationships 360–1, 380–1, 486
respect 167, 220, 252, 361
retention of research participants 389, 390
retrospective interpretation 398
return on investment 373, 374
Revised Edmonton Fatigue Framework 69–70, 72
Reyes-Rubilar, T. 126
Reynolds, D. 178
Rhoten, D. 67
Ricoeur, Paul 78, 535, 550
Riessman, C. K. 270, 272
risks 7, 359, 361, 365–7
Risman, B. 242
Rist, R. C. 376–7

Ritter, S. 432
ritual 165, 166, 221
Roberts, Mary 260
Robertson, M. H. B. 206, 208
Robinson, R. 422, 424
Rodney, Patricia 453, 459, 460–2
Rodriguez, R. 237
Rogers, Carl 15
Rogers, Martha 217, 321, 326
Romanow, Roy 451
Ronquillo, C. 457
Roper, N. 441, 520
Rorty, R. 149, 150, 151
Rose, L. 455
Roth, Philip 154, 155
Rowan, M. 195
Roy, B. 461
Royal College of Nursing (RCN) 420
Ruland, C. M. 555
ruling relations 243–4, 246, 247
Ryan, S. 236, 237

Sacks, Harvey 285
Said, E. 458
Saiki-Craighill, Shigeko 9, 597–609, 627
Salantëra, S. 533
Salmon, A. 321–3, 324, 327
Salovey, P. 610
sampling 75–6, 87; amplified 399; focus groups 310–11; interpretive description 299–300; Latino childhood obesity 105; mixed research 348–9; network 324; theoretical 34, 175–6, 308–9, 316, 606
Sandelowski, Margarete 7, 21, 22, 26, 177, 332, 338, 347–56, 568; data collection 403; fabrication 396; generalizability 413; grounded theory 33, 35; mixed research 625; research evaluation 584; truth 409
Sandström, U. 374
Sanhueza-Alvarado, Olivia Inés 8, 478–99
Santa Fe Institute 193
Sarter, B. 206
Sartre, J.-P. 151
saturation 173, 372, 569, 605, 606; ethnonursing 223, 226; Internet research 389, 390
Saussure, Ferdinand de 283–4
Schachman, K. A. 140
Scharer, K. 177
Schatzman, Leonard 3
Scheper-Hughes, Nancy 240n3
Schnepp, W. 176
Schofield, J. W. 413
Schön, D. 553
School of Health and Social Science, University of Edinburgh 429
Schoot, T. 178
Schreiber, Rita 5, 183–202, 624

Schumacher, K. L. 77
Schutz, Alfred 455
Schwartz, M. & C. 204
science 192, 217–18, 298, 326, 411, 419, 433;
    concept of 429; human science paradigm 214;
    interpretive description 304, 305;
    non-neutrality of 480; Participatory Action
    Research 320, 328; research funding 374; as
    truth 327
Scotland 8, 419–36, 626; see also United Kingdom
Scott, H. 474
Scott, P. A. 447–8
Scott-Findlay, S. 532
secondary data analysis 7, 34, 95, 96, 97, 393–404,
    586, 626
segregated research design 352–3
selection bias 389
self-esteem 77, 80
self-organization 193, 196
self-organizing maps (SOMs) 197
Selikoff, I. J. 119
sensitive topics 314, 365–6, 367
sexual abstinence 314–15
sexual abuse 26–7, 48–9, 53
sexual orientation 49, 457; see also lesbians
Seyle, H. 67
Shamdasani, P. M. 307
Shawler, C. 177
"shell words" 252
Sheridan, V. 208
Sherr, L. 387
Shih, H-H. 178
Shin, H. S. 139
Shin, Kyung Rim 9, 577–96, 627
Shortell, S. M. 411
Shyu, Y-I. 177
signs 286
Sikhs 178
Silva, Abel 521–2
Simpson, Majorie 420
Sims, L. 183–4
Singapore 613, 614, 616, 620
Singer, Merrill 240n3
Singleton Jones, D. 177
Sinkkonen, Sirkka 532, 533
situated freedom 151
situational analysis 187–92
situational maps 188–9
Sjöström, B. 531
Skär, L. 79
Skinner, Quentin 455
Sköldberg, K. 409, 411
Skott, C. 530, 531
Skovdahl, K. 532
Slow Science Academy 374
Smith, B. H. 269
Smith, Dorothy E. 242–4, 246, 250, 252, 458

Smith, G. 248
Smith, L. N. 139
Smith, M. 218
Smith, M. J. 3
Smith, Richard 376
smoking 397, 429
Smyth, W. 238
Snow, Nicole 251
Snowden, A. 186
So, W. S. 139
social determinants of health 116, 456, 458
social environment 53
social frameworks 260–1
social interaction 65, 69
social justice 55, 178–9, 239, 461, 627; Canada
    452, 456, 463; critical ethnography 230;
    interpretive description 305; Spain 511
social structures 371, 406, 461, 462; critical
    ethnography 237; discourse analysis 287;
    ethnonursing 215, 221, 222; situational analysis
    188
social support 23, 332, 385
social worlds/arenas maps 189, 191
"societal discursive practices" 285, 288
sociology 16, 163, 236, 283, 307; ethical and legal
    issues 396; ethnography 204; human science
    paradigm 214; Portugal 514; Spain 509
Söderberg, Siv 4, 75–85, 532
Söderlund, Maud 534
Sofaer-Bennett, B. 422
Soriano, Fabiola Castellanos 8, 478–99
South Africa 135
South-East Asia 9, 610–22, 627
Spain 8–9, 135, 500–13, 626–7
Spiers, J. 237–8
spirituality 178, 461–2
Spivak, G. C. 458
Spradley, J. 204, 207, 297, 583
Sprague, J. 242
Spray, S. L. 196
St. John, W. 177
Stajduhar, K. I. 457
Stegenga, K. 140
Stengers, I. 193
stepfamilies 167
Stern, Phyllis Noerager 5, 162–8, 183–4, 578,
    623
Steve, P. 21
Stevens, P. E. 195
Stevick, E. L. 138
Stewart, D. W. 307
Stewart, N. 459
Stickley, K. 423, 427
Stockbridge, J. 317
Storch, J. 324–5, 459
stories 269–70, 271, 272–7
Stranger to Trusted Friend Enabler 221–2

Strauss, Anselm 3, 5, 15–16, 27, 162–3, 166, 169–82, 184, 405–6; bracketing 187; Canada 455; coding technique 297; complexity 192; constant comparison 119; context 187; core concepts 194; data collection 604; Japan 601, 602, 603; Korea 583; metasynthesis 332; modifiability of theory 39; Netherlands 564; Portugal 518–19, 522; quantitative and qualitative data 34; translation of books 20

Street, Annette Fay 236, 238, 432

Strengthening Capacity to Limit Intrusion (SCLI) 32–44

Streubert Speziale, H. 245

structural analysis of stories 272

structural equation modelling 351, 352

structuralism 284, 291

Study of Patient-nurse Effectiveness with Assisted Communication Strategies (SPEACS) 97, 98, 99

subjectivity 263, 298, 347, 491; discourse analysis 282–3, 284, 291, 292

substance abuse: Feminist Participatory Action Research 322–3; Hispanics 177; Ireland 441; Mexico 492–3; ventilator-dependent patients 95; women 26, 37, 50–1, 52, 54–5, 57

substantive theory 33, 40, 119, 120

suffering 25–6, 531, 565–6

Suhonen, R. 533

Sun, F. K. 176–7

Sunrise Enabler 221

Svedlund, Marianne 531

Swansea University 428–9

Swartz, A. L. 196

Sweden 9, 527–32, 533–40, 627; descriptive phenomenology 135, 139, 140; interpretive phenomenology 146; postpartum depression 127; qualitative research methods books 19, 20

Switzerland 139

symbolic interactionism (SI) 162–3, 164, 170, 184, 187–8, 406, 492

systems thinking 192–3, 195

tactful monitoring 166–7

Tahereh, B. 178

Taiwan 9, 615–16, 621; descriptive phenomenology 135, 139, 140; grounded theory 177, 178; postpartum depression 127

Tanaka, C. 459

Tappan, M. B. 272

Tate, B. 246

Tate, Judith 95

Taverner, T. 331

Taylor, B. 471

Taylor, Stephanie 283, 284–5, 287

technologic access 88–9

Temple, B. 362

ter Meulen, R. 178

Terragni, L. 553

texts 244, 251, 253, 287, 288, 290, 299

Thailand 614, 615–16, 617, 621; grounded theory 166–7, 177; interpretive phenomenology 146; qualitative research methods books 18, 20

thematic analysis 272, 315, 408, 470

thematic synthesis 337, 339

theoretical codes 164, 166, 424

theoretical sampling 34, 175–6, 308–9, 316, 606

theoretical sensitivity 36, 424

theoretical traditions 298–9

theory construction 169–70, 174, 180, 409

Theory of Technique 71

Thifault, M-C. 257

Thomas, J. 230, 231

Thompson, R. 459

Thorne, Sally 6, 7, 21, 32, 162, 270, 295–306, 360, 393–404, 457, 624–5, 626

Thorngate, W. 375

Thorpe, A. 209

Thoun, Deborah 165

"thrownness" 149

Tierney, A. 441, 520

tiredness 65, 66, 68, 72, 81

Tiwari, A. 457

Tobin, Carolyn 8, 437–50, 626

Tobin, G. A. 446

Todres, L. 422, 423, 425

Toman, C. 257

Torheim, H. 551

Toto, R. 387

Tracey, M. P. 447–8

training 43, 99, 360; Brazil 479; Japan 607; Mexico 493, 494; Spain 502; United Kingdom 429; see also education

Trangenstein, P. A. 77

transcripts 315

transcultural nursing 16, 213–14, 216, 218–19, 227

transferability 33, 50, 223, 315, 539

transitions 77, 78, 519, 520

translational research 413

translational science 218, 226, 227

trauma 48, 51, 123, 140, 141

Traynor, Michael 6, 282–94, 442, 624

treatment interference 86–91

Trentini, Mercedes 482

triage 249

triangulation 206, 314, 339, 411, 508

Triscari, J. S. 196

Trochim, William 197

Troyan, P. J. 178

trustworthiness 315, 339–40, 399

truth 327, 409, 428, 471

Tsai, P. L. 139

Tschikota, S. 456

Tuhiwai Smith, L. 458

Turkel, M. C. 195–6
Turkey 135, 140
Turrill, S. 190

Udry, J. R. 373
the unconscious 291
United Arab Emirates 127
United Kingdom 8, 419–36, 626; descriptive
    phenomenology 135, 139, 140; managerialism
    287; postpartum depression 127; see also Great
    Britain
United States 374, 406, 408, 455–6; critical
    ethnography 237; descriptive phenomenology
    135, 139, 140; dissemination of methods 20;
    ethnography 209–10; historical research 260,
    264; Internet research 389; interpretive
    phenomenology 146; politics 373; postpartum
    depression 126; qualitative research methods
    books 17, 18, 19; spirituality 178
University of Edinburgh 429
"unknowing" 153, 154, 155, 158
usability of findings 51
Utrecht model of developing interventions 567

Valaitis, R. K. 386
validity 51, 206, 271, 528, 584; participatory
    approaches 327; Postpartum Depression
    Screening Scale 125; secondary data analysis
    401
Välimäki, – 533
Valmari, G. 530, 531
values: Canada 452; critical ethnography 231;
    cultural 104, 222; ethical conduct 359;
    ethnoscience 68; peer review 375–6
Van der Bruggen, Harry 563
Van der Lyke, S. 566
Van Dijk, T. A. 283
Van Hecke, Ann 9, 560–76
Van Kaam, A. 135–8, 142, 582, 583
Van Maanen, H. M. T. 568
Van Manen, M. 20, 146, 150, 157–8, 550, 551,
    578, 582, 583
Van Meijel, B. 567
Van Staa, A. 565
Vancouver School 550
Vandall-Walker, V. 177
Vandenberg, H. 238–9
Varcoe, Colleen 4, 32–46, 327, 459
Varma, M. 459
Vasquez, J. 177
ventilator-dependent patients 4, 86–102, 550–1
Verhaeghe, Sofie 9, 560–76
video recordings 97
Vieira, Margarida 522
Viney, L. L. 270
voicelessness 88, 89–90, 98
Voils, Corrine I. 7, 347–56

Voloshinov, V. N. 286
voluntary consent 362–3
Von Post, I. 531
Vossos, H. 214, 223–6
vote counting 351
vulnerability of research participants 365

Wagner, L. 553
Wales 8, 419–36, 626; see also United Kingdom
Waletzky, J. 272
Walker, A. 178
Walker, J. 422
Walshe, C. 423, 426
Walthew, P. 474
Ward-Griffin, C. 458
Ward-Smith, P. 140
Warren, J. 422, 424
Wasserman, J. A. 188
Waters, A. L. 209
Watson, Jean 218
Wax, R. 204
Weatherbee, D. 248
Webb, C. 316
Weber, M. 549
Wehbe-Alamah, H. 214, 223–6
Weiss, S. M. 459
Wellard, S. J. 474
Werezak, L. 459
Wester, F. 83
White, G. 140
Whitehead, L. 432
Whittemore, R. 432
widows 138–9
Wiklund-Gustin, L. 534
Wilkinson, L. 471
Willis, D. G. 149
Wilson, Holly 163
Wilson, K. L. 188
Wilson, M. 214, 223–6
Wilson, M. G. 377
Wiltshire, J. 271
Winters, R. 474
Wishart, Paul 163
Wittgenstein, Ludwig 217–18
women: benefits of participation in research 365;
    Canada 457; childhood abuse 26–7, 48–9, 50,
    52, 54; chronic pain syndrome 76–82;
    Colombia 488; contraceptive strategies 177,
    440; domestic abuse 4, 32–46; Feminist
    Participatory Action Research 321–3; fetal
    abnormality 444–6; focus groups 310, 317;
    HIV/AIDS 26, 188–90; Internet research 384,
    387; lesbian 47–8, 54–5, 56, 457, 459;
    narrative inquiry 275–7; negative core beliefs
    56; Netherlands 560; postpartum depression
    119–29, 152, 471, 620; Spain 500, 509;
    substance abuse 50–1, 52, 54–5, 57; tobacco

reduction 397; traumatic childbirth 140–1; women's movement 260; *see also* feminism; gender
Women's Health Effects Study (WHES) 34, 37–8, 39
Wong, M. 457
Wong, S. 457
Wong, T. K. S. 176
Worrall-Carter, L. 178
Worster, B. 140
Wright, K. 459
"writing culture movement" 233
Wu, M. 140
Wu, N. 265

Wuest, Judith 4, 32–46, 183–4

Yamashita, M. 398
Yang, T-C. 176–7
Yearwood, E. L. 177
Yin, R. 323–4
Young, Lynne 6, 319–30, 625

Zaforteza, Concha 8, 500–13
Zahourek, R. P. 178
Zarchin, Y. R. 384, 389
Zizek, Slavoj 283, 291
Zoffmann, V. 177
Zuelzer, Helen 257–8

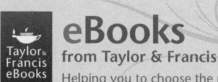
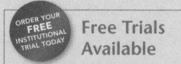
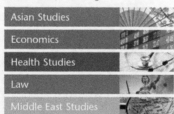